Yoga Anatomy Made Simple

Your Illustrated Guide to Form, Function, and Posture Groups

Yoga Anatomy Made Simple

Your Illustrated Guide to Form, Function, and Posture Groups

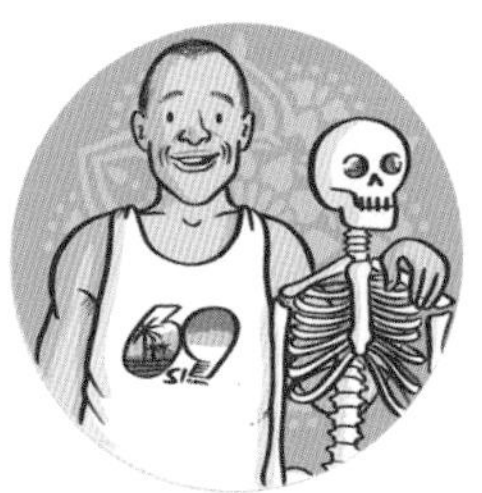

Author

STU GIRLING

Illustrator

BUG FAWCETT

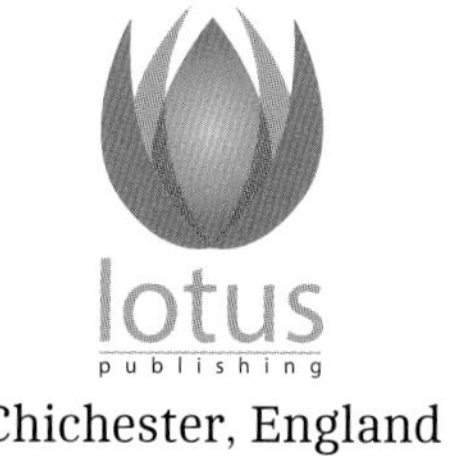

Chichester, England

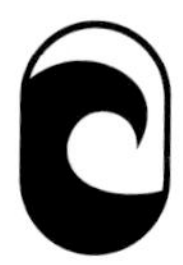

North Atlantic Books
Huichin, unceded Ohlone land
aka Berkeley, California

First published in 2021 (ISBN 978 1 8383556 1 6) by Stu & Bug Books
This revised edition published in 2023 by
Lotus Publishing
Apple Tree Cottage, Inlands Road, Nutbourne, Chichester, PO18 8RJ, and
North Atlantic Books
Huichin, unceded Ohlone land
aka Berkeley, California

Illustrations Bug Fawcett
Models Victoria, Doug, Dave, Vihan, Stu, Skelly, Aren, Ben, Betty, and Zane,
Wendy, Jasmine, Bug, Myra, and Sasha
Text Design Medlar Publishing Solutions Pvt Ltd., India
Cover Design Jasmine Hromjak
Printed and Bound in India by Replika Press

Yoga Anatomy Made Simple: Your Illustrated Guide to Form, Function, and Posture Groups is sponsored and published by North Atlantic Books, an educational non-profit based on the unceded Ohlone land Huichin (*aka* Berkeley, CA), that collaborates with partners to develop cross-cultural perspectives, nurture holistic views of art, science, the humanities, and healing, and seed personal and global transformation by publishing work on the relationship of body, spirit, and nature.

North Atlantic Books' publications are distributed to the US trade and internationally by Penguin Random House Publishers Services. For further information, visit our website at www.northatlanticbooks.com.

British Library Cataloging-in-Publication Data
A CIP record for this book is available from the British Library
ISBN 978 1 913088 35 4 (Lotus Publishing)
ISBN 978 1 62317 906 9 (North Atlantic Books)
ISBN 978 1 62317 907 6 (Ebook)

Library of Congress Cataloging-in-Publication Data
Names: Girling, Stuart, author. | Fawcett, Bug, illustrator.
Title: Yoga anatomy made simple : your illustrated guide to form, function, and posture groups / Stuart Girling ; illustrations by Bug Fawcett.
Description: Revised edition. | Berkeley, CA : North Atlantic Books ; Chichester : Lotus Publishing, 2023. | First published 2021 by Stu & Bug Books. This revised edition published in 2023 by Lotus Publishing and North Atlantic Books. | Includes bibliographical references.
Identifiers: LCCN 2022044903 (print) | LCCN 2022044904 (ebook) | ISBN 9781623179069 (trade paperback) | ISBN 9781623179076 (ebook)
Subjects: LCSH: Yoga. | Human anatomy. | Posture.
Classification: LCC RA781.67 .G57 2023 (print) | LCC RA781.67 (ebook) | DDC 613.7/046--dc23/eng/20221004
LC record available at https://lccn.loc.gov/2022044903
LC ebook record available at https://lccn.loc.gov/2022044904

Contents

Introduction ... 7
List of Abbreviations ... 9

PART I—KEY CONCEPTS

1. **Fundamentals of Yoga Postures** ... 12
   - Making Shapes ... 12
   - Individuality ... 14
   - Gravity ... 17
   - Alignment ... 21
   - Fighting Own Restrictions ... 26
   - Balance ... 29
2. **Movement Basics** ... 38
   - Range of Motion ... 38
   - Flexibility ... 43
   - Stretching ... 49
   - Multi-Segmental Movement ... 59
   - Moving in Patterns ... 61
   - Compression ... 63
   - Fundamental Movements ... 66
   - Relational Movement ... 68
3. **Muscles and Fascia** ... 71
   - Neurophysiology ... 71
   - Open and Closed Kinetic Chains ... 75
   - Polyarticular Muscles ... 78
   - Strength ... 81
   - Variety ... 86
   - Opposing Muscles Restrict ... 89
   - Secondary Action of Muscles ... 92
   - Fascial Considerations ... 94
   - Recommended Reading ... 100
4. **Breath** ... 101
   - Breath ... 101
   - Breath and Posture ... 104
   - Breath and Trauma ... 109
   - References ... 114
5. **Other Personal Considerations** ... 115
   - Environmental Influences ... 115
   - Lifestyle ... 117
   - Personal History ... 118
   - Psychology ... 119
   - Risk Factors ... 121

PART II—BODY BITS

6. **Foot and Ankle** ... 130
   - Construction of the Foot and Ankle ... 130
   - Muscles that Move the Foot and Ankle ... 132
   - Arches of the Foot ... 134
   - Foot Alignment ... 137
   - So How Do We Start Working on This? ... 138
   - Putting Things into Context ... 139
7. **Knee** ... 143
   - Construction of the Knee Joint ... 143
   - Muscles that Move the Knee ... 144
   - Putting Things into Context ... 146
8. **Hip** ... 152
   - Construction of the Hip Joint ... 154
   - Muscles that Move the Hip ... 155
   - Putting Things into Context ... 161

9. **Spine** 164
   Construction of the Spine 164
   Muscles that Move the Spine 174
   Putting Things into Context 176

10. **Sacroiliac Joint** 179
   Construction of the Sacroiliac Joint 179
   Muscles that Move the Sacrum 180
   Putting Things into Context 181

11. **Shoulder** 184
   Construction of the Shoulder Complex 184
   Muscles that Move the Shoulder Complex 186
   Putting Things into Context 194
   A Bit About Moving the Head 198
   Putting Things into Context 198

12. **Elbow and Wrist** 200
   Construction of the Elbow 200
   Muscles that Move the Elbow 202
   Putting Things into Context 204
   Construction of the Wrist 206
   Muscles that Move the Wrist 207
   Putting Things into Context 207

PART III—POSTURE GROUPS

13. **Forward Bends** 210
14. **Hip Rotations** 228
15. **Backbends** 242
16. **Twists** 257
17. **Postures Involving the Shoulders** 265
18. **Inversions** 282
19. **Arm Balances** 289

APPENDICES

1. Anatomical Language and Movement Terminology 302
2. Stu's Simple Model of Infinite Complexity 317
3. Names of Poses/Postures (Asanas) 334

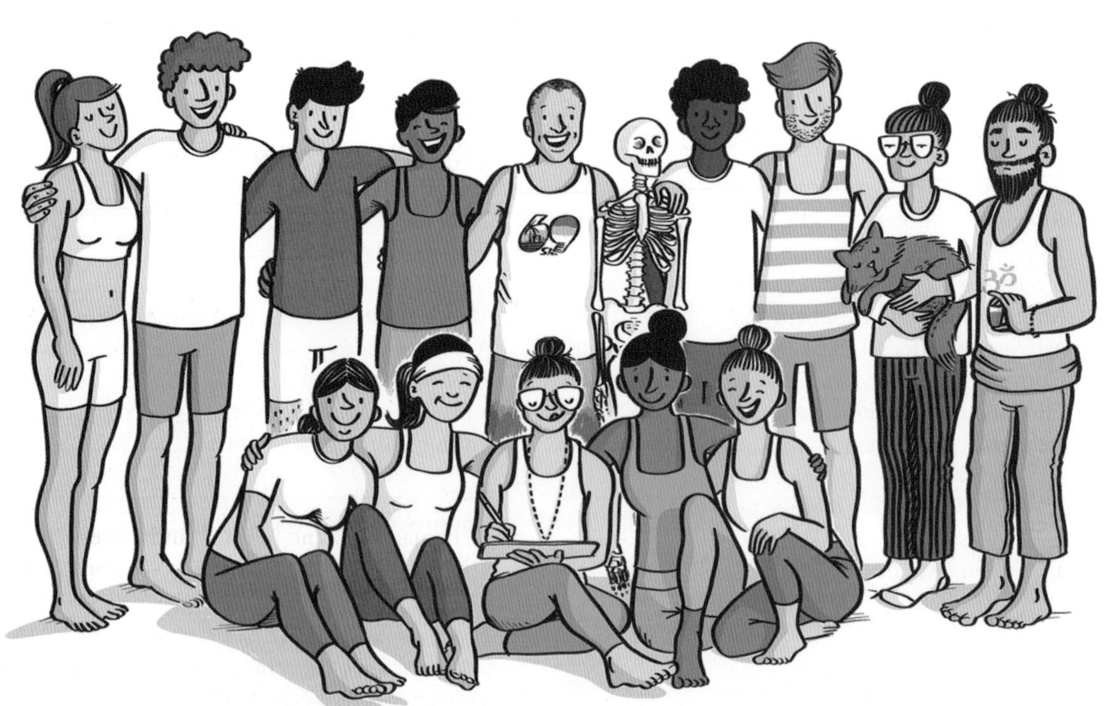

Our gang of yogi demonstrators—notice we come in all shapes and sizes.
From left to right back row: Victoria, Doug, Dave, Vihan, Stu, Skelly, Aren, Ben, Betty, Zane.
Front row: Wendy, Jasmine, Bug, Myra, Sasha.

Introduction

The focus of this book is to present what I see as the "Key Concepts" of functional yoga anatomy in an accessible and usable way, which will provide you with the tools to make informed decisions about the way you or your students might practice. I have teamed up with the incredibly talented visual artist Bug Fawcett, who will pipe those ideas straight to your frontal cortex with plenty of amazing supporting images!

My God, anatomy can be a dry and dull subject in the wrong hands, and it is so easy to be turned off the subject to such an extent as to prefer to rely solely on intuition. While this may take us so far, with a little additional information, the possibilities are vast.

The human body is both amazing and incredibly complex, and the key to successfully working successfully with it is not to get lost in unnecessary detail but to maintain the focus on what we love to do, yoga. I want to make this book as accessible as possible, so throughout, I will give both simple language and that which is more anatomically correct. The style will be relaxed yet with sufficient detail for you to understand the key points and how to implement the ideas given.

If you understand these concepts clearly, you will be able to analyze yoga postures from a physical perspective, sequence more effectively, understand practitioner limitations, and appreciate the importance of individuality in the experience of postural yoga.

Structure of Contents

There are four main parts: *Key Concepts*, *Body Bits*, *Posture Groups*, and the *Appendices*, including *Stu's Simple Model of Infinite Complexity*.

I use the Sanskrit name for each yoga pose throughout the book for ease of reading, but there is a full English translation of each at end of the book. These translations vary slightly depending on which source you use, but I've chosen the most common ones in everyday use.

Then we are going to do things a little different from the norm. Many anatomy books start with a whole load of information about the body that is sometimes difficult to perceive how you are going to use it before they get into the juicy bit, if ever. Instead, in *Key Concepts*, we are going to jump straight into thinking about the makeup of the human body and how that influences movement and our ability to create yoga postures. These concepts give you the tools to understand how to work with the body from a physical perspective within a postural yoga framework. We will consider topics such as individuality, patterns, restrictions, variety, breath, and strength, all, of course, within the context of yoga.

Initially, you won't need to know the names of bones and muscles, but you will want to get them into your head along with some joint movements at some stage. We have put this stuff into Appendix 1 because some of you will already know enough. The details of 20 or so muscles and bones with some associated movements will give you the language you need. A bit like learning a few snippets of conversational French before you travel to Paris for the first time and find out you can't order breakfast!

Although ideally, we want to view our integrated body from a holistic perspective when we are learning about it, looking at one area at a time seems to make the task more straightforward. To this end in *Body Bits*, we will divide the body into the major joints, hips, shoulders, spine, knees, ankles, and wrists. We will consider any influences their construction may have and take into account the muscles that move each joint.

Following on from *Body Bits* are the posture group chapters of *Forward Bends*, *Hip Rotations*, *Backbends*, *Twists*, *Postures Involving the Shoulders*, *Inversions*, and *Arm Balances*. We will be combining the initial concepts with what we have learned about the major joints in the previous section and applying it to the different areas of the body and associated movement groups. Everything is brought together with examples so that you can use the same ideas to consider any posture or sequence.

In Appendix 1, you will find definitions, learning tools, and question and answers.

In Appendix 2, *Stu's Model*, we will endeavor to bring everything together within a more holistic framework that takes into consideration lifestyle and environment influences, as well the student's life up until the present moment.

Appendix 3 is a list of all the asanas/postures included within the book, with an accompanying illustration, Sanskrit name (in italics), and English translation.

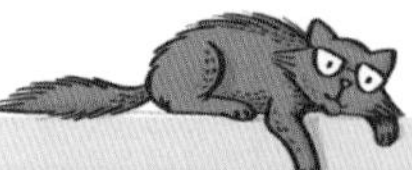

Whenever I am teaching in person, I try and have a mix of about 50 percent theory to 50 percent practical because I have found for many people, experiencing things physically greatly improves understanding. So, I have placed quite a few exercises throughout the book for you to try, and I would definitely suggest that, if appropriate for your body, you have a go. Also, I have added some extra detail for the anatomy geeks among us, but don't feel you have to digest these bits if it makes your brain boil.

These sections will have colored backgrounds to differentiate them from the surrounding text and make them easy to find. I have a feeling Betty's cat Gerald will make an appearance too. He'll have his glasses on if it is a geeky section.

There is also no index! This is deliberate. I would like people to read the book, not just dip in and out and read a sound bite. It's useful to know everything in context.

Inside the front cover, you will see the usual disclaimer relating to physical activities and the ideas put forward in this book. We get so used to seeing this sort of thing nowadays that it almost doesn't sink in. However, it is vitally important that you take responsibility for your own body, both when reading this book but also whenever participating in physical exercise, whether led or self-guided.

The aim of this book is to assist you in making informed decisions about how yoga could be practiced, but these are not blanket recommendations. If in any doubt about the appropriateness or medical issues, seek out professional medical advice, don't just risk it.

List of Abbreviations

ACJ acromioclavicular joint
ACL anterior cruciate ligament
AIIS anterior inferior iliac spine
ALL anterior longitudinal ligament
ANS autonomic nervous system
APA anticipatory postural adjustments
ASIS anterior superior iliac spine

BOS base of support

CAR controlled articular rotation
CNS central nervous system
COG center of gravity
CPA compensatory postural adjustments

DOMS delayed onset muscle soreness

GHJ glenohumeral joint
Gmax gluteus maximus
Gmed gluteus medius
Gmin gluteus minimus
GTO Golgi tendon organ

HRV heart rate variability

ITB iliotibial band

LCL lateral collateral ligament

MCL medial collateral ligament
MTU musculotendinous unit

PCL posterior cruciate ligament
PIIS posterior inferior iliac spine
PLL posterior longitudinal ligament
PNF proprioceptive neuromuscular facilitation
PSIS posterior superior iliac spine
PSNS parasympathetic nervous system
PTSD post-traumatic stress disorder

QL quadratus lumborum

ROM range of motion

SCJ sternoclavicular joint
SCM sternocleidomastoid
SIJ sacroiliac joint
SNS sympathetic nervous system
STJ scapulothoracic joint

TFL tensor fasciae latae

UHP *Utthita Hasta Padangushtasana*

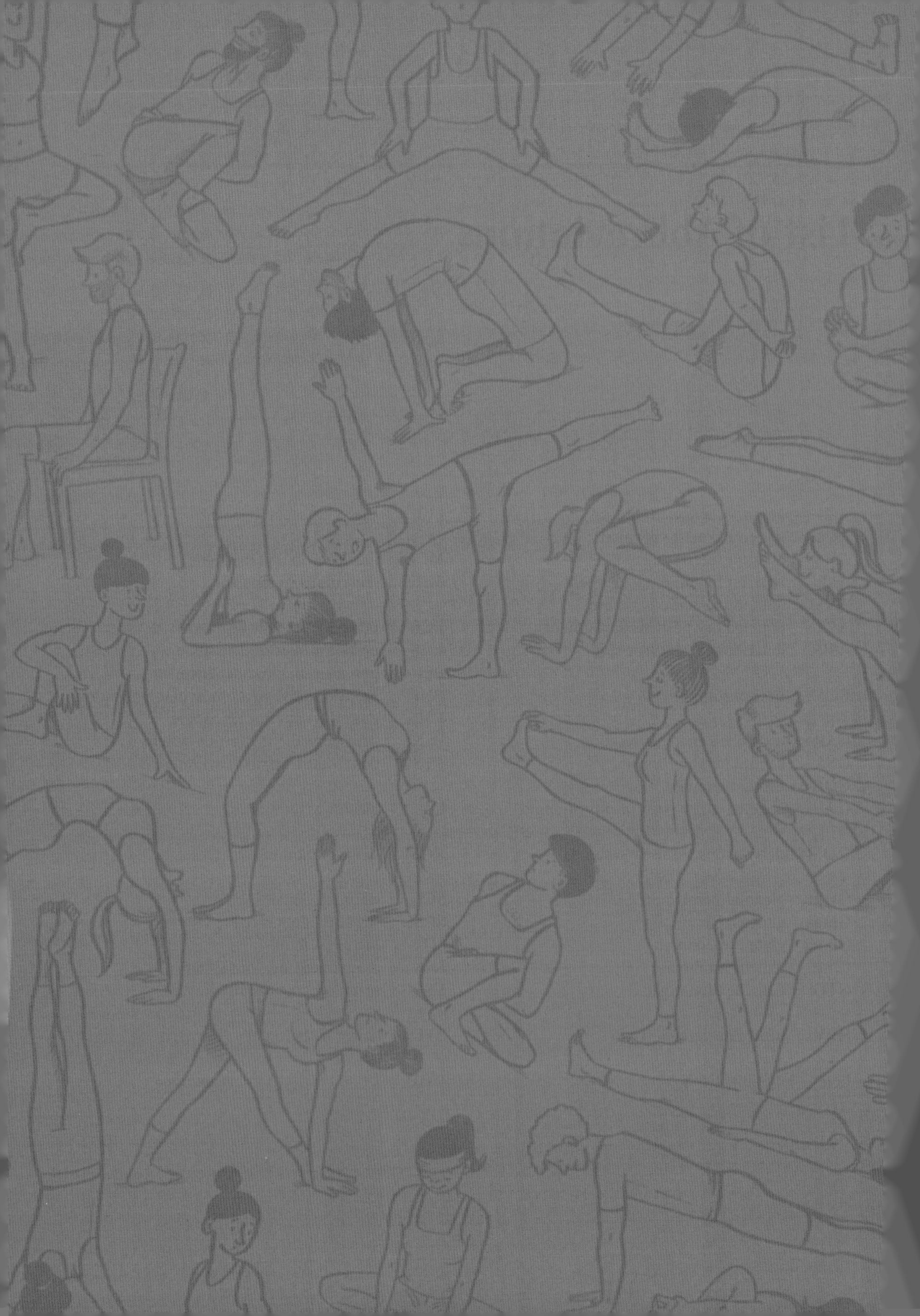

PART I

KEY CONCEPTS

"Key concepts interact with one another differently depending on the requirements of the posture and for each individual. This interaction also changes over time."

CHAPTER 1

Fundamentals of Yoga Postures

Making Shapes

How do we go about making a yoga posture with our body? Well, we have to move our body into a three-dimensional position that closely resembles, or not, the picture in our mind, book, or teacher's instructions. This involves placing our body parts in a particular relationship to one another, our mat, or environment. Arm reaching toward the ceiling, legs so far apart, front leg doing this while back leg does that, standing, sitting, face up, face down, on one leg, on your hands, it doesn't matter, we are making shapes. It might be more than that energetically or mentally, but physically we are making shapes. What that does to us will depend on what shape we are making, how mindfully we are doing it, and if we have any vulnerabilities, as well as how long we hold it for, our foundation, intention, whether we are being active or passive, and what context it sits within.

Now, this might sound a lot like alignment and, of course, it is related. However, alignment is about achieving the essence of the posture by positioning the body most appropriately (see *Alignment*). Making shapes is about where you have to move from to make that shape or achieve a particular alignment. Through understanding the shapes, you can determine the necessary movements, the muscles that will actively create them, and from where a restriction might come.

You might have noticed that it is not always possible to create a shape or posture in the way that you envisage or there might be variations that change how you experience it. Some positions might be comfortable, while others are difficult or maybe even seemingly impossible. This very much relates to the components of each shape. You might consider yourself good at a whole group of postures, while others are a constant challenge.

The parts we need to move to create these shapes are the joints, and several factors influence if we

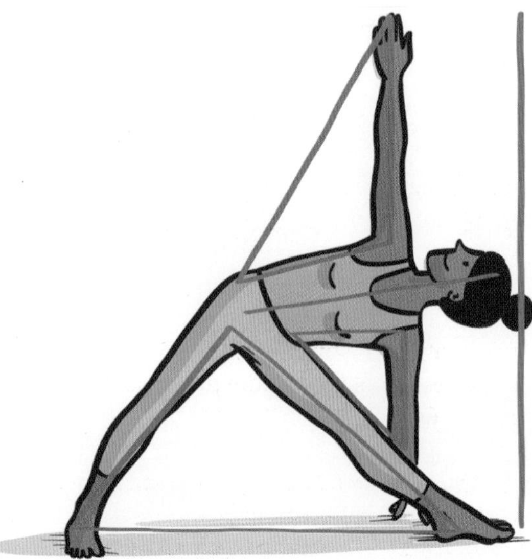

Figure 1.1 Every yoga posture is made up of sub-shapes.

can move the desired amount in the necessary areas. Proportion, flexibility, strength, stability, coordination, bony structure, and technical knowledge are just some of the considerations, and we will explore them later.

We can go one step further and say that each posture is a collection of sub-shapes and that because we live in an integrated body, they have a relationship with each other (Figure 1.1). In short, if we can't move in one area enough, we will generally try and make up the difference somewhere else. Often this is the neighboring sub-shapes, but not always. Whether happening subconsciously through lack of attention or even willingly, then we are likely to be escaping out of the intentions of the posture or, worse still, placing stress on a particular area.

In Figure 1.2, *Natarajasana*, can you decide where in the body our yogi is compensating the most? If you look at the angle of her pelvis, it is still pointing down, and there is a minimal amount of hip extension (leg moving backward relative to the hip). She is mostly making up for this in the lumbar area, but also in the shoulders. As you will find out later, for the majority of us, there is not very much hip extension available, which means that for postures like this, there will always be an area that has to facilitate a lot of the movement. From that perspective, we might decide that this full expression of the posture might not be sensible for everyone to do.

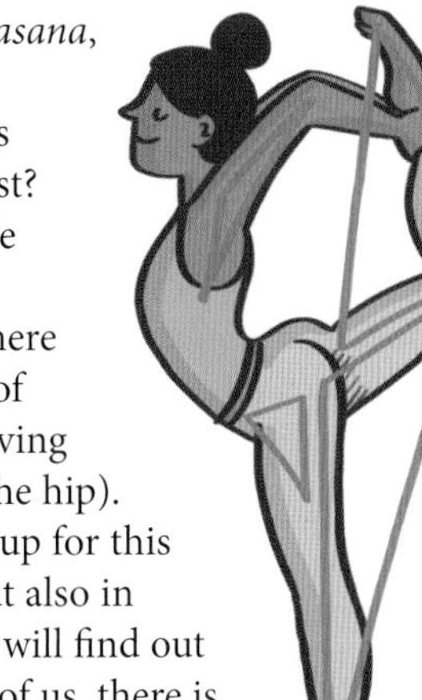

Figure 1.2 Natarajasana *and its sub-shapes.*

Students who have a range of motion (ROM) restriction in a particular area, or excessive freedom in another, often show compensation patterns in many related postures. For example, in *Virabhadrasana A*, students who find extension (bending backward) in the lumbar spine easy often avoid the work of hip extension in the back leg by anteriorly tilting the pelvis to compensate and increasing the backbend (Figure 1.3). Because the spine is between the hips and the shoulders, it is often the site for compensation. Similar exaggeration of the lumbar curve also frequently happens when students are restricted in shoulder flexion (that's taking the arms overhead).

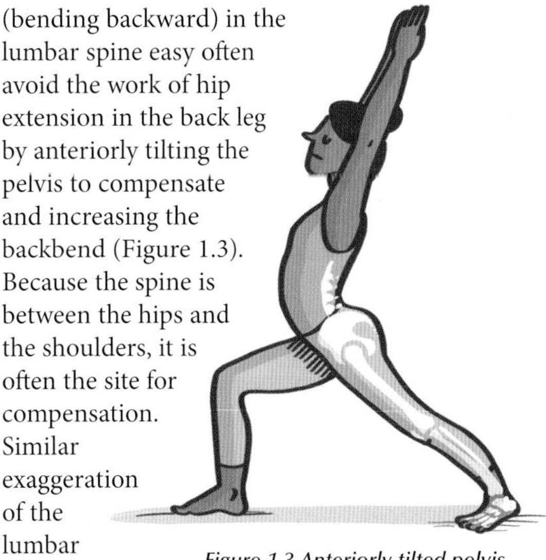

Figure 1.3 Anteriorly tilted pelvis, exaggerated lumbar curve.

Many of those shapes or postures that you find hard or easy will be linked by the commonality of the areas from which you are required to move. There are fundamental movements that need to occur to facilitate the successful completion of a posture to a specific depth, with different ones calling for varying amounts of these from minimal to lots. Should you, for instance, want to create the flat shape of the torso on straight legs, whether standing or seated, you will need tons of hip flexion (Figure 1.4). The ability to create that particular shape is probably one of the fundamental movements that make most postures attainable.

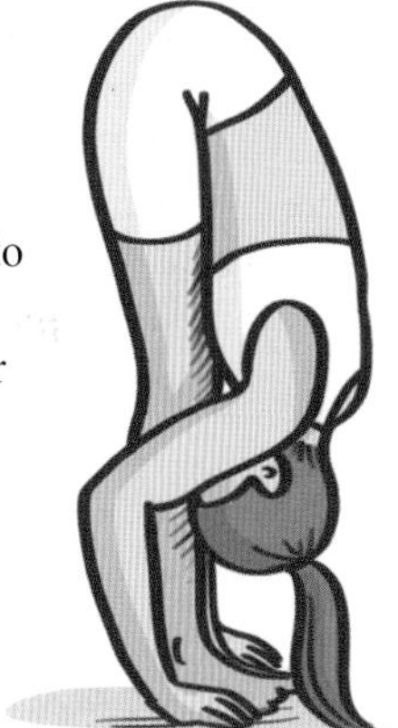

Figure 1.4 Straight-legged hip flexion, a fundamental movement.

You can see now that we also want to be able to consider a posture by the fundamental movements that it includes.

Individuality

We may look similar, but we are not clones of each other (Figure 1.5). Even if we put aside psychology, work, eating and sleeping habits, exercise preferences, relationships, ethnicity, and anything else you can think of, and only contemplate the physical components, we are still not the same. Just consider for a moment the variation in your friends, family, and work colleagues. Tall, short, wide, thin, long arms, short arms, long torso, thick legs, broad torso, narrow shoulders, sporty, couchy, long neck, no neck, the potential combinations are immense.

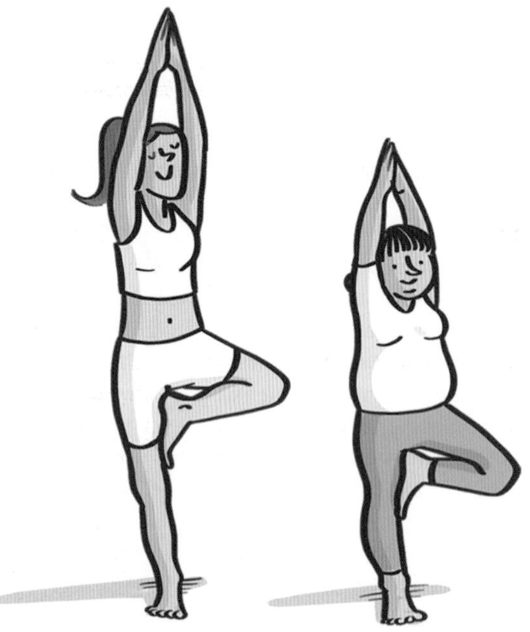

Figure 1.5 We're not all the same.

Let's add some attributes to that, strong, weak, coordinated, clumsy, flexi, stiff, energetic, lazy, fit, unfit, calm, relaxed, stressed, agitated, etc. (Figures 1.6 & 1.7).

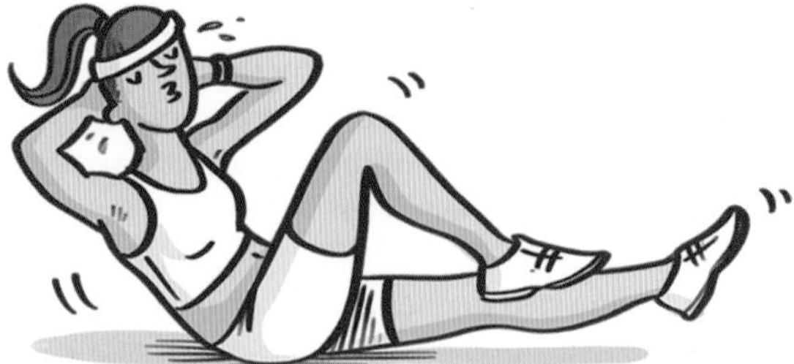

Figure 1.6 Yoga makes me feel so calm, but ....

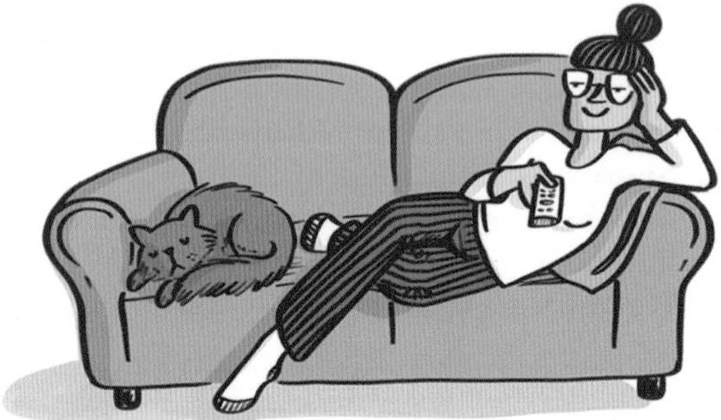

Figure 1.7 Maybe I'll skip yoga today and sit here with Gerald instead.

The human body is fantastic, and we don't want to underestimate our potential, but we are not all made in such a way to be able to do precisely the same or in the same way.

> Try this simple experiment: Can you get your index finger and thumb to meet if you clasp around your wrist? I can't.

This is a proportional relationship. I have neither pianist's fingers nor substantial wrists, and no amount of repetition or daily practice will change the outcome. This sort of body part relationship is repeated everywhere, and some will be beneficial to making yoga postures, others detrimental, and the rest of minimal consequence.

One example of proportion we see a lot of is arm length relative to torso length (Figure 1.8). This might make moves such as L-sits and jump throughs more difficult as the natural clearance will be reduced. A lot of this can be made up for with good engagement of the abdominal area and shoulder girdle, but it will be harder. Shorter arms also have some relevance to the potential pressure on the head in *Sirsasana*, and we will discuss this later.

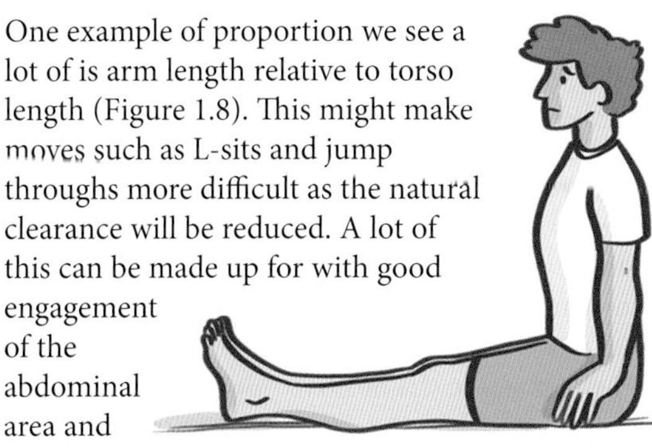

Figure 1.8 Doug has a long torso, but not such long arms.

Any specific yoga posture may itself accentuate the need for particular proportions, or it may not matter. If we think of the posture *Kurmasana*, then nothing gets in the way of anything else. The legs are apart, and if there is the freedom in the hips, the torso comes down between the legs. It doesn't matter how long your legs are if you have a large body.

On the other hand, if you take a posture like *Supta Kurmasana* and you have thick thighs, wide torso, and short arms, your hands won't be able to touch. You may still have enough ROM available in the hips and shoulders, but your proportions are stopping you (Figure 1.9). So, of course, you should hold a strap. Similar obstacles could be easily experienced in many binding postures. Conversely, a student with long arms and slender body can often escape the work in these types of postures, by letting their proportions make up for missing ROMs.

It might not be a case of being unable to do the full expression of the posture but rather that it would be healthier to do it differently. Let's consider a person with a long torso and average length legs. If they prepare to do a posture like *Marichyasana C*, you may see that when they fold in their leg and get ready to twist, the knee is below the height of

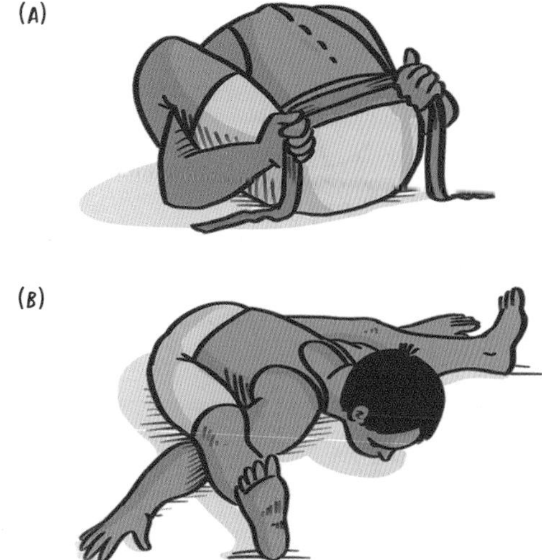

Figure 1.9 (A) Want longer arms? Just use a strap, (B) Vihan has good hip flexion but is stocky.

the armpit. The temptation is often to round the spine so they can bind around the leg. However, this is not very healthy as they are twisting in that rounded spine position. It would be much better for them to hug the leg and keep the spine long (Figure 1.10).

Other times, all we may need is a block to even out the proportions. In, for example, *Ardha Chandrasana*, a student with long legs may well find that they need to tilt the torso toward the floor to place their hand down. This requires greater freedom in the hip of the standing leg and may trigger a compensation somewhere else. Simple solution, block under the hand (Figure 1.11).

Maybe you can sense some physical disproportion in your own body. I feel I have a large ribcage that comes down a long way, stopping only a thumb-width from my iliac crests (the rounded upper ridge of the pelvis). I remember as a young teenager going to a posh school where I had to wear a blazer, and I could never get them to fit—they would burst open at the chest and flap around with too much material around the waist. In workshops, I often get students to feel how much space different students have between the bottom

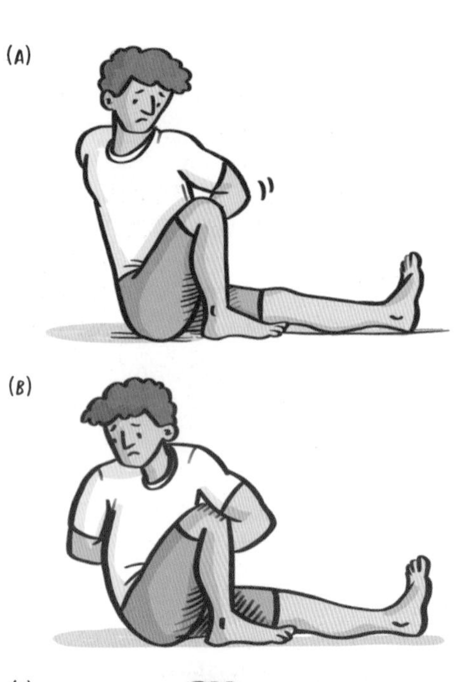

Figure 1.10 (A) Oops, there's that long torso again, (B) look at Doug's low back when he tries to bind, (C) for Doug, leaving the bind is healthier.

of the ribs and the top of the pelvis, and it varies from a hand-width to someone like myself with almost nothing. One of the things I find is that if I don't sit up tall when twisting, the bones rub on each other (good form reminder). You would be amazed at how many below-par maneuvers I blame on this particular physical attribute. Back bending, side bending, foot placement in *Marichyasana B & D* (ribs get in the way), and, of course twisting, are just a few. On the positive side, if some gangster gave me a punch to the kidneys, they should be well protected.

In some styles such as Ashtanga, jumps, lifts, and presses feature highly. In my opinion, not only will someone's proportions greatly influence the ease with which these are performed but may also indicate if it would not be healthy for the body to do too many. If, for example, you have wide hips and a disproportionate amount of your body mass is situated below the waist, then the wrists and shoulders will have to deal with that load as you transition, and they are relatively unstable joints.

Perhaps instead you would like to think about the most suitable yoga practice for someone suffering from anxiety or stress, for a person in their teens or their 80s, new to exercise or an athlete. We are individuals, and our yoga practice should reflect that. Generic cueing is a starting point but is not sufficient in most cases to deal with a class full of individuals adequately.

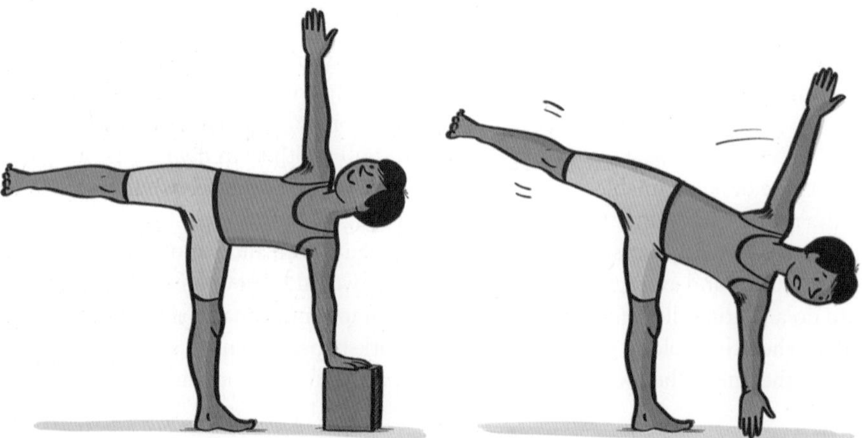

Figure 1.11 For Vihan, a block under the hand brings the body into a much better alignment.

Gravity

The force of gravity is pulling us toward the floor and our yoga mat constantly. It might not be enough to get us on the mat on a dark winter's day, but without it, we would drift off over the trees. Understanding how gravity influences us in yoga poses will give you numerous eureka moments. Ok, I know it wasn't Sir Isaac Newton that first said that, but I'm sure he often had reason to use Archimedes' famous exclamation (Figure 1.12).

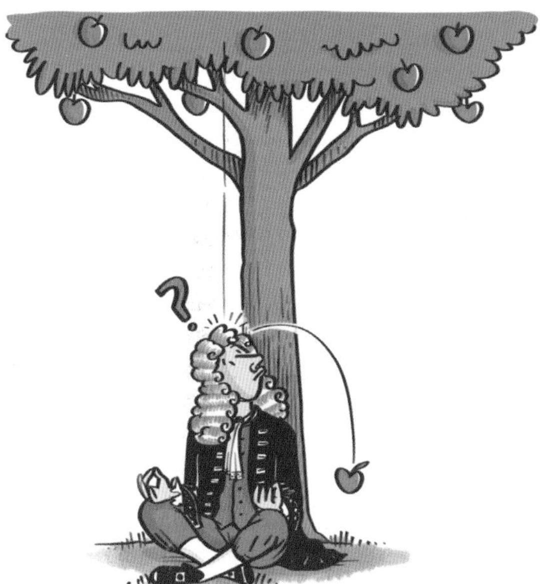

Figure 1.12 Sir Isaac Newton under that famous apple tree.

Gravity can take us deeper into a pose or prevent us from getting deeper, make us feel rushed or grounded, and influence our positioning, balance, and strength requirements. It will be an element of everything we do on the mat, with its influence varying from negligible to considerable. It is also responsible for confusing many students regarding which muscles are needed to perform a particular movement as the orientation changes. So, let's have it, I hear you say.

Lifted-Arm Experiment

Lift your arm for me and then relax all your muscles. Surprise! It doesn't stay where it was, it falls back down. Every time you repeat it, the result is the same, and it will fall at the same acceleration, as would the rest of you, approximately 9.807 m/s^2. Now place your hand on your leg. You can feel the weight of it pressing into your leg.

That's as much pseudo-science as we need to appreciate that whatever we are doing on the yoga mat, gravity is taking us toward it. We then use that knowledge to decide how it relates to the things I mentioned above.

Let's start by considering how gravity helps or hinders us in relation to the depth of a pose. We will use three examples of a V-shaped body position. For simplicity, we won't worry about giving them names, muscle actions, or joint movements, just think of where bits of us are inclined to go and the consequences.

In Figure 1.13, gravity will draw the upper body toward the lower body, helping to deepen the pose. If we chose not to use any muscles to pull the upper half to the lower half, we would still go that way. It would be possible to be very passive

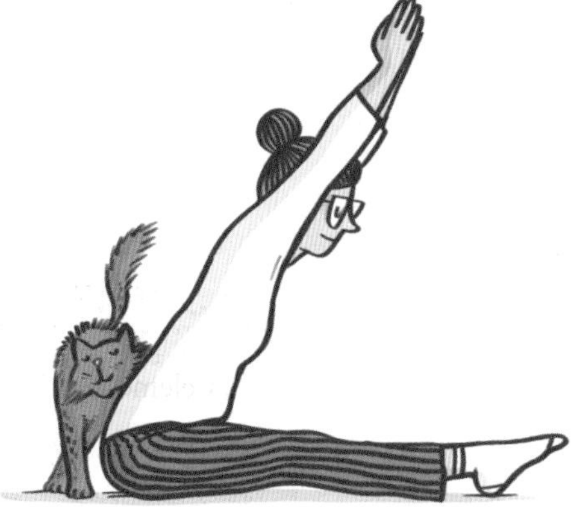

Figure 1.13 Gravity helps to deepen the pose.

and hang out for a while. We can call this a gravity-assisted position, which can certainly make things easier if we can find the right orientation.

In Figure 1.14, gravity will be pulling both the upper and lower halves of the body away from each other and toward the floor. No chilling out here, muscles would need to be engaged to maintain the shape. If we wanted to deepen the pose, we would need to have the strength available to overcome gravity and our soft tissue restrictions. This is against gravity positioning and as such, more strengthening.

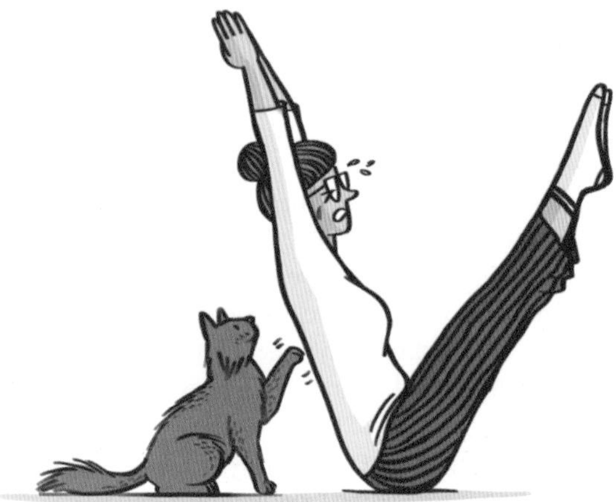

Figure 1.14 Gravity will pull the upper and lower body toward the floor.

In Figure 1.15, the body is in a side-lying gravity-neutral position. Of course, gravity is still pulling on the body, but it is neither taking us deeper nor pulling us apart. Muscle engagement would be needed to deepen the posture, but now we only need to work against the soft tissue restriction and some friction with the floor.

This can be a nice orientation to test out some active work.

The easiest thing to think of next is the potential confusion with joint movements and muscle actions. When a joint is moved, some muscles contract to take it in any direction available, and then others bring it back again. In gravity-neutral travel, muscle contraction will be needed to move the joint in both the opposite paired directions, for example, moving a limb away from the body and then back again. But as we can see from the examples and our "lifted-arm experiment," sometimes the orientation is such that gravity can do the work for you, and what we need to do is control the movement.

We will expand on this more in Chapter 3, *Strength*, but for now, imagine you were turned upside down and raised your arm to point toward the ceiling (Figure 1.16). You would this time need to engage muscles to bring the arm by your side, whereas in our previous example, it just fell by your side. Now, as you release your arm, it free falls above your head, whereas before, you needed to use muscles to bring it above your head.

Now you might think I am pointing out the bloody obvious, but you would be surprised, nearly everyone falls into the trap of not considering gravity when they are thinking of what muscles are needed to get into a pose. If I cut a finger off every time I was told by a student that the biceps were used lowering from High Plank to *Chaturanga*, I would either not have any fingers left, or there would be one hell of a lot of students with missing fingers. Think it through for yourselves now, decide why the biceps are not being used, and we will cover it later in the book.

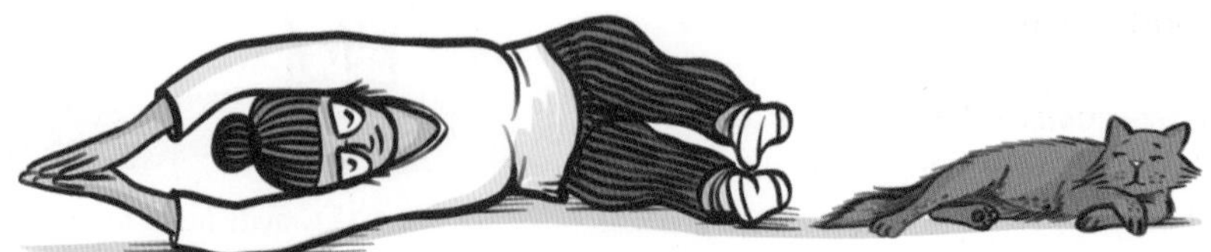

Figure 1.15 Here, gravity is neither taking us deeper nor pulling us apart.

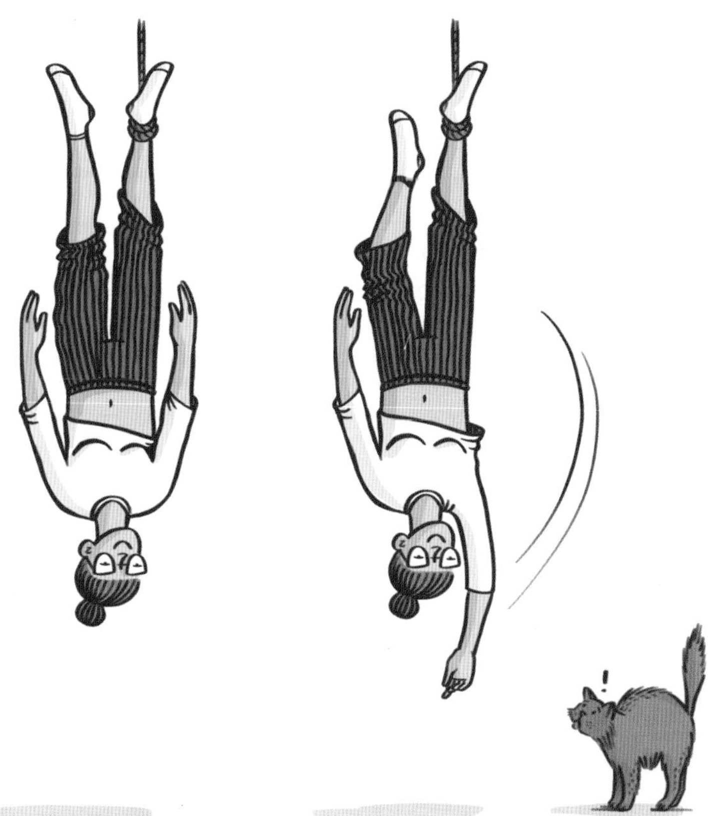

Figure 1.16 This is not what Betty envisaged when she signed up for aerial yoga, but at least she got to demonstrate the concept for us. Your orientation in gravity will determine if muscle contraction is needed to create a movement or to resist one.

Did you notice how quickly your arm fell if you didn't try and slow it down? Well, that's the same as if you are doing any jumping transitions and don't try and control your speed by resisting gravity. The quicker you are traveling, the more rushed you will feel. As momentum is directly proportional to mass and velocity, more strength will be required to bring the body under control the longer you allow gravity to accelerate you toward the mat. The key to grace and fluid movement is to start controlling your descent as soon as possible and don't wait until you are almost at your destination.

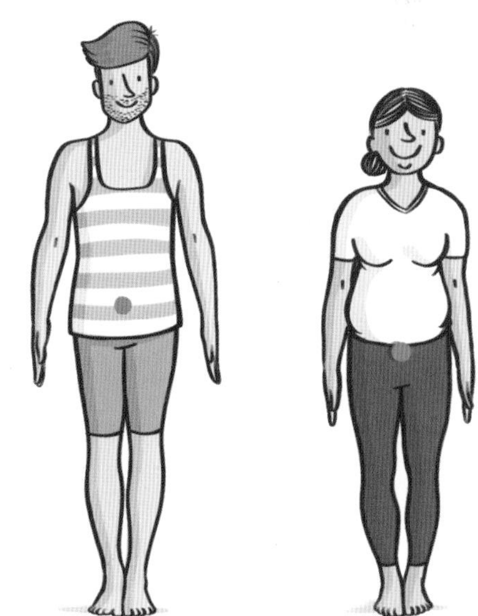

Figure 1.17 COG will shift up and down depending on your overall proportions and weight distribution.

A person's center of gravity (COG) is the point around which their mass is evenly distributed. In an adult, COG is at the level of the mid-pelvis when standing in anatomical position (think *Tadasana*), but as there is a difference in mass distribution between individuals, it will move somewhat up or down (Figure 1.17). Females tend to have more flesh on the hips and thighs, so their COG tends to be a little lower than males, who also generally have bigger shoulders. I have always felt that my legs are really heavy, and my suspicions were supported when Lorraine (my wife) and I signed up for a Thai massage course in Chang Mai. She spent the whole two weeks saying that lifting my heavy legs were knackering her out and that it would be better if she lay down visualizing the moves as I ran through the massage on her. Anyway, to get back to my point, my heavy legs mean that I may have to adjust my positioning in some postures to bring my COG to a place where balance is more easily achievable. Everybody will need to carry out their own fine-tuning according to their individual proportions.

COG is not a fixed point in the body. As we change the shapes we make with the body to create yoga poses, so too does the body's COG shift (Figure 1.18). Depending on how we are positioned, the COG may even be outside the body. A student's COG and its relationship to their base of support (BOS) will determine how they need to position their body to maintain balance. When we come to *Balance*, later in this chapter, we will continue this theme. You can see how gravity feeds into so many other topics, and you will find that I frequently refer to or consider gravity throughout the book.

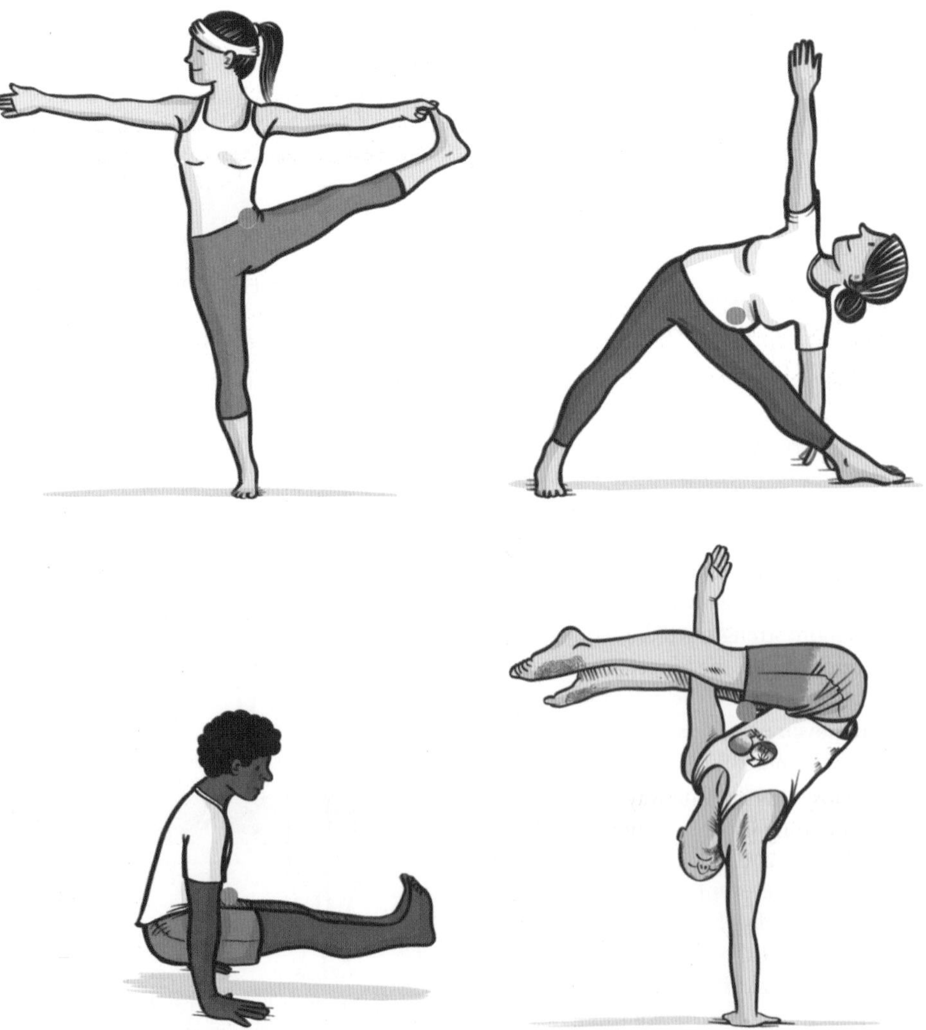

Figure 1.18 As we change the relationship of body parts, the COG will shift.

Alignment

"Alignment is the purposeful orientation of the body in space informed by the intention of the posture and the requirements of the individual."

I came up with this definition a few years ago when I was trying to clarify in my own mind a broader concept of alignment. For many students, the first thing they think about when mentioning this topic is often stacking joints and looking out for wayward knees, or prescribed asana positioning. Let's aim higher.

I think alignment underpins everything we do in yoga but maybe not in the straightforward way that might be easy to jump to, as underpinning alignment itself is intention. The other key elements I blend in as well are health, adaptation, foundation, and mind. I'm sure you know by now that no way am I going to suggest that everybody does the same thing, so how can I be such a stickler for alignment?

Let's forget for the moment about doing a posture the way Iyengar, Ashtanga, or any other school suggests, and think of making the posture in the way that feels right for you. Move organically, flow, feel where you need to be, use your intuition. Can you sense where you are, what is happening in the body, or why you want to be there? Would you do it the same next time?

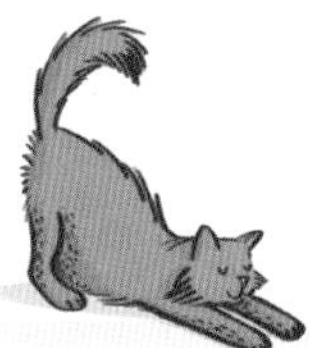

Do it now. Pick a posture or two, put the book down and have a play.

You're back. How close was it to the way you usually do it, was anything in a dodgy position? In Chapter 2, *Moving in Patterns*, I will discuss some of the reservations I have about free movement, but for the moment, I'll say that I think it's hard to learn from a form without guidelines. So, does that mean that I think we should always perform a posture in the way somebody has detailed? No.

Every style of yoga has some recommendations about how we should place our body when doing a particular posture. I call this an "Asana Blueprint." By positioning ourselves in a certain way, there will be a corresponding emphasis on something specific. It might, for example, be the twist, inner thighs, the rotation of the back hip, the symmetry or asymmetry, strength, balance, mental calmness, or ROM. Whatever it is, as we change our position between styles, the emphasis will change too. As the body thrives on variety, mixing it around would probably make the most sense, but how hard should we try to stick to the prescribed shape when our body doesn't want to cooperate? I think it is the essence of the posture that is important, and if we must distort ourselves so much to make a shape that is not available, then that essence is likely to be lost. Adjust the posture for yourself as an individual. If it is meant to be a twist, make sure you are twisting in the thoracic spine; if it is a hip rotation, make sure you are getting some action in the hip and not accommodating it in the knee, and so on.

Do these asana blueprints serve any purpose? I think they do because, by trying to make the shape as detailed, we uncover the reality about where we are restricted (Figure 1.19). However,

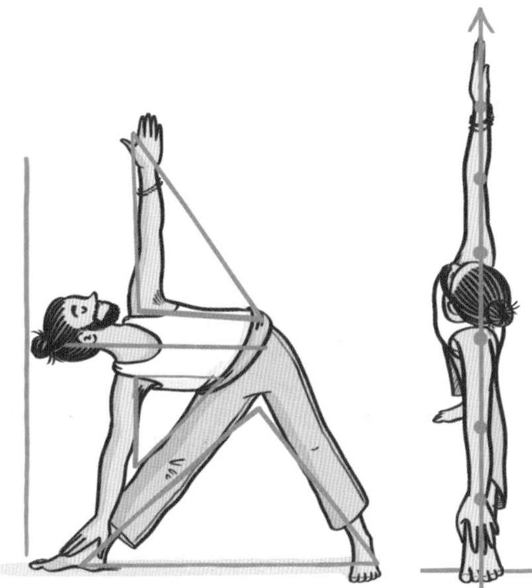

Figure 1.19 Utthita Trikonasana *aligned in a single plane.*

quite often, we have to be present enough to notice we are not doing what we think we are. I feel the best approach is to start off trying to perform a posture in whichever style is your preference. If it is easy, then try adjusting it, maybe a wider or narrower stance than you are used to or a different angle of the feet. If it is too hard and you are losing that essence, use a prop or change your position enough that you can realize the work in the posture. Now and again revisit the blueprint to see how things are changing.

It is the purposeful orientation of the body that allows us to challenge our restricted or weak areas. What is the intention of the posture, what is our intention? For example, twisting is something I find hard, so when I do *Parivrtta Trikonasana*, I often keep my top hand on my hip so I am not tempted to fake the twist by moving at the shoulder more than the spine (Figure 1.20).

In *Parshvakonasana*, I like to have a very wide stance with my front thigh parallel to the floor to work on leg strength. I also put my bottom hand inside the foot rather than outside because I feel that I access the groin better in that position. We can do the same posture, but by changing things slightly, work on different aspects.

One of the things to consider when placing ourselves purposefully in space is whether there are any potentially detrimental outcomes. In other words, how healthy is it for us? This is where we start thinking about the position we have placed certain joints and if they are now vulnerable. As with most things to do with the body, the conclusions are far from straightforward.

Let's use the example of placing the knee in front of the ankle in a lunge or similar posture. The idea behind this contraindication is that it can give rise to an amount of stress on the knee joint that, in some individuals, might cause injury. Although this might be a good starting point, nothing exists in isolation. If we are taking our weight backward rather than forward, the forces into the front knee will be reduced. What about the amount of bend in the front knee, or the proportion of weight in the back leg? Our vulnerability may be more related to our strength in the muscles that cross the knee and those that stabilize the leg than the position itself.

We may even choose to place the knee in a more challenging position if we have built up the strength to control it, especially if we might encounter that position in some other exercise we do and want to prepare the body for it. We will look at some more of these possible body placement contraindications in subsequent chapters.

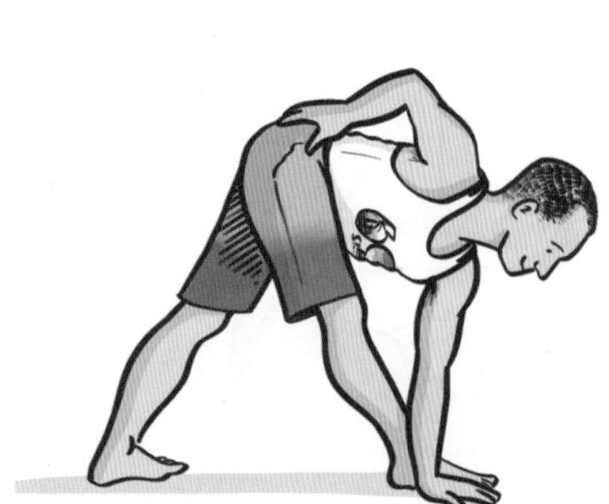
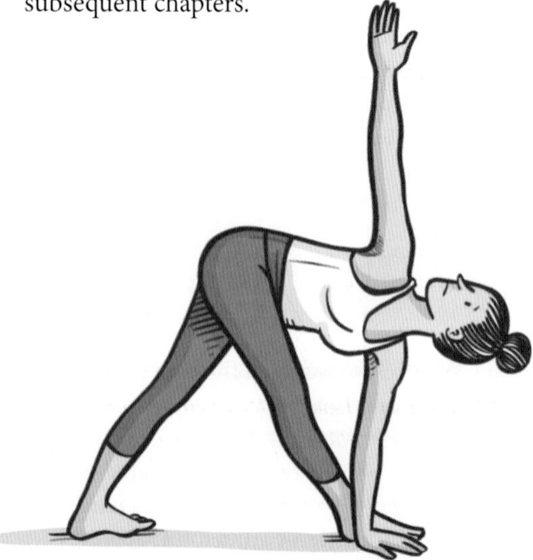

Figure 1.20 One possible adaptation for Parivrtta Trikonasana *to suit the individual.*

Certain postures require that we place ourselves in a potentially vulnerable position. Taking straight-arm *Bakasana* as an example, a substantial degree of wrist extension is necessary to move our COG far enough forward to maintain balance, especially if you have plenty of junk in your trunk. That positioning can place a lot of strain on the wrist, particularly if you have a less robust bony framework (Figure 1.21). In these situations, we must ask ourselves if this version of a posture is sensible for us to do. Generally speaking, the more flamboyant and fancy a pose is, the greater the risk involved.

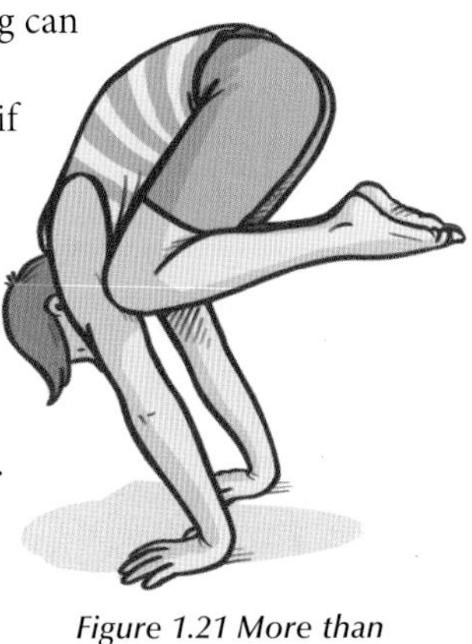

Figure 1.21 More than 90 degrees wrist extension required.

Sometimes, deceptively simple shapes provide an almost too enticing opportunity to put ourselves in harm's way. For example, *Paschimottansana* is near enough just a flexion at the hips with some spinal flexion once your ribcage touches your thighs. However, so many students faced with a pelvis that doesn't want to tilt anteriorly due to uncooperative hamstrings (oversimplification, but it will suffice here), round the spine, consciously or not, excessively placing detrimental pressure on the low back (Figure 1.22).

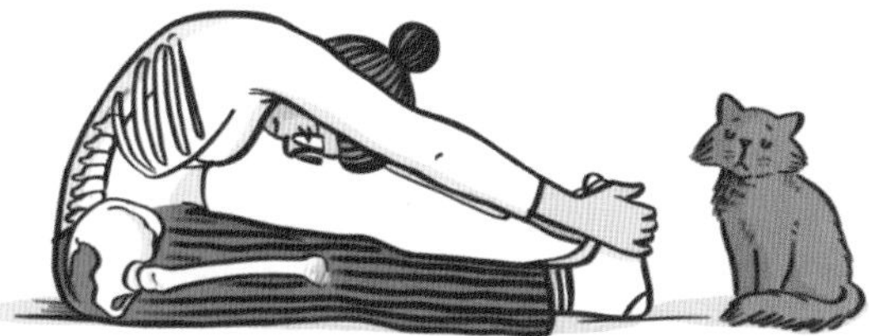

Figure 1.22 Stick your head in almost any yoga room and you will see this dubious form.

There may be times when a healthy alignment is just not available for a particular individual. If, for instance, we take someone with a hyperkyphotic thoracic spine performing *Sirsasana*, I would suggest that they can't align themselves in a way that their cervical spine would not be vulnerable in a weight-bearing position. In these situations, it is better to seek the essence of the posture in something else entirely. You could use a headstand stool, or if it is the inversion that you are after, maybe just put the legs up the wall in *Viparita Karani* (Figure 1.23).

One of the most useful tools we have available to us is adaptation. We can access an otherwise unattainable posture by making suitable adjustments to our position or by using props to provide necessary support or foundation. We can also alter the emphasis of a pose by making subtle changes to the alignment. We might choose to challenge the ROM of a different area or to work more on balance, strength, or coordination.

For example, students who are hypermobile need to find the strength work in a posture and not just hang out, which, of course, will be a lot easier. On the other hand, those students whose bodies veer toward stiffness might need to find a way to do a posture where they can work more slowly toward the proposed shape, deciding on more passive or active flexibility depending on how well they respond to each.

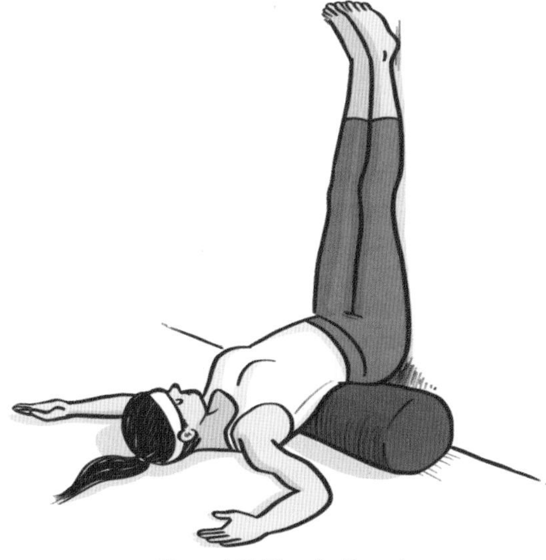

Figure 1.23 Viparita Karani.

Adaptation also gives us the incredible potential for variation, the real food that the body thrives on. As the human body is such a fantastic organism, it responds to new challenges by adapting, getting stronger, more agile, resilient, flexible, or stable. Adaptation for variety is as essential as adaptation for accessibility.

One of the most important adaptations to make is aimed at accommodating an injury. I think there is much confusion around this area as there is a great deal of talk around practicing through an injury, or the yoga practice helping to heal. If you are in pain and you continue to do things that hurt, then you will just turn your issue into something that, at best, is a chronic problem and, at worst, is something that will stop you from practicing altogether for some time.

With most injuries, it is a particular area of the body that is affected and then usually only specific directions or movements. Generally, it is possible to continue to practice, but only if you adapt what you do by removing or modifying those postures that cause irritation or pain. It may be that you feel pain whenever you use an area or only when you stretch or use strength, in which case, modify accordingly. This might mean you need to adapt the width of a stance, complexity (such as removing the bind), the number of times you repeat something, the amount of support, or the number of foundational elements or distance between them. Sometimes, if an injury is severe or happens to be one that is difficult to adapt for within a dynamic practice—e.g., an intercostal strain—then you may temporarily need to change the way you practice completely and do something more supported, such as restorative or Yin.

This brings me nicely to the use of blocks and props. These aids are actively discouraged by some styles of yoga or teachers, but often they are just what the student needs to find an alignment that is right for their proportions and ability level. It is, for example, much better to sit on a blanket or block in a seated forward fold if the alternative is to have the pelvis in a posterior tilt (dropping backward, Figure 1.24). As we have mentioned already, there is such a variety of body proportions and tension patterns that no singular asana alignment will suit all individuals. We don't need to go through all the ways that props can be used in different postures, but suffice to say, that if their use enables a better foundation, more desirable body positioning, helps to control wayward limbs, or allows the student to access areas that would otherwise be bypassed, then it is definitely worth considering their use.

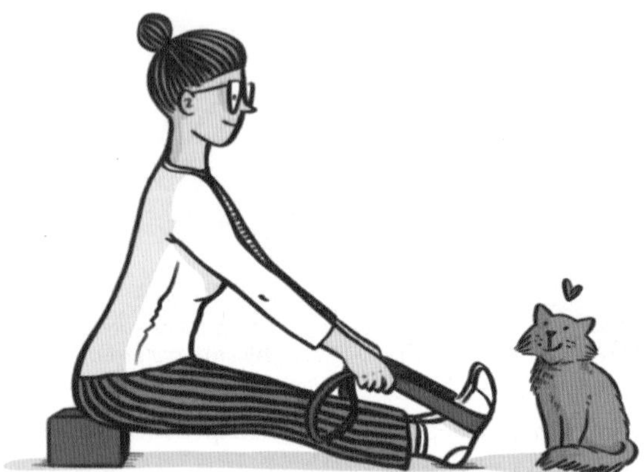

Figure 1.24 Use props to get rid of that crappy technique and everyone will be happier and healthier.

If your chosen style of yoga is dynamic or fast-moving, then the use of props can be seen as disrupting the flow. It is better to think of this as a temporary phase that will assist you in keeping a healthy position in challenging postures while you are waiting for your body to open or get stronger. The idea of an adaptation that changes over time is important; as our ability progresses, we need to continually assess what we really need so that what was enabling us does not become a crutch.

Our foundation is the base upon which we build our posture. It might be two feet, one hand one foot, two hands, forearms, backs of the legs, or whatever comes into contact with the mat or floor. Much like building a house, if the foundations are shaky, it's not going to last long. The quality of the foundation will influence everything else above it. The smaller the foundation, the less stable, and as we work within gravity, the greater the forces that will be experienced in that area.

As a starting point, some postures are symmetrical and others are not. It may seem simple, but if the posture is symmetrical, so too should be our foundation. How often do you see, or even notice in yourself, hands that are not level in Down Dog (one a little further in front of the other), a foot turned out more, one shoulder coming down lower in *Chaturanga*, or one elbow wider in Shoulderstand? Is the head twisted or tilted in *Sirsasana*? I know I see it a lot. The reason is often muscular tension patterns, but has the practitioner noticed and are they trying to actively re-establish symmetry.

Proper alignment won't be established from a misaligned foundation as compensation will be occurring higher up the chain. Of course, the problem arises that, as you try and align your foundation, those same tension patterns will pull something else out of alignment, so it is a constant interplay between pieces. If you are a vinyasa practitioner, now would be a good time to look at your mat and see if the wear patterns are symmetrical. Generally using more effort from one leg will result in differences.

The forces generated by gravity and body weight will be directed down to our foundation, so we need to be actively lifting out of that foundation. We also want our weight distributed evenly over our separate foundational elements (foot, hand, etc.) as well as somewhat equally between those elements. I say somewhat because depending on where our COG is, that will not always be possible or desirable. For example, if you are doing *Ardha Chandrasana*, there will be more weight on the foot than the hand.

Sometimes we may want to take our weight forward or back, but that is a conscious decision, not an unconscious pattern. We may also find ourselves favoring a stronger side (Figure 1.25) or protecting a vulnerable area by shifting more weight into one side more than the other. With asymmetrical postures, depending on which one it is, there will be a tendency (even necessity) for more weight to be in either the front or rear leg. The idea would be to distribute the weight more evenly and not dump it all into one foundational element.

As far as the individual elements go, we want to spread the load. Common mistakes would be taking too much weight toward the outside of the hand, placing strain on the wrist or the inside edge of the foot due to collapsing arches, over pronation, etc. Spreading of the fingers and toes can help toward having a foundation that is more stable and responsive to the fluctuation of alignment above it.

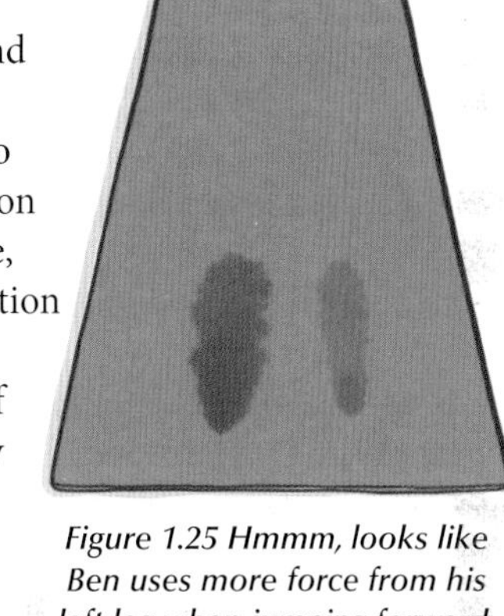

Figure 1.25 Hmmm, looks like Ben uses more force from his left leg when jumping forward.

From that strong and stable foundation, we should be able to maintain our position more easily, balance, and move our attention inward. We often mention stacking of joints, and the body indeed uses less energy when the gravitational forces can be directed down through the bones. But although this might work well in postures such as *Tadasana* and High Plank, once we start to shift our COG, we need to change our minds. Later in the book, we will explore *Chaturanga* and return to this discussion.

When I'm exploring this topic, I like to add in something about aligning the mind. We often talk about being present, but that is not always easy to achieve. We can spend whole chunks of time moving our body this way and that as we go through our practice but at the same time thinking about something completely different (Figure 1.26). In the same way as driving a car and suddenly thinking, "I don't remember going through such a place." We can be on autopilot. The problem with that is we are relying on established movement patterns and neglecting the daily fluctuations of physical performance. Have you ever been adjusted in a posture and thought, "That can't be square?" It feels wrong, even though you are told you are now aligned. We get used to our ways and imperfections, and we cannot rely on feel alone as our spatial awareness can be flawed.

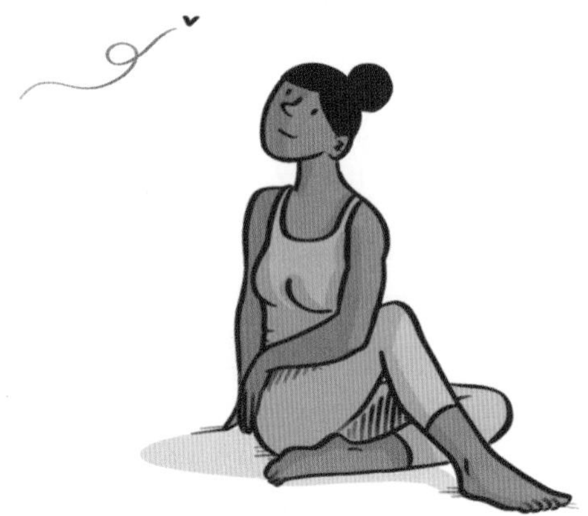

Figure 1.26 The mind loves to wander and wonder.

I don't think that we will naturally find good alignment over time. If we are not consciously aware of what we are doing, we will continue to repeat existing patterns indefinitely. If we have tension patterns, muscular imbalances, or even structural variations (e.g., a shorter leg on one side or scoliosis), we will be pulled in different directions and, after a short time, that position will feel "normal."

We also need to be tuned into how our body feels at that moment. An alignment that was fine yesterday may not be available now. As our practice develops, new opportunities will present themselves; going deeper into a posture will change the alignment options. As different parts of the body open or get stronger and more stable—we often forget it is not all about gaining greater and greater ROM—it will change the alignment possibilities for other areas. It is always worth revisiting your gross alignment. On numerous occasions, I have found that I could do something I didn't think I could. If I had not been present, I would not have discovered that.

When explaining some of my ideas about alignment, students sometimes say, "I like to flow and just do what I do, not be thinking about the details all the time," and depending on what your intention for your practice is, it may be a valid point. It is possible to get wrapped up in certain things at the expense of others. However, the problem with not addressing alignment issues adequately is that you may not get the physical change you desire, and particular aberrant movement patterns may set you up for repetitive strain injuries. If you are a flow- or meditation-based practitioner, you can have it all ways, just spend some time to establish new patterns when necessary, returning to check on them at regular intervals. Practice with fluidity but also sensitivity and awareness.

The key for me is always to know why you are positioning yourself in a certain way. Sense if you are altering a posture, without realizing, in order to escape a restriction. If you have always done a pose in a particular way, then try it slightly differently to see how that changes the way it influences the body. If you have a vulnerable area or injury, adapt the shape to keep you from aggravating the problem further.

Fighting Own Restrictions

Do me a favor and scratch your head. How much effort did that take? Not much, I hope, or we have a lot of work to do. Have you ever been wearing tight clothes and tried to do something and either had to exert more effort to do it or couldn't achieve what you wanted? Maybe you felt the springiness of resistance pulling you back. There are, for sure, some yoga postures that require strength to do, but for the most part, there is not so much needed.

So, what is it we are experiencing when we think we are not strong enough? Mostly it is ROM restriction in the necessary joints and directions, and more often than not, this is muscular. Often the same thing is going on in different positions, but we don't realize because of our relationship with the floor and that wonderfully useful, but at times, frustrating force of nature called gravity.

Let's explore this with a simple example:

If you are sitting in *Dandasana* and decide to fold forward but can't, it is quite easy to accept that some restriction to hip flexion is preventing your desired repositioning. We might instinctively say, "my tight hamstrings are stopping me," but, of course, it's often not quite that straightforward. We may observe some students flop forward onto their legs with close to zero effort, even though, hopefully, they are still being active (Figure 1.27).

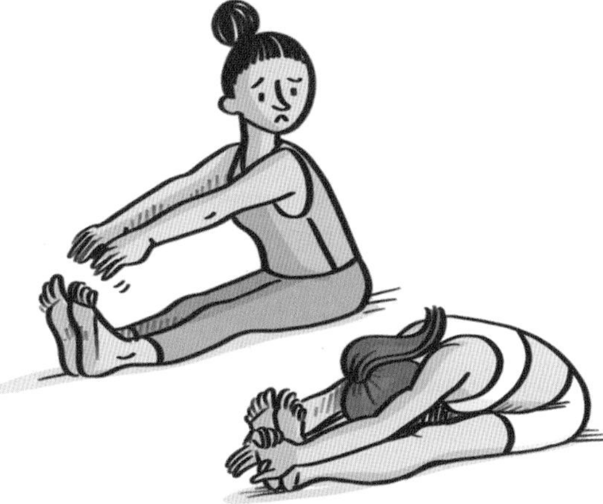

Figure 1.27 Some students find forward bending much easier than others.

Now instead of going forward, we decide to do *Navasana*. We may choose to make a beautiful sharp-hulled boat by raising our legs higher, but they may not cooperate. We are contracting everything that can help us to do hip flexion, but our boat still looks like a rowing boat, not a speed boat. Our groin and legs may then get tired from the effort, and it is easy to think that you need more strength, but the same restrictions that stopped the seated forward fold are again at play here (Figure 1.28).

No amount of extra strength will help if the fundamental movement of straight-legged hip flexion is not available. The same person that had that comfortable forward flop will undoubtedly have a relatively easy sharp *Navasana*. But, what about gravity, long legs, heavy legs, big belly?

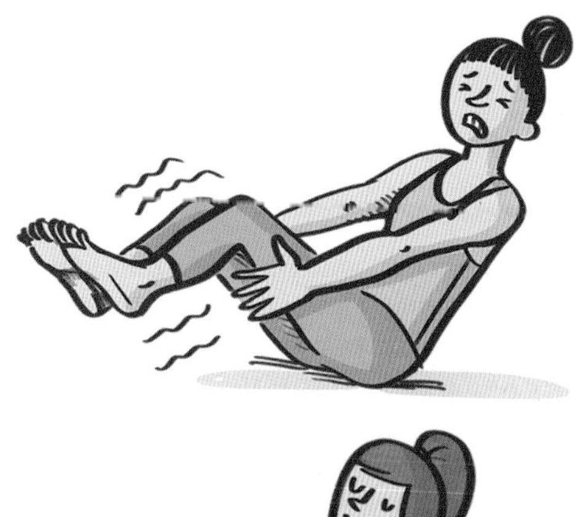

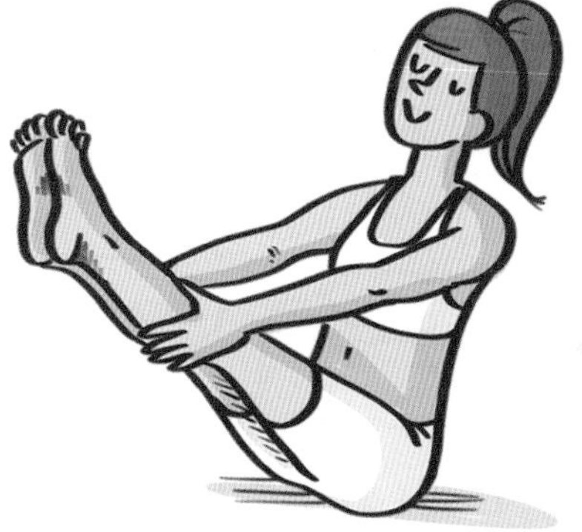

Figure 1.28 Navasana *requires easy straight-legged hip flexion, not so much hip flexor strength.*

Yes, they are also factors, but the major one is the limited hip flexion ability.

In the posture *Urdhva Dhanurasana*, some students will, again, have the feeling they are not strong enough to push themselves up off the floor. Only very occasionally is that the case; it is usually resistance in the shoulders or hips to the necessary ROM (Figure 1.29). So how do we know which it is? If the student can perform the required joint movements for the posture independently but still

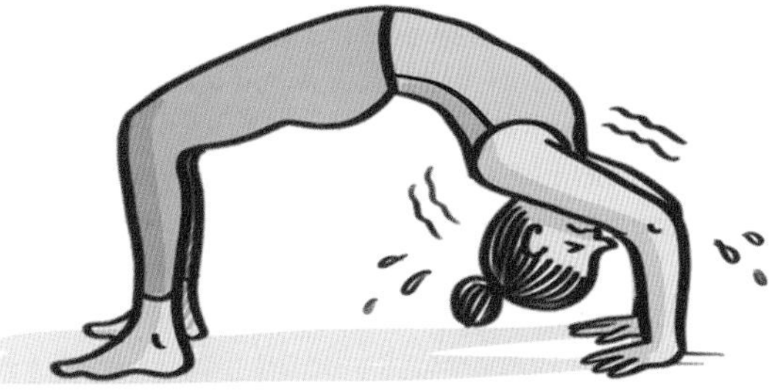

Figure 1.29 It is not often that lack of strength is the reason students can't push up into Urdhva Dhanurasana.

can't push up, then maybe it is a strength issue. However, I would again look at the technique first.

Sometimes in class, to illustrate this point, I get someone who finds *Urdhva Dhanurasana* easy to demonstrate, and then while they are up, engage them in a conversation to show how little effort they are expending (Figure 1.30). On the flip side, a student with severe restriction may feel they are trying to lift a car as they attempt to push up, go red, and veins might pop out on their forehead. You can't overcome your restrictions with willpower alone. Ease of creating postures comes from lack of limitation and the strength to control your ROM.

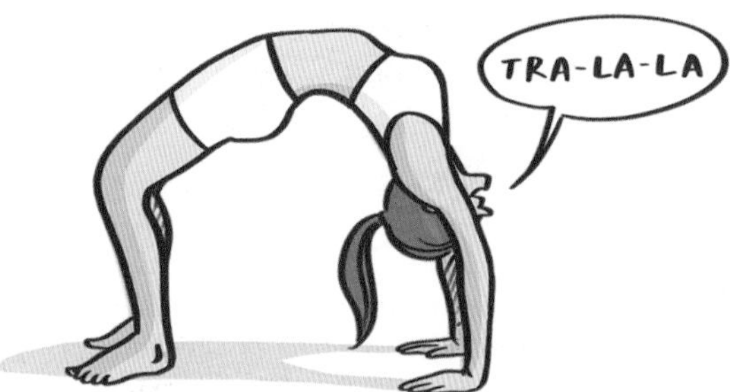

Figure 1.30 The less muscular restriction you have, the less strength you need to push up.

One more example introduces polyarticular muscles (Chapter 3). If we have changed the angle at one of the joints that a muscle crosses to facilitate a greater ROM at another, then we may experience what seems like a strength issue when we try and move the original joint back to its starting place.

To illustrate this, I will use the example of *Tittibhasana*, which, in essence, is a very deep straight-legged forward bend. If you are not sure, take a moment to think about what the finished posture looks like and where you would have to move from to create it.

There are many ways to enter *Tittibhasana*, sometimes as a separate posture or maybe as a transition, but the essence is similar. The knees are bent as much as is necessary to flex the hips deeply, resting the backs of the legs on the arms.

Now comes the fun of straightening the legs. Because for most students, the resistance to straight-leg hip flexion needed for this posture comes from the hamstrings, many students find that they are unable to straighten their legs once they have them in position on their arms. To straighten the knees, we can contract the quadriceps, but it may again seem that they are not strong enough to do that.

The reason for this sensation is that our hamstrings have already lengthened quite a bit because of the deep bent-knee hip flexion that was used to initiate the move. As we now try to straighten the knees, the attachments of the hamstrings on the lower leg move away from the upper leg, further lengthening the muscle. If we have no more lengthening available, the legs won't straighten, no matter how much strength we have (Figure 1.31). Why? Because you can't fight your restrictions! Again, our student with comfortable straight-legged hip flexion will have little resistance to having straight legs in this posture (Figure 1.32).

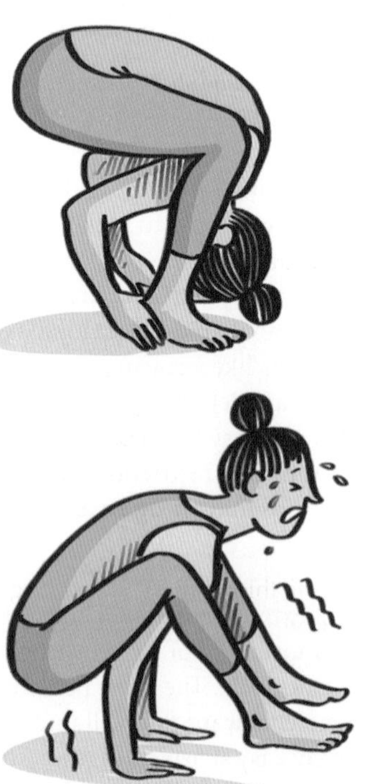

Figure 1.31 Straightening the legs is not a strength issue.

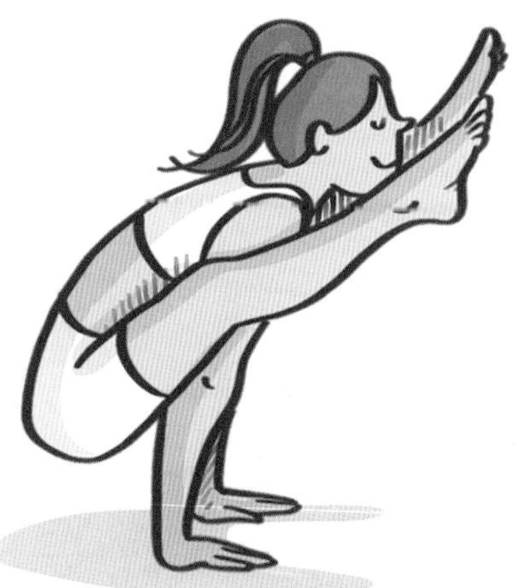

Figure 1.32 Easy peasy lemon squeezy.

If you want to test this idea out in a sample way without the need to try the posture, you can have a go at this . . .

Therefore, this concept involves examining a posture to see what moves need to be performed at which joints. Check that you or your student has that ROM freely available before deciding it's a strength thing that is the problem. Relax, don't force.

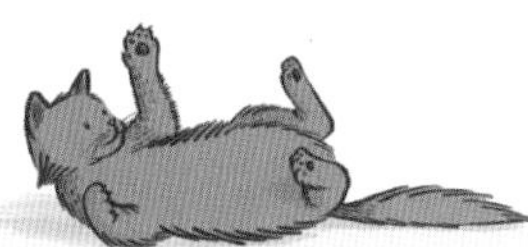

Lay on your back with both legs straight on the floor. Now bring one straight leg toward your head—you can gently pull it if you want. Make a mental note of where it comes. Keep the leg in the air and now bend the knee. The leg will travel toward you, increasing the hip flexion.

Keep bending the knee and bringing the thigh down until you land up in *Ardha Ananda Balasana*. If the thigh is past your ribcage, it approximates the amount of hip flexion needed for *Tittibhasana*. Hold the thigh and keep it where it is while you try and straighten the leg. Unless you have a relaxed straight-leg forward fold, you won't be able to straighten the leg. This is exactly what is happening in *Tittibhasana*.

Balance

When we think of balance, we generally visualize some variation of a single-legged standing posture, but of course, our foundation could be on our hands, head, elbows, knees, or, in fact, any body part. This view of balance involves us placing our body in such a way that we can maintain its position relative to our foundation. The wider the foundation and the closer our COG is to our BOS, the easier it is to balance. If we have multiple foundations, aligned primarily in one plane, we will be more stable in that plane but probably less stable in other planes.

In Chapter 5, *Psychology*, there is an image of me doing a *Sirsasana* variation. Balancing is more achievable in this posture if you have your hands not directly in line with your head, but where's the fun in that? Have a go and see what you think, not really!

If you tune into your body when standing in *Tadasana*, you will feel that you sway slightly back and forth (postural sway), Figure 1.33. With our high COG, just maintaining this upright posture requires the constant interplay of muscular effort and regulatory control loops. Static stability is not enough (standing rigid). Usually, when you observe someone in a static pose, you don't notice these continual small corrective movements, but record some video and then play it back speeded up and the constant movement will jump out at you. When you have time, video yourself in a standing posture you feel really solid in, but don't forget to speed up the playback though.

Even though we feel pretty secure standing still on both feet, our body is using proprioceptive feedback to keep the body upright against the force of gravity. If you start to lean to one side, a tilt of only a few degrees will begin to bring about instability.

Figure 1.33 Tadasana *from the side.*

We can think of the space between our foundational elements (our feet in this case) as the critical area of support (BOS). The vertical projection of our COG is called the line of gravity, and as it moves further away from the BOS, the higher the rotational force and the less stable we become (Figure 1.34). Our BOS is fundamental to maintaining position, and the body will try and keep our COG within it, either by moving our body relative to our feet, or our feet relative to our body. This is regularly demonstrated in *Utthita Hasta Padangusthasana* when we observe students succumbing to a hopping reflex as they lose their balance, and the body tries to reposition the foot under the COG.

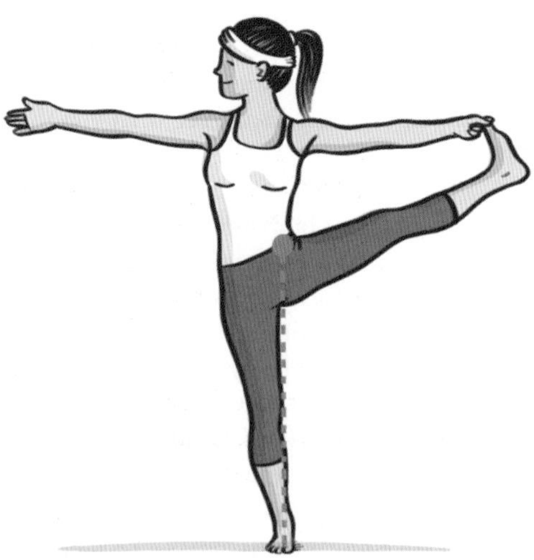

Figure 1.34 COG shifts because the leg is out to the side. The line of gravity then needs to be kept over the BOS for easy balancing.

The greater the area covered by our BOS and the more foundational elements that make it up, the easier it will be to balance. I have often used this principle when trying to learn a new balance by using an extra foundational element, such as a hand, and then gradually reducing the weight in that part until you can do the balance without that additional help. ROM allowing, you can make any shape you want with your body and the same principle of keeping the line of gravity over the BOS, will apply. As we mentioned in *Gravity*, sometimes the COG is actually outside the body because of the way it is positioned (Figure 1.35).

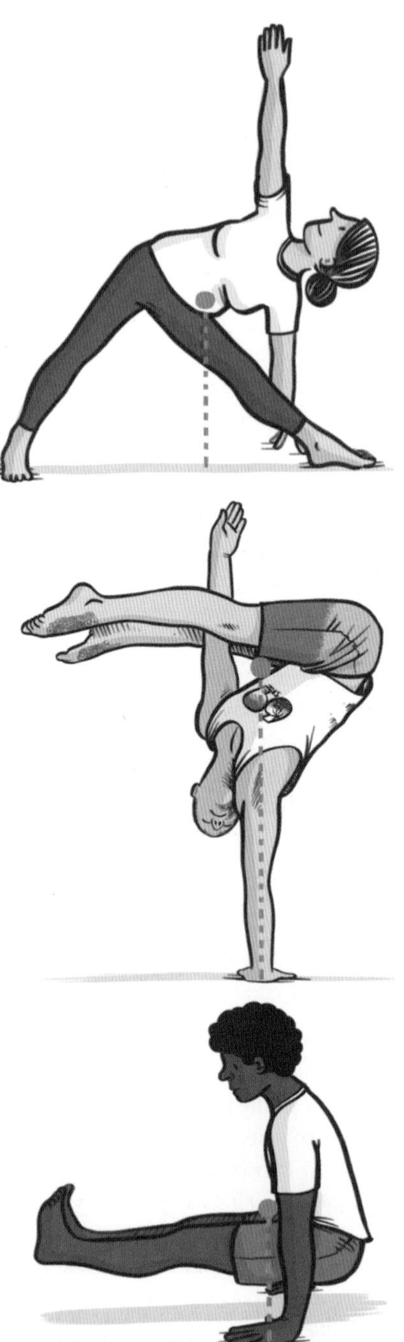

Figure 1.35 Sometimes COG lands up outside the body because of its position. It still needs to be placed over the BOS.

The more we shift our COG away from our foundation, the more strength we need to use to maintain the position.

The mass (body weight) of the individual will also play a role in the way the body needs to be aligned to maintain balance, and a good strength-to-weight ratio will help a lot. Not only is the total mass a factor but also the distribution of that mass. A good example is how the body has to adjust its posture when pregnancy causes a significant distribution of weight to the front of the body. The back tends to extend, bringing the head and shoulder back as a counterbalance.

The same can be seen with the male equivalent of the substantial beer belly. Often backache will result from this repositioning as the back muscles have to work extra hard to try and stop the body tipping forward.

In *Mayurasana*, your hands are the foundation of balance, and your elbows are the pivot point for your body weight. It will require less strength to position yourself parallel to the ground if you can have roughly the same amount of weight in front and behind the elbow, and the elbow over the wrist. If you have a heavy lower body compared with your upper body, you will probably need to move the elbows toward the groin. However, where you can place your elbows will be mostly dependent on the length of your upper arms relative to your torso. If you try and move them further down and your arm is not long enough, your shoulders will be pulled down, shortening the front of the body, and causing it to round toward the floor. So, instead you can try and shift more weight forward of the wrists (Figure 1.36).

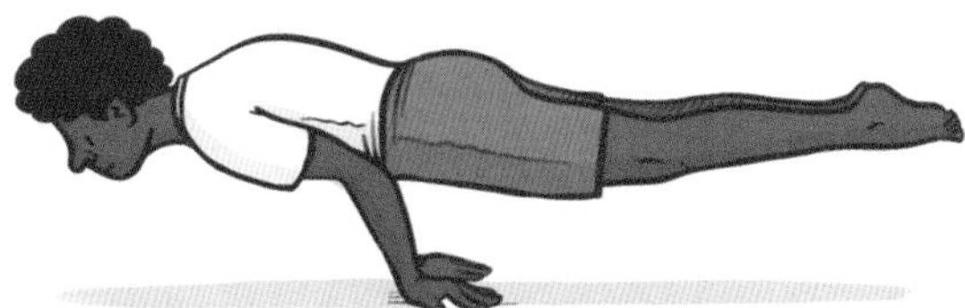

Figure 1.36 Aren has shifted his elbow forward of the wrists to find balance. This is also kinder on the wrists as less extension is required.

If the upper arm is kept parallel to the ground and the angle at the elbow is increased, the body will move forward slightly. The downside is that if the fingers are pointed forward, the movement described will increase wrist extension, which (a) must be available, and (b) could make the wrist vulnerable. If the fingers are pointing toward the toes, then this is not a problem because the movement can be combined with decreasing wrist extension. In *Padmasana*, more weight is brought closer to the COG, so finding balance will be easier (Figure 1.37).

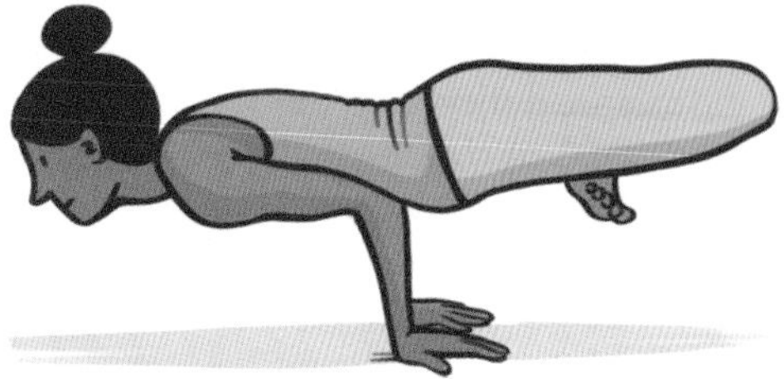

Figure 1.37 When the legs are folded in, balance should be easier as the lever is shorter.

Balance can be either static (held) or dynamic (transitioning). In any balancing posture, you will notice there is a constant interplay between the muscles as they work to maintain your balance, even having to account for your inhales and exhales. With dynamic balance, there is an even greater need for sensitive motor control. You are contracting some muscles and relaxing others as you move, while all the time, holding some static. We can often see that those students we might consider as more mobile (especially in the spine) have a hard time with balancing, particularly in inversions.

If we take a Handstand as an example, I have come across many students who can do very advanced backbends (Figure 1.38) but cannot hold a static Handstand even though they may be able to transition through it such as when performing tic-tacs. They can find it hard to stabilize that mobile spine and hence the relationship of the upper body to the lower body (Figure 1.39).

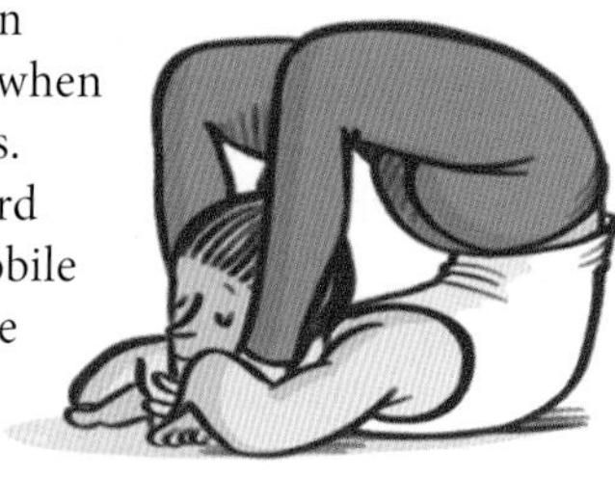

Figure 1.38 Sasha is so content in deep backbends.

I often teach that more flexibility can lead to less stability at joints in the absence of the appropriate strength to control increases in ROM. It is that last bit that plays an integral part in balance. Students, such as the ones mentioned previously, will see dramatic improvements in their ability to maintain this sort of static balance if they focus on strengthening their core area and shoulders. If you watch videos of performance artists, such as those from *Cirque du Soleil*, you will observe that it is possible to have both properties in abundance.

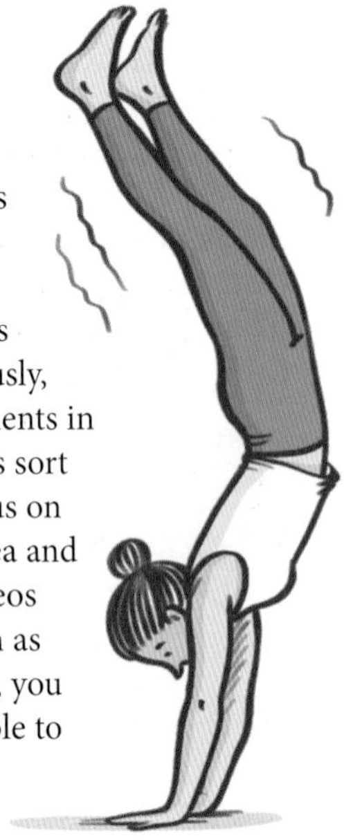

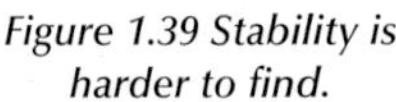

Figure 1.39 Stability is harder to find.

I am going to suggest that balance extends beyond just maintaining our position in space with minimal foundation. I'm not sure where the line is that separates balance from alignment, but many fibers blur the edges. If we don't have our foundation or COG nicely positioned, successful balancing will be fleeting.

I was reminded rather ruthlessly the other day that balance resides in many of the less precarious postures when I spectacularly fell sideways out of *Parivrtta Trikonasana*, landing on my backside. After 19 years of doing this posture, I am obviously still a klutz! When you start yoga, you can have trouble sometimes lengthening into a standing pose because you feel you are going to lose your balance or fall over. So, we need this stable base and balance in many poses that we don't consider balancing postures per se, so we may focus on other elements.

Attaining high levels of proficiency in balancing postures is heavily dependent on not only the necessary strength and available ROM but also the development of superior neuromuscular control and the processing of sensory information. These last two items are strongly associated with learning. I think most of the gains in neuromuscular control come from doing the posture or easier variations repeatedly. Initially, we often overreact to the smallest wobble or movement, almost trying to hold ourselves rigid in case the slightest movement throws us off our balance. Over time, we gain a sensitivity of voluntary and reflexive muscle activity—allowing us to correct our position more smoothly—as well as relax and move other parts of the body almost independently of the main work of the balance itself. Hand in hand with the need for better motor control is a smooth flow of neural information and the subsequent processing and interpretation of it. The sensory systems of importance are visual, vestibular, and somatosensory.

The visual input we receive helps to give us spatial orientation within our environment as well as the speed of movement and direction through that environment. The fixing of the gaze on a point of reference is a common example of using visual input to steady our balance. I have noticed in the past when doing yoga outside, that even something as straightforward as *Trikonasana* can present a balance challenge when your reference point is a clear blue sky. Try closing your eyes in a posture and see how the balance falters.

The inner ear contains the vestibular apparatus, which is responsible for providing information about the head's movement in relation to gravity, building up the picture of how we are positioned at any moment. It is particularly important in dynamic stability. The stimuli from the vestibular system provide information independent of the visual system, which must be how we can still balance when we close our eyes. I am not sure if it can tell if we are upside down or not because I remember an incident when I was diving in zero visibility and, without a point of reference, got confused as to which way was up or down.

Somatosensory refers to information from sensory receptors in the muscles, tendons, ligaments, and joint capsule (mechanoreceptors) that provide feedback on muscle state (contraction, length, and tension) and joint position. Sensors in the

In standing balancing postures, one of the primary sources of information is coming from the mechanoreceptors in the soleus and gastrocnemius muscles. They are responsible for controlling a lot of the postural sway and play a major role in our orientation relative to our foundation. Golgi tendon organs (GTOs) give information about muscular tension, and muscle spindles on muscle length and speed of stretch. With our feet in contact with the ground, pressure sensors help to let us know our distribution of weight across the feet. The vestibular sensory system gives us information about the position of the head in space (Figure 1.40).

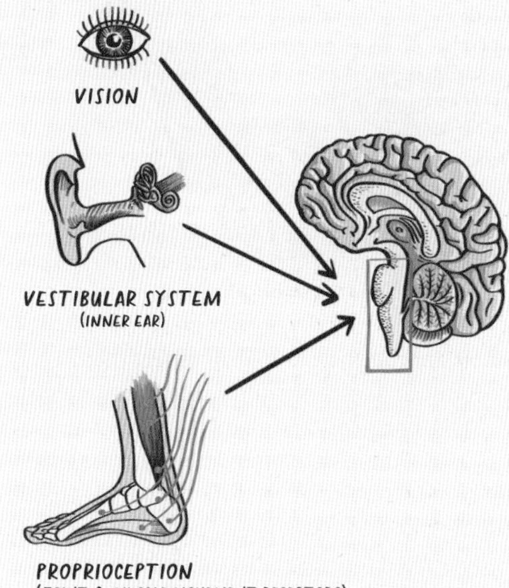

Figure 1.40 The vestibular sensory system.

To know how our body is situated, we need to be aware of the positioning of the head relative to the body. This information comes from proprioceptors in the neck muscles and around the cervical vertebrae. Through sensory input, we are continually monitoring the positioning of our body and any internal forces generated. We are also sensing external forces, such as gravity and from a teacher.

An excellent way to improve your balance is to do yoga outside in the wind (Figure 1.41), necessitating a constant adjustment to these forces. Coming back inside you will find that you are rock solid. Just make sure you are on stable ground and clear of obstacles so that you don't land up coming back with an injury instead.

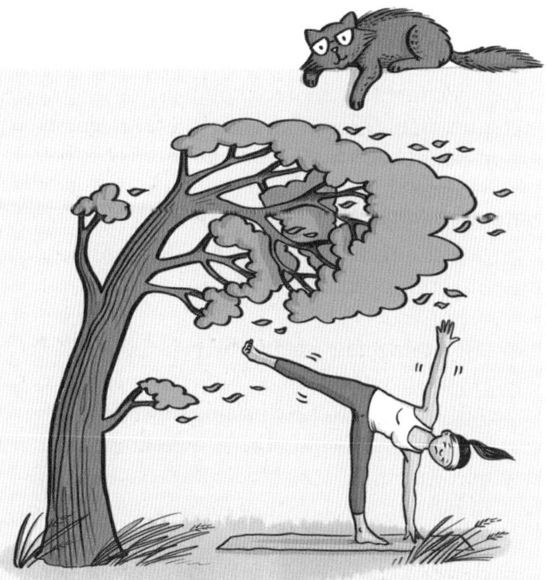

Figure 1.41 Practicing in adverse conditions can help you improve your balance.

All this collected information is what we might call feedback, and what we decide to do about it is called compensatory postural adjustments (CPA). However, so we are not just playing catchup, the body doesn't just wait for something to happen and react. It also thinks ahead using what it has learned so far and makes anticipatory postural adjustments (APA) using feedforward mechanisms. These include taking into account the expected magnitude of the disturbance to balance, associated voluntary action, postural configuration, and any additional tasks being performed.

I would like to suggest you take the time to watch the YouTube video with Andrey Moraru called "Fragment." One of the impressive things about his control is not necessarily how much time he spends on his hands or how easily he goes up, but all the extra movement going on once he is balanced. It is seemingly utterly independent of the balance itself (watch those feet!).

skin and fascia provide additional information on temperature (thermoreceptors), pressure, vibration, tactile sensation, and pain (nociceptors). All this input helps build a picture for the brain as to where one body part is relative to another (proprioception), as well as how fast it is moving in a particular direction. For instance, we don't need to see to bring our finger to our nose.

This last bit might be useful when cueing someone while in an inverted balance. I often come across students who have trouble placing unviewable parts of their body within their environment. For example, you might ask a student to take their hips toward the wall. Because they can't see their hips or the wall, they are not sure which way that is even though they know the wall is behind them. Often, some reference to other body parts instead can achieve the desired movement. An example would be the instruction, "bring your pubic bone toward your ribcage."

These inputs provide continuously updated information and feedback on our spatial positioning. The body needs to learn how to filter out the most useful information and react with more sensitivity, either through voluntary or reactive movement. If you started practicing Handstands next to the wall, you might remember initially giving the wall quite a clunk as you kicked up. Eventually, the body learns how much effort to use, when to put the brakes on, and how to engage the right muscles quickly to maintain balance. It is not too long before you find yourself kicking up and finding the right place without having to touch off the wall first.

Based on the experience of similar situations, the body guesstimates what is going to happen and gets ready to do it. I think this is what happens with my wife, Lorraine, in *Sirsasana*. She knows she gets scared when I help her because I straighten her up, so more often than not, when seeing me get up to help, she somehow is already on her way down. Joking aside, there is a lot of learning involved in balance, particularly when finding that right spot quickly. Repetition, familiarity, and not overreacting to small fluctuations of steadiness, are vital principles to finding proficiency in balancing.

When we looked at alignment, I brought up the point of being focused and fully present. Balancing is one of those areas that is unforgiving if you are thinking about what you will have for breakfast (Figure 1.42).

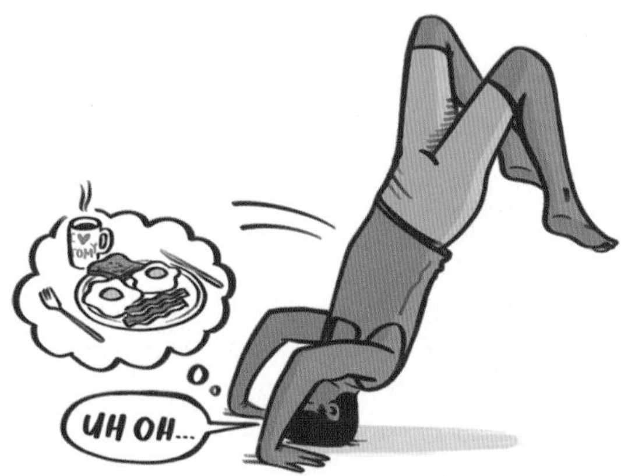

Figure 1.42 Focus on what you are doing.

There is another psychological aspect that I have found makes a big difference in achieving the riskier balances, and that is to know you have a way out. I remember when I first started Handstands in the center of the room, I was afraid of falling like a tree flat on my back. Consequently, I tended to keep my weight too much toward the safe side (called under-balance). Once I learned that I could pivot and cartwheel out if I felt I was going all the way over, I felt safe to explore the limits of my balanced position. So maybe practice how you will fall out of a balance, much like you learn to do an Eskimo roll when starting with canoeing.

We have postures that challenge us to maintain a position in whatever orientation, but we can also think of balance in terms of evenness. Is our weight spread across a foundational element in a balanced way?

If we use the foot as an example, we could ask if it is distributed evenly between the inner and outer heel, base of the big toe and little toe, and then between front and back. Expanding from there, we could consider are we taking too much weight into one foundation compared with another. If the posture were some form of asymmetric standing forward fold, we could try and feel how evenly our weight is between our front and back leg. Even in a seated posture like *Paschimottanasana*, it would not be uncommon to feel a difference between how your sit bones, calves, or heels contact the ground.

If we went to the foundational extreme and lay in *Shavasana*, I wonder if we scanned our body whether we would feel we made contact with the earth evenly. Try it at the end of your next practice and see if you notice one heel more as it presses into the ground, a shoulder blade, or uneven head. This pose is an excellent time to routinely perform a body scan on yourself, as in this relaxed position, we can pick up on tight, light, heavy, or even achy areas. As a teacher, you will often observe students in *Shavasana* that are completely wonky. It is a perfect time to square people up while they can process the altered body alignment in a supported position. If you are going to adjust someone in *Shavasana*, don't leave it too long. I made the mistake of quietly approaching someone and placing my hands on their head, only to have them jump out of their skin with a shriek. The student must have been on the verge of nodding off, and my intervention sort of spoiled that peaceful feeling until another day. Still, you only make that mistake once!

We can even think about balance in our body as a whole. Are we tenser on one side compared with the other, and is one part of the body disproportionately tighter or more open than another? I know many people who come to see me for my bodywork suggest that one side of their body feels completely different from the other. It also seems that any issues they get also reside on that same side.

If we are applying our model from this angle to a particular posture, we could consider how it addresses that balance in ourselves or in itself. Most asymmetric postures are repeated on both sides, but some considered symmetrical are only done once. For example, poses that involve the legs in *Padmasana* are invariably only done the once. If we always take the same leg in first, that could not be considered balanced. Long-term practices like this create differences between the two sides of the body.

Transitions are another area that we tend to have a favorite way and, as such, can lead to imbalance. If you are a student who jumps through and back, do you always cross your legs the same way or are you taking care to even things out by changing the cross? Those of you that do the former will be astounded at the difference between the sides if you have a go the other way around. Do you always kick up with the same leg into a Handstand or *Pincha Mayurasana*? If we wanted to get picky, do you always do the same side of a posture first? As a teacher, do you always put the same leg forward to take someone into drop backs?

Recently I cracked off half a back tooth eating some bread with hard grains in it (or maybe it was a stone) and was reminded how even subconscious tasks can create imbalance. I had to try and chew on the other side of my mouth, which turned out to be surprisingly awkward as my renegade tongue kept throwing the food back to that side. This simple preference is bound to create some muscular imbalance around the jaw. I know chiropractors and osteopaths often locate the jaw as a root cause to problems. I even noticed I have a crooked smile. I wonder if that comes from the one-sided chewing! I know we have got way off the point here with my eating habits, and it would be a bit of a stretch to link it to my tighter right shoulder. Still, I reckon even small repetitive deviations will create patterns of movement that will land up as imbalances in either strength or ROM.

If we return to our first view of balance, that of maintaining our position relative to our foundation, in many instances, how we achieve it will also be heavily dependent on joint ROM. We will take the forearm balance *Pincha Mayurasana* as our example. If you do not have sufficient shoulder ROM in the required directions (flexion and external rotation), you will be placed in a position where you have to take your legs further over your head to be able to balance.

Because balance is so heavily reliant on strength, ROM, and learning mechanisms, it is also posture variable. Just because you can balance in one way doesn't mean you will be good at another (although I imagine your learning curve won't be so steep). In Chapter 3, *Variety*, we discover that Ashtangis who go to a vinyasa flow class and experience *Ardha Chandrasana* or *Virabhadrasana C* for the first time, wobble around incredulously. We can now add variety to our shopping list of things to do to attain excellent balance skills.

You may feel that magic has no place in such a serious textbook as this, but I can't leave *Balance* until I have introduced the *Magic Fist* (Figure 1.43). Ideal for those practitioners that struggle with balance routinely or as an emergency "save me" go-to movement for those unexpected lapses of concentration. You'll be glad to know I haven't patented this move, so you are free to share and use as you wish. Easy peasy, as you start to wobble (Figure 1.44), make a strong fist with a free hand, and reach the arm toward the floor, feeling the body brace (Figure 1.45).

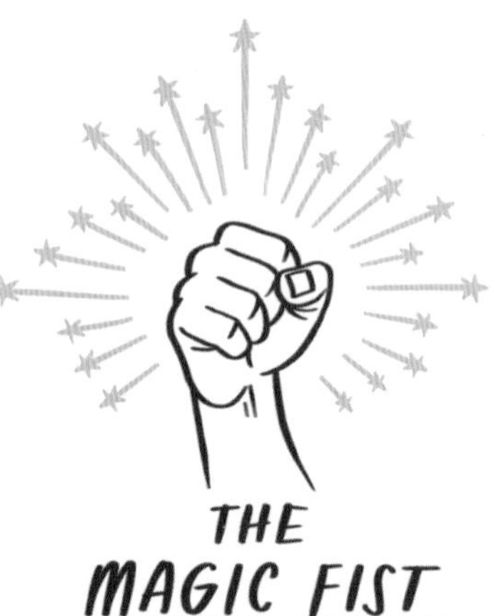

Figure 1.43 Magic Fist.

Only use the magic fist for good!

From this rather long topic, we can begin to think of how to improve our balance prowess. First, consider how you are going to move your COG before you remove one of your foundational elements. Experiment with an exit strategy if needed, and then let your body learn what is

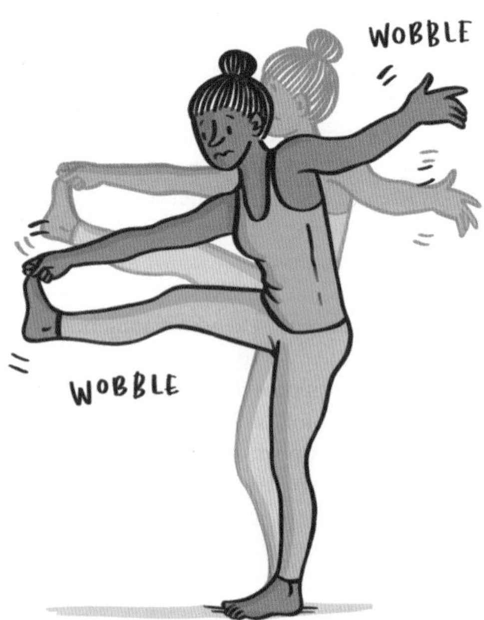

Figure 1.44 Starting to wobble!

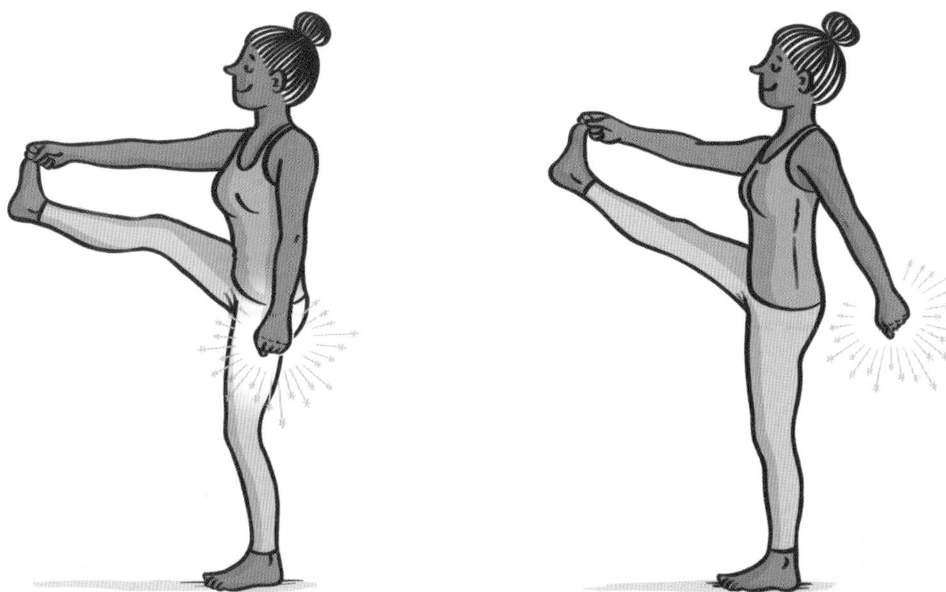

Figure 1.45 For that extra secure feel, take the arm back behind the body.

required of it by practicing a lot. Keep the mind focused and gaze still, tune into your foundations, and sense the distribution of pressure. Work on building up any specific strengths required, especially around the core, and, last but not least, add in lots of variety.

If in trouble call on the magic fist!

CHAPTER 2

Movement Basics

Range of Motion

"Range of motion is joint-specific and direction-specific."

I call range of motion (ROM) the king of concepts, and getting to grips with this one undoubtedly opens up an excellent, straightforward way to view the components of postures and the movements required to perform them. You'll start to be able to predict with which poses a student will have trouble, sequence more effectively, and give individual adaptations while still maintaining the essence of the posture. As such, this section will be a bit longer, so give yourself time and go over anything that's not entirely sticking. Remember you can look at Appendix 1 if some of the terminologies are troublesome.

ROM refers to the ability of a joint to move in a particular direction. In a scientific setting, it is measured in degrees. We might say that a specific student has 120 degrees of hip flexion so should have no problem with their forward folds as it is the major movement required in that group of postures. As a comparison, a person that has an average amount of hip flexion would be able to achieve about 90 degrees, and a severely restricted person maybe 70 degrees. If you were to look at charts of joint ROM, they measure hip flexion with a bent knee, here I am considering a straight leg. For our purposes, we want to differentiate between hip flexion available with a straight leg or bent leg, but more on that later.

Flexibility is directly associated with the ROM through which you can move. So, we could say as far as hip flexion is concerned, the student who has 120 degrees of movement is flexible, 90 degrees has average flexibility, and 70 degrees inflexible (Figure 2.1).

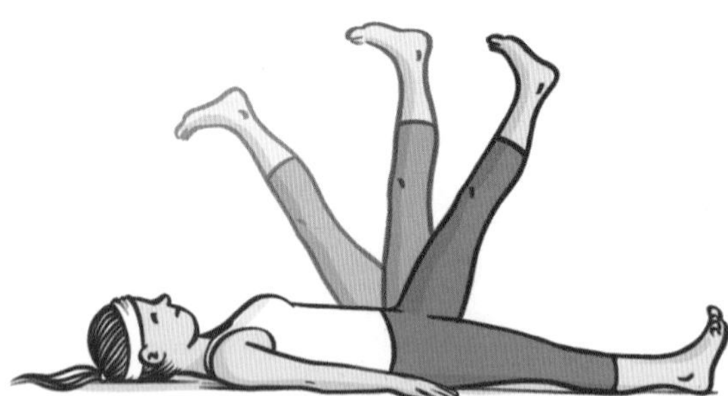

Figure 2.1 Example of straight-legged hip flexion from left to right 120, 90, 70 degrees.

Although I often say 90 degrees rather than leg straight up, perpendicular, or something similar, in a yoga setting we are much more likely to say that a student has a lot of a particular movement or that the movement is challenging. The availability of specific ROMs directly relates to our ability to make those fundamental movements and related yoga postures. Don't worry if I have thrown a lot at you, it will all become clearer.

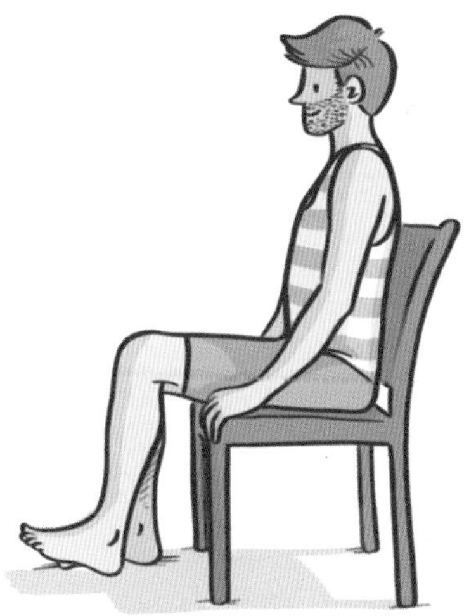
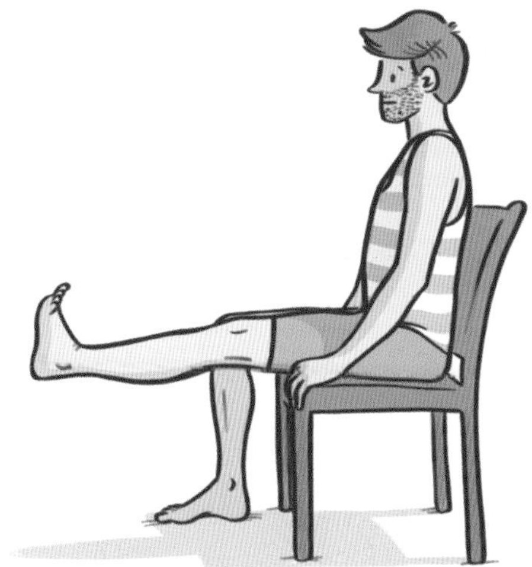

Figure 2.2 The hinge action of the knee, flexion (left) and extension (right).

When we are thinking of ROM, we have several things to consider. We can start by saying that each joint has only specific movements that can be carried out because of its design. So, for example, I'm sure you know that a ball-and-socket joint, such as the hip, has many more directions it can go in than a hinge joint, such as the knee. Nothing is straightforward when dealing with a human body, so although we call the knee a hinge joint, it is not really like a door that opens and closes; it is more of a modified hinge as it can also rotate a bit. Try it out for yourself now. Straighten (extend) and bend (flex) the leg at the knee (Figure 2.2). Now with the knee bent to 90 degrees, turn the lower leg externally and medially while keeping the upper leg still (Figure 2.3). This movement has also happened at the knee. While you're at it, just notice if you rotate one way more than another and we will come back to that.

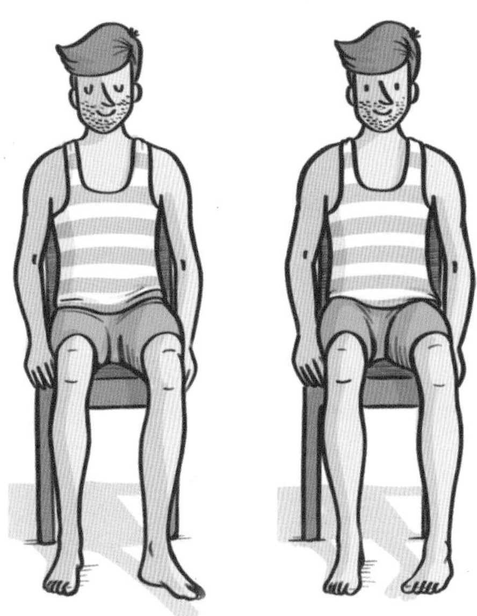

Figure 2.3 The knee is a modified hinge that also rotates.

What all this means is that we want to know what movements should be available at different joints, so we don't try and get them to do something they are not designed to do. The knee, for instance, is designed to flex, extend, and rotate a little, but is not intended to move side to side. We want to make sure that when we are doing yoga postures, we don't find ourselves levering the lower leg in such a way as to place a negative force into the knee. This sort of thing can happen, for example, when we don't have enough external rotation in the hip and try and put our legs into *Padmasana*.

This same information also helps us understand what movements are required at certain joints to perform a particular posture. We can even group poses by the necessary actions, so we might say this collection of positions requires good hip flexion and another group requires external hip rotation. Of course, you will have postures that are members of more than one group.

Everyone will have some potential for a degree of variation in the design of their joints, and those slight differences might make some movements easier or more difficult. If, for instance, my hip socket is deeper than yours, it might be more stable. However, let's say that the big lump of bone on the side of the femur (greater trochanter) is larger than average, this might mean certain movements are restricted by bone coming in contact with bone (hard compression).

So far then, we can say that:

- Not all joints are designed to have the same movements available.
- There may be some slight variability between individuals.
- A posture will require a certain amount of particular movements.

We declared in our initial statement that ROM is direction-specific, so when we are talking about ROM, we are referring to a singular movement available to a particular joint. We are not designed in such a way as to have the same expected ROM in all possible directions. They can be vastly different. Think back to when you rotated your knee, mine rotates further externally than medially, what about yours? Apparently, on average, there is about 45 degrees external and 25 degrees internal rotation when the knee is flexed between 30 and 90 degrees. This reduces as the leg straightens until there is no rotation available when the knee is fully extended. Again, try it now if you want, just hold your thigh still so you don't get confused by introducing some hip movement. Also, keep the ankle still relative to the lower leg, as that can throw you off too. The knee doesn't rotate the same in both directions, and that is how it is meant to be. We don't need to set about trying to even this up.

As we use hip mobility so much in the yoga, let's use this joint's movements to explore the idea of direction-specific fully. The movements we have at the hip joint are, flexion, extension, medial and external rotation, abduction, and adduction. There is also horizontal adduction and abduction, but we won't worry about that for the moment. Each of these directions will have its own ROM

Time for another practical. We will work with active ROM for the moment, which is how far you can go using your muscles to move the joint.

- Stand up and take your weight into your left leg.
- Now keeping your right leg straight, raise it as high as possible out in front of you, moving only at the hip (straight-leg hip flexion). (1)
- Bring it down, and then without tilting the pelvis forward, take the straight leg behind you as far as you can (hip extension). (2)
- This time, bring a bent knee up in front of you, thigh parallel to the ground, knee at 90 degrees. Moving only at the hip and keeping the knee facing forward, start rotating the hip externally. This will result in the instep traveling toward the ceiling (external rotation). (3) Rotate as far as you can and then come back to starting position to try the other direction.

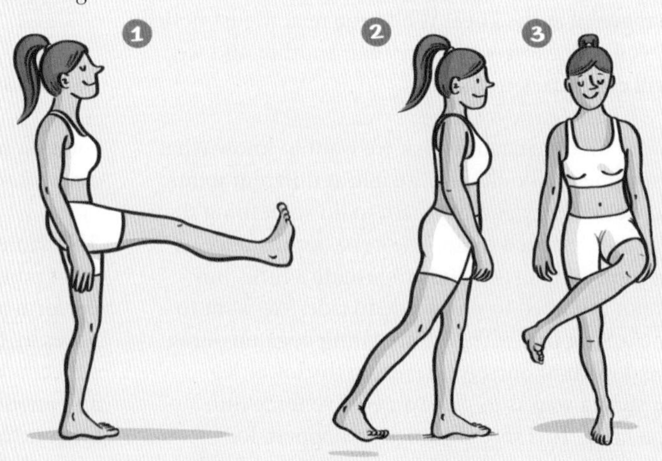

- Rotate the hip medially this time, the outside edge of the foot will travel toward the ceiling (medial rotation). (4)
- Starting with a straight leg, take it out to the side only (abduction). (5)
- Lastly, take it across the front of the supporting leg (adduction). (6)
- Now swap and try the same movements with the other leg.

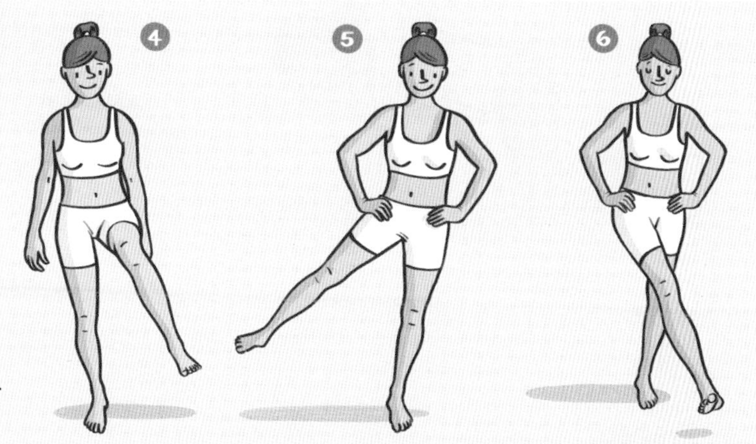

with the potential for a lot or a little change in joint angle. Everyone will be better at some of these than others, and from that, we can tell what postures they will likely find hard or easy.

I bet you found a lot of difference between the movements, maybe were even a little surprised by how little of something there was. How far did you manage to extend the hip? The average is roughly 20 degrees. Not much compared with hip flexion. There will be more abduction than adduction, and generally more external rotation than medial. Although, some people will find the inverse true for the rotation.

Think for yourself how those movements you performed relate to postures that you are familiar with and if they represent a fair relationship to the level of difficulty you have with them. It's not unusual to see examples of students moving very freely in one direction and be extremely restricted in another. I often encounter students who are entirely happy forward folding but have great difficulty with any posture involving external hip rotation (Figure 2.4).

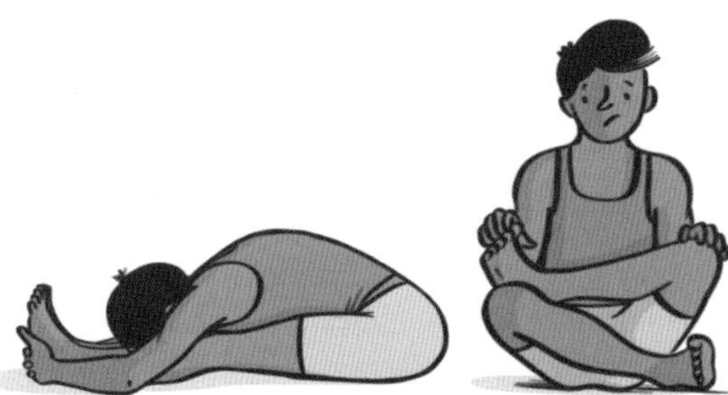

Figure 2.4 It is extremely common to find some movements very much easier than others.

Armed with this knowledge, we can work toward increasing the ROM in the directions we require more of while respecting those inbuilt differences that are meant to be there. So don't think you can ever get 90 degrees of hip extension because the hip is heavily ligamentous to resist that movement. Achieving 30 degrees would be an awful lot.

Q. What is happening to allow a student to do *Hanumanasana*?

So now we know we can't say, "I've got tight hips" because the answer would be, "In what direction?"

Earlier, I introduced the fact that different joints allow for various movements because of their design (ball-and-socket, hinge, etc.). This refers to the "joint-specific" part of the initial statement. There is another element to this and that is to do with joint independence. Just because I have trouble flexing my hip, it doesn't follow that I will have difficulty flexing my knee, hip, shoulder, spine, or elbow. Each area will be influenced by the factors they have been exposed to, such as sport, work, previous injury, stress, etc. It's even relatively common to see students that have extreme differences between collections of

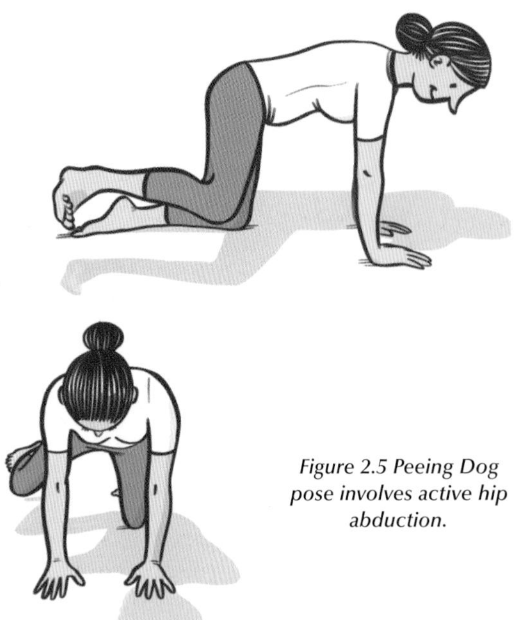

Figure 2.5 Peeing Dog pose involves active hip abduction.

movements, for example, finding backbending postures easy and forward folding postures hard or vice versa.

Now would be an excellent time to contemplate your yoga practice and joint ROMs. Don't fret though, we will be bringing all the concepts together later in the book when we look at each major joint in turn. In the hip practical earlier, I mentioned that we were testing active ROM (Figure 2.5). It will always be less than the other form of ROM, which is called "passive" because you have to use your muscles to overcome any tensional resistance, rather than an external force.

Examples of passive ROM would include being gravity-assisted, pulling yourself into position, or being helped by a teacher (Figure 2.6). The opposing muscles to the ones you are stretching are relaxed when passively moving through a ROM and contracted when actively moving. Ideally, we want to think of closing the gap between active and passive ROM because it is desirable to be able to control the ROM we have. Strength would be an essential factor in improving active ROM, and we will talk more about it in a coming chapter.

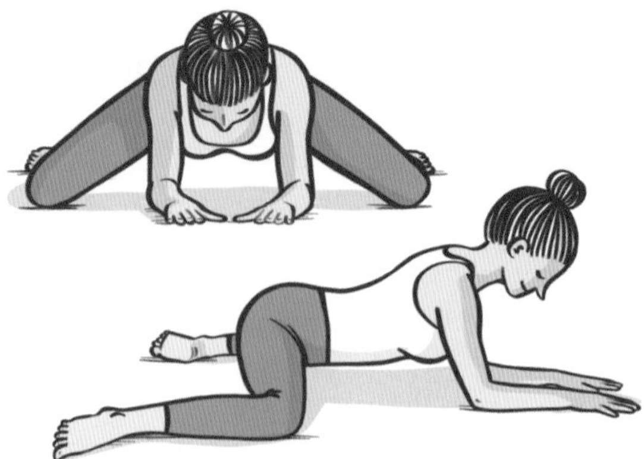

Figure 2.6 Bhekasana *involves passive hip abduction.*

It's time to think of some of the things that influence ROM. We are going to restrict the discussion to some of the physical things, tension, compression, proportion, and orientation. There are also other influencing aspects, such as temperature, time of day, aging, psychology, lifestyle, work, sleep, and many more. All the highlighted factors apart from orientation are covered in Chapter 1, *Individuality*; Chapter 2, *Compression*; and Chapter 3, *Opposing Muscles Restrict*; so we will just introduce the ideas here.

When trying to move deeper into a yoga posture, it's common for students to reach a point where they feel they can't go any further. They have moved through a certain ROM at one or more joints and now something has stopped them. The first distinction we can make is whether the sensations being experienced are in front of or behind the direction of travel.

We will use ankle dorsiflexion (shin toward the top of the foot) as an example (Figure 2.7). Postures such as Down Dog, *Pashasana*, *Utkatasana*, and squatting all require the ankle to dorsiflex. The more we take the knee in front of the ankle, the more dorsiflexion we create. If, as we try and go further forward with the knee, we experience a stretch

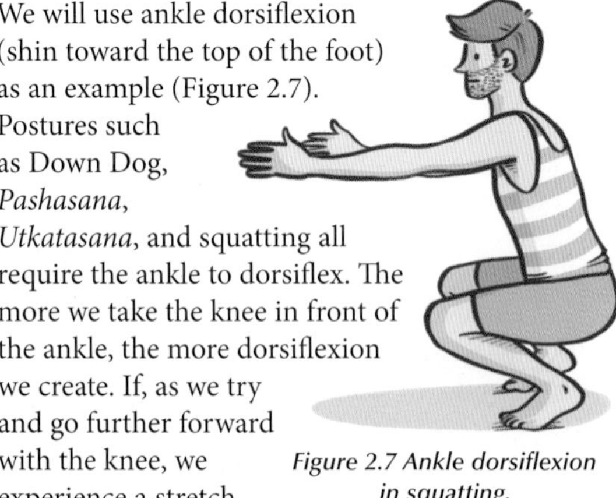

Figure 2.7 Ankle dorsiflexion in squatting.

sensation in the back of the lower leg or ankle, then we are encountering a tensile resistance. We tend to immediately think of muscle or myofascia (muscle and fascia), but it might also be tendon, ligament, or joint capsule. Often, the restriction is coming from the muscle or muscles that do the opposite action to the one we are trying to perform. In this example, that is plantar flexion, and the muscles responsible for that movement are the gastrocnemius and the soleus. The important thing is that we are feeling the sensations behind the way we are trying to go.

If, on the other hand, we experience some discomfort or pressure at the front of the ankle, usually the joint crease, then that is likely to be the tibia coming into contact with the talus bone. We have encountered bone on bone restriction, hard compression. In this example, there is no soft tissue (flesh) to get in the way but read Chapter 2, *Compression*, to understand that, in other situations, it might be medium or soft compression. With compression, the sensation is experienced in front of the direction of travel.

Another consideration might be that our proportional relationship makes it hard for us to travel in the direction we want. Maybe it has caused a shift in our COG that is taking us in the wrong direction or has created a disadvantageous lever or positioning in space. In our example of dorsiflexion, when the knees are also well flexed (as in a squat or *Pashasana*), long femurs or a hefty butt can mean that the COG moves backward, making it hard to go forward enough to balance.

To check if this is the problem, we could ask the student to hold onto something in front of them and pull themselves forward. If by doing this, they can increase the amount of dorsiflexion, then it is not the direct ROM at the joint that is the issue but not being able to access it because of positioning.

Bones are not straight sticks, they twist, turn, change direction even. Think of the top of the femur. At certain joints, the orientation of the adjacent bones can influence the degrees of motion that will be available at the joint in specific directions. In our example of dorsiflexion, it is not relevant, but we will encounter this factor when we talk about the hip later in the book.

Q. How is dorsiflexion at the ankle influenced differently depending on whether the knee is extended or flexed? Think Down Dog versus squat.

Flexibility

"Flexibility is the range through which it is possible to travel at a joint or series of joints."

You can see how many of those words in the definition are familiar with our understanding of ROM. That is because it is really the same thing but viewed from a slightly different perspective. Flexibility is a measure of how far through a particular ROM it is possible to go. So, in that way, it is joint-specific and direction-specific, the same as ROM. If someone has good ROM, they would be considered flexible as opposed to inflexible. We can be precise and say that someone has excellent hamstring flexibility, inferring that they can travel through an extensive range of hip flexion, or with a broader scope, we can say someone is flexible. The latter doesn't really tell us much because there will be some joints and directions that move more freely than others. The same would apply if considering a single joint, such as the hip.

Working on flexibility means trying to increase the range through which we can move at a specific joint in a particular direction. Well, that is the reality of the language even if the intention was broad. Flexibility will be changed only for the joints and directions worked on.

Although many yoga teachers would like to promote the spiritual aspects of yoga, it's often not why people start. If we are to believe some of the studies, apparently the majority begin yoga for physical exercise and to become more flexible. So why do people want to be more flexible? Research now suggests that being more flexible doesn't help prevent injury, can reduce performance (depending on the exercise type), and above-average flexibility is not of any use unless you have a need for that ROM in the tasks you want to perform. So, from that perspective, all those hours of bending and stretching could be a waste of time.

As it happens, if we are going to move deeply into many of the yoga postures, we will need above-average ROM at most major joints. That is the nature of what we, as postural yoga practitioners, choose to do. But at some stage, we will need to say, "OK, I have enough" (if you reach that point), or without the necessary strength, there is a risk of increasing instability. I know many seasoned yoga teachers who have eventually come to this conclusion. After decades of looking for greater and greater ROM, they sense this instability in their body and put the brakes on, holding back from their edge and working on strength and stability, even at times, actively seeking to reduce their available ROM. Depending on your body constitution, that might need to be your thought process right from the word go.

I have met many hypermobile students that, after a brief honeymoon period with yoga, feel that it hasn't done them any favors. Bendy newcomers often land up being treated like a new plaything, with the adoption of a let's-see-what-you-can-do attitude by the teacher, particularly if the student also has a striving mindset. It is beyond the scope of this book, but if you feel you might be hypermobile, please do further research into the subject so that you may practice yoga in a beneficial way.

Flexibility for flexibility's sake still gets a tick from me. Primarily because it's sexy, and you can make cool Instagram pics. Joking apart, we might characterize aging as a gradual decline into stiffness and reduced mobility, and youth as carefree fluidity. There is something about being in a flexible body with the ability to move as you wish, that keeps ignited—or reignites—that playful spirit inside. This youthful feeling is beneficial for your overall sense of wellbeing. I continually observe that most yogis seem younger than their age. Even if there are no aspirations to create complicated postures, purely maintaining existing flexibility over time

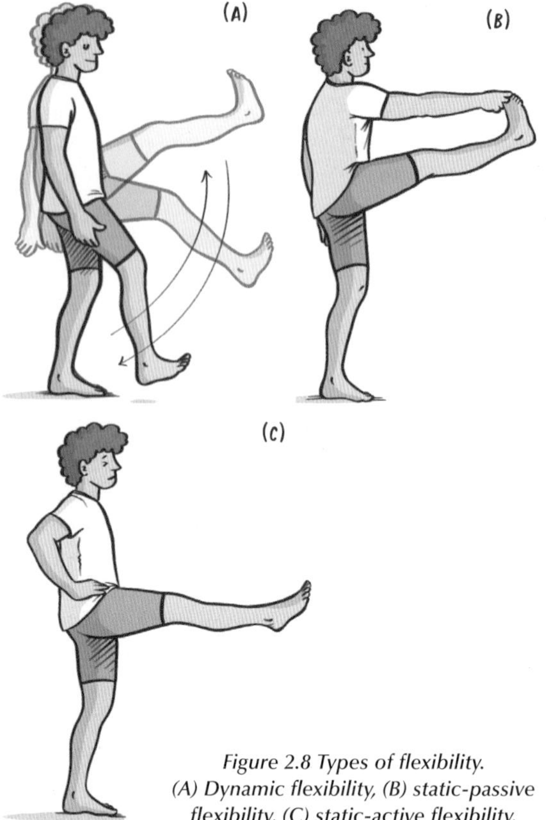

Figure 2.8 Types of flexibility. (A) Dynamic flexibility, (B) static-passive flexibility, (C) static-active flexibility.

is a worthwhile endeavor. I remember watching a documentary on Ido Portal[1] called *Just Move* and thinking, yes, you are so right, just use that fantastic body and don't let it stagnate.

Flexibility comes in a few flavors: dynamic, static-passive, and static-active, none of which are as exciting as Belgian chocolate and coconut, but at least you can make some pretty shapes with them (Figure 2.8). Dynamic flexibility is sometimes referred to as "functional flexibility" because of the inference to usable ROM. It involves movement influenced by the velocity of the moving part or parts. An example would be standing in *Tadasana* and swinging one leg upward to see how high it will go.

---

[1] The Ido Portal method is a physical fitness practice utilizing the practitioner's own bodyweight and movements, rather than external weights and machines, to develop strength, agility, and flexibility, see www.idoportal.com

Static flexibility, on the other hand, involves no use of momentum and can be divided into passive and active. Passive flexibility refers to the ROM achievable with the aid of an external force to create movement at the joint. That could be as simple as using gravity and body weight to just hang out and take you deeper, or to assist yourself by taking hold of a strap or limb and encouraging the movement. Being assisted in a posture would also fit into this category if you let the teacher do all the work. Sometimes we refer to the latter two examples as "assisted ROM."

The difference between passive and active flexibility is that active flexibility involves muscular activity to move and hold the position, again no momentum. Raising a straight leg and keeping it there using only hip flexor muscles would demonstrate active flexibility. Remember these tests only relate to hip flexion. Someone might be brilliant at this but rubbish at other movements at the same or different joints.

In yoga, most of what we do when holding postures relates to static flexibility (either passive or active). It is not desirable to have a large difference between the ROM you can travel through actively and passively because it means there isn't the strength to control the full ROM. Although we are moving in yoga and transitioning from one posture to another, most of the time we are not using momentum, it is done slowly and with control. There are a few times when dynamic flexibility might be useful in yoga, such as when jumping into a posture.

Even though it is theoretically convenient to classify types of ROM in this way, as with most things, there is often a mixture of these elements going on. For example, in all likelihood, in many of the seated forward folds, we will be assisted by gravity and a grip on the foot but also engaging muscles to help take us forward.

What Changes When You Become More Flexible

As it may help us decide how we want to work to change flexibility, we might now want to consider the physiological and neurological changes that may occur during a yoga class (acute) and after months or years of regular practice (chronic). I must admit I like knowing the science behind how stuff works and, on planning this book, I intended to give some tidy explanations in light of current research. However, the more I read, I was convinced that there is still no clear understanding of either the potential physical adaptations or nervous system responses. So, what you are going to get instead is my take on things.

Before that, we need to decide what we are doing in yoga postures as they relate to flexibility. For some yoga poses, the limiting factor may well be strength, but for most of the others, it is having the necessary ROM available. Being flexible enough to do the poses means that as the joint angles change, the attachment points of the muscles will be taken further apart and the muscle will need to lengthen. The muscles are being placed under a stretch. It always seems a bit heretical to reduce yoga down to stretching, but your tissues don't know the name of the pose, how you are breathing, or that you are "en route" to spiritual enlightenment, so they just respond to the changing body position. Or do they?

As it happens, stretching seems to be one of the few modalities used for increasing flexibility, so no wonder many students get more flexible after a program of yoga. As we look at what happens in response to stretching muscle tissue, it will get a bit geeky, so if you don't fancy that, skip past the colored section to where I conclude that we are working to change the nervous system's perception of what is happening rather than physically elongate the muscle.

Stretching Muscle Tissue

First off, I'll introduce some terminology.

A muscle and the related connective tissue, including the tendon, is called an "MTU" (musculotendinous unit), Figure 2.9. When we move a joint through a ROM, we will be influencing the whole MTU not just muscle tissue as it does not exist in isolation, the fascia runs right through it and via the tendon, connects it to the bone. An MTU is **extensible**, which means it can be lengthened (stretched). It also has **elastic** properties, which return it to its resting length after it has been lengthened.

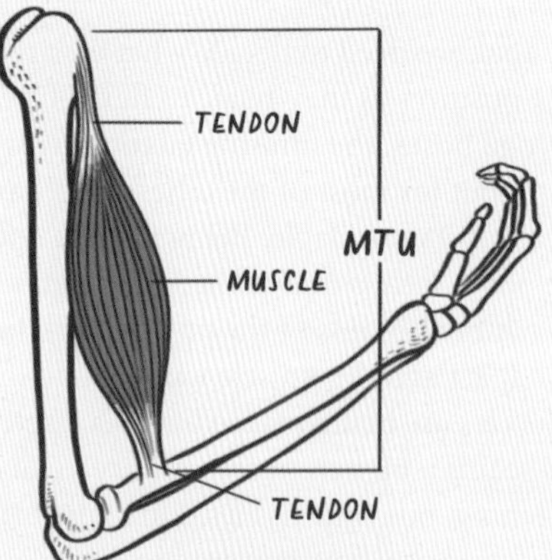

Figure 2.9 Musculotendinous unit.

Although in everyday language, when we use the word **stiffness**, we infer inflexibility; in biomechanical terminology, it refers to how much force is needed to deform a material. So, in relation to the MTU, stiffness is a measure of how much force is required to lengthen it by taking a joint through a given ROM. If it takes a lot of force to stretch the MTU, it would be considered stiff.

On the other hand, if it deforms easily, it would be referred to as **compliant**. Remember that stiff is not the same as inflexible—it is possible to go through a considerable ROM but, at the same time, need a substantial force to achieve it—that would be stiff but flexible. MTU stiffness has both **passive** and **active** components. Passive refers to the mechanical properties (physical structure) of the MTU, and neurological muscle reflexes, such as tone (resting tension) and contraction to active.

One nervous system response to the stretching sensation is called **stretch tolerance**. In other words, at what intensity of stretching force is an individual going to say, "That's far enough?" As you can imagine, everyone will have a different experience of what determines their limit, often related to the type and intensity of exercise they have done in the past as well as their overall pain sensitivity.

Viscoelasticity is when a material displays both elastic and viscous properties. Translated, that means a sustained load will create a deformation of the material (viscous), and it will then return to its original state (elastic) but over time. This is a property believed to be present in MTUs, so when held in an elongated position for a period of time, it will lengthen but then, after a time, recover back to normal again. So, there is a time-dependent deformation (if a stretch is held), referred to as muscle **creep**, followed by a time-dependent return. Greater viscous deformation is thought to occur in prolonged low-load stretching compared with shorter durations at a higher load. This might help explain the gradual sense of increasing depth felt in those long holds found in Yin yoga.

Finally, we have the term **stress relaxation**. Don't be misled by the word stress, it is not the same as, "How the hell am I going to pay for those six-inch red stilettos the missus has just bought?" It is the resistance to the load (stretch force) exhibited by the tissues. Stress relaxation is the phenomenon whereby if the MTU is held under a constant load for a period of time, the tissue's resistance to the load reduces. This is closely linked to viscoelastic deformation. Imagine it in this way. If you go into a deep gravity-assisted stretch and support yourself with a bolster or blocks so that you can't go deeper, then the load that is gravity will remain the same.

After muscle creep has occurred, the lengthened MTU will then provide less resistance, and the intensity of the stretch sensation will reduce.

Not all the reduction in intensity will be due to the muscle creep, as any constant sensory stimulus is likely to undergo sensory adaptation. In massage therapy, I used to use this response when wanting to apply deep pressure to a trigger point. Rather than make the client squirm in pain, you could hold back from the desired pressure until the client got used to it and then go deeper. Try it for yourself now if you want. Squeeze the tip of a finger between the thumb and finger of the opposite hand, applying enough pressure to get a level of discomfort. Now wait, keeping the amount of pressure exactly the same. It won't be too long before the pain subsides. You can let go of the finger now.

If you get into some technical reading, you will also come across the terminology **stress** and **strain**. In our context, stress is the resistance by the MTU to the load placed on the tissues by the stretching, and the strain is the change in length of the MTU. So, when we thought of stiffness earlier, high stiffness would infer a low strain-to-stress relationship, and high compliance, a high strain-to-stress relationship. If this is one step too far, I don't blame you, it makes my head ache also. Just skip merrily along.

Now we can apply some of that language, physiology, and neurology to the body being placed under a stretch while in a yoga pose. Muscle tissue is made of building blocks called **sarcomeres**, but contrary to what might seem likely, research agrees that when ROM has been increased, there is no change in the physical length of a muscle. No more sarcomeres have been added. So that means when we are stretching, we are not trying to stretch the muscle (make it longer). Bizarre right!

There is also disagreement as to whether viscoelastic deformation even happens to the MTU. If it does and is responsible for stress relaxation and muscle creep, it would not be a lasting effect as, sometime after the stretch, it would just return to normal. Therefore, if there is no lasting mechanical change, sustained increases in flexibility and a reduction in active tension must live in the realm of neurological responses. That brings us to the popular **stretch tolerance** theory, which suggests that there is no change in passive resistance but that repetition, either consecutively or through prolonged programs, results in a greater intensity of stretching being tolerated.

Having stretched for many years, I will now tell you why I am not convinced by this explanation. If resistance to MTU lengthening didn't change, then the force required to stretch it a given distance would remain the same. Any increase in flexibility would be down to being less sensitive to the stretching sensation (stretch tolerance). This is not the experience of repeatedly stretching. There is no need to try harder as the joint will easily move through a greater ROM.

Let's consider the common example of someone starting yoga and not being able to fold forward in *Paschimottanasana*. Instead, they find all they can do is to sit upright in *Dandasana*. Sometime later (months or years) they can now comfortably lay on their legs. Imagine the additional effort that would be required to fold flat on your legs if you had to overcome the resistance that once stopped you at *Dandasana* and the additional resistance to traveling through the rest of the ROM. So, something changes the resistance to be overcome. I think this is the nervous system adjusting its perception of what is a safe range through which to let you travel and allowing the increase in flexibility. I also believe we can tolerate greater intensities with training, but this relates to challenging a new resistance more vigorously. When you observe any accomplished practitioner in yoga, dance, or the martial arts, they move with fluidity and grace not as if they are battling to overcome restrictions.

From my point of view, this whole section culminates in the idea that when working on increasing flexibility, we are endeavoring to inform the nervous system of our need to perform certain joint ROMs and the safety of doing so. The intention is to establish a new **set point** that the nervous system is happy to let us go to.

So, for those of you that skipped the geeky section, I can summarize as follows:

- Research indicates that increases in flexibility do not equate to a physical change in the structural length of muscles.
- Temporary physical change may occur during stretching, but the muscle will return to its length after a short period of time.
- Nervous system responses are primarily responsible for the available ROM.
- Therefore, when working on increasing ROM, we don't need to bully the target area into submission, but instead work with the nervous system to demonstrate the need for greater flexibility.

Working on Flexibility

When you put a search into google for increasing ROM, nearly everything that comes up relates to stretching, and it is probably the method most frequently used, however, a few other options exist.

Controlled articular rotations (CARs) involve moving joints through end-range circles or rotations, using control and active muscular work. The aim is to improve **mobility** (controlled flexibility) by increasing strength and precision at the limits of ROM. Figure 2.10 is not to follow but just to give you the idea.

We have talked about the importance of strength already, but now we are introducing the term mobility (functional flexibility). For example, the difference between having your hands on the floor to support your weight and sliding the legs away into *Hanumanasana*, as against controlling yourself down into the pose from standing using only your leg muscles (Figure 2.11). Better still, being able to come back up again. The nervous system will sense that you are safe in what you are doing, and it is more likely to let you build on your achievable ROM from there. I'm sure that there are many other derivatives of the same idea.

As another option, how about just doing what you need to do? What I mean by that is if you want to be able to squat, start incorporating it into your daily routine, and spend more time squatting (Figure 2.12). It might seem a bit silly, but what better way to demonstrate to the nervous system that you need to be able to do something than trying to do it a lot. You will find out later that squatting is something we refer to in this book as a fundamental movement, and I happen to know

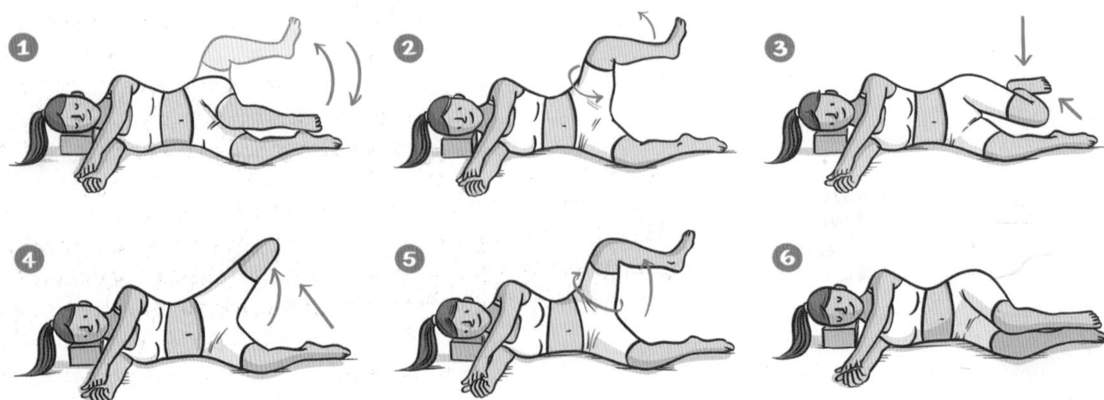

Figure 2.10 Controlled articular rotations.

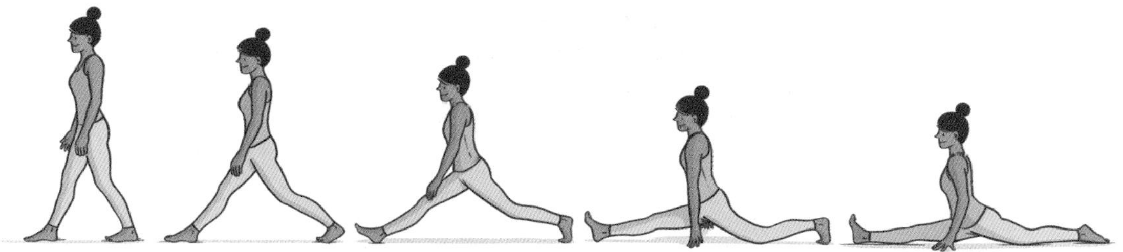

Figure 2.11 Sliding the legs away into Hanumanasana.

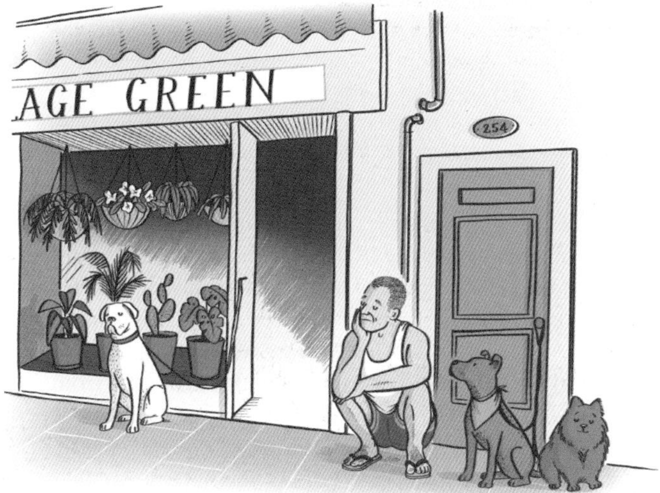

Figure 2.12 Squatting as part of your daily routine.

many yoga teachers that squat during breakfast, reading, or waiting for the bus. I do remember, on many occasions, squatting outside a shop with the waiting dogs while my wife was inside, apparently making in-depth decisions about the right product to buy.

If you have ever watched women planting rice in the paddy fields of Asia, you will observe that most have fantastic Standing Forward Bend. They do it all day, every day, they need it, it is useful, they have it. Of course, it doesn't mean they have good shoulder flexibility. The problem with repetitive action for flexibility gains is that it is very specific in its targeting. But as a rule, the more you can use strength and flexibility within your regular life, the more easily these movements will be incorporated into the body.

Stretching

This brings us to stretching. Hopefully we've established that we are, for the most part, stretching in postural yoga, so a deeper understanding may give methodology choices within the poses as well as for homework.

Types of Stretching

You won't be surprised to find that the same categories of flexibility feature in stretching as well, because flexibility is a measure, and stretching is the work. So, we have static and dynamic, but we can also add to this precontraction and resistance stretching (Figure 2.13). Because I am saying that many yoga postures are also stretching, I will use this as the basis for the following discussion. In this

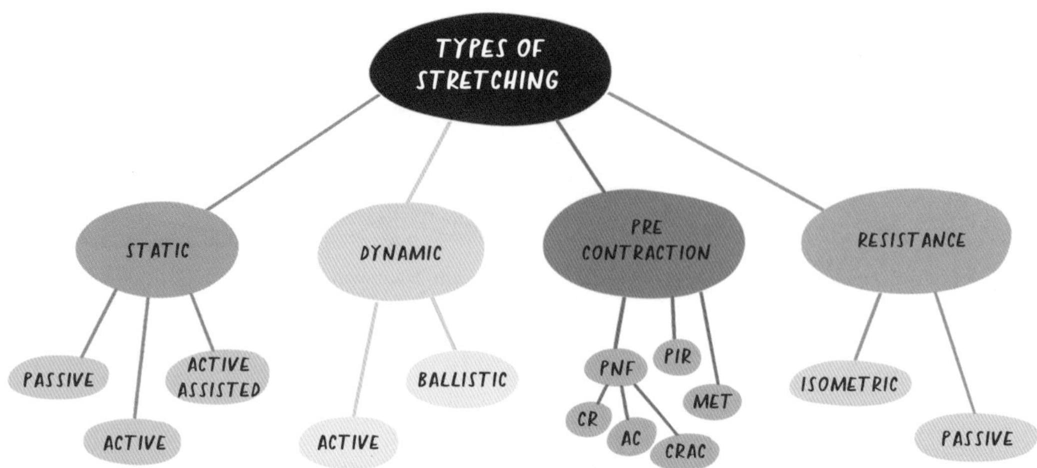

Figure 2.13 Types of stretching.

way, it may give some ideas of how you could work within a pose, but you may also apply the same information to more traditional stretching scenarios.

Static

Static stretching is very straightforward. You go into a position or posture and hold it there at a particular intensity for a chosen time. This might be for as little as five seconds to several minutes, but around 30 seconds is often thought to be optimal. In yoga, time is usually measured in breaths, so most likely between five and eight slow breaths. I will add more about stretching times toward the end of this chapter.

Under the static umbrella, there are three modes: passive, active, and what I will call, active-assisted. The last one you won't find in classical breakdowns of stretching, but I have added it because this is often how I work, and I feel that it can be beneficial for particular body types. The difference between the modes is how you get into position and what you do while you are there.

With a passive stretch, you are either holding yourself in the position by using muscles not related to the targeted joint movement, someone is helping you, or gravity is doing the work. In active mode, the muscles that perform the movement are being used to travel through the ROM and keep you in position. With active-assisted, you are working as in active mode, but supplementing it with a little help from either gravity, friction, pushing, or pulling.

As you have probably experienced, the distance you can travel through a ROM passively is less than that when working actively, sometimes considerably less, especially if gravity is against you. Available strength is associated with active range, but it is also influenced by how easily the passive range is achieved. If very little assistance is needed to reach the individual's deepest position, then when the same movement is done actively, it doesn't require too much strength to perform almost the same ROM. However, you may be in the type of body that can go pretty deep in postures but only when plenty of help is available, either from grabbing stuff or a friendly assistant.

In the geek section before, I introduced the idea of potential resistance to stretching arising from body type. The word I used was stiffness, but this is not the same as inflexible. In this context, it means the myofascial (muscle and fascia) construction where the individual has a greater resistance to being lengthened. Imagine different thicknesses of

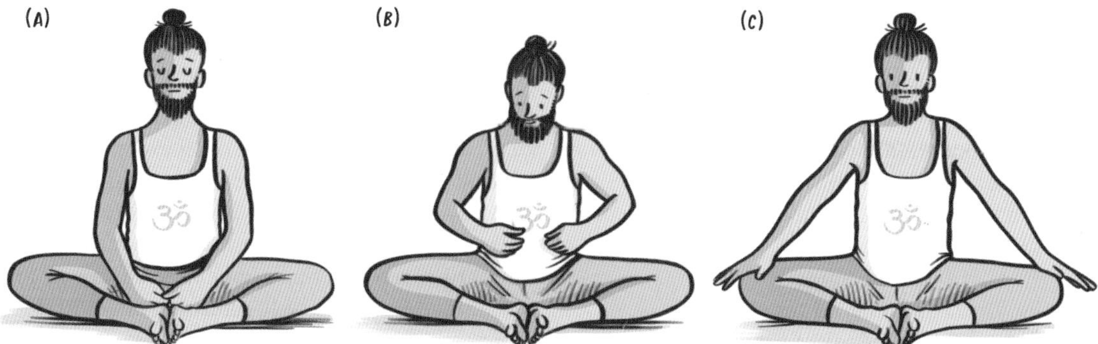

Figure 2.14 Types of static stretching in Baddha Konasana. *(A) Passive, (B) active, (C) contracting and help is active-assisted.*

rubber bands. With this type of body, there will be a more significant difference between active and passive ranges, and it is unlikely that the sort of strength needed to overcome the resistance could be developed. This scenario is where active-assisted can be useful.

Have you ever been in *Paschimottanasana* and heard the teacher say, "Let gravity take you deeper?" For some students, the passive assistance that gravitational force provides will do exactly that. But in the stiffer body type, the downward force can be too little to overcome the tissue's resistance, and they will stay exactly where they are, even when adding active hip flexion. This is my type of body. I can hover over my legs in *Paschimottanasana* all day unless I use a little help from the hands on the feet. We are not thinking here of how much stretching intensity you can bear, just some people are naturally more stretchy than others.

I will use *Baddha Konasana* as a working example of the static stretching modes (Figure 2.14). Assisting the depth of the pose by opening the feet with the hands, resting the hands on the legs, or having someone press down on the legs is all passive. As the movements that primarily make up this posture are hip abduction and external rotation, to work actively, those are the actions that you would need to try and do. In poses like this, it is sometimes hard to visualize or single out the external rotation, so the focus is likely to be on the abduction. As it is easier to get the right muscles to work through movement intention, even if you know which ones to use, trying to pull the thighs closer to the floor using only the hip muscles will do the trick. If that active muscular work is kept going and a little encouragement is added with the hands as a downward force on the thighs, we are in the realm of active-assisted.

Dynamic

Dynamic stretching is characterized by repetitive rhythmic movement rather than holding one position. The general concept is that the motion will take the subject through a greater range and that the combined time of the repetitions equates to a longer overall duration spent in a deeper stretch. I mentioned before that we might use dynamic flexibility when jumping into a pose, but that is a one-off movement to transition, rather than working on ROM increase. Dynamic stretching is often the method preferred during sporting warm-ups because it can generate more heat in the muscles if active contractions are used. However, it doesn't generally seem appropriate in a yoga setting, so it's included here more for the homework potential because it can often return better ROM results than traditional static stretching.

Do you remember those old style football warm-ups where they used to bounce up and down trying to reach their toes? Well, that comes under the dynamic heading because of the movement and is termed ballistic. Inconsistent terminology is such that what is not thought of as ballistic is often called dynamic, but I prefer to avoid confusion and separate those stretches using controlled movement into a subcategory called active. I usually associate yoga with stillness and internalization in the postures, but some styles may add things like pulsing in and out, which would be an example of active dynamic stretching.

Basically, for the most part, I think ballistic stretching is rubbish, because of the lack of control, use of a lot of momentum, and the high chance of taking the stretch into the wrong area. If you look at *Multi-Segmental Movement*, this is precisely the type of thing that can happen in ballistic stretching. The target area stops moving and, where there is less resistance, continues the movement. If we stick with the footballer bouncing in a Standing Forward Bend, what you will see is that during the downward movement, the resistant hamstrings will stop the pelvis moving, resulting in no more hip flexion and the spine flexing instead. The brunt of the momentum is taken in the lumbar spine. In this culture of rehashing and rebranding, physical trainers may finesse the technique to try and create their own marketable style, but generally what I see is the same: the introduction of unintentional joint movements. There are also issues relating to the triggering of nervous system reflexes (Chapter 3, *Neurophysiology*).

The lack of specificity found in ballistic stretching is a potential problem for any stretching method using momentum. Whereas ballistic stretching often relies predominately on gravity to generate momentum, active dynamic methods focus on using a muscular contraction to create the motion. This affords a certain amount of control, but there is still a need to be vigilant for unwanted movements. Apart from maybe the pulsing mentioned earlier, I can't see an appropriate use of dynamic stretching within postural yoga, unless the class draws heavily from dance and exercise. However, I have used this style of stretching with beneficial results myself as homework to improve the depth in particular postures.

It isn't necessary to replicate yoga poses when doing homework stretches, you can instead think of the particular ROM to improve. If you are not sure how to break down a pose into movements yet, hopefully, you will by the end of the book. A dynamic stretch, such as standing straight leg kicks, is an excellent example of an exercise that is relatively easy to perform strictly and with control. When I am at home, I often do this before I start my practice. *Upavistha Konasana* is what I would call a crossover pose that can be used effectively for dynamic stretching as well, returning direct ROM improvements into the yoga practice (Figure 2.15). There will be a bit of help from gravity, but the focus is on generating the hip flexion with muscular engagement and the pushing of the arms further away to create length in the torso and challenge the depth of the forward bend. It works well with rhythmic pulsing as well as returning to the top position between each repetition, as this will use strength as well.

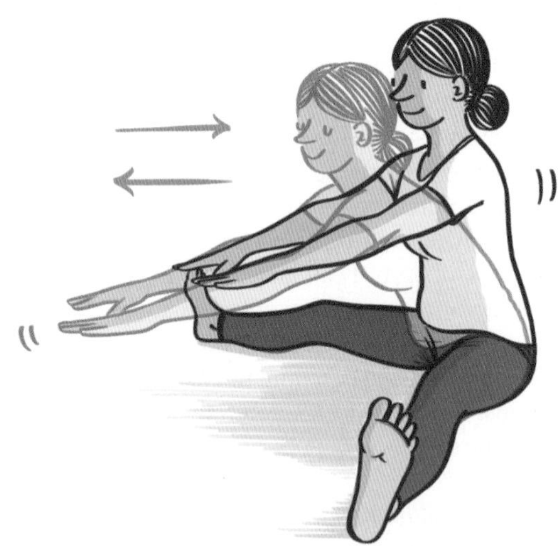

Figure 2.15 Contraction and momentum is active dynamic.

Precontraction

You will observe in the flow chart (Figure 2.13) that there is a myriad of acronyms under this heading, some of which might be considered technique variations or subcategories. As the name suggests, they all involve muscular contraction before the stretch, which may be either the target muscle group, the opposing muscle group, or both at some stage, depending on the particular protocol. Research isn't fully decided on the underlying process by which this group of stretching techniques returns ROM increases, but it is regularly reported as the most effective, both short and long term. The two leading theories are an increase in stretch tolerance (mentioned in the geek section) and a nervous system reflex called the "inverse stretch reflex" or "Golgi tendon reflex" (Chapter 3, *Neurophysiology*).

If I were to go over every variant, we could be here all day, so I will let you do your own research if this category interests you. I will, however, introduce PNF stretching because it is a style that I use a lot myself, both as a diagnostic tool and to achieve permanent ROM change.

PNF stands for proprioceptive neuromuscular facilitation, so a hint toward nervous system involvement is in the name. There are a number of variations, but the most straightforward is first to contract the muscle you want to stretch. It can also be beneficial to contract the opposing muscle (think active stretch) during the stretching period. There are usually three rounds of the stretch completed, as it is felt the additional gains in ROM from further repetitions would be minimal and not worth the time spent performing them. If you haven't tried this kind of stretching before, use the

Lying in *Supta Padangushtasana*, pull on the foot or ankle with the hand to take the leg in the air through as much passive hip flexion as possible, bringing the foot toward the head. You should feel a comfortable but intense stretch on the back of the upper leg (hamstrings). The position the leg is in should be close to your individual end range of hip flexion.

Keeping a good hold on the foot or ankle, actively extend the hip by contracting the hamstrings as if you were going to take the leg back to the floor (A). However, don't let it go anywhere, resist the movement with the arms. Only use about 30 percent effort for this isometric (static) contraction. Maintain the work in this position for around eight slow breaths. The muscles are now allowed to relax, and with gentle encouragement from the arms, passively move the leg toward the head (more hip flexion).

The second round of contraction is started at this new range, and after the eight breaths, the leg is again moved closer to the head (B).

Round three again starts from the new position (C), but this time, after the work and relaxation, the hands are released, and only the hip flexors are used to move into greater hip flexion actively. This position can be held for a further five to eight breaths, after which I like to add assistance from hands. The active-assisted stretch can be maintained for a final 5 to 10 breaths (D).

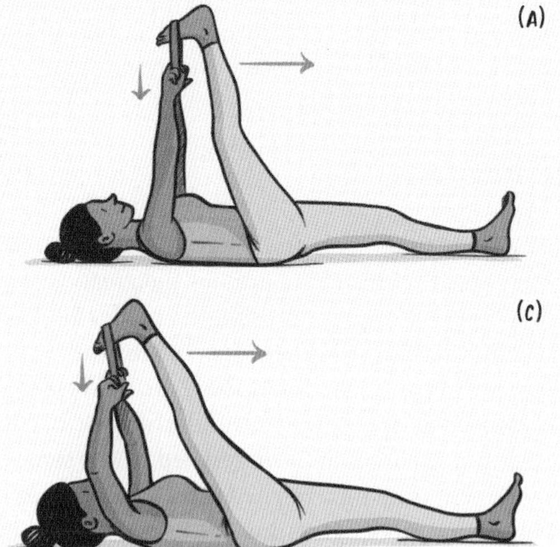

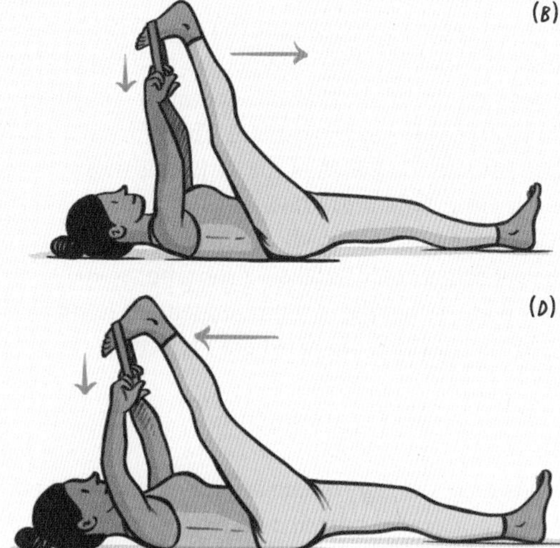

sequence on the previous page to get the idea of how it feels.

I know you're probably thinking that after all that bloody work something better change, and it will, as long as the restriction is myofascial. Even though the acute change in ROM can be quite dramatic—as with all stretching—if it is only done once, the gains achieved will evaporate within an hour or so, never to be seen again. However, regular PNF style stretching should elicit more permanent changes to ROM.

I mentioned above that I use PNF as a diagnostic tool, and it is precisely because of this immediate change to ROM. When trying to determine which restrictions are providing the greatest resistance to a student going deeper in a pose, a systematic testing of the relevant muscles can be performed, and the pose retried between each step. If a change in joint ROM also results in a change in depth or comfort in the posture, then homework stretching or additional postures can be given with the relative certainty that they will make a difference.

In later sections in the book, we will cover how to target particular joint movements, so for this next example, I will talk a little superficially. Returning to the earlier used pose *Baddha Konasana*, we know (or might know sooner or later) that the primary movements are abduction and external rotation of the hip. From a myofascial perspective, insufficient amounts of either of these ROMs will result in the knees or thighs being off the floor. Rather than keep repeating the pose in the hope that it will change, it may be more effective to target the individual movements. But there is also no point in stretching stuff that doesn't need stretching. Therefore, it is better to decide which of the actions is most troublesome. Looking at how easily a student can perform the isolated ROMs of hip abduction and external rotation separately is a start, but we will want to know that the extra time spent on homework will be worthwhile. This is where PNF comes in.

The protocol would be as follows:

- Ask the student to repeat *Baddha Konasana* a few times to establish a body placement that gives a true representation of their usual depth of the posture.
- Make a visual note or take a picture so that you can compare later.
- Pay attention to the height of the knees but also the overall positioning of the body, for example, the angle of the pelvis.
- Elicit a subjective experience of where the most significant restriction is felt, and general level of comfort.
- Perform a PNF stretch to increase the external rotation of the hip.
- Repeat *Baddha Konasana* and make a note of physical and subjective changes.
- Perform a PNF stretch for hip abduction.
- Repeat *Baddha Konasana* and make a note of physical and subjective changes.

Systematic deconstruction and testing of a pose in this manner should uncover the areas a student needs to work on to make improvements. The homework doesn't then need to be PNF stretching—any appropriate poses or different forms of stretching or strengthening are fine. The same information can be used to decide on appropriate sequencing, targeting the most significant ROM with the right postures prior to reaching the pose of interest. Taking our example of *Baddha Konasana*, if it was determined that hip abduction was the student's major restriction, then postures that stretch the adductors, e.g., *Mandukasana* or *Samakonasana*, could be placed before it. Of course, the analysis might suggest that more than one ROM needs to be improved. The homework or sequencing would then be adjusted accordingly.

Resistance

I would say that this is a relative newcomer to the world of stretching but has the great advantage of working on strength and flexibility together (mobility), without just relying on active movement. No doubt there are all sorts of technique variations, but the underlying principle is that the stretch is actively resisted by the same muscle that is being stretched. Yes, a muscle can be contracting and lengthening at the same time—it is called an "eccentric contraction"—and we will cover it in more detail in Chapter 3, *Strength*.

The other tenet of this style is that the depth of the stretch is determined by the range that can be controlled. It is also popular to add a shortening contraction after the stretching phase.

Resistance stretching is believed to allow for a subsequent greater ROM because of neural responses to the many muscle fibers being lengthened and contracted at the same time. If a shortening contraction is also performed afterwards, then a similar response, caused by the isometric contraction used in pre-contraction methods, may again come into play.

We will return once again to *Baddha Konasana* and hopefully reusing the same posture in a number of different ways will help you appreciate how many options there are.

For this example, the setup will be at the wall, as I feel it helps make the work stricter by preventing the pelvis from dropping back. Let's think through the principles and then detail how it will work. That way, you will be able to apply the same thought process to any ROM that needs addressing.

If the knees are up in the air when sitting in *Baddha Konasana* with the pelvis against the wall, then it is a no brainer that they need to travel toward the floor to deepen the pose. We know that it is a combined action of abduction and external hip rotation, but we won't be separating out the movements, just thinking in terms of toward or away from the floor. If the thighs are already on the floor, obviously no greater ROM is needed for this posture, but also the workable range would be stopped by the floor, meaning a different position would have to be used for ROM increases. However, the exercise would still be useful for building strength. Placing the hands on the thighs or knees can provide a variable resistance to work against.

The starting position for the first resistance stretch is with the knees high in the air and the hands in place on the knees (Figure 2.16). The knees are pressed toward the floor using shoulder and arm

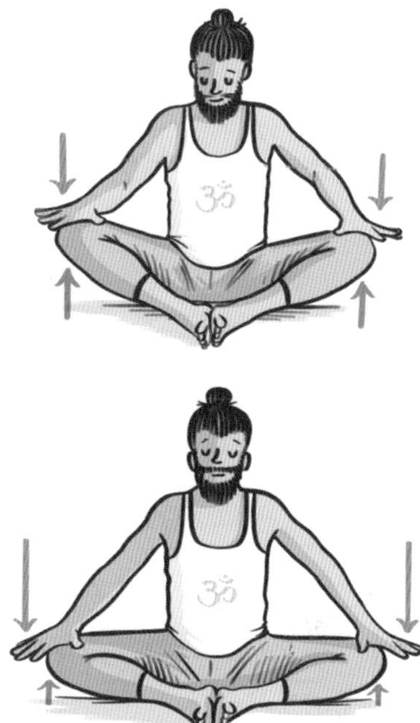

Figure 2.16 Even though the legs are pushing up, the arms push down with greater force. The legs move toward the floor.

strength, but at the same time, the movement is resisted by the inner thighs (adductors). So, the hands are pressing down on the knees, and the knees are pressing up against the hands. However, this is a fixed competition, and the hands must win.

The aim is to allow the downward force to overcome the upward force in a controlled way, allowing the hips to move through the available range of abduction smoothly. Don't use maximum force but something where there is work but not risk. Remember that it is important to build up the strength toward end ROM gradually. On the way down, the adductors are contracting but lengthening (eccentric).

Once at the end of the controllable range (which is probably not the floor), the rules of the game change and now the legs must win. The force pressing down must be reduced enough so that it can be overcome by the legs, and the knees can travel back under control to their starting position (Figure 2.17). On the way up, the adductors have contracted and shortened (concentric). That is one repetition, and somewhere between five and ten should be sufficient. It is essential to start gently

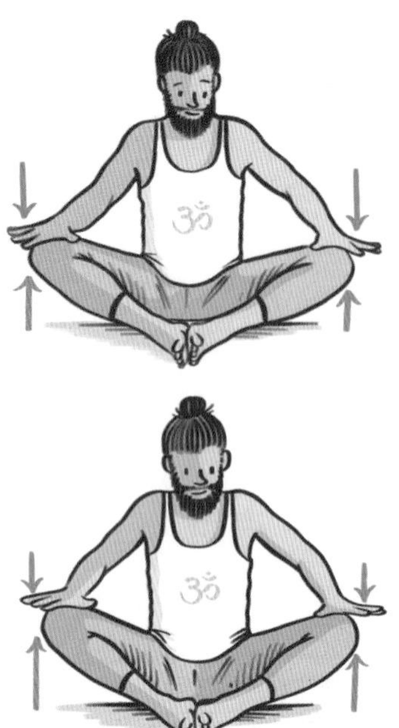

Figure 2.17 This time the legs push up with greater force than the arms are pushing down. The legs move away from the floor.

and build up the force of contraction slowly over many weeks.

Stretching Time and Frequency

In a yoga setting, students may be in a posture for as little as one inhale or exhale up to several minutes. As longer holds will tend to elicit a temporary and reversible physical change, what is important is whether the additional time also has a more beneficial influence on the nervous system.

I would say that research is unclear on this point. Remember we are not trying to stretch what we are stretching, as bonkers as that may sound. There are some studies that suggest longer holds are likely to be more effective on older bodies, which is not surprising as everything else seem to take longer too. Just kidding, but I do think the stretching time is a very individual thing and that it is good to experiment to find out what suits you. It will always be a balance between heat, flow, lightness, grounding, concentration, stretch tolerance, and intention. I have a slow breath and prefer to hang out in postures between 30 seconds and a minute, but for others, that would be way too slow, maybe even frustrating. Generally speaking, the more compliant the body tissues, the less time will be required in the stretch.

The duration of many studies I have come across is often within the range of two to six weeks, so almost irrelevant to a regular yoga practitioner. The type of program that can be maintained for a few weeks is not the same as what can be done for many months or years. Consistency and patience are what return lasting results. Quick hacks are rarely the answer. This is the reason why it is essential to find not only the techniques and times that suit your body but also what interests you.

Frequency is also very dependent on the individual. Some people can take much higher training intensity than others, even flourish on it, while the same program might exhaust someone else. Many yoga styles suggest students practice up to six times a week, but this is probably not the best if you are always doing the same poses or sequence because it doesn't leave much time for recovery.

Repetition is good to initiate change, but too much is likely to heighten the chance of experiencing repetitive strain injuries. The body needs rest to mend and repair, especially if you are challenging it. It is easy to fall into the trap of more must be better, when it really isn't. If you are hitting a plateau in your practice, instead of loading up the intensity to try and breakthrough, see what happens if you introduce another day off.

Whether we are talking about postural yoga or homework stretching, the same principle applies: the higher the intensity, the more rest between sessions is needed. If you love doing your yoga every day, have days when you go for it, interspersed with days that you just flow with the breath, or remain in the comfy zone. Don't go hell for leather every day—something will bust sooner or later.

Of course, the frequency can also be too low. Once or twice a week is probably too little to experience a significant change in flexibility, particularly after the honeymoon period. If you are continuing a regular yoga practice and thinking of introducing additional homework stretching, the number of weekly sessions will be dependent on energy levels and the body's response to higher intensity work. That said, it would be sensible not to target the same area more than twice a week.

Stu's Mega Mix

Hip flexion is another one of the ROMs that I will refer to later in the book as a fundamental movement. A good dollop will go a long way to creating numerous pretty shapes, but it is also a movement many students find challenging. So, to round up *Flexibility*, I thought I would share with you a practical focused on increasing hip flexion that incorporates quite a few of the ideas covered here.

Unless you are already very flexible, you will need a strap for this exercise. Make sure you have warmed up the legs by practicing yoga first or by performing several minutes of graduated straight leg kicks.

The stretching will take place in *Supta Padangushtasana* so lay on your back and take one straight leg into the air (A) flexing the hip to bring the leg to the end of your active ROM (that means no hands).

Stage 1 is to pulse the leg backward and forward using the hip flexors and extensors to generate the power. Aim for a travel distance of about 12 in (60 cm), or 1/4 of total ROM, repeating smoothly about ten times. The intention is to see if you can move deeper into hip flexion with each pulse.

(A)

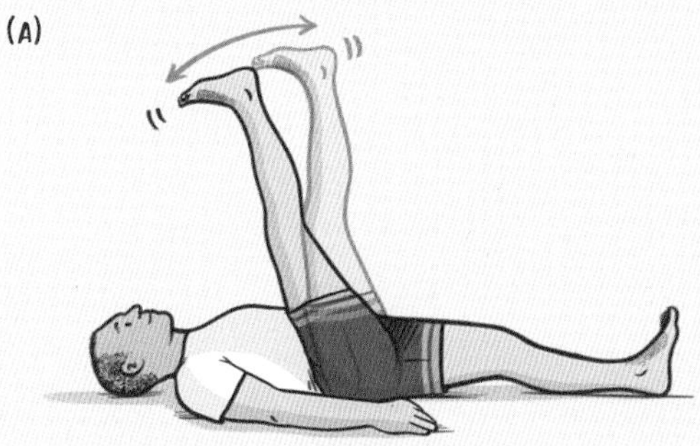

Now loop the strap around the foot so you can keep your head and shoulders on the floor while you complete **Stage 2** (B).

You are going to draw small circles (approx. 8 in [20 cm] diameter) with the foot, again using muscular work, but this time with a little assistance and resistance from the hands and strap. You will continuously be pulling on the strap, but somewhat less as the leg moves away from the body. The top of the circle is the deepest hip flexion you can go to with help, and the bottom of the circle is moving back from that point.

(B)

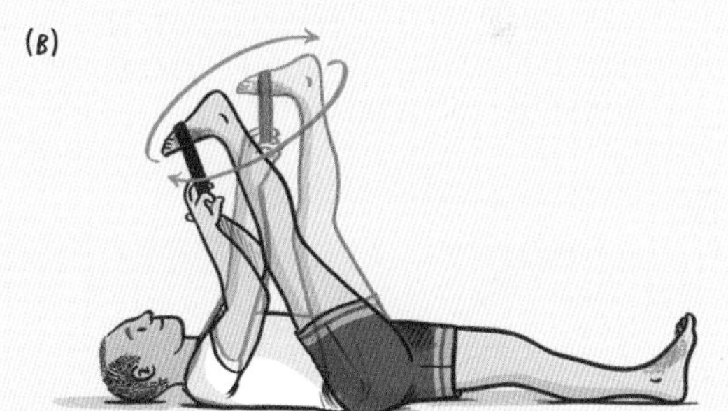

As the leg moves away from the body, the hip extensors (hamstrings) work against the resistance provided by the strap. As the leg circles toward the body, the hip flexors are engaged to assist. Draw about ten circles clockwise and then counterclockwise.

(C)

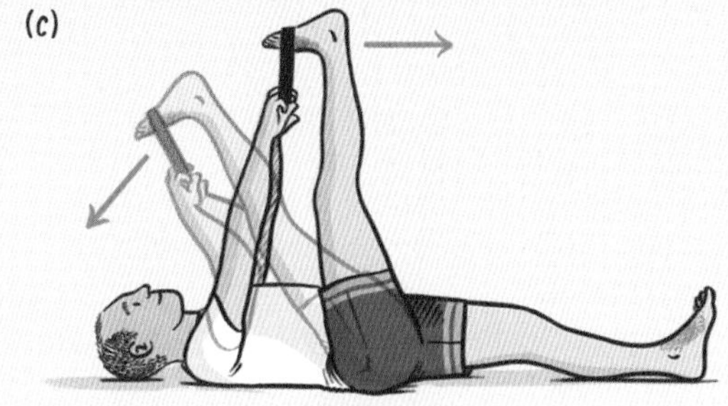

Next comes some resistance stretching (**Stage 3**). Keeping the strap in place, bring the leg toward the body until the end range of hip flexion has been reached (C). Contract the hip extensors (hamstrings) to take the leg back away from the body, providing a bit more resistance than you did with the circles. Aim to travel about 12 in (30 cm) or whatever is available before the shoulders get pulled off the floor.

You may need to set up with a bit of slack in the strap that can be taken up by the arms. On the leg's return toward the body, the pull of the arms continues, but this time the hip extensors try and resist. This technique is the same as the alternating tug of war detailed using *Baddha Konasana*. The hamstrings are therefore contracting continuously, shortening as the leg moves away and lengthening as it moves toward the body. Aim for completing ten return trips.

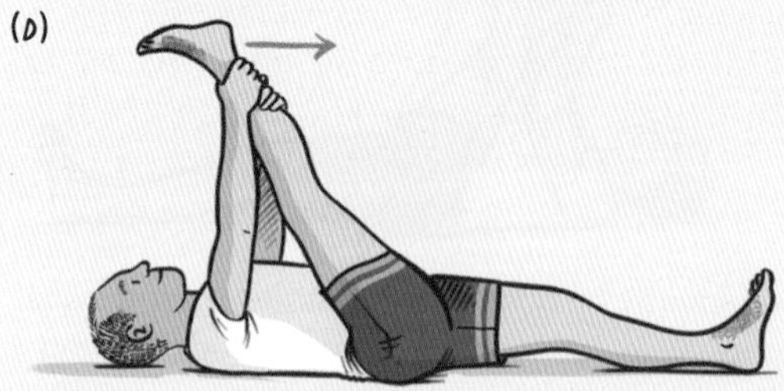

In **Stage 4**, the hands take hold of the shin (or still use the strap if the leg is out of reach) and the leg is taken toward the body, as far as is comfortable (D). Maintain a firm grip, keeping the leg exactly where it is, as you build up the effort in the hamstrings to pull the leg away from the body.

Continue this work for about 30 seconds, and then relax but keep the leg where it is ready

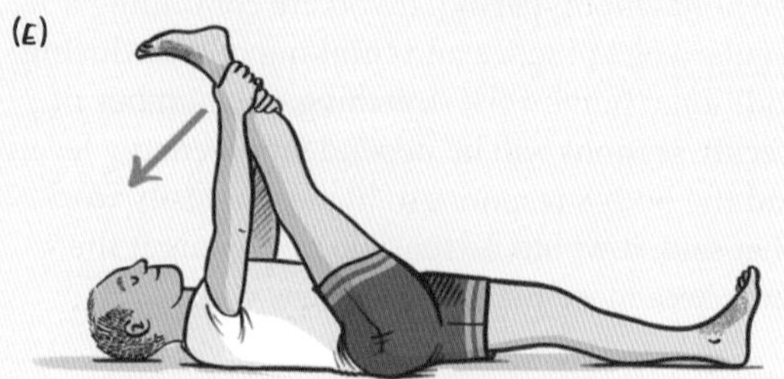

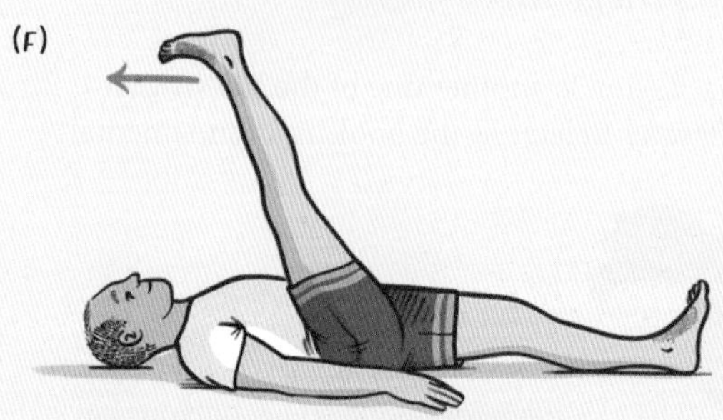

for **Stage 5**. If this sort of exercise is new for you, don't overdo the effort—think of around 30 to 40% of maximal effort. As you become stronger at working near the end of range, this exercise can be used as an opportunity to build strength as well, and the work intensity can gradually be increased. However, I still wouldn't exceed about 80% max. The static contraction should have created a neurological release, and you might now find the leg can easily be brought closer to the body.

Take up any slack and then see if a little encouragement with the hands will bring the leg any closer (E). Hold there for 30 seconds.

The final thing to do is to release the hands from the shin and try and maintain the position of the leg using active hip flexion (F).

As a quick reference we have:

- **Stage 1:** Pulsing—active dynamic stretching
- **Stage 2:** Active and resisted circles—CARs adaptation
- **Stage 3:** Hip flexion and extension—resistance stretching
- **Stage 4:** Static hold work—precontraction stretching and strength work
- **Stage 5:** Static stretch—static passive followed by static active stretching

This exercise combo is a bit of a blast, so to start with, don't be overzealous. Also, this is a once or twice a week thing, maximum.

Multi-Segmental Movement

"In a multi-segmental movement, forces will find the area of least resistance."

If you look at your fingers, it is easy to get the idea that they are made up of three distinct pieces. Flex them, and you see the sections straight away (Figure 2.18). Under that flesh, we have bones and where the ends of each bone meet, there is a joint. We can think of a segment either as a body part bounded by joints on both ends or with one free end, as in the last part of your fingers. A lot of the time, when we move or position our body, we have to change the position of several joints: a multi-segmental movement.

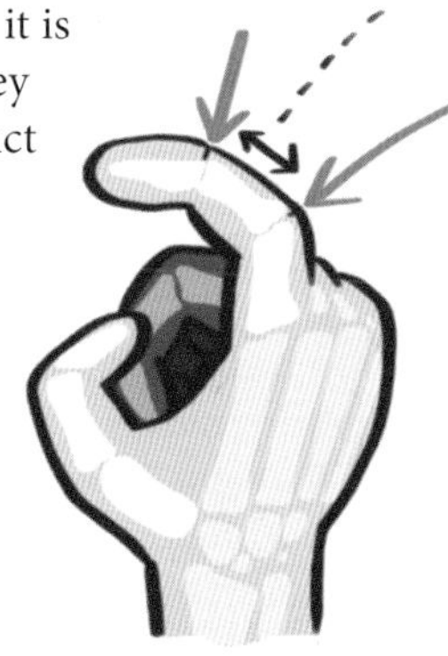

Figure 2.18 See the three distinct sections of your fingers by flexing.

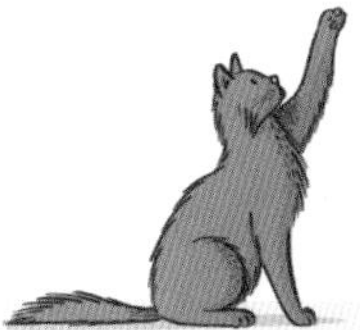

I come from a background in massage, and excessive mobility in the last segment of the thumb can be a problem because it is hard to keep your thumb straight when applying pressure through the tip of your thumb. If you let it bend and apply pressure using the pad of your thumb instead, you will land up hurting your thumb. In a yoga context, if you perform poses where you support yourself on your fingertips and repeatedly let the last segment of your fingers or thumb bend back too much, you would, again, risk hurting that joint. I happen to observe this quite a lot when I am flicking through Instagram. Strength is an essential aspect of controlling excessive mobility, and we will also talk about that in Chapter 3.

The fingers are lovely and straightforward to look at because we just bend and straighten them (flex and extend), and we don't have expectations greater than that. But when it comes to other parts of the body, there are often more movements available at the joints. As we place the body in more challenging positions, such as with many yoga postures, it may be harder to discern when we are moving excessively in a particular place. We may also be less clear about what movements should be

Let's try a little experiment. Place one hand palm down and straighten your index finger (Figure 2.19). Using the other hand, gently pull the tip of the finger toward the ceiling. You will probably notice the last segment of your finger is where the finger bends more into extension. In this example, it is the joint or area of least resistance. I am not counting where the finger joins the hand.

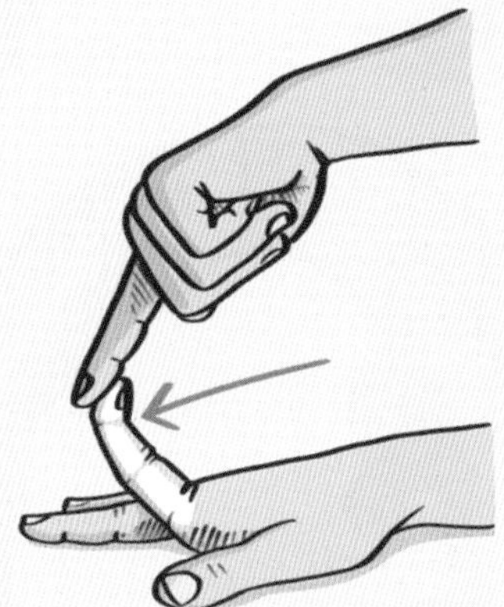

Figure 2.19 Place one hand palm down and straighten your index finger.

If you kept pushing on your fingertip, it would probably start to hurt in that spot. If you did that every day, the likelihood is that it would become more mobile at that site of movement but also less stable. The joint that moves the most might be different, and individuality is also an important concept.

You can try the other fingers and thumb if you wish. Notice any differences? Now compare the other hand. For myself, the last section of the little finger is the most mobile, and the last section of the right thumb moves more into extension than the left thumb.

happening where. The following example might help clarify the idea.

When we place the foot in *Ardha Padmasana,* we need to perform a multi-segmental movement of the lower body. Upper leg, lower leg, and foot need to be positioned in a specific way to allow the lateral edge of the foot to be placed in the opposite hip crease. The movements happen at the associated joints of the hip, knee, and ankle. The upper leg needs to roll outward and move away from the body (external rotation and abduction of the hip). The lower leg needs to close fully against the upper leg (knee flexion) and the foot points, the sole of the foot facing toward the ceiling somewhat (ankle plantar flexion and inversion).

If the desired movements don't happen because of restriction at one or more of those joints, then the foot won't be in the right position, and forces will find the weak areas of the knee and ankle. Often, the movement missing is either external rotation of the hip or knee flexion, sometimes both. Unfortunately, it is not uncommon for yoga students to hurt these vulnerable areas by trying to pull the foot into position against the restrictions of the hip or knee. In this example of a multi-segmental movement, the forces in question are a torquing action and depending on an individual's less stable area, ankle, or knee, that is where the damage will be done. Pain experienced on the medial aspect of the knee or lateral aspect of the ankle is a sure sign that the required ROM is not available, and the student needs to back off (Figure 2.20).

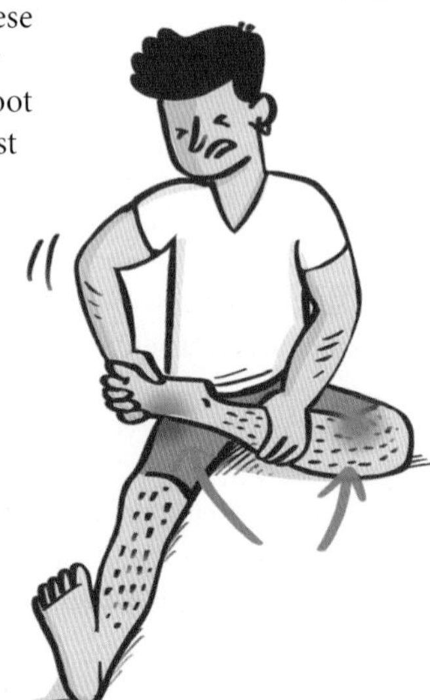

Figure 2.20 Yep, Dave is levering his knee and ankle by indiscriminately pulling on his foot.

If we broaden our perspective further, we can see that often we are using our whole body to make a particular shape, and the same law will apply. There will often be a place that moves more freely and tries to accommodate our restrictions, for example, the low back. If we don't control that area, two things can happen: (1) we will overstress that mobile area, and (2) we will also not effectively access our areas of restriction. Therefore, our progress in freeing up the body will be impeded.

Again, a specific example would be someone who comfortably moves into extension in the lumbar spine. The same students often have trouble with hip extension because they fail to work on that movement when they allow the low back to make too much adjustment (Figure 2.21A). To work effectively, they need to firm the belly, stabilizing the low back, and allowing them to access the restriction at the front of the hip and possibly the shoulders too (Figure 2.21B). The spine itself, of course, is a highly segmented area and we will

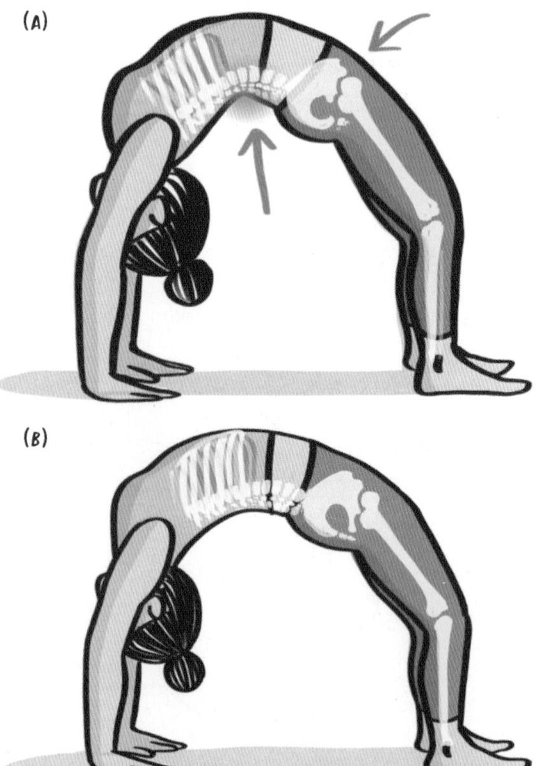

Figure 2.21 (A) Lucy has let her spine hinge, (B) firm belly and more hip extension.

look specifically at what may happen there in later chapters.

When we are positioning ourselves in yoga postures, we want to make sure we are moving in the right places and not trying to accommodate our restrictions by stressing joints. This force can be introduced either by taking the joints in directions they are not supposed to go or by taking them beyond their stable limit.

Q: The elbow is another area where many students can move excessively in a particular direction. Can you think of a few postures where you are moving the arms intending to access the wrist or shoulder, but that can be accommodated in the elbow instead if the student is not attentive?

Moving in Patterns

Whatever we do, we move and interact with our environment in patterns. The body can react more quickly and efficiently if desirable neural sequences are established. We adopt movements or combinations of moves that have been repeated and deemed as successful, less stressful, or more energy efficient by the body. That might mean predominantly emphasizing one side of the body, avoiding weak areas, using open areas, and avoiding restrictions, using strength rather than technique or anything else you might have noticed in yourself.

In a yoga setting, we might even include combining specific movements or postures in particular combinations. For example, being an Ashtanga practitioner, we have a set sequence. I don't have to think about what is coming next; the body is moving to the following posture almost independently of conscious control because that combination has been repeated so many times. On the flip side, ask me to do a pose out of the blue, and I can have trouble thinking about how to go about it. Even if you don't practice a set sequence, you may find you favor particular combinations of moves, or always do a chosen side first.

I think this idea of patterns is also present in what we might consider the anti-pattern modality of organic movement. In trying to break free of the rigidity that comes from a set sequence or guided practice, the aim is to move in spontaneous and original ways and directions. I would like to suggest that you will witness plenty of repetition of patterns that the individual finds easy and the exclusion of directions and positions that are more challenging (Figure 2.22). Left to do your own thing, you may well inadvertently bypass the parts that need work altogether.

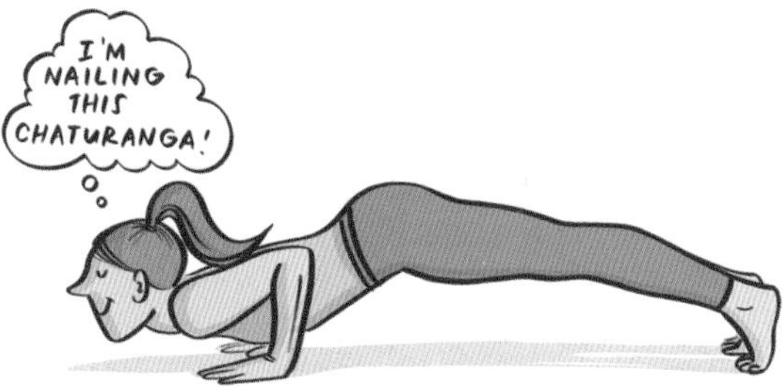

Figure 2.22 It is possible to be completely oblivious to the positioning of your body.

Don't believe me? Put this down right now and have a little organic move around. Try and remember what types of moves and combinations you did afterwards so you can assess it.

If we are not observant in our yoga practice, many of these patterns can go unnoticed and create imbalance, such as relying on our strengths and avoiding our weaknesses. I've heard it suggested that if we just keep doing something, the body will bring us into proper alignment or adopt sensible movements. I think the opposite. For the most part, I consider that patterns are so deeply ingrained that we will just keep repeating them unless we actively intervene. I have seen an example of this in my wife's *Chaturanga*, as she tends to drop one shoulder more than the other when lowering down, but is reluctant to do some serious work on it. Consequently, I have seen the same pattern repeated for as long as I can remember. You may have noticed similar traits in yourself.

We will bring patterns from daily life onto the mat, and yoga gives us the ideal opportunity to recognize them, but only if we are observant. More importantly, we can establish healthy movement patterns on the mat and transfer them to everyday life, but it won't just happen (Figure 2.23). I have seen plenty of yogis with advanced asana practices that have crappy posture (Figure 2.24).

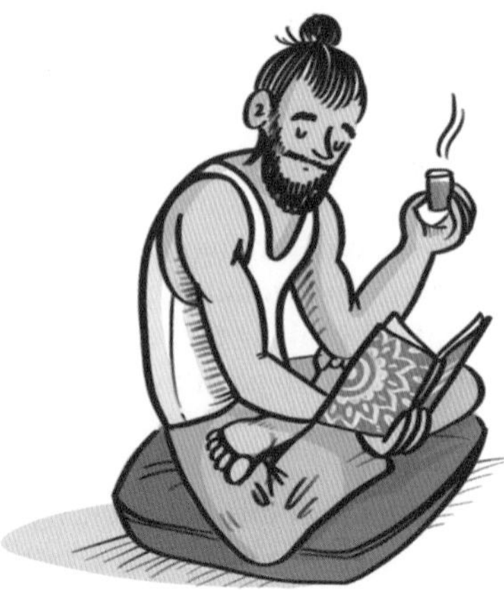

Figure 2.24 We don't want to see that slumped low back on or off the mat.

Many sports use this idea of neural patterning by repeating a specific sequence of moves so often that the body instinctively moves that way. Examples would be throwing the javelin, jump combinations in gymnastics, or ice skating, even power-key combinations on the PlayStation or Xbox. The difference between this repetition and mindless replication in the hope that things will change is that analysis has been undertaken to decide which move should follow which.

The body may also learn to predict what needs to happen when the body is positioned in a particular way. As is the case when starting to find balance in a Handstand, eventually the body reacts to changes in balance intuitively because it has come across that same situation many times and has learned what to do to stop you from falling. Moving in patterns can be both a positive and negative thing.

The key then is a constant awareness of what you are doing, and why you are doing it. Notice how you are moving—if you favor a particular side, transition slightly differently between sides and how you place your feet and hands. Sometimes we can even think we are working on changing something but are still just repeating the same movements.

My last point here would be to apply this idea to adjusting students. If you just reposition a student in a particular posture once, it's doubtful they will replicate the new position next time you see them.

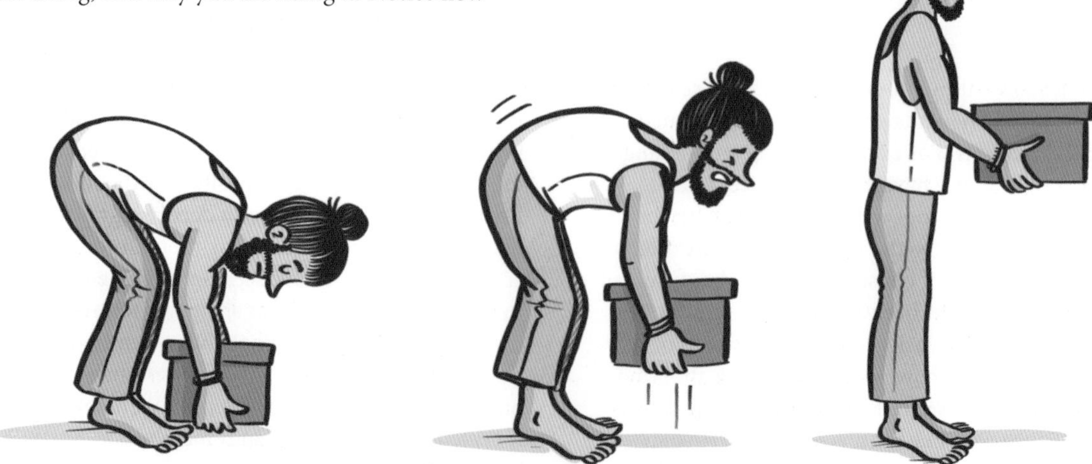

Figure 2.23 This doesn't look so sensible, but his Utthita Trikonasana *looks awesome.*

This is not due to stubbornness, but because their existing pattern is so well ingrained. Therefore, repeat an adjustment until a new position has been adopted rather than chop and change. It is even better when the student is more active in creating the new position themselves. If we just shove them into a position, they are only a passive recipient and not so likely to feel and remember the new placement. Compare the difference between driving a particular route for the first time or being the passenger on the same journey. I'm sure if you drive it, you will remember the way better.

The real last point is that we can't rely on what feels symmetrical or aligned because if we have been adopting a particular position for a while, that is what we will feel as right. When trying to adopt a new placement of the body in three-dimensional space, feedback is necessary either visually by way of mirrors, video, etc., or by a teacher guiding you to a more balanced position.

Your placement of the body in postural yoga needs to be a conscious decision. Being present lies at the core of a yoga practice.

Compression

"In my opinion, there are no marks for getting into a posture by any means, it is all about the quality of the chosen positioning."

Compression in this context means when two bones or associated soft tissue come into contact preventing further joint movement in a particular direction. Within exercise fields, you may also have heard the term compression used when talking in relation to active ROM and the ability to close a joint.

In the first interpretation, compression has a negative implication. It's not something we want to move against as it may well cause us injury, and if experienced, it will stop us from going as deep into a posture as we may like. In the second interpretation, compression may be deemed necessary as well as desirable. An example would be a straddle Handstand press; good compression of the hip is required to close the distance between hands and feet, get the hips high, and press without having to jump up. Don't get confused by the two meanings of the same terminology.

Compression comes in three flavors: soft, medium, and hard, and will be experienced in front of the direction of travel. Each will stop us moving further in that given direction, but the sensations and hazards will be different. Because things must come into contact with one another, we will only experience compression at certain joints and in specific directions at that joint, dependent on the shape of the bones and overlying tissues.

We will restrict ourselves to considering the main joints where most of our movement occurs, spine, hips, shoulders, knees, ankles, and wrists.

Soft compression is when flesh comes in contact with flesh—we could be referring to fat or muscle—the outcome would be the same. Think of a tennis player's or footballer's muscular leg shape. They have well-developed backs of the legs, and if you laid them on their belly and tried to bring their heel to their butt, you would probably find it didn't want to go. The calf muscles would come into contact with the hamstrings, preventing enough knee flexion to close the gap (Figure 2.25). In this instance, it might not be tension in the quadriceps that is the problem, but soft compression (Chapter 3, *Opposing Muscles Restrict*).

Now think of the seated forward fold *Paschimottanasana*—the ability to travel forward

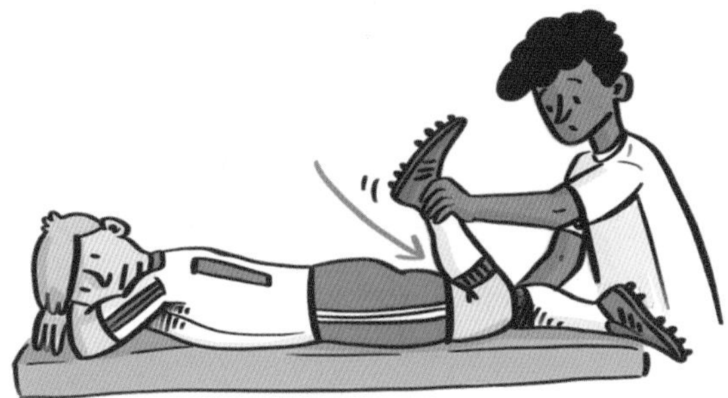

Figure 2.25 An example of soft compression. The calf muscles meet the hamstrings.

is determined by the hips' ability to flex. If you had some spare flesh around the waist, as you fold forward, the belly would hit the fat or muscles on the tops of the legs, stopping any further movement forward, irrespective of how flexible your hamstrings are (Figure 2.26A). If you moved the legs out of the way by taking them apart as in *Upavistha Konasana*, then if it was only flesh stopping you, your travel forward should continue (Figure 2.26B). That is as long as you don't have tight adductors (inner thighs), which would be put under a stretch in the new legs apart posture and, again, influence your positioning. Pressing into soft compression wouldn't cause any damage unless, in doing so, you are prizing a joint apart; it will generally just feel like a broad squishing sensation.

Medium compression happens when some soft tissue gets trapped between two bones. You might say that there must be bone under the flesh in the previous example, but this is more to do with a bony prominence and is experienced as a pinching sensation. One of the most common examples is when individuals experience this pinching in a deep lunge or twist with the hip flexed (Figure 2.27A & B). Here, what happens is that the pointy bit at the front of the pelvis, the anterior superior iliac spine (ASIS), squashes some flesh between it and the femur (upper leg bone). A quick fix can be to get your thumb and pull the

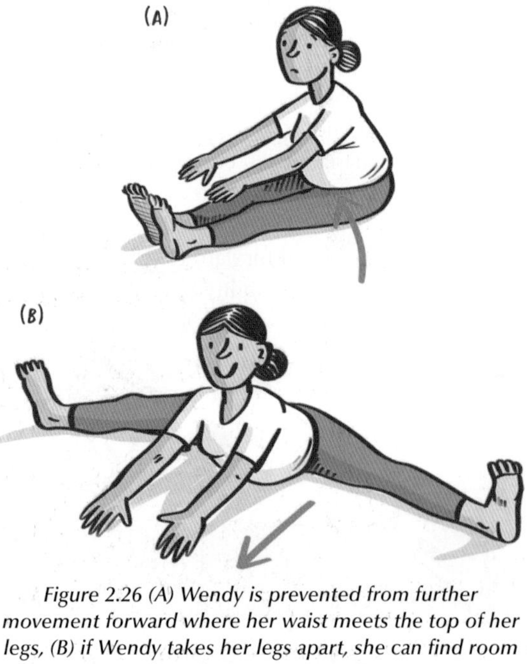

Figure 2.26 (A) Wendy is prevented from further movement forward where her waist meets the top of her legs, (B) if Wendy takes her legs apart, she can find room for her tummy.

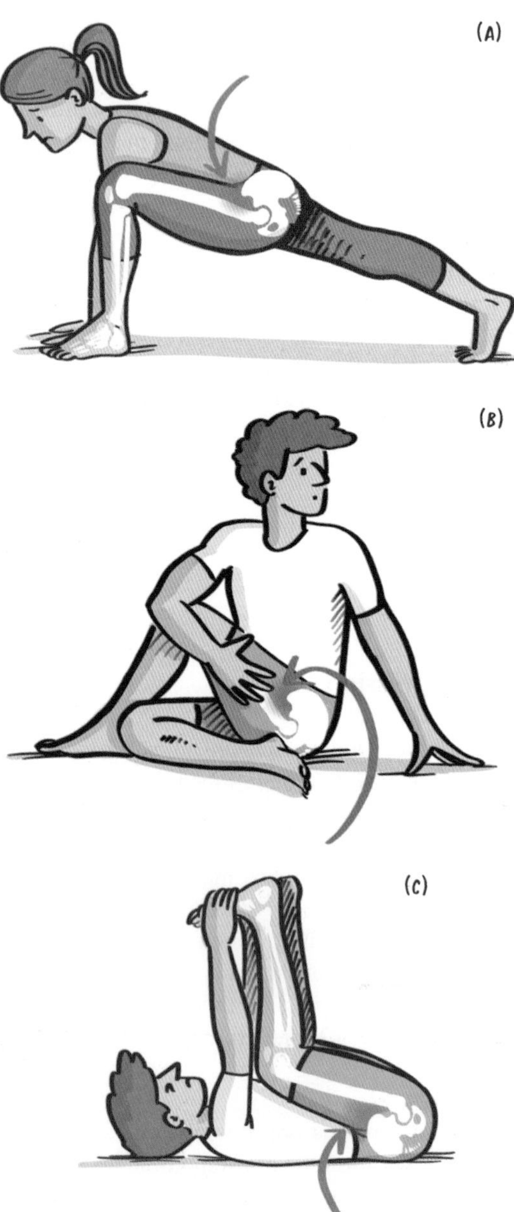

Figure 2.27 (A) A very common spot to experience medium compression, (B) pinching sensation due to medium compression, (C) medium compression in Happy Baby.

muscle or fat out of the way before closing-up the hip joint.

Some students experience the same thing in Happy Baby (Figure 2.27C). In any of these positions, you wouldn't want to put up with the discomfort because you will just cause some bruising and make the area more sensitive.

With both soft and medium compression, I think it is possible that things may change over time. Soft is easy to understand; lose some muscle bulk or flab and the restriction will diminish (I am not saying that this is what we should do, by the way). The bony prominence causing the pinching in medium compression won't change, but sometimes muscular tension pulls the joint in a particular travel path, and this may change as our yoga journey unravels. Of course, the opposite may also be true, where once there was no pinching, now maybe there is. Newfound freedom may mean we are going deeper than before into a posture, and now we find something is being squished.

Hard compression is not going to change over time, and we must understand when this is the case to avoid potential injury. This type of compression is due to bone coming into contact with bone, so you can appreciate that forcing into this will more than likely cause some damage over time. Usually, the individual will experience discomfort at a distinct spot, in front of the direction of bone travel. Typical sites while performing yoga asana would be:

- Wrist when moving deeper into wrist extension.
- Ankle when moving into dorsiflexion.
- Shoulder when moving into shoulder flexion.
- Hips when moving into abduction.
- Spine when moving into extension.

All of these we will consider individually later.

Let's consider *Samakonasana*. The student reports that on the way down, they experience discomfort deep in the hip, pointing above the leg where it meets the pelvis. The first thing to think of is where the leg is moving in relation to the pelvis. The individual may wish to sink deeper down, but the leg is, in effect, going up as the hip moves into greater abduction. If muscular tension were the issue, it would be felt on the inner thighs because the adductors are there, and they do the opposite action to where the leg needs to go. Pain, then, in front of the direction of travel, as is the case here, is likely to be hard compression—there is no flesh getting in the way, so the head of the femur is banging on the hip socket or greater trochanter on the pelvis (Figure 2.28). Therefore, it would be inadvisable for the student to attempt to go deeper if keeping the legs and pelvis in the same orientation.

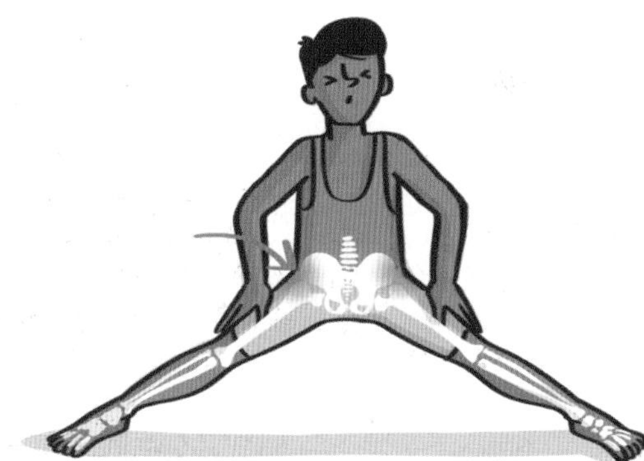

Figure 2.28 Vihan is experiencing hard compression.

Generally, you will find that if you change the relationship between the pelvis and the femurs, the compression can often be avoided. For example, if the student bends forward at the hips or points the toes toward the ceiling, they can usually take their legs much further apart (Figure 2.29). The reason is that the hip flexion in this position rotates the

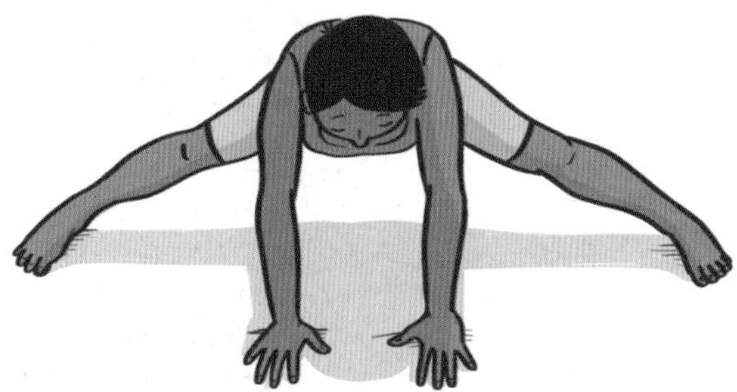

Figure 2.29 By bending forward at the hips, Vihan can avoid the hard compression.

pelvis around the femoral heads, and by pointing the feet to the ceiling, the hips rotate externally. Both examples find space.

For the moment, remember that compression is experienced in front of the direction of movement and muscular tension behind. It would be felt toward the expected end range of movement because that is when bones might come in contact with one another or squash soft tissue between them.

Compression will also be direction-specific to a particular joint—most movements won't offer the opportunity for the two parts to come in contact.

Fundamental Movements

"We might consider that there are fundamental movements that need to occur to facilitate the successful completion of a posture to a specific depth, with different ones calling for varying amounts of these from minimal to lots."

If you want to poo in the woods or many places in Asia for that matter, it will be especially handy to be able to squat. I once took my mum and her friends for a sightseeing trip in the Kerala backwaters, after their cruise ship dropped them off in Kochi (formerly Cochin) for the day. They were all in their early 80s at the time, so it wasn't long before the loo was needed. None on the boat,

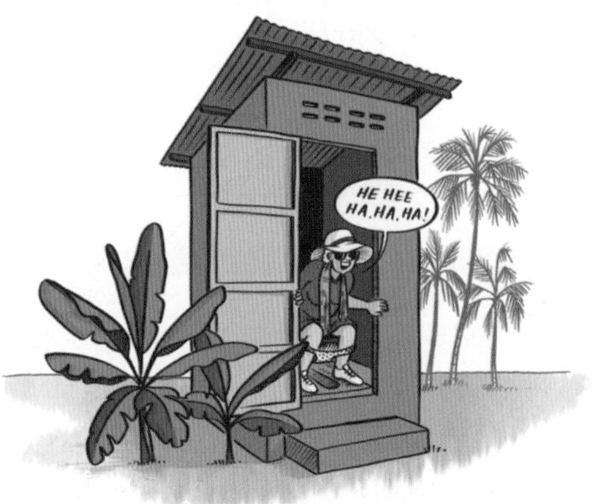

but luckily the captain had a friend with a house on one of the tiny islands. Much hilarity ensued when the garden squat loo was revealed, and they tried to get their tight old Western hips and knees to lower them anywhere close without almost falling over. In their comfy lifestyles, there was no need for the necessary ranges of motion or leg strength to squat, so they had lost the ability to do it.

If we could think back as far as hunter-gatherer times, we would have also wanted skills such as running, climbing, jumping, and throwing to add to our squatting. These are examples of compound movements (involving multiple muscles and joints), which were necessary to perform many of the tasks the day provided successfully. We need the ROMs, coordination, and strength to accomplish what we want to do, and if we choose tricky yoga postures as that thing, then the demands can be quite high, body-wide. Common movement patterns we will need are, for example, to bend forward and backward, lunge, stand up straight, twist, reach up and behind, cross the legs, push our body away from the floor, and, of course, to squat.

In exercise circles, this same idea is often encompassed by variations of the movement groups of Push, Pull, Squat, Lunge, Hinge, and Rotation. Notice pulling is missing from our yoga-related movement patterns, and that is because it is a hard movement to find in yoga. For this reason, I would say that for bodily health and balance, it is worth supplementing your yoga practice with some dedicated pulling exercises.

Earlier in this chapter, *Range of Motion*, we introduced the idea of needing to know the movements available at the major joints. Now, rather than think of the compound movements in the previous paragraph, we can combine these ideas and consider individual joint actions that crop up a lot in the yoga practice. This makes it easier to recognize the movements necessary to perform a yoga posture (compound movement) as well as see the similarities between poses.

We can regard these important joint movements as our fundamental movements for making yoga

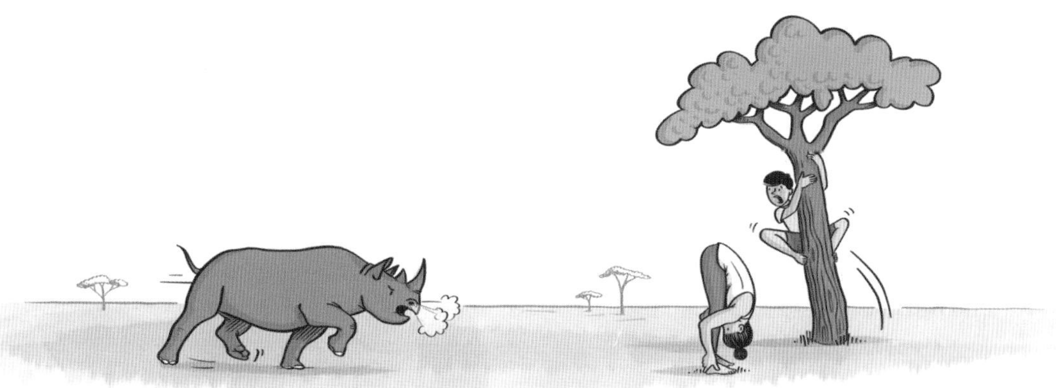

Figure 2.30 There may be some things more useful to be able to do than forward bending.

postures. Of course, all joint movements will be required to some extent in one pose or another, so it's not that any are unimportant, just that they impact fewer postures. Because the hips feature highly in both seated and standing postures, most of the movements available there could be considered fundamental.

Keeping the language simple for the moment. Essential movements at the hip would be: rolling the hip out (external rotation), moving the leg from the hip toward the front (hip flexion) or back (hip extension) with the leg straight or bent, and taking the leg away (hip abduction). Out of those, straight-legged hip flexion and external rotation of the hip would be the most useful. Hopefully, those of you that are getting to grips with these concepts will already be thinking, "Hmm, only if the posture includes those movements." Many do.

Other fundamental joint movements we might consider elsewhere in the body would include reaching forward and up from the shoulder (shoulder flexion), rolling the arm inward (medial rotation of the shoulder), all the spine movements of forward (flexion), backward (extension), side to side (lateral flexion) and rotation, deep knee bending (knee flexion), and top of the hand toward the lower arm (wrist extension).

Here's an example of this idea in use. Let's say you have a problem placing your foot into *Ardha Padmasana*. The main movements required to do this are: good knee flexion, plantar flexion of the foot, some hip flexion, a little bit of hip abduction, and a lot of external rotation of the hip. So, the first thing to do is establish if this is the ROM that you have difficulty with, and we will be detailing how to do this in later chapters (Figure 2.31).

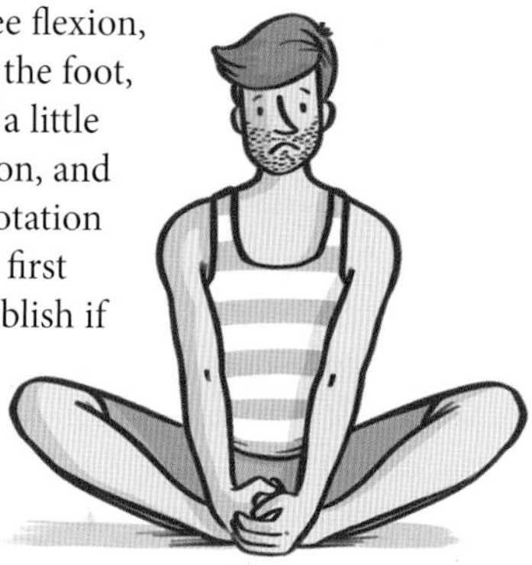

Figure 2.31 Ben's knees don't want to go down.

If you decide that you have difficulty in the fundamental movement of rolling the hip out (external hip rotation), any posture that calls for a lot of that movement will also be problematic. You can expect that other postures such as *Padmasana*, *Baddha Konasana*, *Kapotasana*, and *Agnistambhasana* will also present difficulty. This restriction will also make you more likely to try and make up for this somewhere else, primarily the knee or ankle joints (Figure 2.32).

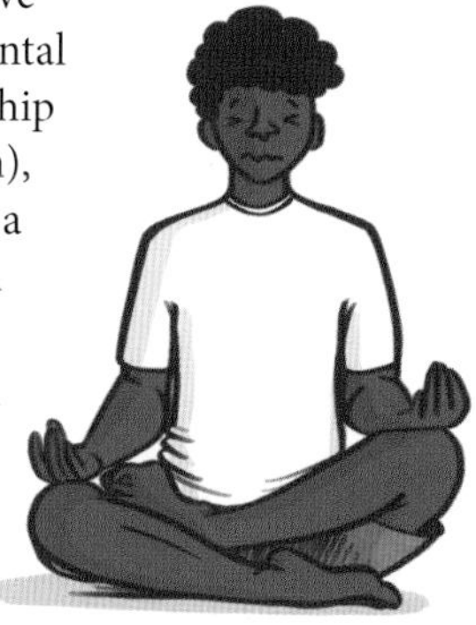

Figure 2.32 Aren has trouble with external hip rotation; in this position, he is compensating at the ankle.

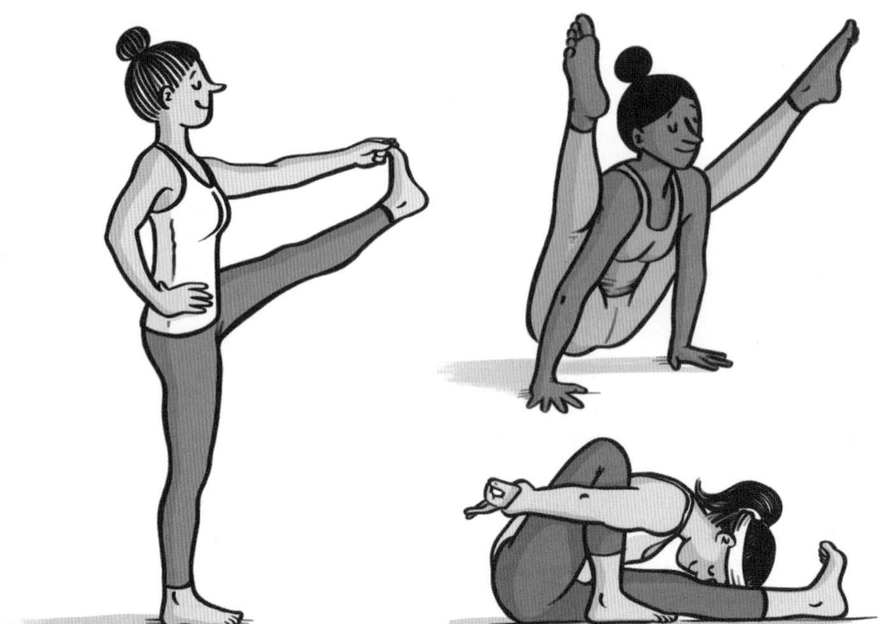

Figure 2.33 Straight-legged hip flexion is a movement that features highly in yoga postures.

If you take time out to work on that fundamental movement of external rotation of the hip, the increased ROM you achieve will not only make *Ardha Padmasana* more easily attainable but will also help you to find comfort in all those postures that contain the same movement.

At the extremes of your posture do-ability, you might have a shape that requires all the fundamental movements that are your most challenging or, at the other end, all your easy movements (Figure 2.33). You can see now that we want to be able to consider a posture by the fundamental movements that it includes.

Relational Movement

Whenever we move at a joint, it is possible to move one segment relative to the other or vice versa. Let's use the upper leg and pelvis and the movement at the hip in a couple of examples to illustrate the point.

From a standing position, we lift a straight leg toward the ceiling until the thigh is parallel to the floor. Only the leg is moving, and that movement is hip flexion. This time, we keep the legs straight and instead, bending at the hip, we bring our pelvis and upper body parallel to the floor. Again, this movement is happening at the hip and, likewise, is hip flexion. In the first example, we moved the leg relative to the pelvis and in the second the pelvis relative to the leg (Figure 2.34).

Even this level of understanding can help us realize what movement needs to happen in a posture, but let's now go one step further.

We are standing in front of a ballet bar and raise our leg, placing the heel on the bar. We have just done hip flexion, leg relative to the pelvis. Now we wish to move forward to lay our chest on our outstretched leg. Our pelvis needs to move relative to the leg to do this action, also hip flexion. If we have used up all our available hip flexion just getting our foot on the bar, then we will be stuck, not able to come further forward. If we have a bit more hip flexion available, we will be able to go forward a bit more, then further forward, and so on. We may well try and fake it by rounding the back, potentially placing stress on the back. What we need is more hip flexion.

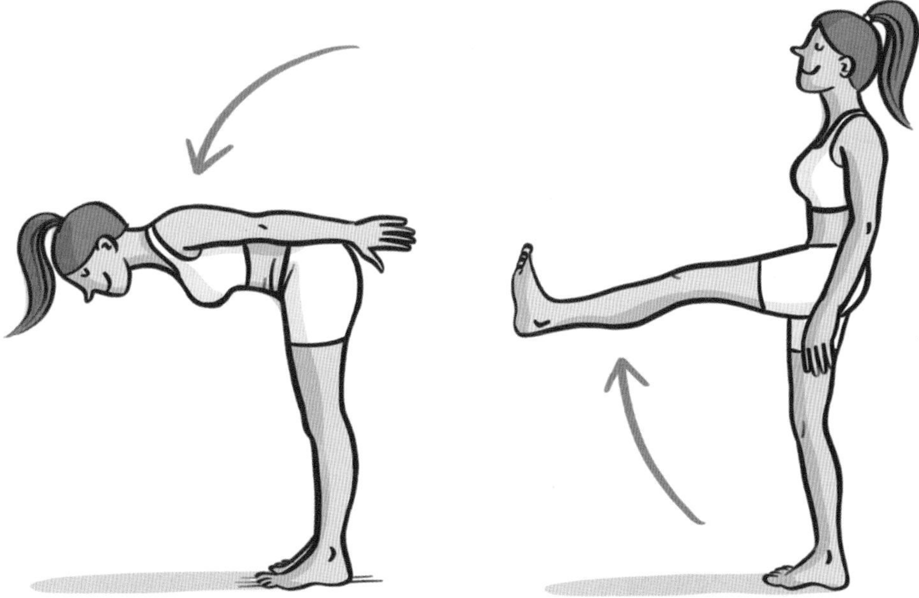

Figure 2.34 Victoria has done 90 degrees hip flexion in both these positions.

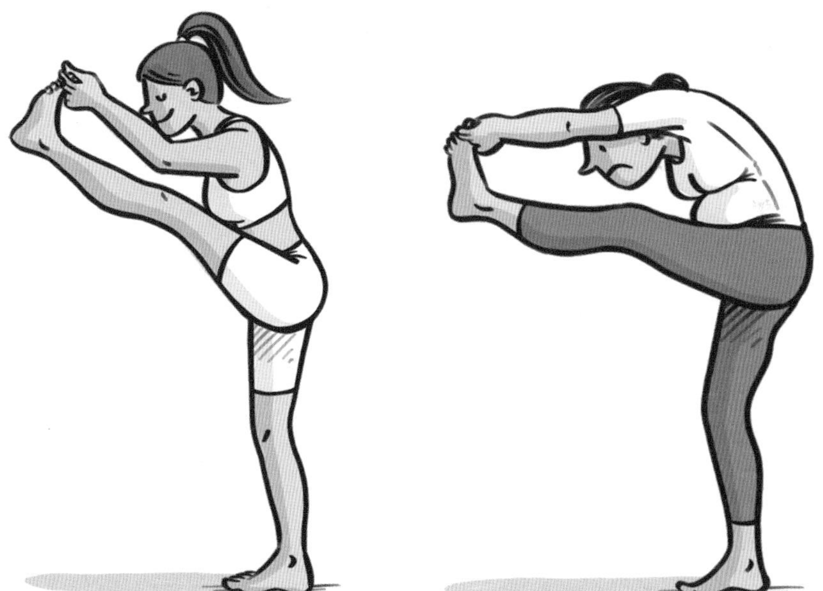

Figure 2.35 Victoria (left) has plenty of hip flexion available. Wendy (right) used all her hip flexion taking the leg up, so rounds her back trying to go forward. Not good news!

This is exactly what can happen in *Utthita Hasta Padangushtasana (UHP)*. If all the available hip flexion is used up when bringing the outreached leg into a position parallel to the ground, then the student would either not be able to fold toward the leg or would accommodate the restriction by rounding the back to do so (Figure 2.35).

Here is another example. In *Janu Sirsasana A*, we start from a seated position. The first action is to take the sole to the inside of the thigh. To achieve this, the major movement required is the rolling outward of the hip (external rotation of the hip). The upper leg moves relative to the pelvis (Figure 2.36A). From here, we now want to come forward over the outstretched leg. The bent leg should stay where it is and the pelvis move relative to the leg, which also happens to be external rotation of the hip (Figure 2.36B).

If we have no more external rotation of the hip available, two things can happen. The first is we stay put, unable to go forward (Figure 2.36C). The second is that as we try and pull ourselves down and, having no more external hip rotation available, the forward movement of the pelvis will bring the upper leg with it (Figure 2.36D). We will discuss the consequences of this in Chapter 7, *Knee*.

Becoming familiar with this concept and being able to view movement in this way will help you to understand why the full expression of a posture is not always available, as well as where attention needs to be focused, and how easily we can inadvertently place stress on links in the movement chain (remember closed-chain movements).

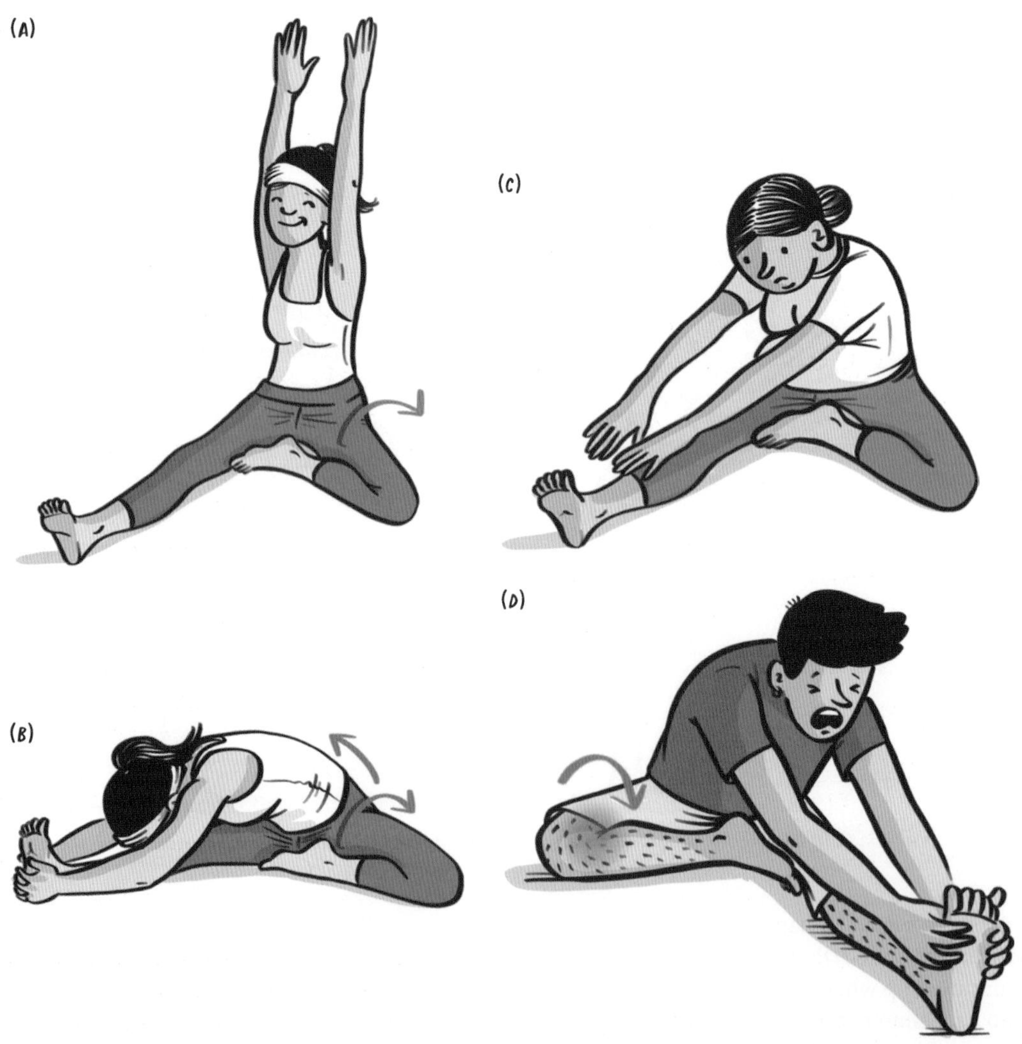

Figure 2.36 (A) The hip is externally rotated, (B) Jasmine has plenty of external hip rotation, so the pelvis tips forward, (C) Wendy gets stuck and wants to round, (D) "Give It A Yank" Dave is pulling the upper leg with the pelvis. More knee pain!.

CHAPTER 3

Muscles and Fascia

Neurophysiology

In this section, I am going to restrict the scope to somatic reflex arcs. If that meant absolutely nothing to you, don't worry, the translation is, "some hard-wired nervous system reflexes that influence the muscles." There are three that are of interest to us: stretch reflex, inverse stretch reflex, and reciprocal inhibition. As stretching is something that we as yoga practitioners do a lot of, I think you will appreciate the relevance.

When we think of the processing of information, we generally immediately think of the brain, but when time is of the essence, it is handy to have a decision-maker closer to the action, even though nerve impulses travel at blistering speeds. The "reflex arc" is one solution, because a set response to a sensory stimulus can be processed at the spinal cord.

Think of a time when you touched something very hot. The hand is away from the object before you have even registered the pain in the brain. The reflex arc responsible for this response is called the "withdrawal reflex," and the action elicited is to contract the flexor muscles and relax the extensor muscles of the limb involved in the encounter. The result is that the appendage gets whipped away from danger before you realize you need to move it. Just as well, because the rate at which some of our brains work would mean we could lose several layers of skin.

Stretch (Myotatic) Reflex

Located within the muscle belly are some sensory structures called "muscle spindles" that detect the length change of muscles, as well as the rate at which it happens. The higher these values, the more excited they are and the greater the number of neural impulses they send to the spinal cord. Their role is to provide proprioceptive information about the muscle, protect the muscle from being overstretched, and control the rate of length change.

The easiest way for the body to ensure that damage doesn't happen to the muscle is to slow down the rate of stretch. The reflex action at the spinal cord is to send impulses to the same muscle to initiate contraction (Figure 3.1). It can also cause an inhibitory stimulus (reciprocal inhibition) of the antagonist muscle (the one that does the opposite action), making it relax. The more signals from the muscle spindles, the greater the reflex action.

The significance this reflex has to yoga relates to how quickly a student goes into a posture. The slower the length rate change of the muscles, the less resistance there will be from the body.

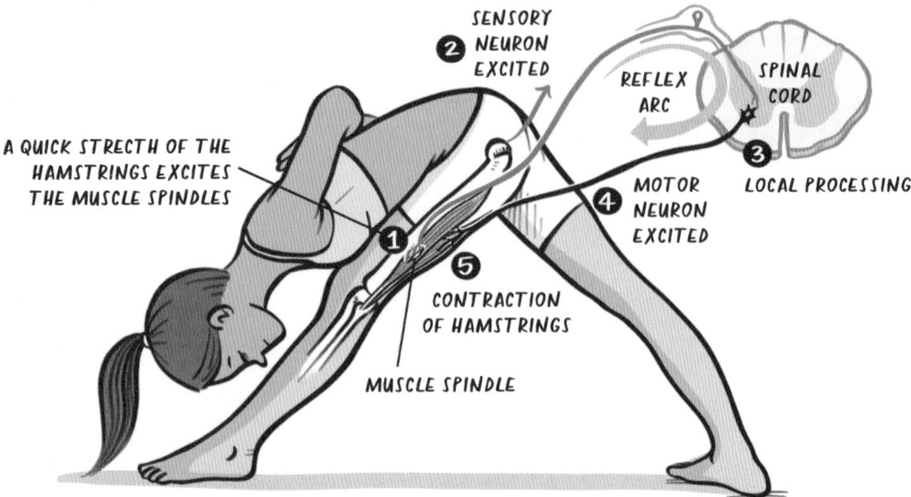

Figure 3.1 The stretch (myotatic) reflex causes a contraction of the same muscle that is being stretched.

The same goes if a teacher is adjusting a student in a way that is too heavy-handed and rushed, the student's body will just tighten up and resist. It is thought that if the initial stretch is not too vigorous, and then followed by a backing off, on re-entry into the pose, the reaction from the muscle spindles will be reduced. All this amounts to not rushing to get to the deepest expression of the posture, but perhaps taking a number of breaths to reach it.

Read "*Flexibility*" and the section on ballistic stretching. Uncontrolled bouncing up and down is likely to get the muscle spindles firing excitedly and create a reflex contraction of the muscle that is the target of the stretching. With the lack of control and excessive momentum often associated with ballistic stretching, this may increase the likelihood of tissue damage.

Inverse Stretch (Golgi Tendon) Reflex

You guessed it—the inverse stretch reflex has the opposite effect to the stretch reflex (Figure 3.2). This time, the structure that triggers the

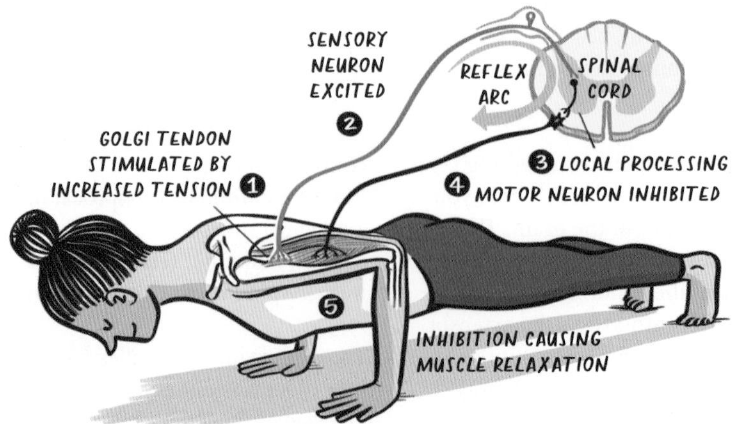

Figure 3.2 The inverse stretch (Golgi tendon) reflex causes a relaxation of the same muscle being loaded.

reflex is the GTO, which is situated near the musculotendinous junction. It responds to the level of tension building up in an MTU due to isometric contraction or stretching. With the same idea of protection, the response from the spinal cord is to reply with inhibitory signals to the same muscle. This causes relaxation or a lessening of contraction and, hence a reduction in tension.

It is the reflex during precontraction stretching that is thought to bring about the change in muscular tension postcontraction. However, as already mentioned, more recent research doesn't support this theory and points toward stretch tolerance instead. For my reasons why I feel this is incorrect, refer to "*Flexibility*", but I will also expand on my ideas at the end of this section.

Reciprocal Inhibition

Imagine a tug of war when both sides are pulling equally—there would be no movement. The idea behind reciprocal inhibition is that when one muscle contracts, its antagonist is inhibited from contracting. Now imagine a tug of war where there are 20 people on one end and only one on the other. There wouldn't be much control, and probably the 20 would land up on their backsides. Therefore, an inhibition is not going to be total because muscles need to work together to create smooth movement. But the idea is, if you are going to travel through a particular ROM, then you don't want the opposite muscle trying to take you in the other direction.

You may have also noticed that I mentioned reciprocal inhibition above in the text about the stretch reflex. I didn't put it in the diagram because I wanted to keep things simple, but reciprocal inhibition can also be initiated when the stretch reflex is triggered. It would make sense if the reason that a muscle was being stretched too quickly was due to its antagonist contracting, then you would want the antagonist to relax (Figure 3.3). Strictly speaking, this is reciprocal inhibition—and, as explained—the same as relaxation, but due to the agonist (prime mover),

MUSCULAR CONTRACTION OF QUADRICEPS
1
2 SENSORY NEURON EXCITED
REFLEX ARC
SPINAL CORD
3
LOCAL PROCESSING
4
MOTOR NEURON INHIBITED
5
INHIBITION CAUSING MUSCLE RELAXATION OF HAMSTRINGS

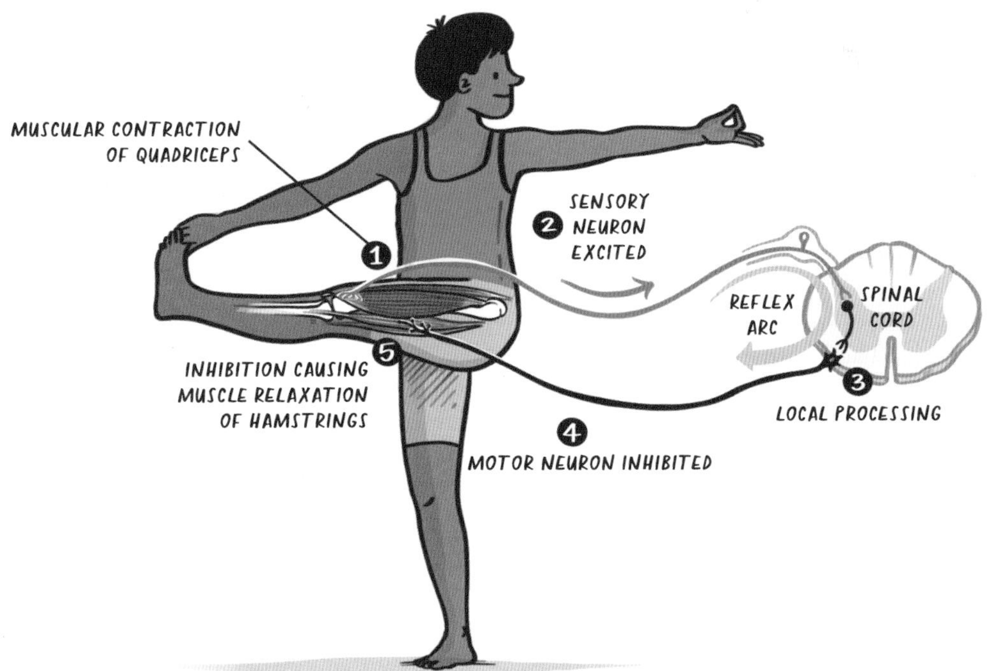

Figure 3.3 Reciprocal inhibition causes a relaxation of the antagonist muscle.

contracting is called "autogenic inhibition." But most of the time it all gets lumped under reciprocal inhibition.

The application of this reflex arc to yoga is to use as much active movement as possible because this will better inform the nervous system of the intent. Be engaged in the postures, not just hanging out or using levering actions.

But . . .

The explanations of these reflex arcs sound so clean and tidy, but no such luck. The body is extraordinarily complex and is receiving multiple stimuli at any one time. The chances are some of these responses will be overlapping, moderated, or combined.

Reflex arcs are involuntary, creating an almost immediate reaction, but that is not to say that there can't be some central nervous system (CNS) override. I'm sure, at times, the local decision making may even be contrary to conscious thought. As an extreme example, think of those unprecedented feats of strength in time of emergency. There must be all sorts of reflexes kicking in to protect the body from damage, but nope, somehow the person does the impossible.

A slightly more down to earth example can be taken from when I used to train rather intensely in the gym, often to failure. Many moons ago, you understand. There were numerous occasions when the muscles had given up and the weight was on the way back down, regardless of my intention of pushing it away. However, on those days when I had greater mental fortitude, I was able to halt it in its tracks and, with focus, send it back up again. I am not suggesting that you will be faced with this level of intensity on the yoga mat, but often with calmness and intention, we can override the body's reflex to jump in and save us. Mind you, it is also important to remember that, for the most part, these reflex arcs are protective mechanisms, so should not be abused.

Stretch Tolerance

More and more research appears to point toward stretch tolerance as the mechanism behind chronic increases in ROM. Frequently, it is reported that the notable differences after a program of stretching, are not a reduction in passive resistance to the stretch from the myofascial (muscle and fascia) tissues, but rather a psychological adaptation to the acceptable level of discomfort near end of range. An increase in tolerance to the stretch amounts to some desensitization by the CNS.

I mentioned already that I feel muscles don't become longer (if we exclude the acute effect of muscle creep) but that it is still possible to move through increased ROM with considerably more ease after months or years of yoga. There is less resistance from the soft tissues. I do agree that it is possible to endure greater intensities of stretching or training with practice, but I want to concentrate on comfortable ROM. For example, when I started yoga, my knees were up in the air when doing *Baddha Konasana*, but now they rest on the ground without having to push them down. The range through which I can travel with minimal resistance has increased considerably in many places.

I will put forward my idea behind chronic ROM changes now and wait for studies to back it up. The starting point is that different bodies will have more or less resistance to stretching, dependent on their tissue makeup. At one end, there are those with stiffer tissues due to greater muscle density or less elastic connective tissue, and at the other, those verging on hypermobility due to greater elastic qualities in their connective tissue (oversimplified, but it will do here). I'm convinced that the majority of resistance to change in ROM comes from the nervous system, and I think a reworking of the concept of stretch tolerance may be the answer.

We know the body constantly adapts and re-evaluates what is worthwhile and useful. Need more strength, your muscles will grow; stop using that strength, they will diminish again. Become sedentary and your mobility and fitness will reduce. The body is both an energy conservationist and a self-protector. In that respect, it is much easier to look after the body if there isn't ROM available well above what is needed. It is much less likely that a joint will be moved through a range where it will become unstable or at risk if movements are kept well within the safe zone. To that end, I feel the CNS has ranges through which it will happily allow us to move after which neural activity will resist further muscle lengthening. We could refer to these as set points. From this perspective, we may like to redefine stretch tolerance as the amount of stretch the CNS will allow before it is resisted, rather than how much discomfort can be withstood.

Once the muscle has been lengthened (stretched) past the set point, the intensity of discomfort felt will increase to discourage further lengthening. If, through regular yoga (stretching), it can be demonstrated to the CNS that greater ROM is a useful commodity and that severe damage has not occurred, then on re-evaluation, it will change the set point. This will result in the ability to travel further through a ROM before it is resisted. Therefore, a greater stretch (change in length) is tolerated, rather than being able to tolerate a greater stretch. As far as I can discern, this is not the accepted interpretation of stretch tolerance, but after years of practicing yoga, it is what makes the most sense to me.

Open and Closed Kinetic Chains

A kinetic chain refers to the idea that muscles and joints work together to create movement and that forces will be distributed between them.

There are two types of kinetic chain: open and closed. The distinction refers to whether the most distal (furthest from the body) segment in the chain is free or fixed in place. Usually, we are talking about the feet or hands as they are often the base for support or the end of the extremity in motion. A particular exercise could then be considered either open- or closed-chain dependent, on the way it is performed. The different kinetic chain movements are considered to be better for certain types of outcome, such as isolating muscles and working on stability. In exercise training and rehabilitation environments, closed- or open-chain exercises would be prescribed based on the desired outcomes.

To give you the idea with yoga postures, a closed-chain posture combination would be moving from a squat back up to *Tadasana* because the feet are fixed in place (Figure 3.4).

If on the other hand, we were thinking of the arms and shoulder girdle in a Sun Salutation, that would be an open-chain movement because the hands

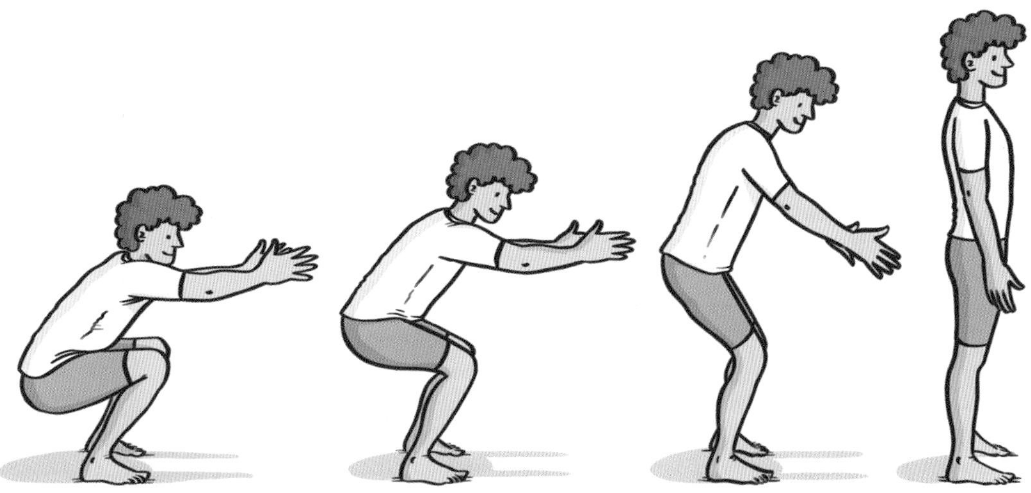

Figure 3.4 Doug is demonstrating a closed chain movement, where the feet stay in place.

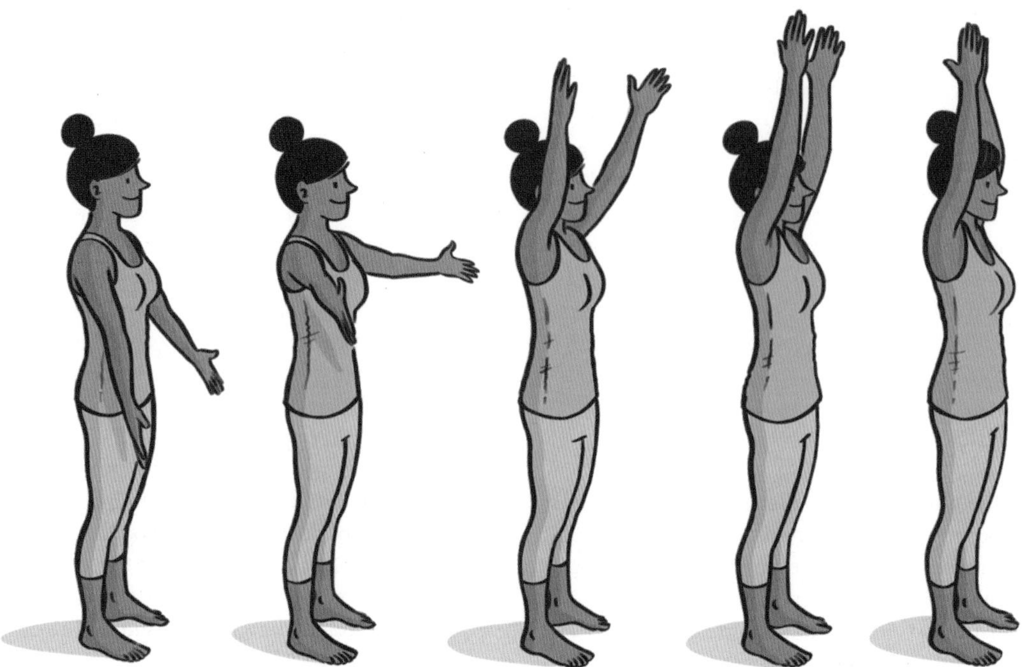

Figure 3.5 Here, Myra is doing a Sun Salutation with the arms, which is an open-chain movement.

are not fixed in place (Figure 3.5). I think you'll be glad to know that we are not going to try and apply this kinetic chain idea to multiple postures. What I want to do is modify this idea slightly and add it to the previous concept of *Multi-Segmental Movement* (Chapter 2). You will have already noticed that we mention segments in both.

The essence of the multi-segmental concept is that weak areas within a chain of joints will be the ones that land up experiencing the most significant negative forces while trying to accommodate the energy introduced to that chain. If we are using our muscles to create the movement and one end of our chain is genuinely free to move, it is unlikely that enough force will be introduced into the complex of joints to be problematic. Think of something like an active twist where you are using the strength in your obliques to rotate (Figure 3.6).

Another example might be active hip rotations either lying or standing, with the rotation muscles in the hip doing the work (Figure 3.7).

However, we are not always out of harm in an open-chain movement or position. We can add an external force, such as an assist or gravity. In something like a standing backbend, we can still allow the movement to be accentuated in a particular place because gravity is taking us toward the floor and the lever can be long and the body heavy (Figure 3.8).

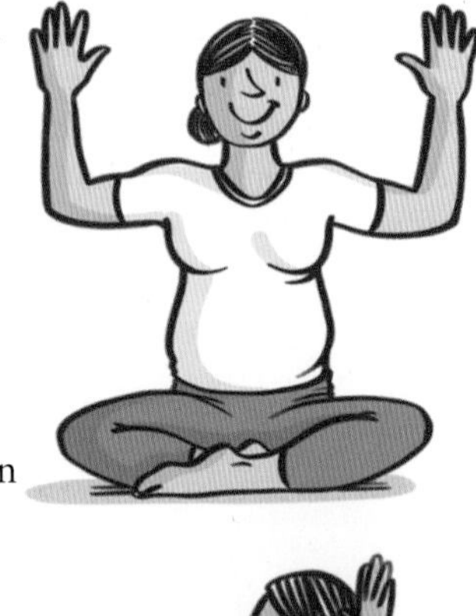

A lot of the time in yoga postures we have our hands or feet in contact with the ground, closing the kinetic chain. In *Urdhva Dhanurasana*, both ends of the whole-body kinetic chain are fixed on the floor, and the forces introduced come from pressing into the ground and gravity.

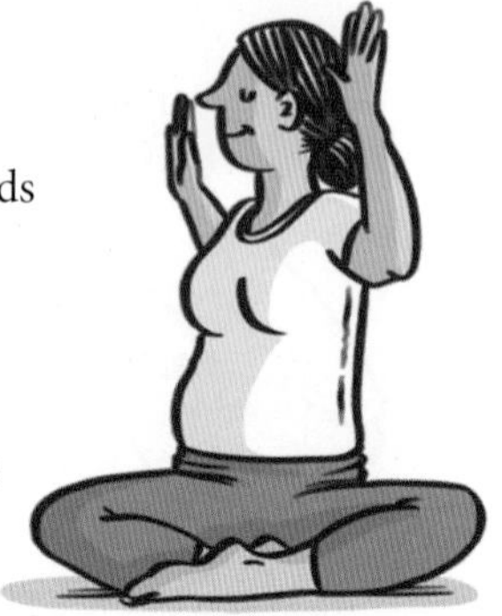

Figure 3.6 Nice active twist by Wendy, no levering to add an external force.

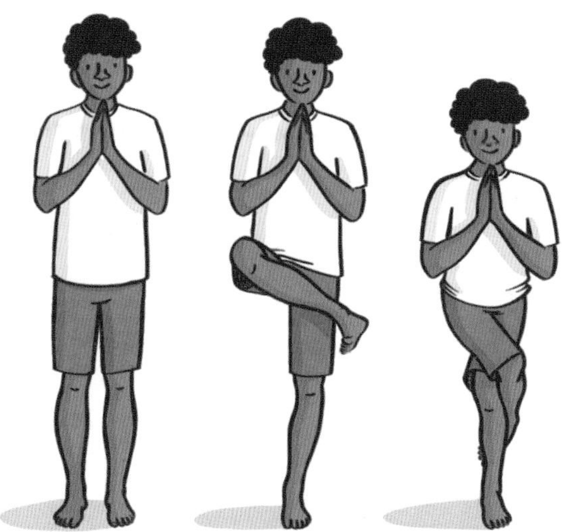

Figure 3.7 Aren is using his hip muscles to move his leg into position, also great for building strength and control.

Keeping with the twisting example, if we placed our hands on knee and floor and used that contact to help us rotate, I would consider this a closed chain and much easier to place forces where we don't want, such as lumbar spine and sacroiliac joint (SIJ), Figure 3.9. In *Eka Pada Rajakapotasana*, the foot is fixed on the floor, so again, is a closed-chain hip rotation; we can take pressure into the ankle, knee, or pelvis if we are not positioned correctly (Figure 3.10).

An active movement combination—sometimes called "windscreen wiper"—that crops up in yoga classes but originated in functional movement circles, is one of my least favorite positionings of the body. It can so easily place stress into the menisci of the knee, especially if you are challenged with medial hip rotation (Figure 3.11). Because the feet are on the floor, it is a closed chain.

Figure 3.9 With the hands on the floor or the legs, this pose becomes a closed-chain movement.

Often the hip is in the air of the medially rotated hip, so you also have that weight bearing down. As well as that, if the feet are dorsiflexed, you have the potential for a lever to rotate the lower leg relative to the upper leg. The vulnerable area in this closed-chain multi-segmental movement

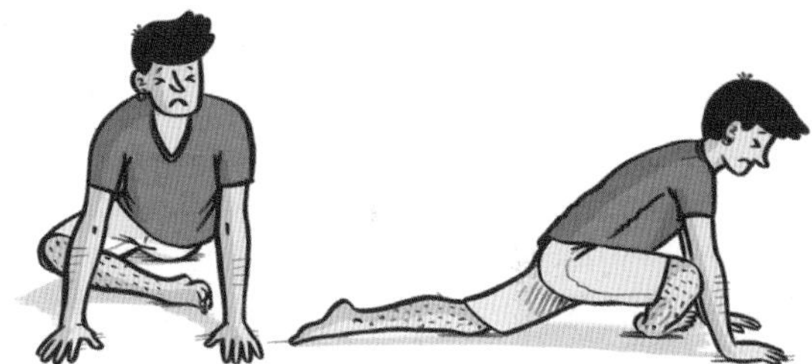

Figure 3.10 Contact with the floor can allow more force to be introduced into a movement.

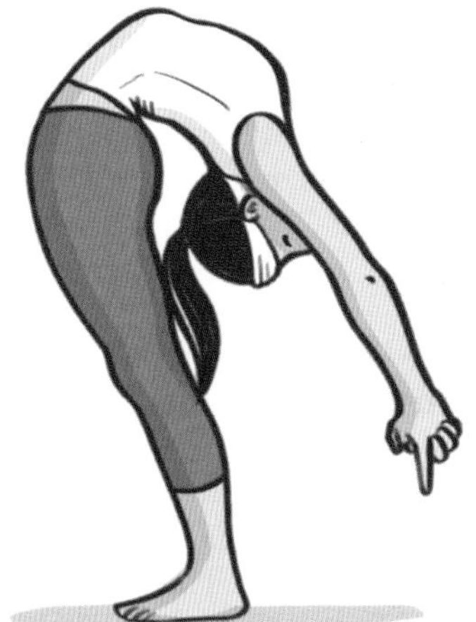

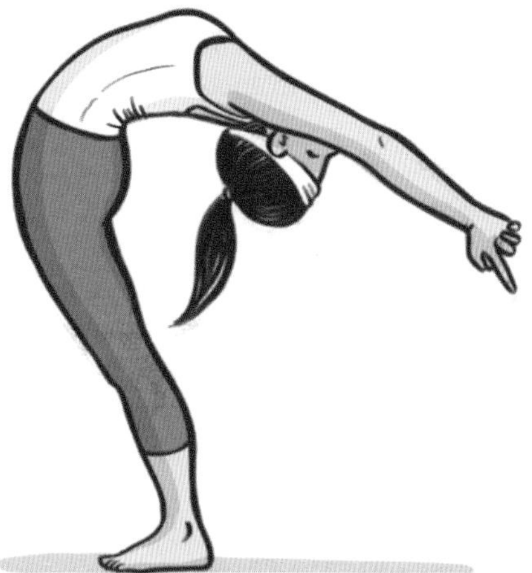

Figure 3.8 On the left, Jasmine let gravity take her too deep and landed up hinging in her spine.

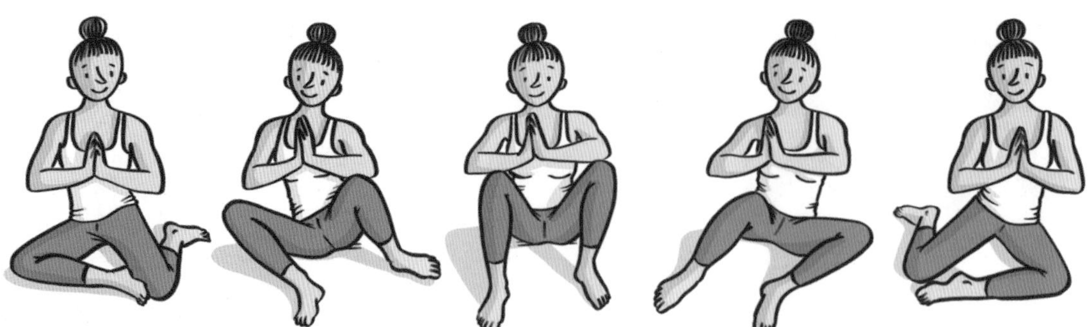

Figure 3.11 I feel active movement sequences like this one can be more detrimental than beneficial.

is the knee, but if alternate hips keep lifting off the floor, the chances are the SIJ won't be thankful either.

I often take ideas and bend them to help me get to grips with what is going on with the body, so this next bit is probably not a strict interpretation of a closed kinetic chain. However, I think for all intents and purposes, when we take hold of our foot and start pulling on it to try and access the hip, we have created a closed chain.

The end segment of the complex is no longer able to move freely. It might just as well be on the floor. Not surprisingly, then we can apply forces into the weak areas of ankle and knee if the hip stops rotating and we keep pulling. I see this action happen so often when students are trying overzealously to get into *Padmasana*. I apply the same logic to any instance where we lock one body part with another and use that as a lever. Again, we can go back to a twist example and think of a prayer twist using the force of the elbow or back of arm pressing into the knee to encourage more rotation in the spine.

The idea of adding this idea of open and closed kinetic chains was to get you thinking of all the different ways we can inadvertently place stress in vulnerable areas when performing yoga postures, multi-segmental movements. What I would like you to take away from this chapter is that the more we can use the proper muscles in the making of our postures, the healthier they will be. If you want to twist, use your twisting muscles, don't just lever yourself around (Figure 3.12).

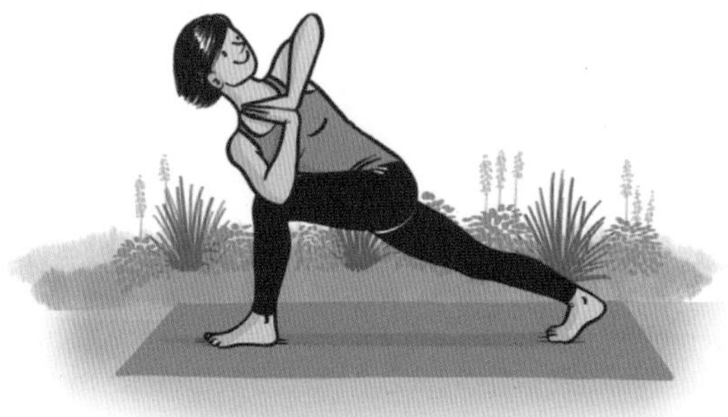

Figure 3.12 It is very easy to overuse contact with other body parts to generate forces that may have negative consequences. It is fine to place your hands in prayer with the arm next to the thigh, as Kathi is demonstrating, but don't also use this position to force yourself around.

We also need to be in tune with how our positioning relative to the floor has the potential to add unwanted stresses to joints, especially if we are then using our body weight and gravity to elicit a change in ROM. It's not that we only want to do active movements because it can feel very nice to be in a long hold and gently release further; we just need to be in our bodies and experience what is happening and where.

Be present.

Polyarticular Muscles

A polyarticular muscle crosses more than one joint and directly influences the movements of those joints and will be affected by the positioning of those joints. There will always be other muscles that perform the same individual actions as the polyarticular muscle, but each of them will only cross one of the joints.

If, for example, we consider rectus femoris (one of the quadriceps), it crosses the hip and the knee, performing the actions of hip flexion and knee extension (Figure 3.13).

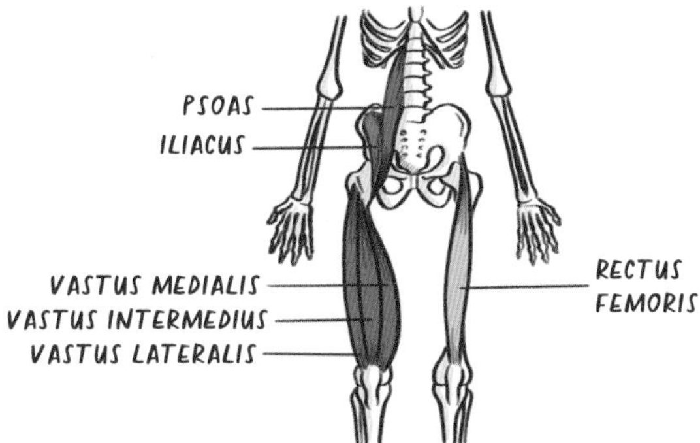

Figure 3.13 Rectus femoris can do both hip flexion and knee extension.

The psoas and iliacus can perform hip flexion, and the other quadriceps that don't cross the hip can do knee extension. There is then a backup plan for when a polyarticular muscle is in a position where it can't work effectively. We therefore need to consider the positioning of all the joints a muscle crosses when aiming to stretch or strengthen it.

Let's continue with the quadriceps as an example of stretching a polyarticular muscle. As the name suggests, four muscle bellies make up the quadriceps. Three only cross the knee, and as mentioned above, the other one (rectus femoris) also crosses the hip. The job of the three that cross the knee is to do knee extension and, of course, stabilize the knee. To stretch those same muscles, we need to take the knee in the opposite direction to the job they do, in this case, that means knee flexion.

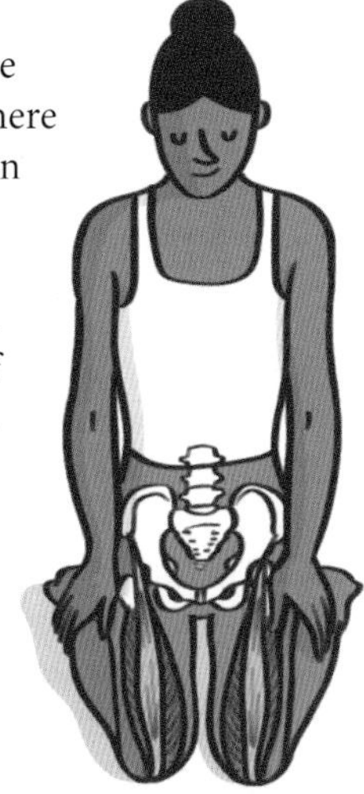

Figure 3.14 Virasana.

If we take the heel to the butt or butt to heel, as in *Virasana* (Figure 3.14) or *Triang Mukha Eka Pada Paschimottanasana*, then we are putting a stretch on all four of the quadriceps.

However, this is not very effective for rectus femoris because it crosses the hip, and the hip is flexed in those seated positions. To give attention properly to rectus femoris, we would need to lie back and in so doing, take the hip out of flexion (Figure 3.15).

If we want to make it more intense, then we could go for a kneeling version. In a low lunge, we can take the heel to the butt and move the pelvis forward while resisting it from going into an anterior tilt. This creates both the knee flexion and hip extension required and, because the floor doesn't get in the way, allows for deeper hip extension (Figure 3.16).

When we want to strengthen a muscle that crosses two joints, then again, we must think of the positioning of both joints. Polyarticular muscles are ineffective at moving a joint if the other joints it crosses are not already in a position that lengthens the muscle. In other words, in a position that is opposite to the action that it performs at that joint. We will use the example of gastrocnemius because it will be easy for you to experiment and see for yourself as there is not much fat covering it.

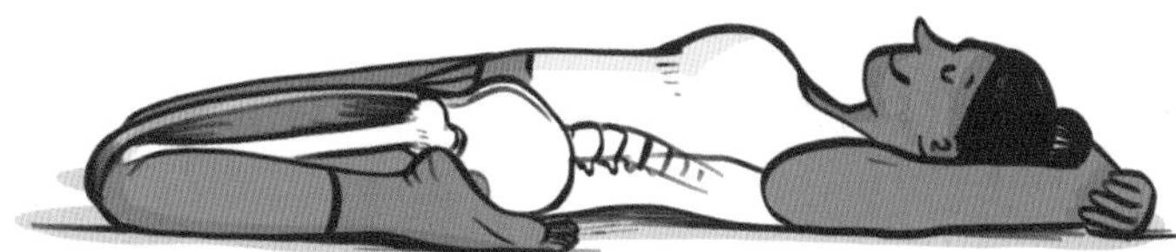

Figure 3.15 To place rectus femoris under a stretch effectively, the hip needs to be extended and the knee flexed.

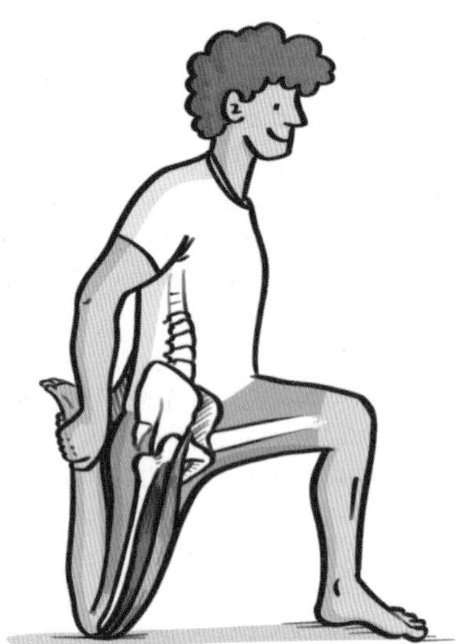

Figure 3.16 Low lunge, taking the heel to the butt and moving the pelvis forward.

The gastrocnemius is on the back of the lower leg and does both ankle plantar flexion and knee flexion. If we use this muscle to plantar flex the ankle, then we need to have the leg straight (opposite to knee flexion, the other action it performs).

If we roughly know where muscles go to and from, we can also use this concept to help understand what we see happen to the body position in some yoga postures. For example, if we think of the posture *Supta Virasana*, it's quite common for a student to feel they can't lie back. If they do, we may see their spine curving away from the floor, ribs cage flaring or adaptation at the other end, with knees off the floor and inner thighs coming apart (Figure 3.18). Why is this happening?

Try this for yourself. Stand close to a wall so you don't have to worry about the balance and, with straight legs, come on to tiptoes (Figure 3.17). You have plantar flexed your foot with a straight leg, and if you look down, you will quickly see the two bellies of gastrocnemius hard and contracted.

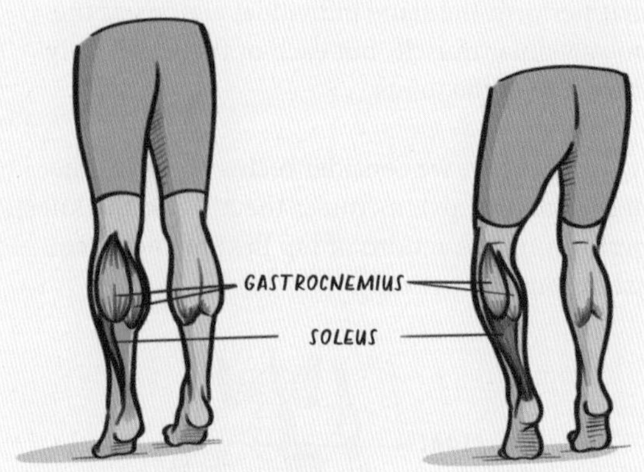

Figure 3.17 When the knee is bent, soleus will do most of the work of plantar flexion.

Now place your heel down on the floor again and bend the knee. This time, come onto your tiptoes, keeping the knee bent. Even though you have risen, if you take a look, the gastrocnemius will be relaxed. Soleus, the muscle that lies underneath and only performs plantar flexion, has done the work.

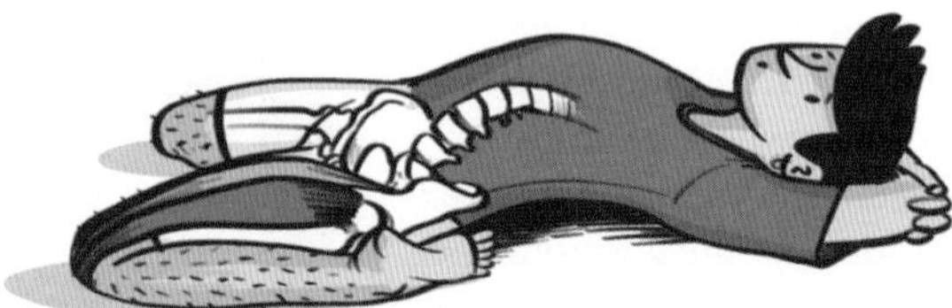

Figure 3.18 Supta Virasana *is not Dave's happy place.*

We start this posture in *Virasana*, a seated position with both knees flexed maximally, and the hips flexed. There is a stretch in all the quadriceps but not a very good one in the rectus femoris because the upper attachment is not on the femur as with the others but beyond the hip on the anterior inferior iliac spine (AIIS). In this position, the upper attachment point is closer to the attachment at the other end, and hence there is less strain on the muscle.

As the student reclines, the proximal attachment moves away, and the rectus femoris can reach its maximum stretch and prevent the pelvis from moving further toward the floor (hip extension). If the student continues down to the ground with the pelvis in this relationship to the femurs, then the shoulders will come down to the floor, but there will be an exaggerated lordotic curve in the lumbar spine (Figure 3.19).

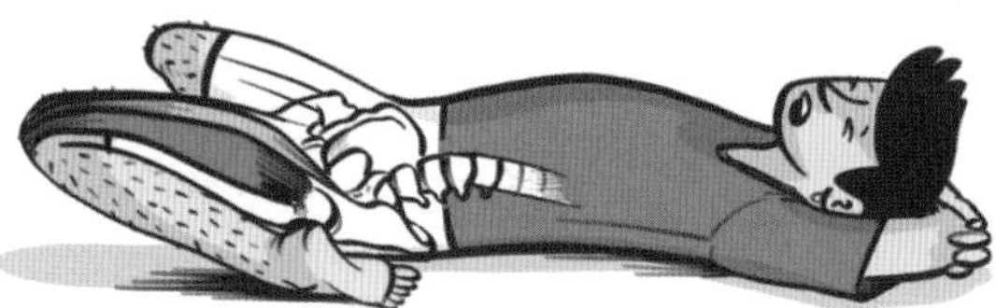

Figure 3.19 Like a seesaw, if the low back goes down, the knees go up.

If they maintain their natural curve instead, the knees will be pulled off the floor and apart. The reason for both body positions are the same—restriction in the rectus femoris is stopping sufficient hip extension from happening, and the body is adapting in other places to accommodate the position you are trying to place it in.

We will cover it later, but now try yourself to think of what you would need to do at the knee in *Salabhasana* if you want to focus on using hamstring strength rather than gluteus maximus (Gmax) to extend the hip.

Strength

"Having the strength to control the full ROM that a joint can move through is essential for the longevity of the yoga practice."

Strength helps us be more stable, integrated, controlled, and reduces the risk of injury, so it is crucial to have a grasp of how to work on it in a yoga setting. Although improving strength is something that gets talked about a lot, in reality, very little is done with this specific intention in many yoga sequences. The reason behind this is probably uncertainty about what we are working on, when, and how to go about it. Because I think, for the most part, students don't want their yoga class turned into a conditioning session, we will focus here on how to work on strength while in yoga postures or when transitioning.

To gain strength, we have to make a muscle contract, and only those muscles that are working will get stronger. If for example, we had a summer job that involved climbing ladders all day, our legs would get stronger but not our upper body. Even then, only the muscles in our legs we used a lot would be affected, anything else would stay the same. For instance, the adductors are on the legs but not used for ladder work. Therefore, their strength would remain the same. Makes common sense, right? But this means we need to know what muscles are used to do which actions, types of contractions, and be able to translate yoga postures into muscle movements. Luckily, I can help you with that.

When we are holding a yoga posture, we are in stillness, but muscles are still working to keep us in position. The amount of work going on will vary between very little to quite a lot, depending on if we are standing, seated, lying, inverted, balancing, how many foundational elements we have, and if we are active or passive. Heat is a waste product of muscle contraction, so if you are getting hot from the work you are doing, that is a good sign.

When muscles are holding us in place, they are working in a stabilizing way, and this type of muscle contraction—where there is no change in the muscle length—is called isometric contraction. Even when we are moving or transitioning, some muscles will be stabilizing in certain areas so that we can move from them. Even when we are still and contracting very little, think of *Shavasana*, the ground is supporting us so theoretically we can relax all our muscles.

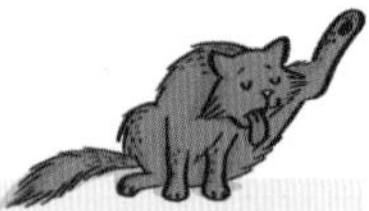

As you are sitting there, straighten a leg out in front of you and then contract the quadriceps, feel the front of the upper leg go hard (1). This is an isometric contraction. Now keep that going, loop your hands under your thigh, and lift the leg off the floor (2). Your leg is straight, and the static contraction of the quadriceps is keeping the knee in extension against the force of gravity that wants to bring your lower leg toward the ground.

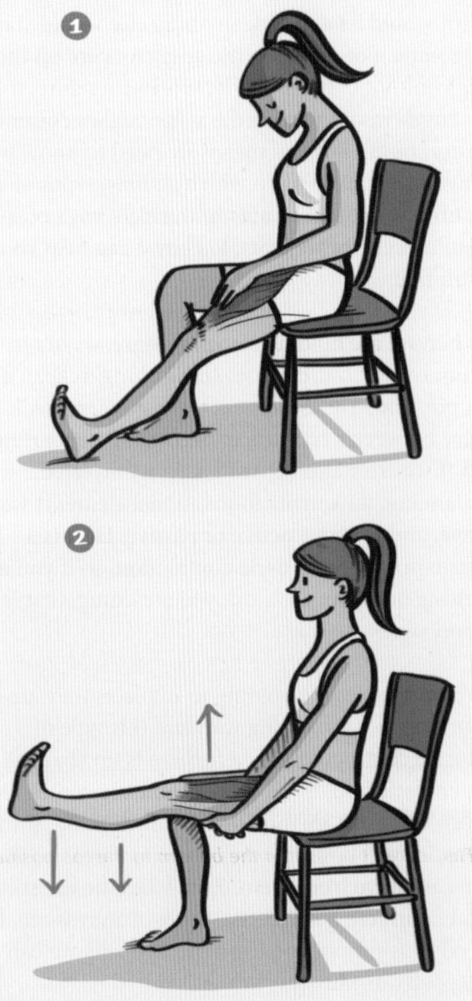

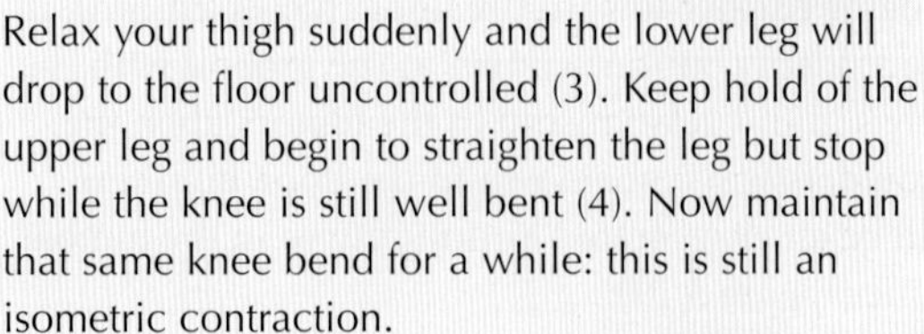

Relax your thigh suddenly and the lower leg will drop to the floor uncontrolled (3). Keep hold of the upper leg and begin to straighten the leg but stop while the knee is still well bent (4). Now maintain that same knee bend for a while: this is still an isometric contraction.

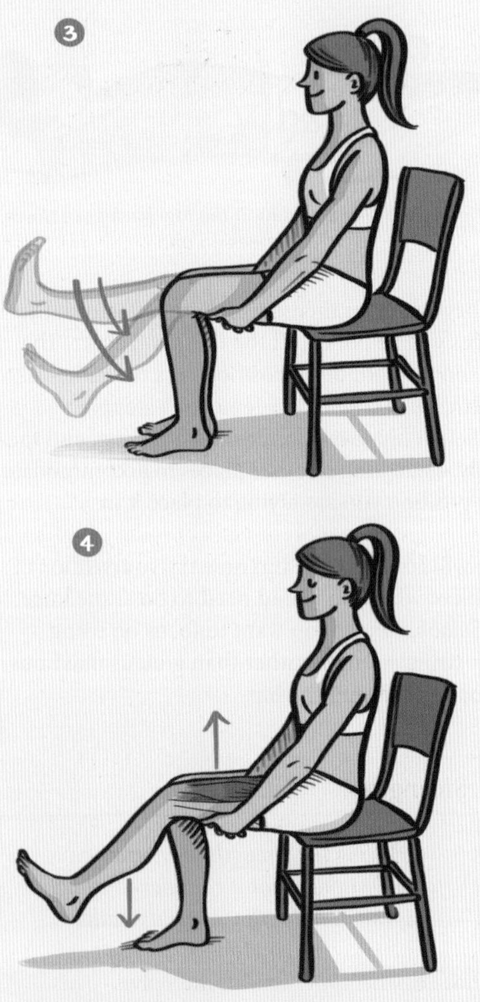

A joint can be at any angle when isometric contractions stabilize it. Many muscles may need to work together to create the stability required in complicated positions.

When you have less support from the ground, you will have to work harder. It follows then that, generally speaking, standing postures will be more strengthening than seated postures. If you reduce your foundation, such as when balancing on one leg, you will have to work harder. If you maintain body parts in a position resisting gravity, you will also be challenging your strength.

Combine these elements into a single posture like *Virabhadrasana C*, and you will have a good example of a strengthening pose (Figure 3.20). However, if we are in and out of it too quickly, the

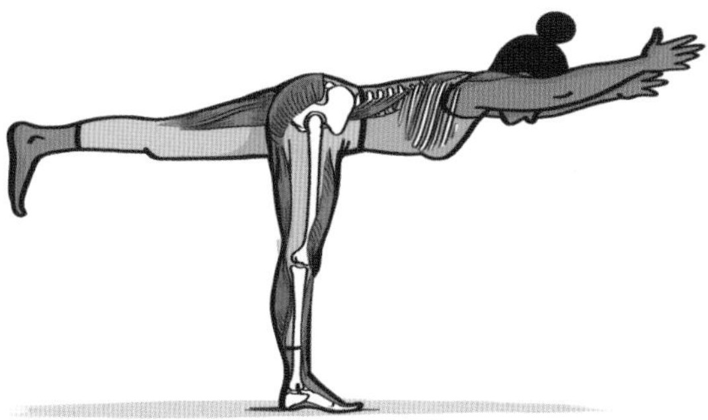

Figure 3.20 Virabhadrasana C *is an excellent strengthening pose.*

opportunity will be lost. Factor one when working with strength is time. The muscles need to be challenged to adapt. If you intend to get stronger, think of holding some of your standing postures for 10 breaths instead of five, or longer still if you find that too easy. Think of adding variations while continuing to maintain the same position if you feel your mind will wander. To consider what happens when we are moving, try the above little experiment for me (see tinted box, top right hand column).

As the quadriceps contract and shorten, their attachment below the knee is being pulled closer to those on the upper femur and pelvis—this type of movement is a concentric contraction. In a gym setting, adding more resistance to the action by weights or cables would make the muscle work harder. In a yoga setting, we have no such equipment, instead we have ourselves and gravity, which sometimes means it is difficult to add enough resistance.

Factor two when working with strength is repetition. If doing something once isn't challenging enough, do it several times. Pressing from *Chaturanga* to High Plank would be an example of a concentric contraction of the triceps because their job is elbow extension (Figure 3.21). Again, move more slowly, as then the muscles are under tension for a longer time and the workload will increase. A top tip—when focusing on increasing your strength—is to find the work in the transitions between postures.

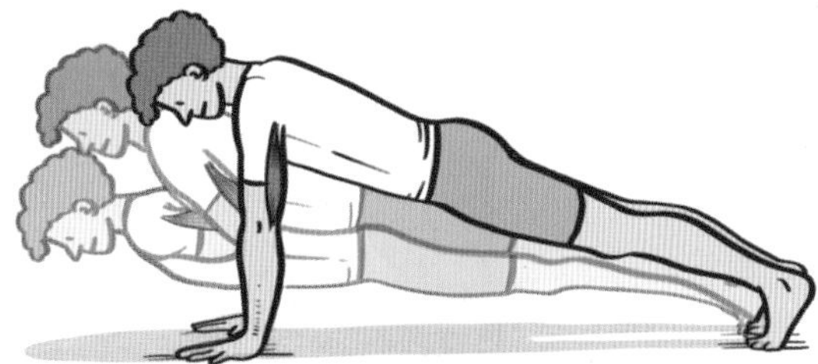

Figure 3.21 Going from the bottom to the top position involves a concentric contraction of the triceps.

What Happens When We Are Moving?

Sitting on a chair or stool with your knees bent 90 degrees and feet on the floor, cross your ankles right over left. The leg that is behind (left) is going to be doing the work, and the one in front (right), will be relaxed and just adding some weight.

Place your hand on your left thigh and keeping the upper leg where it is, slowly start to straighten the leg. Feel the quadriceps working beneath your hand.

Q. What muscles would be concentrically contracting to take us from a squat to standing?

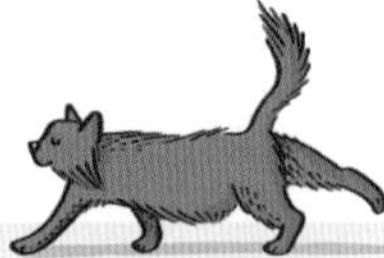

Is your leg still in the air? If not put it back up, hold it at the top for a bit (isometric contraction) feeling the weight of the right leg, which is crossed over the top. Again—with your hand on your left thigh—lower your foot to the floor as slowly as you can.

You should have felt your quadriceps working under your hand as you lowered the leg under control.

This time the quadriceps are lengthening but contracting to resist gravity taking your leg down too fast. This is an eccentric muscle contraction and is very important for you to understand. Without weights and gym machines, it is one of the major ways we can work on strength within the yoga practice. Factor three for working on strength is resisting gravity.

Eccentric contraction mode is often challenging for students to get to grips with because it is tempting to think of the opposite muscle doing the work. For example, in our little experiment, when we had the leg straight and lowered the foot to the floor, the knee is going from an extended position to one of flexion. What muscles control knee flexion? The answer is hamstrings and gastrocnemius. So how come they are not flexing the knee now? Well, because they don't need to as gravity will do the job for them. If we stood up instead, our orientation in gravity changes, and therefore the muscles that are working change. If we balanced on our right foot and took the left heel to the butt (Figure 3.22), the hamstrings and gastrocnemius would need to concentrically contract to flex the knee. Then, eccentrically contract to lower the foot back down again under control.

Q. What muscles control us down from High Plank to *Chaturanga*?

I hope you can see from the discussion so far that working on strength requires some thinking about, and I am just about to add a few more details to the mix.

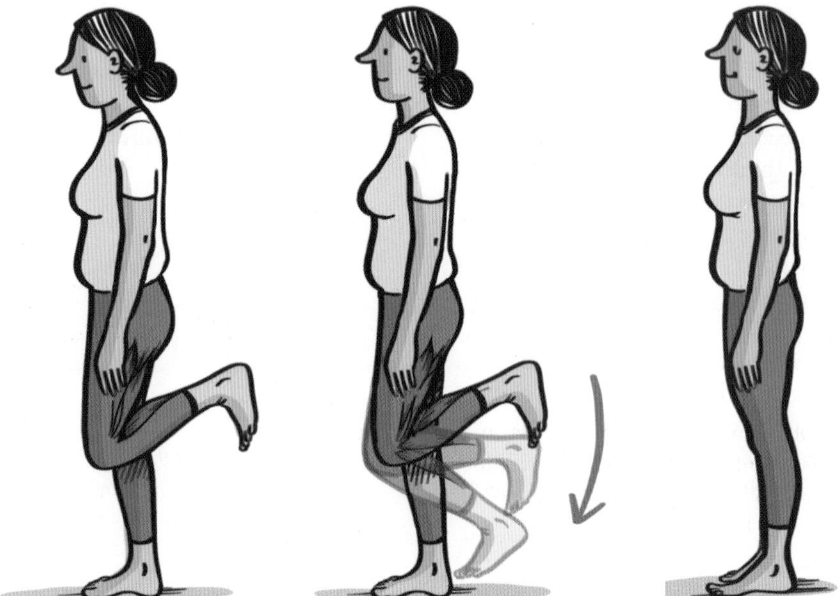

Figure 3.22 An eccentric muscle contraction involves lengthening at the same time as contracting.

Strength work is very similar to ROM in that it is joint- and direction-specific. Therefore, in the same way, we can't think we are strengthening everything around the shoulder just because we do a shoulder-related exercise, and, of course, this is true for every joint. Consequently, much as we said with ROM regarding working on all possible movements at that joint, the same goes for working with strength—different muscles do different actions. Work on strength in all the directions and hence all the muscles crossing that joint. Time for an example I feel.

Let's say you decide you need to strengthen your arms and shoulders and start ramping up the number of *Chaturanga* to High Planks (and reverse) that you do. As you now know from our discussion, you will be strengthening your triceps mostly, as well as the anterior head of the deltoid. This will probably help you with your arm balances because a similar bent-arm strength is required, but it won't help you hold your arms out for longer in *Virabhadrasana B* because there the arms are abducted, and the lateral head of the deltoid does that job. Neither will it help you get higher in *Purvottanasana* because although the triceps help keep the arms straight, the posterior head of the deltoid takes the shoulder into extension. Similar to *Vasishtasana*, which is more to do with the lateral head of the deltoid and shoulder girdle stability.

Strength gain is an adaptation to the stresses placed on the muscles, so continued progress requires increasing the challenge regularly. This is called "progressive overload" and is also related to time under tension. It's probably not practical to keep holding postures for longer and longer, although I have done this myself with a Handstand.

So, what can you do? One way is to compound poses that challenge the same or similar areas of the body. For example, increase over time the number of balance postures you sequence together before you change legs. The strength changes perceived in the first three months of a new program are more to do with increased motor control and nervous system responses than to actual physiological changes in muscle tissue. Therefore, expect to plateau and be prepared to put in the hard work after the honeymoon period.

Have you heard people say that in yoga, there are all pushing movements and no pulling? This is true, Down Dog, *Sirsasana*, Handstand, *Chaturanga*, even going from a squat to standing, all involve pushing away from the floor. Therefore, to create body balance, muscles such as latissimus dorsi and biceps that get minimal strength input, would need supplementation with exercises not found in yoga, such as paddling a surfboard, climbing, or pullups. I will be detailing some possible straightforward exercises later in the book.

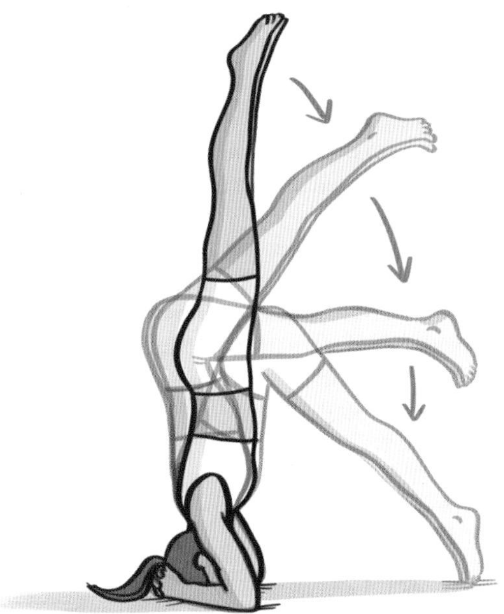

Figure 3.23 Lowering your legs from Sirsasana *to the floor.*

Q. What muscles are you using to lower your legs from *Sirsasana* to the floor (Figure 3.23)?

Successfully work on strength within the yoga practice by:

- Combining the factors of time, repetition, and resisting gravity.
- Reducing foundational elements.
- Doing more standing than seated postures and sequencing several challenging poses together.

- Finding the work in the postures, which might mean sinking lower, shifting your COG, lengthening levers, or reducing support.
- Transition slowly, taking the hardest route.
- Be active rather than passive.
- Know what you are working when you are doing a particular posture or transition, bringing your attention to that area.
- Shut off the music because it will distract your attention.
- We mentioned it on the first point but it is worth mentioning again—use slow eccentric muscle action to resist gravity.
- Memorize the mantra, "Time Under Tension."

Variety

"Adaptation occurs when the body is challenged in an optimal way, not too little and not too much."

The human body thrives on variety, and that is true for psychological stimuli as well as physical input. We are an adaptive organism that needs challenges to flourish, avoid stagnation, and minimize deterioration through repetition.

What happens when you try some new physical exercise? Muscle soreness! Even if you think you are super conditioned to do your regular exercise, when you do something new, magically it finds areas you never knew you had (Figure 3.24).

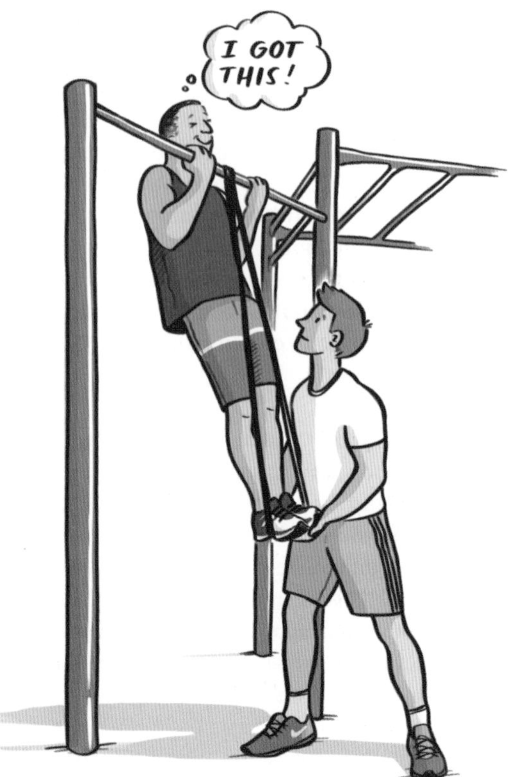

Figure 3.24 Stu tries his hand at calisthenics.

This phenomenon is called delayed onset muscle soreness (DOMS) and is particularly strong the day after the day after. Being a silly arse that just goes for things, after trying a calisthenics leg routine for the first time, I had DOMS so bad I couldn't do yoga for almost a week (Figure 3.25).

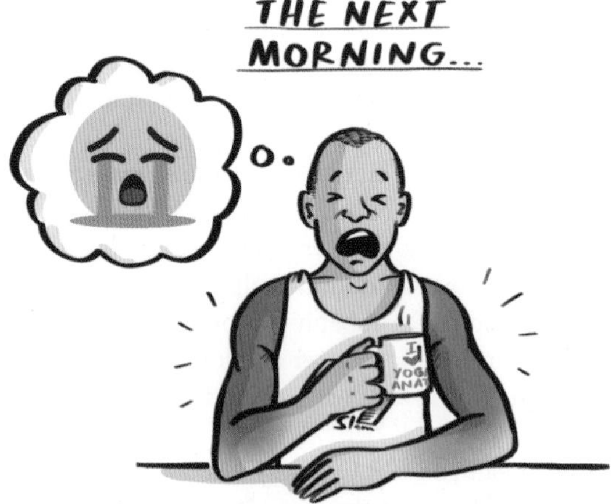

Figure 3.25 Certainly not for the first time, Stu is as sore as hell!

As far as I know, the current understanding of DOMS suggests that what we experience is sensitivity to microtrauma of the myofascia (muscle and fascia). We have used muscles we don't usually, or the same muscles but with more than usual intensity or load. I'm sure you have experienced that the exercise that resulted in the DOMS can be strength-based or flexibility oriented. As long as the challenge is not higher than optimal for positive adaptation, then changes will occur in the form of strength increases, endurance, muscle hypertrophy (size increase), or ROM.

Not everything will necessarily be a physical adaptation of tissue. There will also be a great deal of neural adaptation, more so with flexibility targeted exercise.

As I mentioned in *Strength*, the body responds and adapts only in the muscles and tissues that we use. Well, actually that's not quite true, it also reacts negatively to stuff we don't use by losing strength and ROM. What we use will be determined by the movements we do and the challenges we place on the body.

Ideally, we can analyze our yoga practice to determine which muscles we are using the most and, by swapping postures and changing transitions, work toward balance, whether that is strength or flexibility. However, the more variety we can add, the more likely we will challenge different areas by luck. So, if you have to, just try different postures, pay attention to where you feel the work, and rule them out if it feels like the same as you are already doing.

Plateauing is something students often experience at some stage during their yoga journey. It can be extremely frustrating if you are attached to your physical progress (Figure 3.26). It's not something that happens at the start because everything is so new the body is going, "Wow, what do I need to change." But it is pretty easy for the body to get used to what you are doing and settle into comfy mode, content that what you have will do just fine.

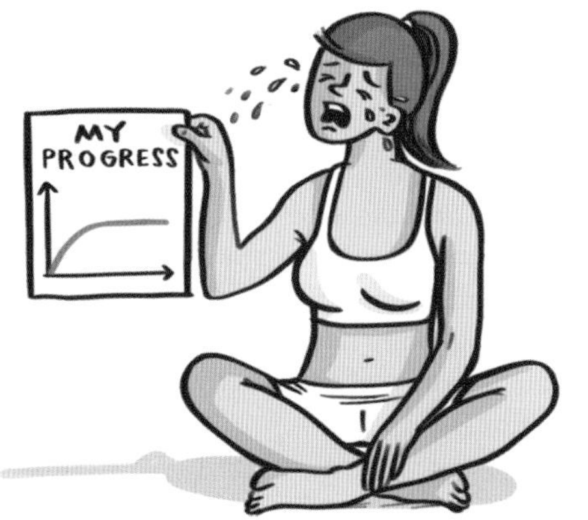

Figure 3.26 Progress can be compromised by plateauing.

As good as the body is at adapting, it is also very good at staying the same unless the challenges placed upon it change over time. If you want to become stronger, you will need to increase the load continually—which means choosing more difficult postures (requiring greater feats of strength)—and if you want to become more flexible, it is no use doing postures your existing ROM allows you to do comfortably. It's much easier for your body to control your movements within a safe range if you are less flexible, so you need to show your body why it should bother changing. You need to coax it into changing the setpoint by demonstrating that you won't hurt yourself at the new ROM, and that it will be useful to have. You may also be doing a posture and still have plenty of room for improvement as far as depth goes, but nothing is changing (Figure 3.27).

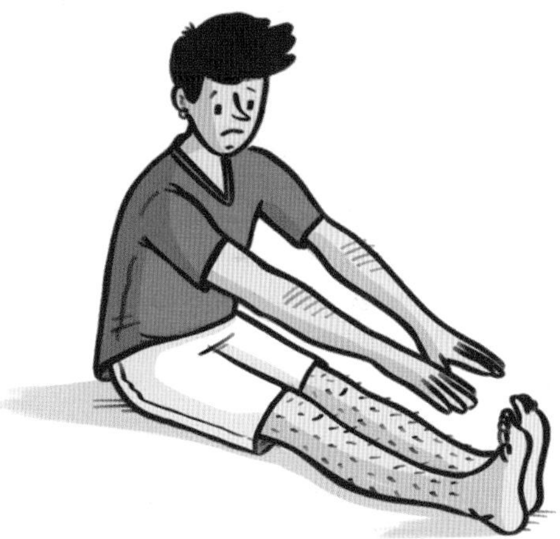

Figure 3.27 Sometimes nothing changes.

So, you have plateaued, but you don't need a harder challenge just a different one. If you keep doing the same posture, the impasse will likely remain. For a month or so, leave the one or more poses that are bothersome and replace them with others that target the same area but in a slightly different position. Often, that is all that is needed to break the deadlock. For instance, if you are having trouble with *Paschimottanasana*, leave it for a while and instead do *Parsvottanasana*, which is asymmetric and has a much more advantageous positioning for assistance by gravity (Figure 3.28).

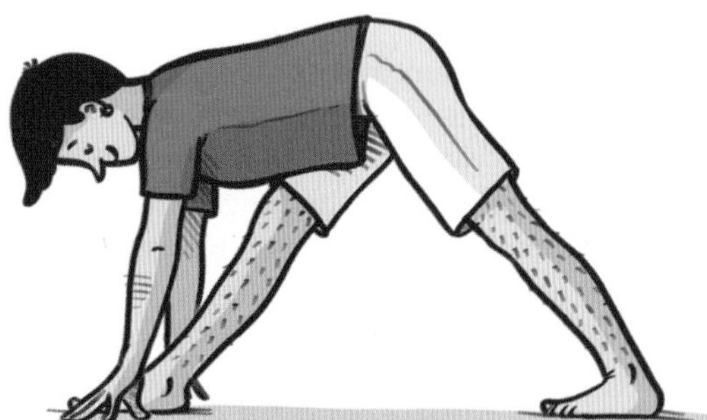

Figure 3.28 Regularly change the postures you do.

Another great reason for adding more variety is to help avoid overstressing a particular muscle, ligament, or joint. Repetitive actions can often result in tissue breakdown and injury, particularly if there is a technique issue. By changing what you do, you are moving the stresses around.

Although I am focusing on the physical in this book, we all know how much the mind feeds into our wellbeing and that feeds into the body. Repetition of the same thing all the time can be comforting because you are staying in your safe zone, but it can lead to a lack of development and increasing imbalance. We tend to like what we are good at and do what we like. This means that you are even more inclined to avoid things you need to be doing as they are probably also the postures you will find the hardest.

Compliance for doing things we should be doing is notoriously low; ask any physical therapist how many clients follow the exercises they are prescribed. Choose postures that interest you, work on something you have been meaning to, set yourself a goal, or draw on some recent inspiration. Then, of course, also slide in what you need to do.

Without diversity, you can also get very used to how your body experiences a particular posture and lose out on that sense of exploration. With variety comes a new stimulus, sometimes that is positive and occasionally negative, but either allows us to learn and develop a better understanding of our strengths, weaknesses, free, or restricted areas.

So how can we introduce more variety into the yoga practice other than trying out new postures? Even subtle changes can make a difference:

- Do the opposite side first.
- Change the order you do the postures.
- Adjust the time you hold positions.
- Add a variation to the same posture.
- If you are used to doing one posture at a time, explore what happens when you sequence some together and vice versa.
- Change your focus in the posture, for example, breath, engagement, awareness, preciseness, or more organic.

If you have trouble trying new postures, don't introduce too many at once and choose ones that are realistic for your current level of strength and flexibility, so you don't get discouraged.

All the above suggestions are easily incorporated into a free form style, but what if you have a set sequence yoga practice, such as Ashtanga? Well, adjusting your focus can add some mental stimuli, but I think it is vitally important to add physical variety too. I'm an Ashtanga practitioner myself and vividly remember that you can get very good and stable in postures you do a lot, such as *UHP* (Figure 3.29), but try something new like *Parivrtta Ardha Chandrasana*, and you can be all over the place (Figure 3.30). The postures may contain similar elements, but the muscles are not used to coordinating in the new position. It is much better to challenge yourself in numerous angles and orientations.

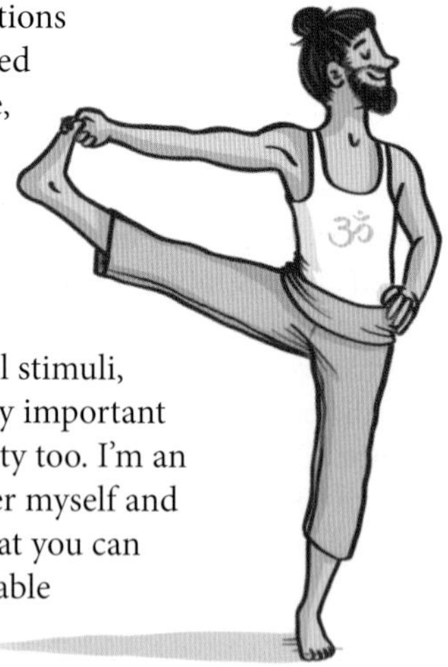

Figure 3.29 Ashtangi Zane is super stable in UHP.

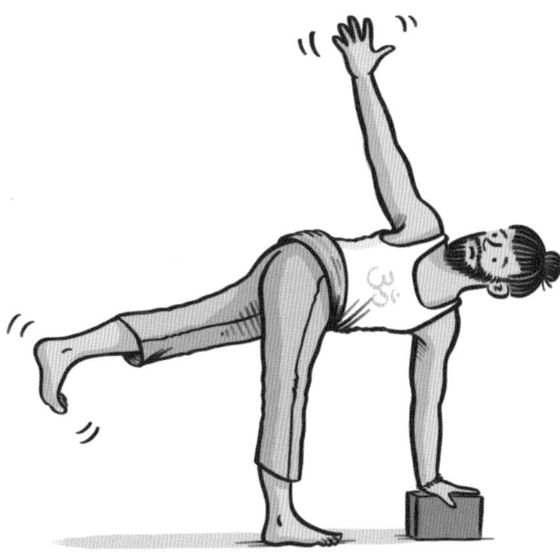

Figure 3.30 Still a single-leg balance, but oh, so different!

Many students will reach a sticking point when their teacher will stop them from advancing through their present set sequence. Although this may be beneficial in the short term, if the student needs time to gain the necessary attributes for the subsequent postures—if it continues too long—it will be to the detriment of the body. This doesn't mean that I think students should do poses they are not ready for, but that other postures should be introduced to supplement their existing yoga practice. This is particularly important regarding physical balance because set sequences will be weighted toward certain areas or movements.

If the student's situation doesn't allow for variety to be added into the sequence, then I would advise that it needs to be addressed at another time during the day or using a different form of exercise.

Take a little time now to consider your yoga practice and decide on something different to do next time you are on the mat.

Opposing Muscles Restrict

There are a few movable joints in the body where there are no muscles whose job it is to move them, but for the most part, we can say that there are muscles to take a joint through all the directions of movement available at that joint. Sometimes a muscle is so big or spreads out such that the directionality of fibers can allow parts of it to do different, even opposite, jobs. However, for the time being, it is more straightforward for us to consider muscles working in pairs or groups. For example, the quadriceps extend the knee and the hamstrings flex the knee (Figure 3.31).

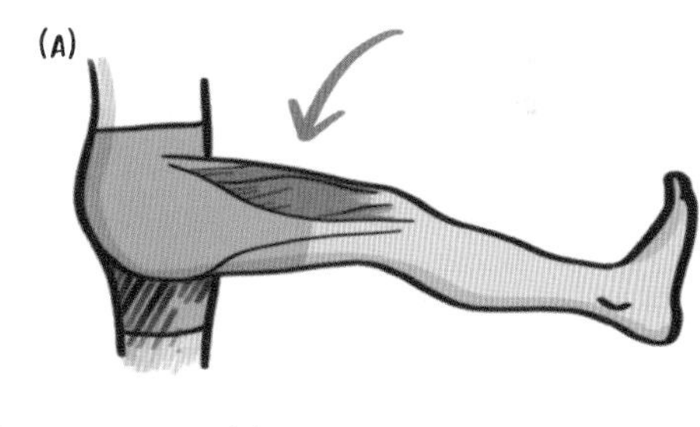

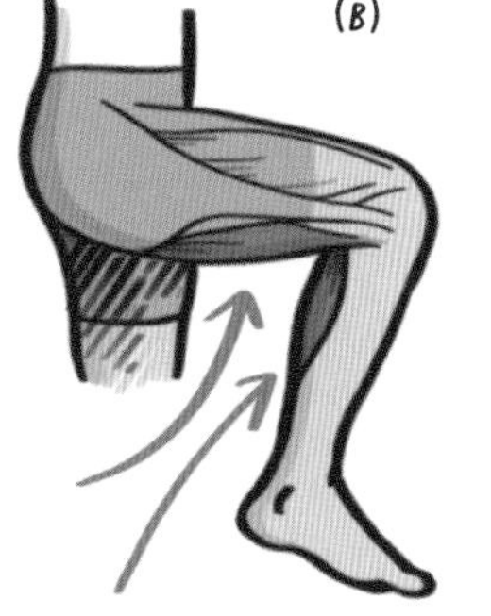

Figure 3.31 The quadriceps and hamstrings form an antagonistic pair, where (A) the quadriceps extend the knee, and (B) the hamstrings flex the knee.

We have a term for these muscles' relationships: "antagonistic pairs." The muscle that is the mover in the direction you want to go, also called the prime mover, is the agonist, and the muscle that creates movement in the opposite direction is the antagonist. If the direction of movement reverses and the previous antagonist muscle is creating the movement, not gravity, then it becomes the agonist and the other muscle the antagonist (Figure 3.32).

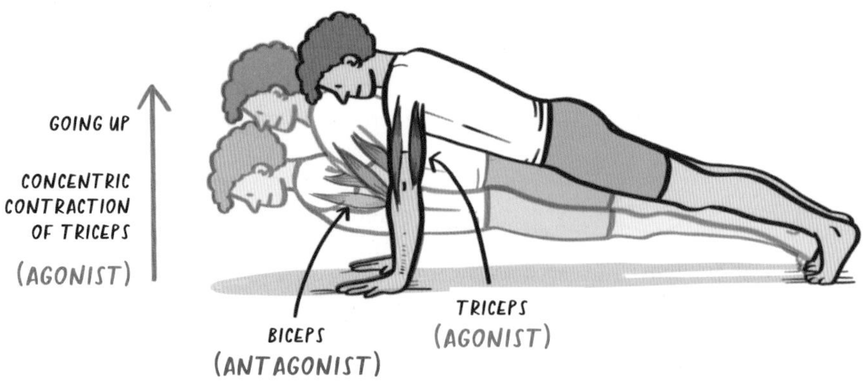

Figure 3.32 The triceps are the agonist on the way up as expected because when they concentrically contract, they perform elbow extension.

You will remember from the section on *Strength* that when resisting gravity, there is an eccentric contraction of the muscle that performs the opposite action. Because this muscle is controlling the movement, it is still considered the agonist.

Previously, we used the example of a High Plank to *Chaturanga* and back up, to consider eccentric muscle contraction. The triceps would be the agonist in both the up and down phases of the exercise (Figure 3.33).

Sometimes, when trying to stiffen a joint, we contract both agonist and antagonist, often referred to as co-contraction.

In a yoga setting, we are often in a position where the movement has stopped and we are resting passively in place due to muscular tension.

Imagine you are in *Supta Padangushtasana B.* On taking the leg out to the side (abduction), you slowed the motion nicely, resisting gravity by using an eccentric contraction of your adductors. In this scenario, the adductors are acting as agonists. Now the leg has stopped moving down but hasn't reached the floor—you have probably stopped contracting the adductors and are relaxing them. Because the leg is a long lever, you will undoubtedly feel the tension in the adductors resisting you from going further. Theoretically,

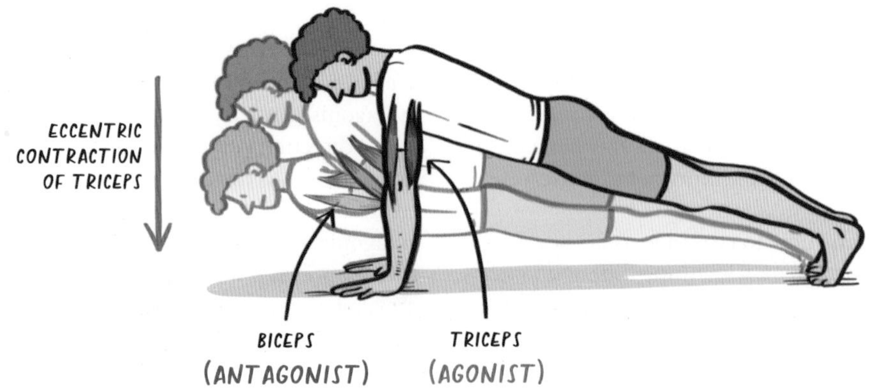

Figure 3.33 The triceps are the agonist on the way down, not the biceps, because they are controlling the descent.

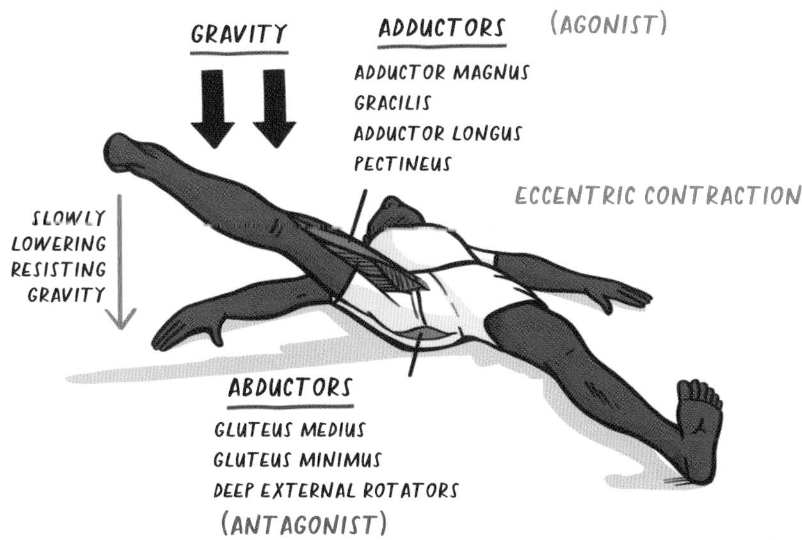

Figure 3.34 Tension in the adductors is likely to be responsible for not moving deeper into abduction.

they are not the antagonist but are responsible for the cessation of further abduction. In this type of situation, it's easiest just to think, "I want to abduct the hip; tension is stopping me." Therefore, it will likely be the muscles that do the opposite action—the adductors (Figure 3.34). This example is an easy one because you will feel it there, but that is not always the case.

If you still want to make sense of the agonist/antagonist concept in this situation, I perceive it in the following way:

Once you have traveled through the gravity-assisted ROM, you will reach a point where the gravitational force is not enough to overcome muscle tension. To go further in the desired direction, you would now have to be active and contract the muscles that would take you in that direction. So, in our previous example, you would need to contract your abductors to move your leg lower. The abductors are now the agonist and the adductors the antagonist (Figure 3.35). Ha! We are back on track.

Incidentally, muscles that help the agonist in the desired motion are called "synergists." They may also control unwanted movements or stabilize an area to allow an action to happen.

As there will often be more than one muscle that does the same job, it is likely to be more

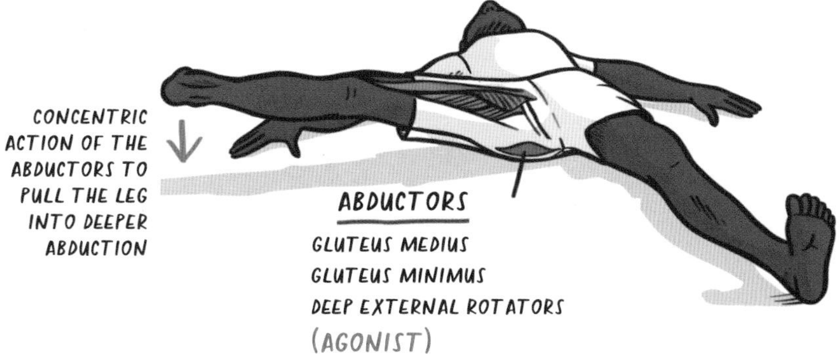

Figure 3.35 If you contract the abductors to actively move into deeper abduction, they now become the agonist.

complicated than just a nice pair of opposites. In the knee flexion example, the gastrocnemius also flexes the knee. Nonetheless, this concept is a useful starting point when exploring restrictions.

In case you got thrown by me adding in a bit of complication, let's finish with something straightforward by returning to the knee flexion example we started with earlier. Think of when someone is lying face down (prone) and wants to bring their heel to their butt, but it doesn't go (Figure 3.36). The knee must flex for this to happen, therefore, the very first thing to think about once you have established there is no pain in the knee is that tension in the quadriceps could well be resisting the action from happening.

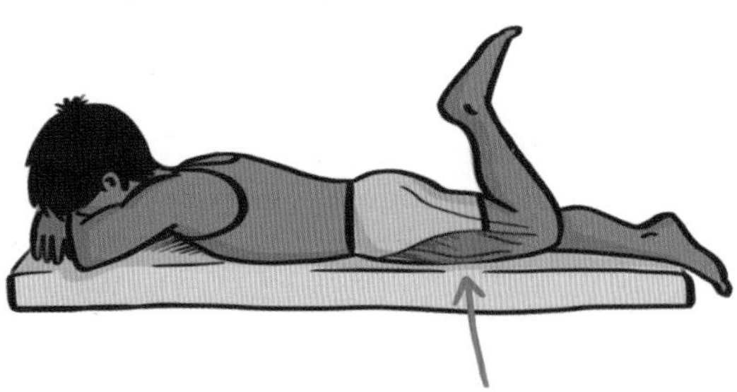

Figure 3.36 Test the most obvious explanation first and explore from there.

Don't get confused by all the terminology. When working out which tensional forces might be stopping you moving through a particular ROM, the critical thing to remember is that the first things to consider are the muscles that would take you in the opposite direction.

In reality, more muscles than just the opposing muscle influence our ability to go in a particular direction. Sometimes other muscles at the same joint that perform different actions can be placed under tension as their attachment points also move further apart.

We might also like to consider tensional chains of muscles or fascial connections. Also, we don't just move in straight lines, one direction at a time; more often than not, we combine joint movements to create our yoga postures. For now, don't worry if you're still grappling to get a handle on this concept, we will call on it a lot when looking at the different areas of the body.

Secondary Action of Muscles

"The knee is particularly susceptible to levering actions, so extra care needs to be taken when performing postures like Padmasana."

I think this concept is fundamental because it helps us understand many of the unchosen alignments in the body when performing yoga. For instance, the elbows going out when doing *Urdhva Dhanurasana* and *Pincha Mayurasana*, or the back leg rolling out in *Hanumanasana*.

You probably already know by now that muscles move, stabilize, and protect joints, and that the movement can be in more than one direction. For example, the psoas muscle does both hip flexion and external rotation. This is possible because of where the muscle attaches on the femur: the lesser trochanter. It is not the landmark itself that determines this but its location, which is posteromedial, meaning around the back but not entirely because it is also some way around on the inner surface (Figure 3.37). The key is the directionality of pull. Let's use a real-world example.

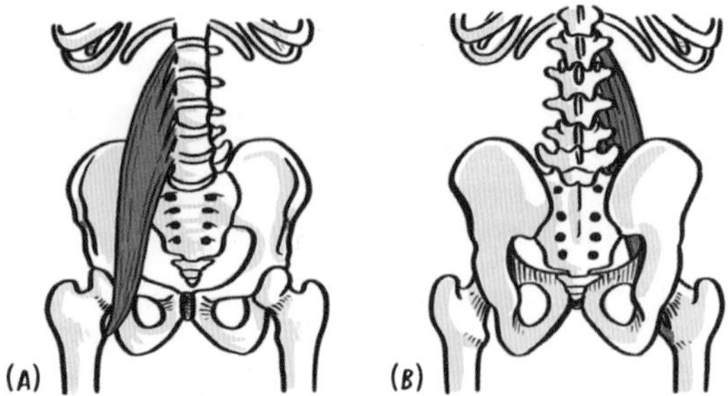

Figure 3.37 Attachments of psoas, (A) anterior view, (B) posterior view.

Imagine yourself languishing on the couch, reading this wonderful yoga anatomy book (Figure 3.38). In one of those eureka moments, you realize that if you could put your feet up on the coffee table, the nuggets of information presented within would be assimilated much easier. Without disturbing your comfy spot, you can only reach one leg of it, so you pull on that to bring it closer. As you pull the coffee table toward you, it doesn't travel squarely, but the corner you are pulling on comes first. You are causing it to rotate. Frustrated with its non-compliance and the fact you pulled it far too close, you ask your beloved to relocate the table, so it's just right. Obligingly, the table is squared up, but in the process of it being pulled further away, your slipper catches on that same corner, and the table rotates again.

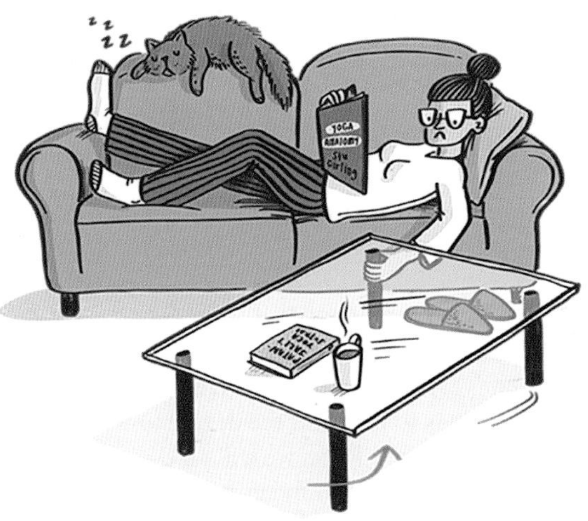

Figure 3.38 Pulling on something unevenly will cause it to rotate.

So hopefully, from this little story, you have gathered that where a muscle attaches will make a difference to the movements that might occur intentionally or otherwise. We introduced the psoas earlier so let's stick with that muscle as a working example of this concept.

The psoas muscle attaches to all the vertebrae of the lumbar spine and then crosses the front of the pelvis attaching to the lesser trochanter of the femur. When it contracts, it will flex the hip, or if the femur's relationship to the pelvis is stabilized, it can help flex the spine. Because of the positioning of the attachment on the femur (posteromedial), when the muscle contracts and shortens, an element of external rotation of the hip will be introduced. This will most often be counteracted by other muscles (e.g., tensor fasciae latae (TFL)) performing the opposing movement of medial rotation to keep the leg neutral (Figure 3.39). Think of when you do *Navasana*. The flexed hip position is initiated and maintained mostly by the psoas (and iliacus). You will notice there is a tendency for the legs to roll out if you don't actively maintain their neutral position.

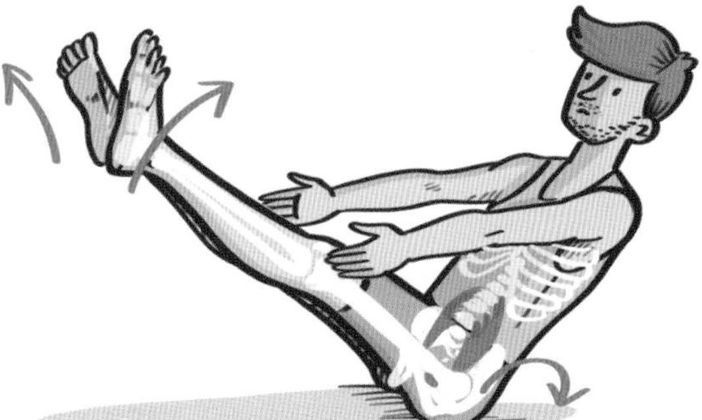

Figure 3.39 To counter the secondary action of the psoas, Ben needs to use the TFL to medially rotate the hip.

Now think of doing *Hanumanasana*—what tends to happen to the back leg if you are not consciously controlling it, is that the leg rolls out (external rotation of the hip) (Figure 3.40). When stretching a muscle, something similar can happen to a muscle contraction even though it seems the opposite. As you move the two attachment points away from each other and reach the point of resistance, you are, in effect, pulling on the attachment points. If those points are not directly in line with each other, then another movement can be introduced, often rotation.

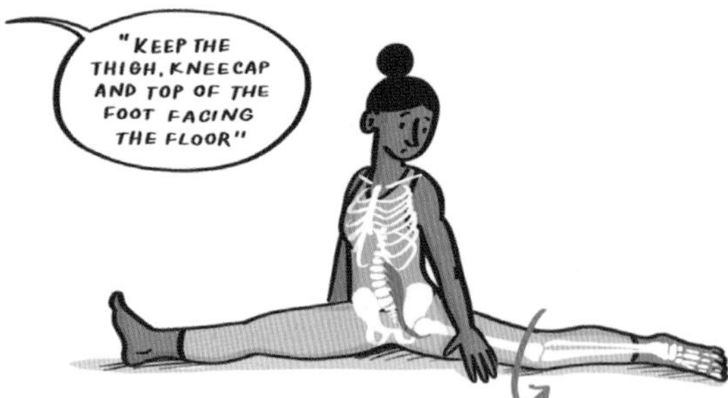

Figure 3.40 Myra has reached the floor, but the back leg has rolled out.

This is what is happening in our example of *Hanumanasana*. The back leg needs to move further behind the pelvis (hip extension), and because the psoas is a hip flexor, it is put under a stretch in this position. As you try and go deeper, the pull on the lower attachment (lesser trochanter of the femur) will cause the leg to roll out if it is not controlled. In understanding this, you can then see how it links in with the cueing of keeping the thigh, kneecap, and top of the foot facing the floor; you don't escape out of the stretch.

On the flip side, you may see students intentionally turn their feet out when preparing to do a drop back (Figure 3.41). If they know it or not, they are trying to avoid the resistance to hip extension. Whether or not this is a good idea, we will discuss when we talk later about backbends.

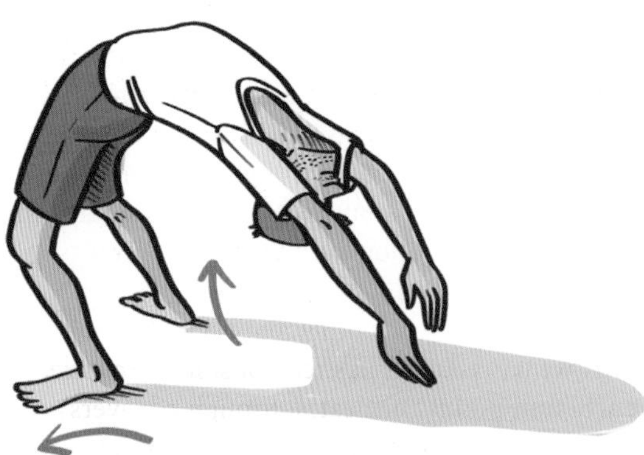

Figure 3.41 Turning the feet out to drop back can place stress on the lumbar spine and SIJ.

Q. Right at the start, we also mentioned the potential for elbows moving out in postures with the arms overhead, and that two common postures where you might see this are *Urdhva Dhanurasana* and *Pincha Mayurasana* (Figure 3.42). This is due to a medial rotation of the shoulder joint. There are two large muscles potentially responsible for this happening, latissimus dorsi and pectoralis major, and two smaller muscles, subscapularis and teres major. Look up now where they attach and see if you can apply the same concept to explain this.

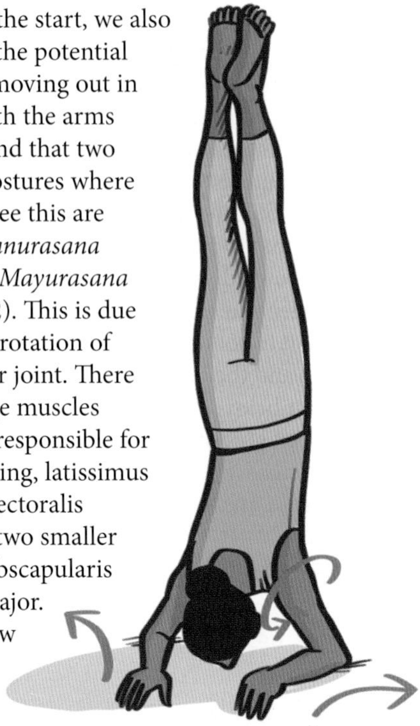

Figure 3.42 Myra's elbows have spun out.

Fascial Considerations

In recent years, interest has surged regarding the role fascia has to play and the degree to which it deserves attention. Here, we will take a foray into the topic and focus mainly on how the emerging knowledge might influence the way we do things in yoga.

I wanted to introduce this topic before we look at the different areas of the body and the muscles that create movements at the joints because we can then take with us a better appreciation for the interconnectedness of body parts and the complexity of movement analysis. As we explore the topic of fascia, you will appreciate that attempting to make sense of joint restrictions and movement patterns by looking at specific areas is problematic. Even though we will take this type of segmented approach in Part II, it can never fully explain what is happening as it fails to take into account the far-reaching interactions through fascial connection. However, muscles do move joints and can also restrict movement, so we can gain a lot of insight by understanding the body in this way. Acknowledgment of the role that fascia has to play allows us to blend ideas of local and global body integration.

I must admit, I am a long way myself from fully understanding everything about fascia and the connected topic of biotensegrity. Still, I will do my best to relay some of the current thoughts and information. A number of leading authors on this subject will be listed at the end of the section, and it is well worth going directly to the source if you desire a more in-depth appreciation of fascia.

What is Fascia?

The body is made of four primary tissue types: epithelial (skin and internal surface linings), muscular (skeletal, smooth, and cardiac), nervous (nerves and associated structures), and connective (supporting, separating, and protecting materials).

Connective tissue is the most prolific type in the body, and fascia is part of this family. Not all connective tissue is fascia, and what exactly constitutes fascia is hotly debated. Blood is a handy example of a kind of connective tissue that isn't considered fascia. Bone, on the other hand, is up for debate with some saying it is starched fascia. The general tenet for connective tissue to be considered fascia is that it must form part of a continuous body-wide tensional structure. Ligaments, tendons, bones, adipose tissue, joint capsules, periosteum, and other enveloping membranes are all considered fascia along with superficial and deep fasciae (Figure 3.43).

Fascia takes many forms, sometimes light and delicate, and in other places, more like a tough band. It can achieve this fantastic diversity by combining the protein building blocks of collagen, elastin, and reticulin in different proportions and

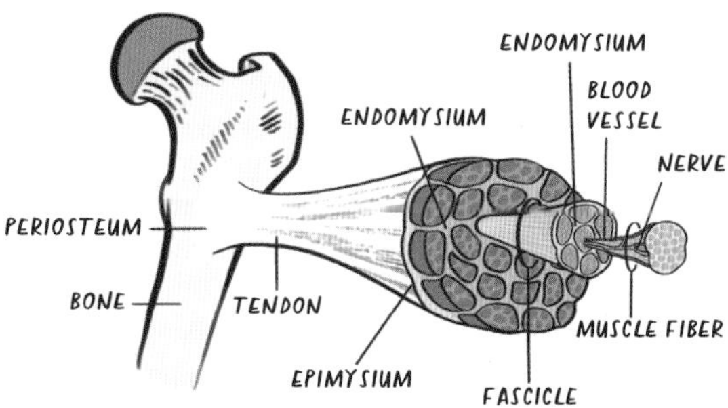

Figure 3.43 Fascia is found at all depths of a muscle and is continuous.

densities, depending on the required function. Fascia plays various roles, such as separating, supporting (as with the thoracolumbar fascia), or providing a particular functional purpose, as with the plantar fascia or iliotibial band (ITB). The fascia of the body can be thought of as a three-dimensional bodysuit because more superficial layers and structures connect to those that are deeper. Somehow it manages to achieve the dichotomy of separating and connecting at the same time. It has been suggested that if we were able to dissolve everything else and leave the fascia, we would still have a clear representation of our body in fine detail.

We can divide fascia into two categories—superficial and deep. The former is just under the basal layer of the skin, and the latter permeates the deeper layers of the body encasing organs, vessels, and bones, surrounding and dividing muscle bellies, forming tendons, ligaments, and much more. The fascia creates three-dimensional connectivity, forming a body-wide tensional matrix. Since it's filled with nerves, some consider the fascia to be a sensory organ. By providing proprioceptive information, the fascia plays a vital role in body awareness.

When we consider fascia's relationship to muscle, we will find that it permeates through all layers of the muscle tissue, separating layers and bellies at different depths, connecting, giving form and shape, as well as merging to create the tendons. It is so incorporated into the muscle tissue that it makes sense to think in terms of myofascial units ("myo" coming from the muscle component), rather than distinct muscle tissue and fascial elements. But of course, the interconnection doesn't stop there. The fascia traveling through the muscle becomes tendon and then continues to merge with the periosteum (the lining around the bone), which is also fascia, and potentially with the fascial components of some adjacent muscles. The idea is that fascia is often continuous but changes its density and properties due to the functional requirements and location.

An example of how this fascial integration might influence adjacent structures can be found when we look at the positional relationship of the diaphragm and psoas (Figure 3.44). The finger-like tendinous projections of the diaphragm called the "diaphragmatic crura," reach down the spine to the first few lumbar vertebrae. The proximal attachments of the psoas reach up the lumbar spine as far as the T12 vertebra. It is easy to perceive that there could be some fascial continuity between them. Building on that perspective comes the possibility of two-way tensional influence. We might hypothesize that tension in the psoas could influence our breathing pattern and, conversely, an aberrant breathing pattern might create tension in the psoas.

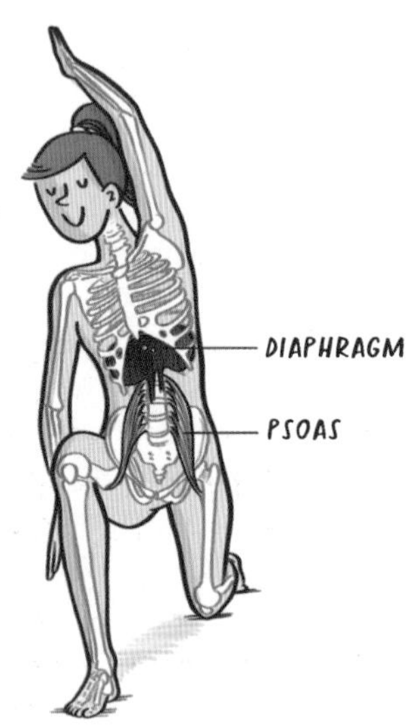

Figure 3.44 There is a potential fascial relationship between the diaphragm and psoas.

Tom Myers provided some groundbreaking revelations when he showed that it was possible to dissect lines of interconnected myofascial units (he coined the term "Anatomy Trains"), sometimes running the whole length of the body. There are some rules that Myers has used to decide if a line of pull can be demonstrated, such as there should be no abrupt changes in direction and there should be no jumping from one depth to another. Of course, although the term "line" is used, these proposed linkages have varying thicknesses and widths. Although this seems to fit nicely with what we may experience when taking our body into a stretch and feeling a connection between one area and another—either energetic or physical—not everyone agrees these lines exist.

We often feel this interconnectedness in yoga poses and may even refer to the experience as "lines of energy." I am not necessarily referring to meridians or other defined energetic routes, but rather the forces experienced between two or more body components changing their spatial relationship to one another. This sensation is most apparent when moving areas in opposite directions toward the movement's end of range. We may even refer to this connectedness by saying, for example, front body, back body, or side body stretch.

If we were to take *Parsvakonasana* as an example, we might like to think of this energy going from the grounded back foot to the reaching hand (Figure 3.45). We might experience interruptions or blockages in the quality of its travel along that route. We could also consider things from a more physical perspective and think in terms of a lateral line of interconnected myofascial units, with those energetic blockages represented by areas of increased resistance or restriction. Are we talking about the same thing just using different language, or are they distinct from one another? Whatever you decide, the experience of yoga is always reminding us of this connection between parts, and maybe this is one of the reasons moving in these whole-body ways feels so good.

The example I used above was linear, but the key principle of fascial connectivity is of a three-dimensional tensional matrix. When we see a skeleton in a book or placed in the corner of a classroom, it is easy to get the idea that these bones are inside us and all the flesh must be held up by that internal structure. This traditional way of viewing the body presents it as a continuous compression structure, one bit stacked on top of another much like you would build a house, with

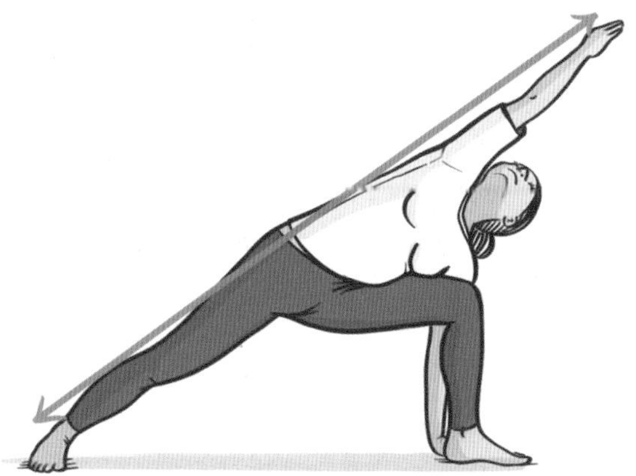

Figure 3.45 What do you think you are feeling with this kind of body positioning?

the segments being moved by muscles using pulleys and levers. To truly incorporate the role fascia has to play as a tensional whole-body network might require a shift from the existing paradigm.

Proponents of the biotensegrity model argue that the current view does not satisfactorily explain the way the body can generate and withstand forces. In a tensegrity structure, there are compression members that are spaced from each other by tensional components. It is possible to build structures that are load spreading and self-supporting, such as the structure depicted, where the compression elements don't actually touch each other (Figure 3.46). If we think back to our flesh-covered skeleton using this model, the suggestion would be that the bones maintain their position not because they are sitting on one another but instead due to the tension in the fascial network. The outer flesh is supporting the inner skeletal framework.

This concept of a self-supporting structure fits nicely with the human body, unlike the house mentioned, we don't have to be in vertical alignment to feel integrated, we can be in any orientation. The other facet of tensegrity structures is that they distribute energy from the local to the global. We find this in our bodies too, one area compensating for another, the strain sometimes spread to distant parts. Even thinking of the positioning of bones, we can observe tensional interplay as a factor in changes to alignment and orientation.

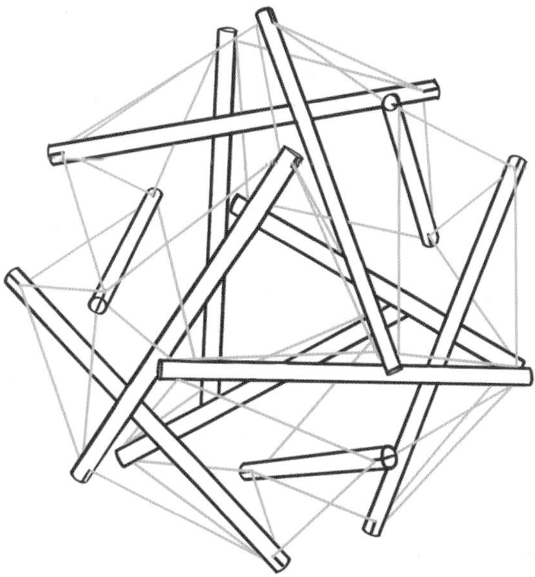

Figure 3.46 A tensegrity model. None of the compression elements are touching.

The biotensegrity model, at this stage, is still in its infancy and can, as yet, not explain everything, but it seems much more promising than the existing biomechanical model. It is likely that the emerging paradigm will lead to an appreciation of a heterarchical system of tensegrities within tensegrities. Encompassing everything from the cellular level to fascial matrix, combining to tension our body in terms of holding parts relative to one another but also allowing elements such as bones to float and muscles to glide within this tensional system. Looking at the way the bones differ in density and size, as more of our body mass is above them, I imagine there will also have to be some appreciation of compression structures involved too. We could explore these topics for days, but to be honest, I am still grappling with my understanding, so instead, I will leave you to read further on this subject if you care.

If the fascia is the tensional component that helps maintain the correct positioning and orientation of the compression members (bones), then having an idea of what keeps fascia healthy should help us practice in a way that makes sense for the body.

Fascial layers can change their properties depending on the forces placed on them. If stresses are experienced locally through repeated patterns of movement, then the fascia may become denser along those lines of pull. This might, in some instances, be beneficial if, for example, we need more structural support. However, if instead, it is due to undesirable postural positioning, then that same reinforcement might be constrictive. Adding variety into our movements and actions is likely to help spread forces around and promote a more balanced system.

When we are younger, the appearance of the collagen fibers seems to be more wavey, something called "crimp." As we age, this crimp reduces and with it the elastic qualities. This elasticity is extremely valuable in energy conservation and fluid movement. We can solely use muscular effort to perform many actions, but if we can add some rebound or spring, then the outcome is often smoother and more dynamic. A lot of the time in postural yoga, we are moving slowly with the breath and then maintaining stillness, so it is not always easy to see how the elastic component can be encouraged within this modality.

I think one of the times it is easiest to see it at work is in the more dynamic transitions, for example, a hop up to Handstand. If you are too grounded and try to jump up just by pushing into the floor, the result can seem very heavy and labored. On the other hand, if you pre-tension the body and then dip down and pop up using more of elastic recoil, the ascent can be much lighter and even floaty, as well as using considerably less muscular effort.

Flexibility and elasticity don't always go together. In many sports, being too flexible may reduce performance as a mechanism of energy conservation is to use the elastic recoil from the resistance of muscular tension to feed into the next movement. I think that when there is more resistance in the system, there will be greater elasticity. At one end of the scale, we can have a tensional system that is too loose, and at the other, one that is too high. In yoga terms, our minimal tension example could be "bendy Wendy" students who can flip and flop between postures but feeling integrated and finding stiffness in poses like the Handstand is hard for them. The other extreme is our strong but inflexible student that struggles to move fluidly but has no problem supporting themselves. We should endeavor to move toward a middle ground of ease of movement but with power and stability when required.

Ballistic stretching movements are recommended in lots of literature on fascia, with the intention of promoting that elastic quality. There are a number of reasons that I am not in favor of this in general and specifically in a yoga setting. The body positioning in the majority of ballistic stretches I have seen incorporates too many joints and, drawing from our idea of multi-segmental movements, often the target joint stops moving and another less resistant in the chain moves instead. An example would be the standing forward fold, bouncing toward the floor with the hands. There are all sorts of specific instructions I have seen, but what I observe is always the same—the hips stop moving, and the low back takes up the slack.

Many ballistic stretches also make use of gravity to generate momentum, which reduces the need for muscular engagement, as well as making the end point less controllable. If a dynamic stretch was going to be used, I would much prefer to see one where the force was generated through active muscle contraction, such as in the standing leg swing. The benefit of this particular example over the previous one is that the low back is also taken out of the equation. Having said that, my view of postural yoga involves slow movements, stillness, and introspection. I know this is not always the case, but within the framework I just mentioned, repetitive bouncing and swinging movements are inappropriate.

So how can we manipulate our tensional system? I think we have to find that balance between strength and flexibility. Working on strength will add to the tone of muscles, and stabilizing actions while doing so will add to integration. Working on flexibility will reduce tension and make fluid movement more accessible. It's not quite that straightforward because, if you remember, it is possible to be flexible but have to apply a lot of force to go through the full range available. Here, it's essential to grasp that strength and flexibility are not on opposite ends of a linear scale; they are different qualities. An individual can be strong and flexible (think gymnast) or weak and flexible, as well as strong and inflexible or weak and inflexible. Of course, they could also be all the in-between stuff, moderately this and that. It's desirable then to tailor your yoga practice to focus on what you need most.

You have already covered *Variety* earlier in this chapter, and this is relevant to fascia too. We are working with a three-dimensional body-wide tensional matrix, so repeating the same lines and combinations over and over again is unlikely to provide fluid movement in all directions and combinations. By exploring the body with movement combinations you are not used to, it will be more likely that areas of dominance, weakness, instability, or inflexibility are revealed. Even in static postures themselves, slight changes in focus and positioning will vary the influence. As muscles and many supporting structures are arranged in spiral formation rather than linear, playing with unconventional shapes might also be rewarding.

One further point on this is that postures incorporating whole-body positioning rather than targeted at specific areas are thought to address the fascial system more efficiently by highlighting the interconnectivity.

The less we move, the more fascia seems to lose the elastic quality that is often associated with youth. Flowing, effortless movement with smooth changes in speed and tempo is aptly displayed in contemporary dance. The great sense of ease and agility that combines both subtlety and power in multiple planes shows the potential of a body in tensional harmony. We can embody some of those same qualities within yoga even though we may be moving more slowly. Effortlessness comes with the synchronization of breath and precision of thought, combined with proprioceptive awareness of where every part of us is positioned in space, which promotes fluidity at any speed.

Fascia exists in a fluid environment, so it is proposed that inadequate hydration has an impact on its glide, responsiveness, strength, and adhesions (bits that stick together). Yes, we need to make sure we are drinking enough, but moving and using the body will also help get the water where it needs to be. So, hopefully, you're doing your yoga, not just reading about it.

Another characteristic of fascia that is worth noting is that the rate of lasting structural change (remodeling) is extremely slow, taking many months or years. So if we are experiencing changes to our posture, grace, flexibility, integration, or physicality in shorter timespans (minutes, hours, weeks), it will almost certainly be to do with the nervous system and the more readily responsive muscular system. I don't know if you are like me, but the way I experience my physical body differs drastically between days. There is a baseline of ability expectation, but sometimes after the first moves I make, I know, "Today, I am going to fly." I am full of energy, springy, light, and more flexible. Then, of course, there is the pendulum swing the other way, of days that are heavy and tight and, by comparison, inflexible. This can't be fascial changes because it happens too quickly, so after everything I have presented here for you, I invite you to question how restrictive fascia might be.

Fascia is integrated into every part of us, so when we are using our body, conscious of whether fascia exists or not, we are also using and moving it. As we mentioned earlier, fascia invests through all layers of muscle tissue and is tendon, ligament, and bone, so whether we stretch, contract our muscles, stay in stillness, or continuously flow, we have the potential for eliciting adaptation of the myofascia. The key question to leave you with is: can we really target one element more than another in the way we practice yoga?

I hope I have managed to relay some of the interesting thoughts on fascia. Below are some suggestions for further reading if this topic interests you.

Recommended Reading

Avison, A. (2021). *Yoga, Fascia, Anatomy and Movement, Second Edition*. Handspring Publishing, Edinburgh.

Myers, T. (2020). *Anatomy Trains: Myofascial Meridians for Manual Therapists and Movement Professionals, Fourth Edition*. Elsevier, London.

Scarr, G. (2018). *Biotensegrity: The Structural Basis of Life*. Handspring Publishing, Edinburgh.

Schleip, R. (2021). *Fascial Fitness: Practical Exercises to Stay Flexible, Active and Pain Free in Just 20 Minutes a Week*. Lotus Publishing, Chichester.

Schultz, L. & Feitis, R. (1996). *The Endless Web: Fascial Anatomy and Physical Reality*. North Atlantic Books, Berkeley.

"Yoga postures are created in all sorts of orientations, so when thinking of joint movements and actions, consider relationships and gravity rather than ups, downs, or sideways."

CHAPTER 4

Breath

Breath

I'll take it that you know we need to breathe and that the inhale brings in oxygen, and the exhale gets rid of waste carbon dioxide (CO_2). The breath is a central pillar of yogic endeavors and is used in many ways. In the asana practice (postural yoga), we can use it to calm the mind, bring lightness, indicate effort, relax the body, and provide focus. We can synchronize breath and movement to give rhythm, attention, power, or subtly. We can choose to alter the emphasis of the way we breathe to create space, provide stability, give energy, or promote stillness. We can decide to control it or just let it be. In this book, we will confine ourselves to considering the relationship between breath and postures. When making our yoga shapes, your breath will influence your position and will also be influenced by it. But before getting to that, we need to know what we're working with.

Often, when I am teaching and have asked students to demonstrate the size of the lungs, they will make a shape that resembles the size of a grapefruit, but wow, the lungs are so much bigger. Apart from the heart and some tubes (trachea, esophagus, aorta, vena cava, and a few smaller ones), the lungs fill the whole space encompassed by the ribcage (thoracic cavity). There is no free space, they extend sideways to the inside of the ribcage, upward to just below the clavicle (collar bone), and downward to a thin dome-shaped sheet of muscle called the diaphragm (Figure 4.1).

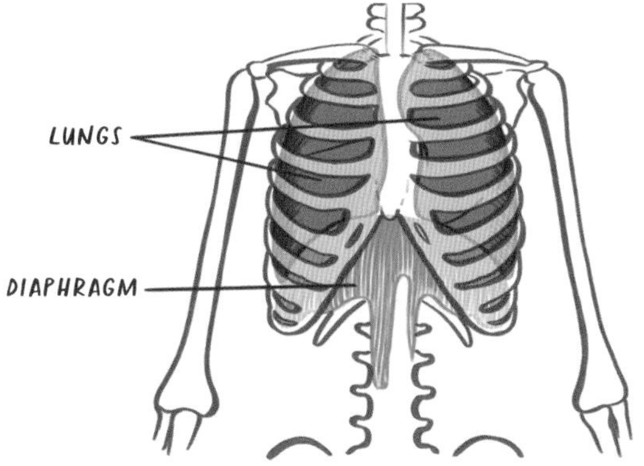

Figure 4.1 Lungs and diaphragm.

The diaphragm is the primary muscle of respiration (breathing) and separates the thoracic and abdominal cavities. It attaches to the bottom of the ribcage and has fingers called "crura" that reach down to the first few lumbar vertebrae. When it is relaxed, it is domed-shaped but flattens as it contracts. It has a central tendon so if, when it contracts, the ribcage is fixed, it will flatten by moving down. On the other hand, if the central tendon is held in position, it will flatten by pulling up on the ribcage. Don't worry if you can't visualize this at the moment. We will be explaining more in a moment. In case you are interested, the phrenic nerve innervates the diaphragm. Rhythmic impulses from the respiratory center in the brain maintain our breathing rate, but as you know, this can be overridden when we choose to hold our breath, breathe slower, or breathe faster.

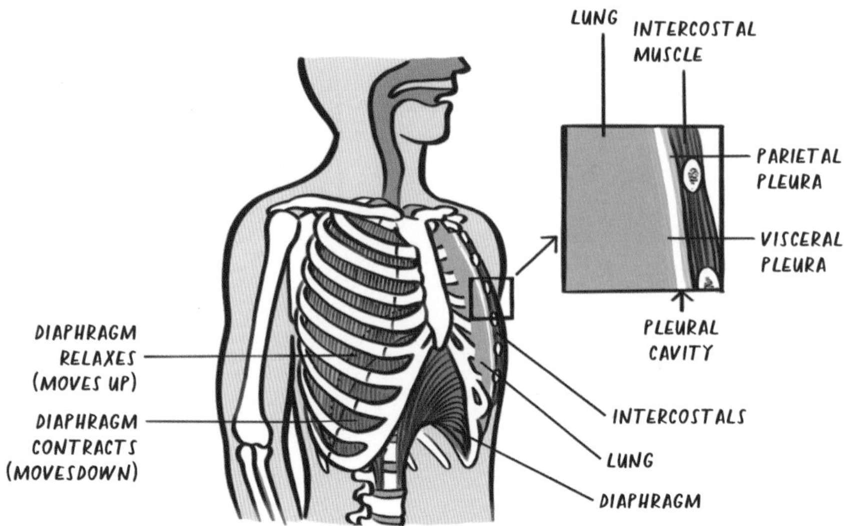

Figure 4.2 The double-layered pleural membrane sticks the lungs to the inside of the ribcage.

Importantly, between the lungs and the inside of the ribcage is a double-layered membrane (Figure 4.2) called the "pleural membrane." This membrane has a thin film of secreted fluid between the two layers that essentially sticks the lungs to the inside of the ribcage and superior surface of the diaphragm. The lungs themselves are not muscular, but they are elastic. These facts will become crucial in understanding the mechanism of breathing.

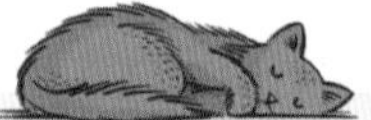

Take as deep a breath as you can now for me and see the ribcage expanding impressively. It seems like the ribcage is being pushed out as the lungs expand, but that is not what happens. I'm super sorry, but to appreciate what is happening, I have to introduce Boyle's Law.

Boyle's Law

Boyle's Law states that there is an inverse relationship between pressure and volume, and here lies the key to how it all works (Figure 4.3). As the volume of a container reduces, the pressure increases, and as the volume of a container increases, the pressure decreases. The ribcage is our three-dimensional container with the diaphragm forming the bottom. If we can change the shape of this container, we can change the volume and, consequently, the pressure. Remember the lungs are going to move with the container because they are elastic and stuck to the inside. So, the pressure inside the lungs can be altered by changing what we do with the ribcage and diaphragm.

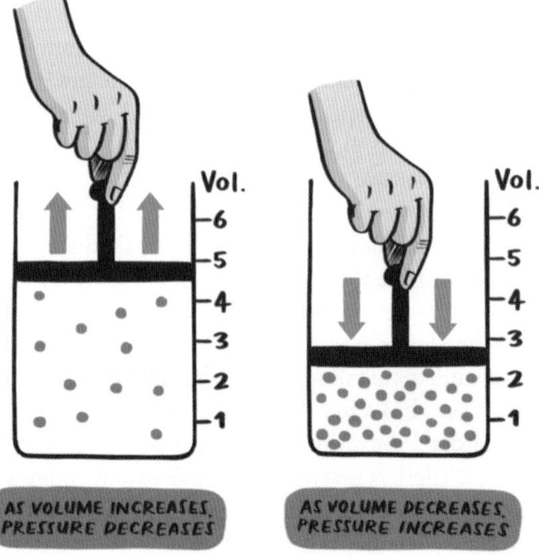

Figure 4.3 Boyle's Law.

So, what goes in and out of the lungs when we breathe is air, which is a gas, and one of the characteristics of gas is that it will move from an area of high pressure to an area of low pressure. Do you see how this is coming together?

Inhaling, we increase the volume in the lungs by expanding the ribcage or moving the diaphragm down. The pressure inside them will drop, causing the air to travel from outside the body to inside. Then for the exhale, we increase the pressure in the lungs by allowing the ribcage to move back and the diaphragm to relax and move up. The inhale is always going to be active, but the exhale can be passive or active if we are trying to get extra air out. So, breathing happens by changing the shape of our three-dimensional container. Take a few more deep breaths and see if you can now perceive the muscles working on expanding your ribcage. If the shape of our body needs to change to accommodate breathing, it will be affected by how we are positioned and vice versa.

The movement of the diaphragm and ribcage can be combined in different ways to create what we refer to as types of breathing. We will consider abdominal, diaphragmatic, and thoracic breathing next. Just be aware that there are other breathing patterns, such as paradoxical, as well as different ways to classify breathing.

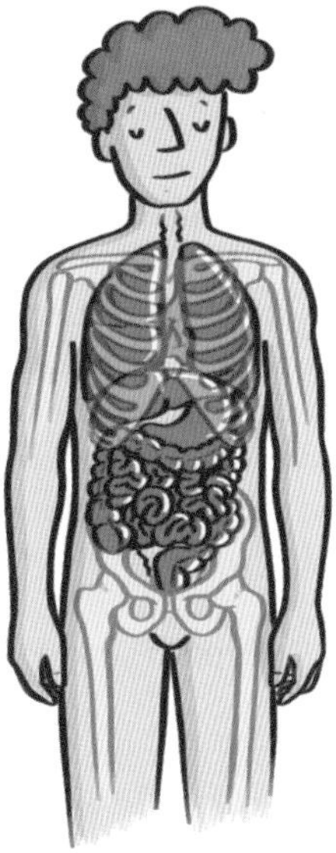

Figure 4.4 The abdomen is crammed with viscera.

When we do abdominal breathing, you see the belly moving in and out. We know it's not air down there because the lungs are up in the chest and the abdomen is crammed full of viscera (internal organs) (Figure 4.4).

So, what's causing the rise and fall? The muscles between the ribs are called the internal and external intercostals, and in this type of breathing, they are kept under mild isometric contraction, holding the ribcage somewhat rigid. When the diaphragm contracts for the in-breath, it flattens and pushes the abdominal viscera out of the way (Figure 4.5). It can't move further down because of the pelvic floor, or back because of the spine, so instead, it moves outward. The belly expands and you see or feel it rising. On the exhale the diaphragm relaxes, going back to its domed shape and allowing gravity and soft tissue tension across the front of the belly to encourage the viscera back to its starting position. You see or feel the stomach falling.

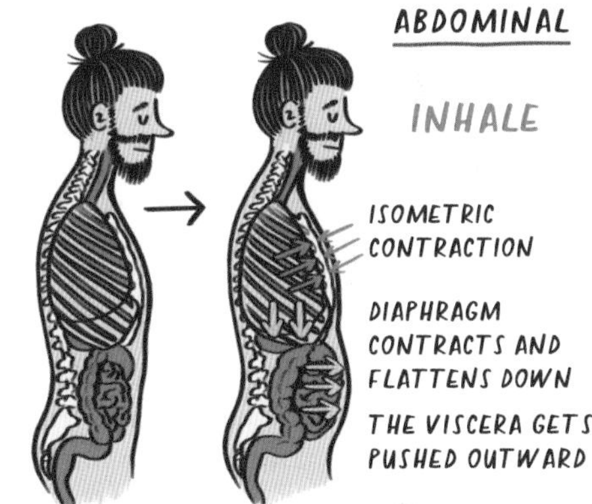

Figure 4.5 The belly gets pushed outward on an inhale.

Abdominal breathing uses the least amount of energy because it is only the diaphragm doing most of the work (Figure 4.5). It is ideal then for postures such as *Shavasana*, where we are trying to let go of effort and promote active relaxation. Also, in this lying position, the abdomen is more relaxed and gravitational force assists the exhale. Some students have trouble letting go of the abdomen sufficiently to allow this type of breathing to happen. If this is the case, it can be worthwhile placing a block on the belly and asking them to raise and lower the block with the inhale and exhale, respectively.

With diaphragmatic breathing, the lower abdomen is kept in a mild contraction (Figure 4.6). This means that when the diaphragm contracts, the viscera can't move out of the way to let the

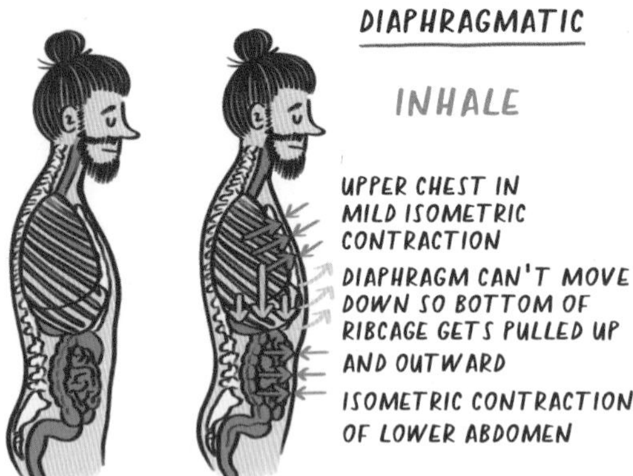

Figure 4.6 The bottom of the ribcage flares outward.

diaphragm flatten downward. So instead, the central tendon of the diaphragm is fixed in place. Its contraction pulls the bottom of the ribcage up. Sometimes this is referred to as a "bucket handle" movement. Imagine a bucket handle laying on the side of the bucket and the arc it creates as it moves up and away a short distance.

If we start with the same lower belly contraction and diaphragm action as diaphragmatic breathing but add to it the contraction of some accessory muscles to draw the upper ribcage out and up, then we have the actions of thoracic breathing (Figure 4.7).

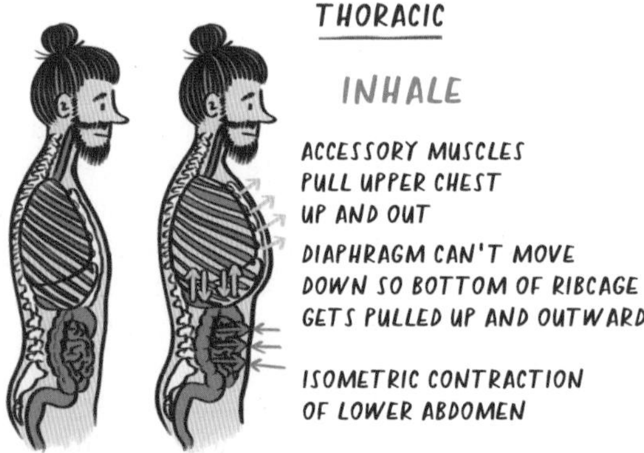

Figure 4.7 The upper ribcage expands and draws upward.

In everyday life, we don't think of imposing a particular type of breath (Figure 4.8). We will naturally do the appropriate one. That is unless we have adopted an aberrant pattern for some reason,

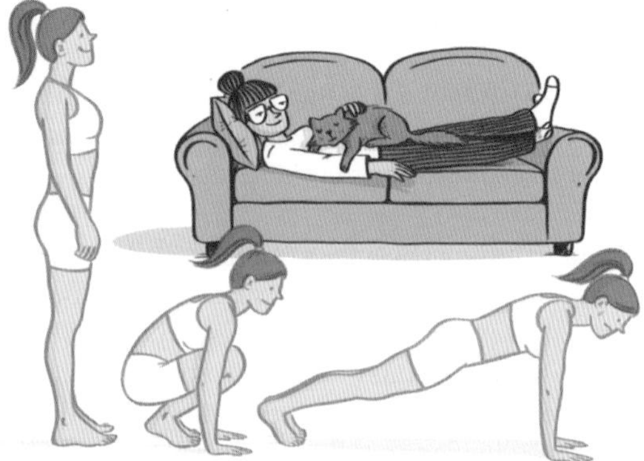

Figure 4.8 Breathing in everyday activities.

like anxiety or insecurity. Furthermore, I would say that we often use combinations of the patterns detailed. For instance, the belly going out as in abdominal but also combined with the lower ribs flaring as in diaphragmatic. We also swap between them continually as we move around, only settling into a particular pattern if we are stationary or in a repetitive situation. The reason for this is that as we move, we will place tension in some of the areas that need to adjust.

If you think about when we bend forward to pick something up, the belly will be squashed, and abdominal breathing is a non-starter. We will have to move the ribcage. If we are reaching overhead, the ribcage will be lifting and there will be tension across the abdomen, encouraging diaphragmatic or thoracic breathing.

Breath and Posture

We can take the breathing ideas outlined so far and start to try and understand their implications in postural yoga. Firstly, we can go back and think of why we breathe. That is to get in oxygen for energy production and get rid of the waste product. So, our breathing volume should be representative of the energy requirement of the activity being undertaken. You will notice that you change the rate and depth of your breathing as you go from sitting quietly to walking around, and so on. Because we can create the greatest expansion with thoracic breathing, it is often associated with the higher oxygen requirements of high energy pursuits.

If you feel like testing this out, do 10 burpees and observe your breath. If you feel so inclined, get somebody else to do it and watch them instead. Actually, yogis are not necessarily very "cardiovascularly" fit because of the lack of prolonged heart-raised activity, so probably five burpees will be plenty. Most of the time, what we do in yoga doesn't call for this sort of volume of air. Occasionally, we will puff a bit after a particularly hard posture but, it is a good idea to use your breath as a barometer of effort and keep it under control if your objective is to calm the nervous system (Figure 4.9). From that point of view, thoracic breathing is unnecessary for yoga unless you are performing a particular *pranayama* technique that uses it.

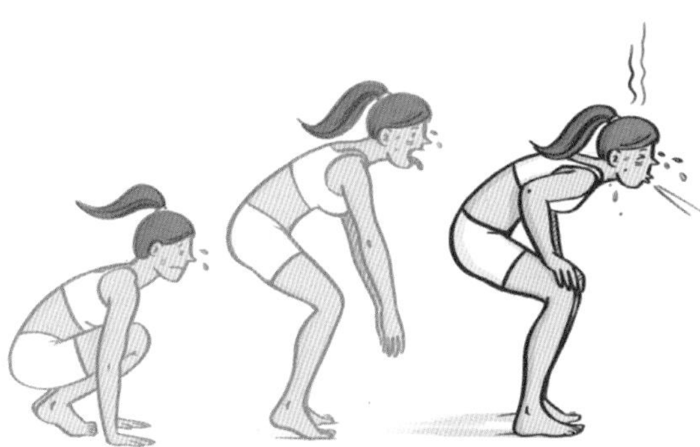

Figure 4.9 "Puffing" after a particularly hard posture!

As you will see from the following section, sometimes we will have to use the lifting of the upper ribcage, which is associated with thoracic breathing, due to our positioning. However, we would not be incorporating this with the same volume of air generally related to this type of breathing.

When thinking about how much air to take in, we might start to get confused with also wanting to slow the breath down. It doesn't follow that just because we breathe in for 10 seconds, we will intake a higher volume of air than in four seconds. It is possible to fill your lungs in a couple of seconds or take much, much longer. Try it for yourself now (see panel above).

> Sit up straight, exhale fully, and then make an inhale through your nose. Draw in a superfine stream of air as slowly as possible. Don't hold it at all but keep it going as long as possible. I tried it myself as I wrote this and quite comfortably managed to drag the inhale out to 60 seconds. With control, you can refine how much air you take in using any of the previously outlined methods.
>
> From a postural yoga point of view, it is not about how much air you need but what is the best way to get it in.

I mentioned at the start of this chapter that, "When making our yoga shapes, your breath will influence your position and will also be influenced by it." This is because, as you now know, our abdomen or thoracic cage must change shape so that we can breathe. Sometimes the breath will dictate what is going to move, and other times the shape will dictate where you are going to breathe from. What we'll do next is to consider this idea within the context of different movement groups.

The ribcage, diaphragm, and abdominal area all share a connection to the spine. We can start very generally by thinking about a gross movement tendency as it relates to breath. The spine tends to extend on an inhale and flex slightly on an exhale. Therefore, it usually seems more intuitive to fold in on yourself on an exhale and expand and reach on an inhale. For example, in Cat-Cow, it feels good to exhale into Cat and inhale into Cow. If you are doing some sort of vinyasa, then it flows with the body's natural movement more comfortably if you inhale into a backbend and exhale when folding forward, twist on an exhale, and lift tall on the inhale.

Sticking with the spine for the moment, we can consider some postures that incorporate spinal extension. In a backbend from standing, your front body is controlling your descent. As the spine extends, the tension will build across the abdomen. The inhale adds to the intra-abdominal pressure and stiffens the lumbar area, restricting the freeness of backbending. On the exhale, the pressure will decrease, and

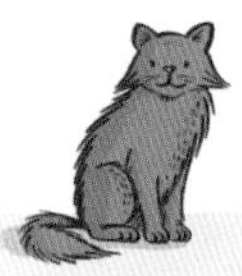

We can easily experiment with how posture influences the quality of breath in a simple seated position. Sit on the floor cross-legged and slump forward, not worrying too much about sitting tall. Now try and take slow even breaths. Compare this with sitting upright while also maintaining your lumbar curve (Figure 4.10).

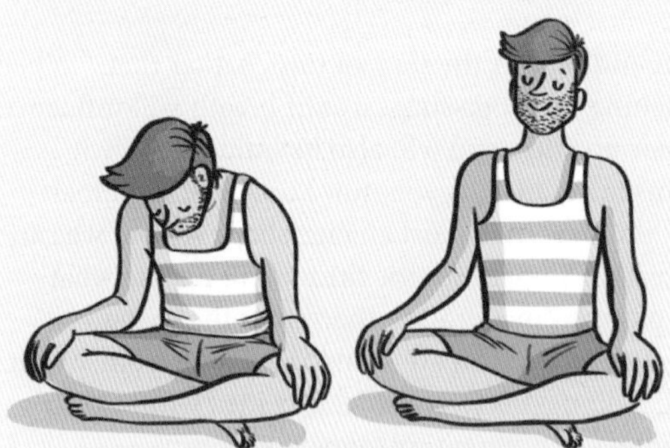

Figure 4.10 If you don't sit tall when doing breathwork, the quality will be severely compromised.

Often students find it hard to find an even inhale and exhale when sitting for meditation or *pranayama*. Most of this can be attributed to the way their spine is positioned. If you are restricted in the hips in such a way that the knees don't rest on the floor, then the pelvis will move into a posterior tilt. The natural lumbar curve will be lost, and the body will round forward.

movement into greater extension will be easier. Of course, you may decide that it is sensible to maintain more intra-abdominal pressure to help protect the lumbar area (Figure 4.11). Particularly as this type of gravity-assisted backbend with the body acting as a long lever can place considerable forces into the lumbar area.

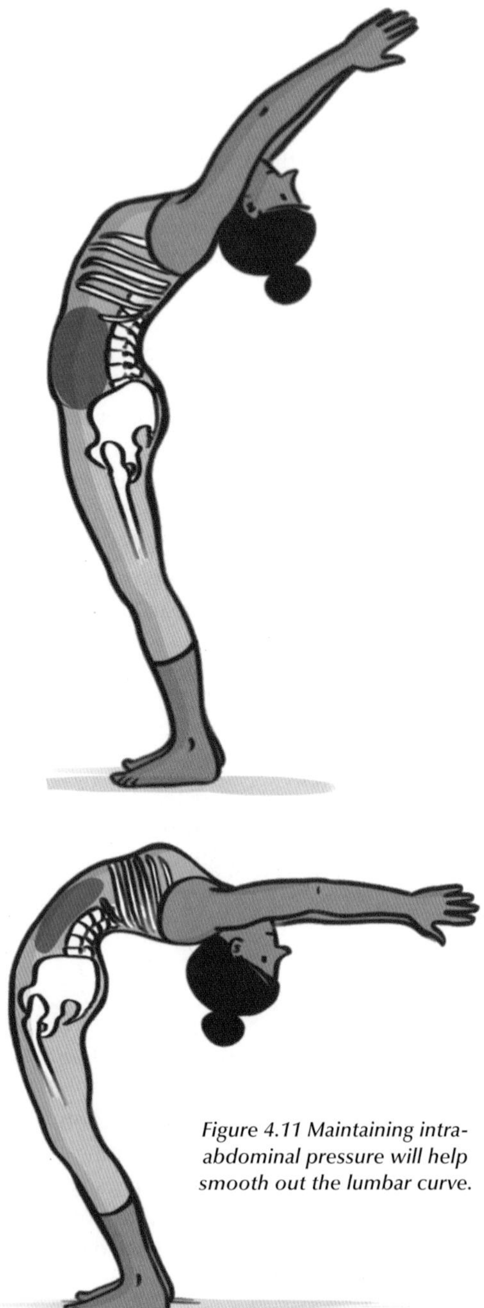

Figure 4.11 Maintaining intra-abdominal pressure will help smooth out the lumbar curve.

The previous example had the spine moving into extension with the hip also extended. This will tend to anchor the bottom of the pelvis and create more tension across the abdomen, making it hard for the abdomen to expand outward on an inhale. On the other hand, in a flexed hip position, gravity and a more relaxed abdomen will mean an inhale can assist the backbend rather than restrict it. However, a soft belly means it's easier to move excessively in one area (hinge), so I would say it is better to keep some tension there and be aware of where you are moving from.

By contrast, in a deep forward fold, we can find the belly squished and unable to move out, so it will be the ribcage that moves more readily. You may sense this rise and fall if your ribcage is resting on your legs, such as a deep *Paschimottanasana*. If you are holding yourself firmly in place on your legs, the ribcage may have to move more upward or sideways (Figure 4.12A).

Sometimes, we are engaging the abdominal muscles to stabilize our position, and this would also fix the belly and encourage the necessary movement to happen in the ribcage. Staying with the idea of forward folding, students who find this group of postures challenging may engage their abdominals to either stop themselves falling backward (if their pelvis is posteriorly tilted) or to help with moving forward. A posture like *Navasana* that uses the stability of the abdominal area to maintain the "V" shape would be another example (Figure 4.12B).

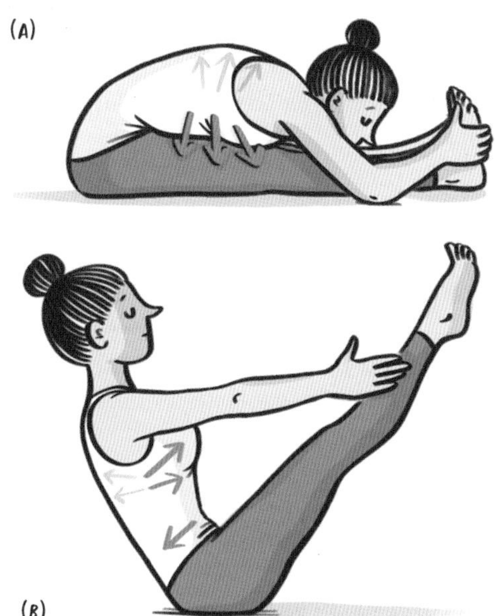

Figure 4.12 (A) When the abdomen is firmed in a pose it means the ribcage must expand, (B) Navasana *uses the stability of the abdominal area to maintain the "V" shape.*

Likewise, twisting is a group of postures that tightens the abdominal area, making diaphragmatic or thoracic breathing the more natural options. That is unless it is an intense twist, in which case it will tie down the bottom of the ribcage, and the breath will need to move higher if it can. We can take this idea one step further with a posture such as *Marichyasana D*. Along with the intense twist, there is a leg in *Ardha Padmasana*. So, we are adding a heel in the belly and a position where the ribcage is squeezed against the other leg (Figure 4.13). This helps to explain why so many beginners find it hard to access a full breath in this posture. Often the suggestion is to seek space in the back of the body and to sit up tall. The ribs are attached to the spine at the back of the body, so there is not much movement available there either.

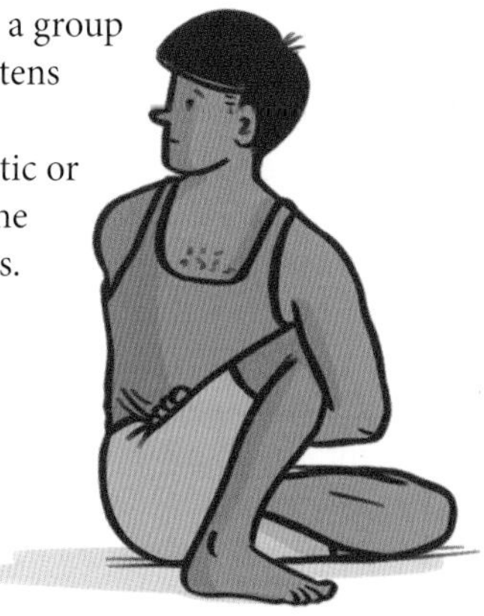

Figure 4.13 Heel in the belly, and ribs on the leg can make it hard to find space to breathe.

Inversions are an interesting group of postures for several reasons. Can you remember which way the diaphragm moves when it is contracting without obstruction? Hopefully, you recalled that it is domed when relaxed and flattens downward if contracting. When standing or seated, gravity is assisting the movement of the contracting diaphragm and encouraging the downward movement of the internal organs. This translates to an outward movement because they can't move down. Turned upside down, gravity has the opposite effect. The contracting diaphragm now has to push up against the weight of the liver, stomach, guts, and other abdominal viscera (Figure 4.14). We can consider inversions to be toning for the diaphragm, like any other muscle that finds itself having to work harder, as much of the success in finding stillness in inversions relies on the stabilization of the shoulder girdle, ribcage, and thoraco-pelvic interface (the abdomen). This tends to limit the ability for the ribcage to expand, and if combined with a stiffening of the abdomen, generally results in a shallower breath.

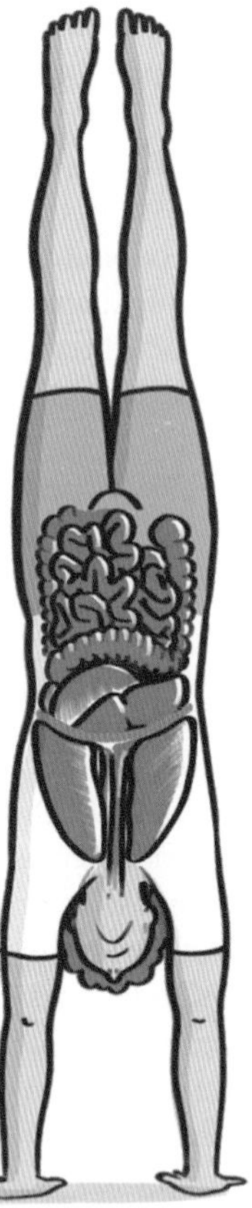

So, we can have influences by the posture and our body parts on the ability for our thorax and abdomen to undergo three-dimensional shape change, but also by the surfaces we interact with. When in yoga postures, we often find ourselves in a position where these areas will not be able to move freely because of our relationship to the floor. For example, when we are in a posture that has us in a prone (face down) position, our belly will be stopped from moving out by the floor. If we are lying there and still encouraging an abdominal breath, we will probably see the low back and hips rising slightly on the inhale and descending on the exhale.

Figure 4.14 Inversions mean that the contracting diaphragm must push up against the viscera.

In postures like *Dhanurasana* or *Salabhasana*, we are adding tension to the abdominal wall (Figure 4.15). This, combined with the resistance of the floor, will lead to the restriction of abdominal breathing and promotion of diaphragmatic. The body is likely to rock or move as the ribcage expands and contracts.

Many yoga styles adopt a diaphragmatic breath with varying degrees of lower abdominal contraction, depending on how they view *uddiyana bandha*. I feel this is sensible if the yoga practice is more dynamic, with a lot of standing and balancing poses, because we want some stability

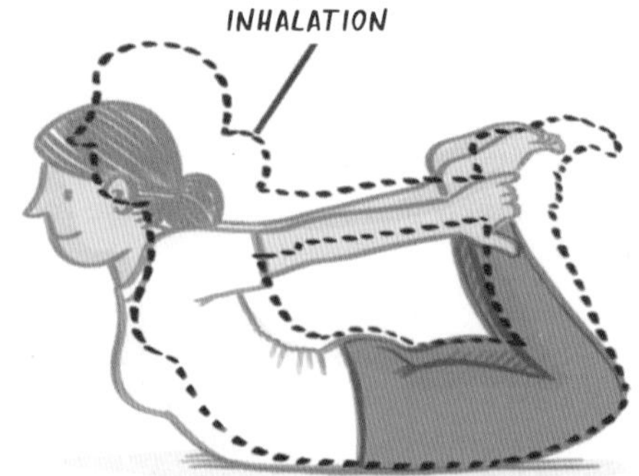

Figure 4.15 Adding tension to the abdominal wall in Dhanurasana.

in the abdomen in many positions. As mentioned, intra-abdominal pressure also helps to protect the lumbar spine, especially in backbends.

Shavasana is the ideal posture to feel supported by the ground and release any control over the breath (Figure 4.16). Abdominal breathing will be the natural breath to assume because the belly can fully relax. If you notice that the belly is not rising and falling with the breath, then you are not letting go of that area. This is fairly common for gym addicts doing plenty of abdominal work, as well as those used to maintaining a drawn-in belly as part of their postural habit. It is important to be able to do all forms of breathing so your body can function with ease in any given positioning, so if you notice you can't let go here, do some specific training.

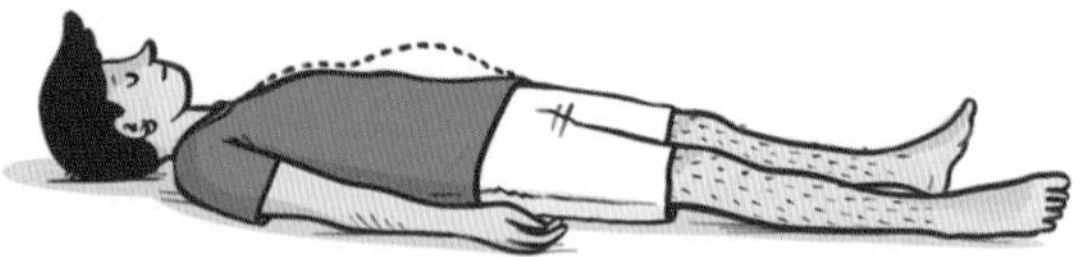

Figure 4.16 When in Shavasana, *abdominal breath is the most relaxing.*

If the yoga practice is more floor-based and supported, then it is probably fine to allow the body to breathe in whichever way seems natural for the position you are in, often an abdominal breath. The main thing that we can learn from this section is that the breath will change depending on our positioning and that we want to be able to have the freedom to modify the breath as required.

Breath and Trauma

Contributor Josefin Wikstrom

Most of the time, we breathe without thinking. It is an ongoing unconscious process that keeps us alive. However, the breath is strongly connected to our emotions. When we are scared, we hold our breath. When we are happy, we breathe faster, also when we are anxious or stressed. If we feel calm, we breathe slow and relaxed. Breathing practices and focusing toward the breath can be challenging to access for someone who has been exposed to trauma and for those suffering from panic attacks, because it can be a reminder of the emotions that are connected to the trauma or anxiety attacks.

What is a Trauma?

The word trauma originates from Greek, and translates as "a wound." A trauma is an event that overwhelms us physically and emotionally. What is overwhelming depends on each person's personality, environment, genetics, history, the individual's unique experience and interpretation, and in general, the interaction between protective factors and stressors.

What is perceived as a traumatic event is dependent on who we are and where we are in our lives when the event is happening. Our usual reaction after the trauma is to be stressed and overwhelmed in an initial period, named "acute stress." Trauma can be a single event, such as an accident, natural catastrophes, or violence, but also interpersonal and emotional, such as abuse, bullying, or neglect, and a lack of love or attention as a child while growing up. One description of trauma can be that you have lost control over the situation and experience a lost sense of self and direction.

The Trauma Response

A traumatic event can trigger reactions for survival in a few different ways, commonly known as the "fight-flight or freeze response." The fight-flight response mobilizes us for moving physically away from danger. This response is initiated by the sympathetic nervous system (SNS), part of the autonomic nervous system (ANS). The ANS controls our bodily functions necessary for survival, for example, heartbeat, breath, digestion, etc.

One reaction of the SNS related to the fight-flight response is to make our heart beat faster, and is also connected to the breath to keep us active and moving. The freeze response is when we perceive that we are unable to move away from danger. It is initiated by the sympathetic part of the nervous system but can also involve an over-activation from the parasympathetic nervous system (PSNS) according to the trauma researcher Stephen Porges. This is normally the rest and digest part of the ANS that allows us to restore, to feel social and relaxed, and it also slows down our heartbeat via the vagus nerve. The body can go into what is called "tonic immobility." The body starts to shut down bodily functions and even slows down the heartbeat as if playing dead to escape the threat. The freeze response can be a psychological response developed as a reaction and defense mechanism from childhood.

Dysregulation

Most of the time, we can calm ourselves down and regulate the traumatic stress response. After all, we are very resilient as human beings. Our most common ways of calming down are via our social connections, such as reaching out to family or friends, being able to calm ourselves down by realizing the danger has passed, and by breath and movement. Depending on our social networks, life situation, genetics, and mental health, sometimes this stress response can be hard to regulate and for us to return to a relaxed state. This can cause a dysregulation in the ANS and in the CNS (i.e., the brain and spinal cord). The brain is continuing to react as if we were in ongoing danger and continues the stress response, with high stress hormone levels even though the danger has passed. There is then a risk of developing post-traumatic stress disorder (PTSD).

Being exposed to one or limited events is categorized as PTSD type 1, and prolonged repeated exposure is called Complex PTSD type 2, with this type of trauma being often inter-relational. Exposure to trauma, such as neglect and abuse at a young age—the time crucial for brain development—affects the person's relationships and mental health later in life. Children growing up with complex trauma are more likely to have concentration difficulties and a higher likelihood for developing depression and anxiety and antisocial behaviors. This is called "developmental trauma" and is not yet addressed in the diagnostic manuals.

PTSD can give rise to symptoms such as flashbacks (reliving the trauma), sleep disturbances, memory processing, concentration, avoiding places and people, social isolation, anxiety, depression, problems with relationships, emotional regulation, and dissociation both mentally and from our bodily sensations. Apart from the adverse psychological effects, it can also contribute to diabetes type 2, heart problems, autoimmune disease, and substance abuse as a way of coping with the strong emotions.

Yoga and Trauma

A combination of physical hatha yoga practices with an emphasis toward a trauma-informed mindfulness-based instruction and relaxation has been shown to be effective in reducing both depression and anxiety and many of the negative symptoms arising from traumatic stress, as well. In addition, improvements in sleep and increases in mental awareness are often experienced.

van der Kolk explains that because regulation of physical movement is a fundamental priority of the nervous system, focusing on and developing an awareness of physical movement can lead to improved synchrony between mind and body (2015). He also published a research study in 2013 showing that 16 of 31 participants (52 percent) in the yoga group no longer met the criteria for PTSD compared with 6 of 29 (21 percent) in the control group.

Yoga is beneficial, he says, especially for those suffering from psychological conditions, such as depression and PTSD, because an improved sense of connectedness between mind and body gives rise to enhanced control and understanding of their "inner sensations" and state of being. By reducing stress and increasing parasympathetic activity, yoga can directly reduce amygdala hyperactivation (the alarm bell of the brain reacting to a perceived threat) and elevated cortisol (stress hormone) levels in patients with PTSD and thereby reduce symptoms.

Interventions that are specific to yoga, breathing, moving, relaxation, and meditation, are thought to be responsible for this shift in autonomic balance to the parasympathetic side of the ANS. Physical yoga, in combination with mindfulness, breathing, and relaxation, are positively affecting many of the areas in the brain that become negatively affected by PTSD.

Stress Resilience

Many mental health issues are linked to a lack of strength and flexibility in the ANS. One of the best ways to strengthen this system is by implementing practices that increase and lower the heartbeat in intervals. This is effective due to the connection with the ANS that is controlling the heart rate. The vagus nerve is the longest and the most important nerve of the PSNS. It sends 80 percent of its signals from the body to the brain and is crucial in mind/body awareness. By engaging and strengthening the signals from the vagus nerve, we can more easily enhance feelings of social safety and calm down after experiencing stress. The vagus nerve transmits signals to the heart to slow down the heart rate, and the SNS sends signals to speed up the heart rate. This happens naturally during the day and keeps the cardiovascular system healthy.

If we are relaxed or excited, the heart rate will move toward either PSNS or SNS, respectively, the heart rate goes back and forth during a day, which is a healthy response, called heart rate variability (HRV). The higher the variation in the HRV, the more resilient we are toward stress. A low-level change indicates difficulties in cultivating energy or calming down after a stressful situation. HRV is mostly mediated by signals from the medulla oblongata in the brain stem, transmitted by the vagus nerve to the heart. The frequency is higher than the signals from the SNS. In a trauma-informed class, we are implementing a gentle pulse increase combined with stillness and postures to bring the heartbeat down again. The aim is to increase HRV and eventually also add some breath practices (Figure 4.17).

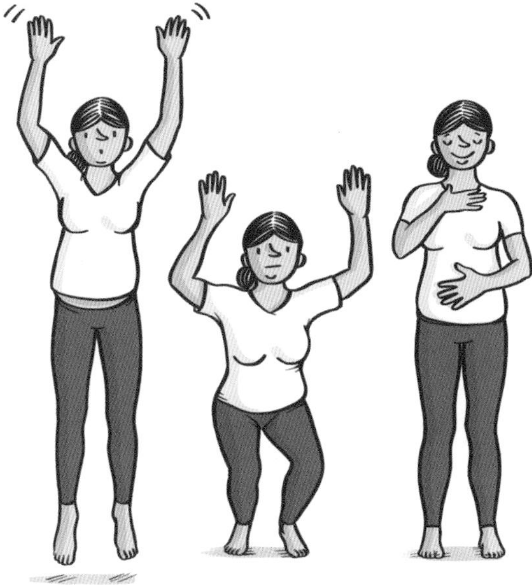

Figure 4.17 Try to move around to gently raise your heartbeat for as long as feels comfortable, then stop. You can try to place the hands on your belly and the center of the chest, slowing the heartbeat down. If you like, you can try exhaling relaxed and long out through your nose or your mouth, perhaps with a "Haa" sound or like you are blowing up a balloon.

Trauma-Informed Yoga

The following are some of the key elements:

- Invitational language for allowing a sense of control and shared power dynamics between facilitator and students.
- Allowing different choices in postures and movements to allow a sense of safety and agency.
- Interoception, guiding the awareness to the felt sense in the body.
- Counting down in challenging poses to provide a sense of control.
- A class that is combining active movements with slowing down to increase HRV.
- The mats are placed with the back free to allow the participants to feel safe.
- No physical adjustments.
- Set routine and a similar program for a long period of time for recognition and safety.
- The teacher is trained in trauma-informed yoga.

Trauma and Breath

Focusing toward the breath can be difficult at the start of a yoga practice, especially if the body is holding a lot of tension in the muscles around the ribcage from prolonged stress and anxiety. Also, it can be quite common that participants have a reversed breathing pattern, where the belly comes in on the inhalation and out on the exhalation.

In addition, they may constantly be pulling in the belly. This can come from posture, habits, as well as prolonged stress. Reversed breathing and faster-paced chest breathing can also be a protection mechanism and something that feels safe. Hence, we go slow when introducing breath focus.

Breathing slower can take us into a para-sympathetic drive too fast too soon and can trigger a lot of emotions. It may as well remind the person of a freeze response. The breath can also be a reminder of the trauma, especially if the breath was restricted during the event (Figure 4.18).

In teaching dynamic classes, a counted, even rhythm of the breath (*sama vritti*) is used. It is a good idea to count how many breaths are left in the posture, as this reinforces a sense of common rhythm and control.

How to Start?

Initially, allow students the time to get used to the yoga program and establish a sense of security in the physical postures, the feeling of safety in the group, and the sequence. Introduce postures and gentle movements into the sequence that can help release built-up tension around the joints and the ribcage that can restrict the breath. For example,

Trauma and Breath—How To Start

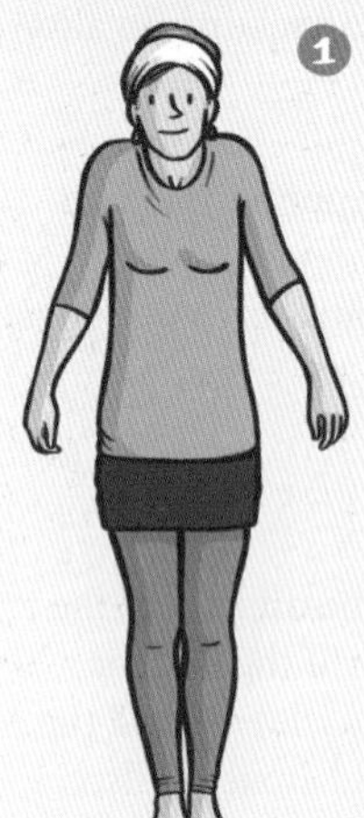

1. Lift your shoulders to your ears and roll the shoulders down with a long exhale out of your mouth.
Move joints—hands, elbows, shoulders, and jaw.
Drop the breath into the belly.
Example for mental awareness:
Inhale mantra, "I am breathing."
Exhale mantra, "I am centered and calm."

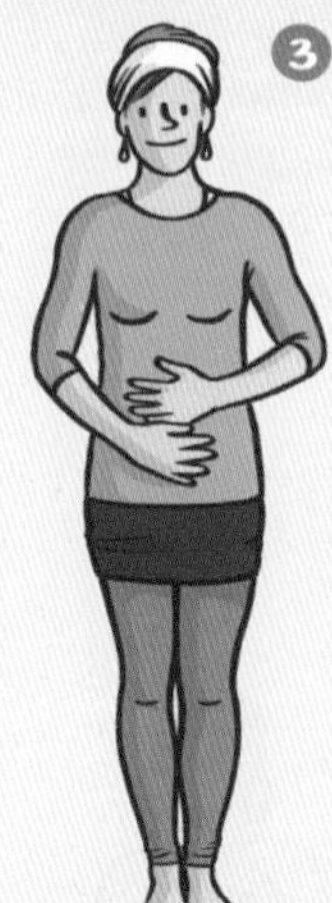

3. Breathe into the hands on the belly. Feel the movement of the breath in your belly and the warmth from your hands. Feel the connection between your feet and the ground. Maybe try to rock forward and back to activate the feet. Imagine that you are breathing from the ground into your belly and back down to the ground when you are exhaling. Empty your lungs completely, breathe through your nose or your mouth.

2. Chair posture. Stay for as long as you can. You can choose to keep bending the arms, engaging their muscles.
Fold forward—long exhales—repeat Chair posture x 3. End with shoulder rolls and release tension from the forehead, eyes, jaw, shoulders, hands, belly, knees, and ankles.

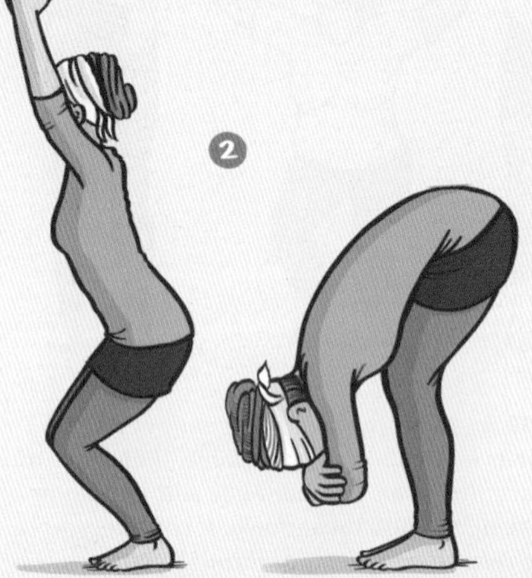

Figure 4.18 Here are some practices and advice if someone feels overwhelmed or is having panic attacks.

Additional Guidance

Try to create tension in your legs and arms as you breathe in, and relax as you exhale. Notice the difference between tension and relaxation. You can try to close one hand when you breathe in and the other as you breathe out. These practices are to bring the awareness into the body, activating the coordination and the muscles in the arms and the legs that normally want to move and engage when we perceive danger.

- If you have cold water, rinse the hands and the face. You can also hold something that is cooler, which can disrupt the panic response.
- Notice five everyday things in the room. Think or speak the name of the objects quietly to yourself.
- If you have a particular smell that you like, you can use it if you start to feel anxious. This has been shown to have a calming effect for many.

side bends, shoulder openers, psoas stretches, such as *Virabhadrasana A* and gentle backbends, such as *Salamba Bhujangasana*, which will help stretch the belly muscles.

When introducing the focus toward the breath, moving and breathing in a synchronized rhythm, especially at the same time as engaging the large muscle groups, seems to be easier to tolerate. These movements can be pushing the hands forward in *Utkatasana* and exhaling at the same time with strong arms and legs. The participants are always invited to include breath focus if it feels right and to breathe through the nose or mouth as feels best for them.

Relaxed Abdominal Breath and the PNS

Eventually, when the participant feels ready to include more breathing practices, a relaxed belly breath can be introduced, which also activates and strengthens the vagus nerve and the peripheral nervous system. Relaxed belly breathing can be a slow progression to implement for someone who has been in sympathetic overdrive for a long time. They can be experiencing tense muscles around the chest and belly, also the psoas (a deep hip flexor) tends to be tense.

To find a relaxed belly breath, it can be helpful to lie down on the back, with the feet placed on a chair, and an object like a book, pillow, or maybe

Examples of Getting Connected With the Breath—Self-Holding

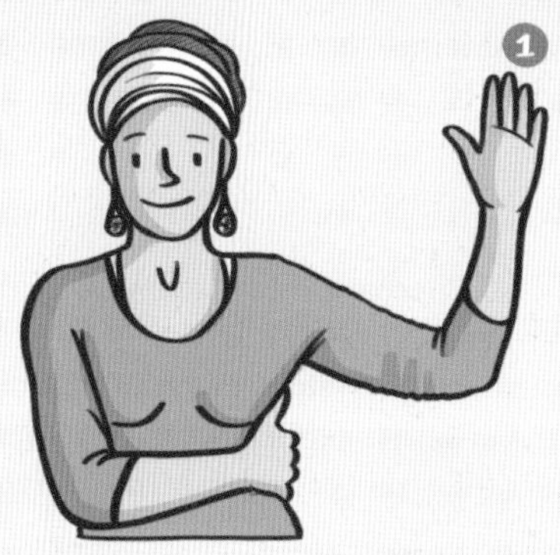

1. Place your right hand around the left side of your ribcage. Relax your left arm. Inhale and notice the movement in your right hand, 10–25 breaths.

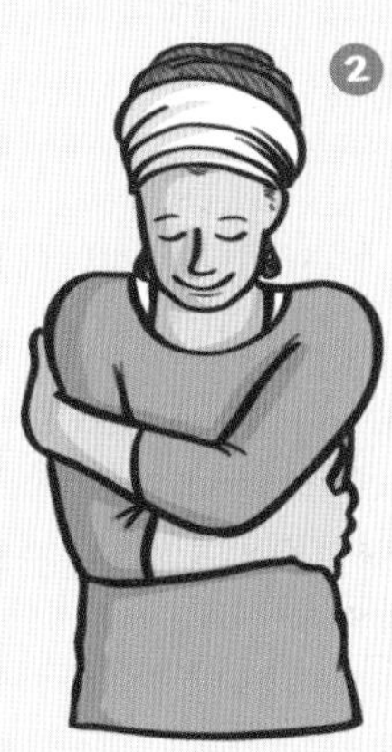

2. Cross your left arm over your left side and hug yourself, relaxing your shoulders. Notice your breathing in the sides of your ribcage and between your shoulder blades, 10–25 breaths.

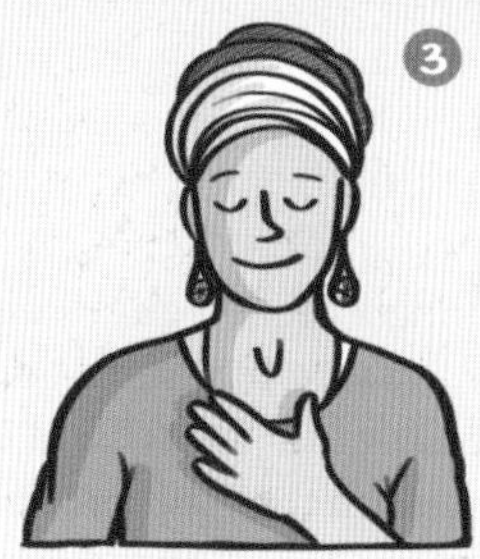

3. Breathe into your hands, on the solar plexus and heart center, 10–25 breaths.

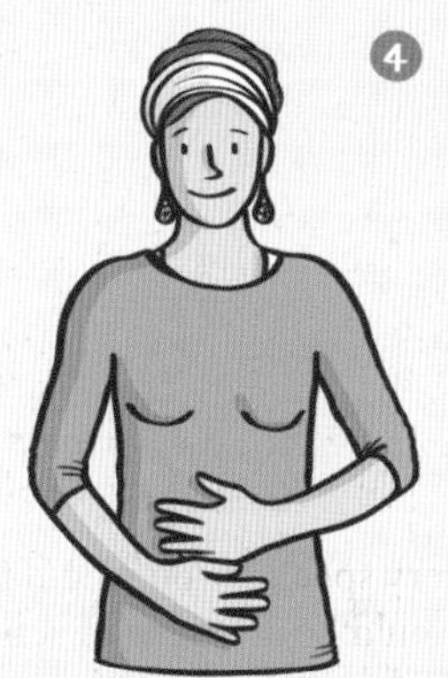

4. Place your hands on the belly, perhaps adding the humming sound on the breath, and notice the vibrating sound in your belly. You can try opening your mouth and moving your jaw in different directions as you make the sound to release tension in the jaw and face. Try to continue for approximately 2–5 minutes.

Lie down and rest for 5–10 minutes.

student's own hands placed on the belly. Then imagine lifting the object gently on the in-breath and relaxing on the out-breath where the object lowers down toward the spine. This can also be done when standing or sitting by gently placing one hand on the chest and the other on the belly to connect with the movement of the breath.

When a relaxed breath is present, it may be possible to add an internal focus point, for example, counting the breath or a mantra/personal word if it feels comfortable. A prolonged exhalation can be used if there are feelings of stress or anxiety, to send calming signals to the brain and increase the vagal tone. A soft humming sound may also be added, or a "haaa" sound, almost like you are fogging a mirror on the out-breath. This can increase the vagal activation further as there is a connection with the vocal cords.

Coherent Breathing

Ultimately, breathing with an equal length on the inhale and exhale, may be tried. It is good to start with a 3-second inhale and a 3-second exhale. When comfortable with this, the length can be gradually increased up to 5-5 or 6-6. The breath is as relaxed as possible. If tension or an increased heartbeat is experienced, the count should be lowered. The asanas, in combination with the breathing techniques, are facilitating a shift from an active state to a passive state, and in turn, increasing HRV.

Caution

Fast-paced breathing techniques, e.g., *Kapalabhati* and *Bastrika*, are contraindicated for these groups because they are too activating and can be a reminder of an anxiety attack. Many may also suffer from high blood pressure. Also, long breath holds, as used in *Kumbhaka*, are not recommended.

References

Balasubramaniam, M., Telles, S., & Doraiswamy, P.M. (2013). Yoga on our minds: A systematic review of yoga for neuropsychiatric disorders. *Frontiers in Psychiatry*, 3:117.

Fried, R. & Grimaldi J. (1993). The Psychology and Physiology of Breathing: in *Behavioral Medicine, Clinical Psychology, and Psychiatry*. American Psychological Association, Washington.

Kerekes, N., Fielding, C. & Apelqvist, S. (2017). Yoga in correctional settings: a randomized controlled study. *Frontiers in Psychiatry*, 8:204.

Mason, H. and Birch, K. (2018). *Yoga for Mental Health*. Handspring Publishing, Edinburgh.

Sfendla, A., Malmström, P., Torstensson, S. & Kerekes, N. (2019). Yoga practice reduces the psychological distress levels of prison inmates. *Frontiers in Psychiatry*, 9: 407.

Streeter, C.C., Gerbarg, P.L., Saper, R.B., Ciraulo, D.A. & Brown, R.P. (2012). Effects of yoga on the autonomic nervous system, gamma-aminobutyric-acid, and allostasis in epilepsy, depression, and post-traumatic stress disorder. *Medical Hypotheses*, May 78(5):571–9.

van der Kolk, B. (2015). *The Body Keeps the Score: Mind, Brain, and Body in the Transformation of Trauma*. Penguin, New York.

Prison Yoga Project

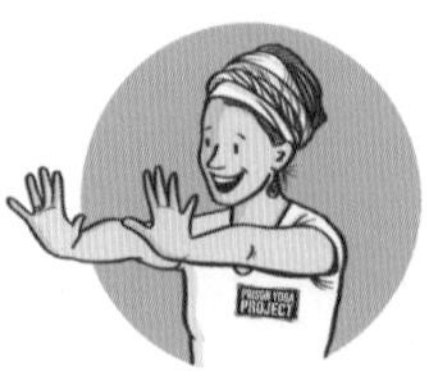

Josefin is part of the amazing Prison Yoga Project. if you would like to find out more, or donate to their worthwhile cause, you can use the following link: https://prisonyoga.kindful.com

CHAPTER 5

Other Personal Considerations

Environmental Influences

It's funny in a way that a practice essentially aimed at drawing the focus inward is often associated with experiencing it in an externally aesthetic place. Almost every picture promoting yoga is set in a beautiful *shala*, or on an exotic beach, looking across the Himalayas or some other scene that draws the senses outward. Having said that, I have practiced in all sorts of places, hotel rooms, parking lots, kitchens, grungy makeshift *shalas*, and the odd sea view platform, and I must admit, there is something special about doing something you like to do in a place that awes or inspires. I think it is more like mood setting because once you start, you hardly notice where you are until, almost by accident, you happen to catch sight again. Besides our view, there are many things that can feed us or irritate us, make things easier or harder, and raise us up or drag us down.

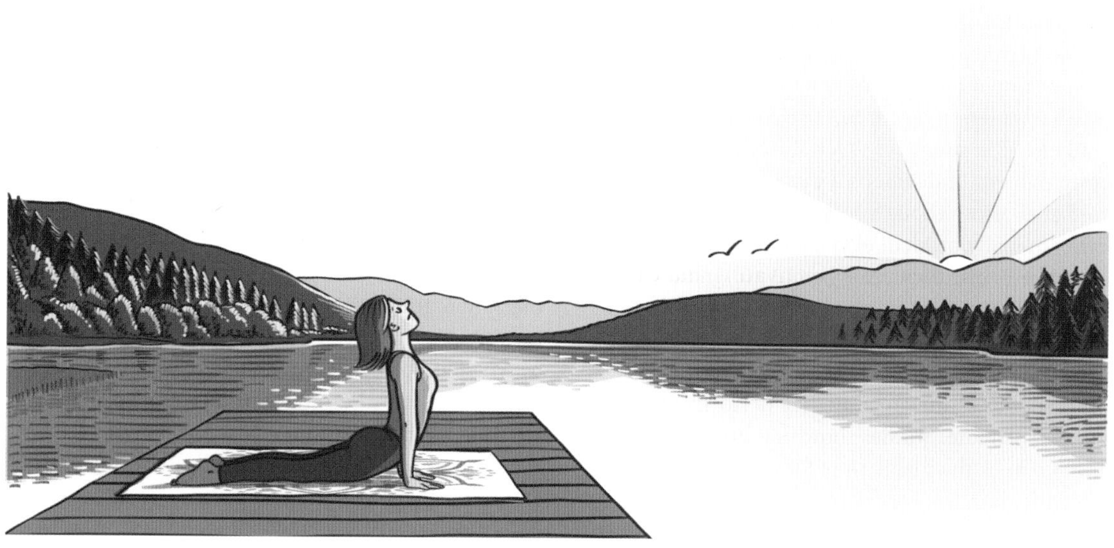

Environmental influences include anything in our direct surroundings, such as the type of mat, flooring, temperature, time of day, noise, and of course, vista that somewhat indirectly influence our mood, pliability, or other physical or mental attributes.

Some would say that we shouldn't even use a mat, but I'm sorry, I love mine. How can you focus or move from your foundation when your foundation is slipping away? What you have under your mat is equally important, too soft like carpet and you risk placing stress into your wrists, uneven like a lovely traditional cow dung floor (horrible personal memories), and you will feel all wonky and find it hard to balance. There might be some psychological appeal to having something soft to land on if you are training something like Handstands on the beach, but really the potential for injury to the wrists outweighs the benefit.

Arriving in India, many students experience an immediate increase in their ROM due to the heat. The tissues soften like any other material. Apparently, a rise of just one or two degrees in tissue temperature is enough to make a difference. Some yoga styles like Ashtanga focus on increasing internal heat by using breath, bandha, and vinyasa. Others heat the room itself. The increase in the pliability of the tissue due to an "x" degree rise in temperature will be the same no matter how the heat was delivered. However, the benefit of heating from the inside is that, at the same time, you are lubricating the joints, establishing motor control, movement patterns, blood circulation, and generally getting the body ready for exercise. Conversely, too cold and the body tightens and stiffens. I don't do well in the cold at all. Even though I was born in the UK, I'm sure I'm really of Mediterranean descent. I don't even like British food. Maybe the milkman was from further south!

Most students find that time of day also makes a difference as to how readily they perform asana as well as meditate. Studies show that between 2:30 and 4 p.m. is the magic time for ease of movement, but early morning for a clear head to meditate.

Of course, you could be reading this thinking the exact opposite. One thing I have tested many times is how long I sleep for. It seems to me that if I am in bed for less than 6 hours (this is not exact you understand), my body feels much more flexible than if I have more, and it is significantly different enough to be enticing. You do have to catch up on sleep with a little siesta later though. Try for yourself, I have spoken to quite a few teachers that feel the same.

The list of potential external distractions for the mind is enormous, but one thing worth mentioning is the presence of other people. They can be a complete nightmare with their flying sweat, noisy breath, constant coughing or sniffing, arm-waving, odor, grumpiness etc., etc., but, like the right mat, neighbors can be inspiring and uplifting. I practice a lot with just my wife, and there is something special about that collective experience. In fact, nowadays, that is what I like the most about yoga.

A good teacher is easily one of the biggest positive external influences. Not only in the way they hold the space but with their guidance, support, and encouragement also. However, it is not always the case, and if you find yourself with a teacher that is too controlling, narrow-minded, or unsupportive, seek out someone new.

Even the wrong sort of clothing can impact us. I mean, how can you possibly practice in something that is not color-coordinated! Joking apart, not wanting to be somewhat self-conscious displaying my clutter in figure-hugging lycra, I used to wear regular sports shorts, but they always restricted many of the forward folding postures. Then I found four-way-stretch surf shorts—perfect. Another side issue that popped into my head when I started to think of color is that even the color of your mat makes a difference. I hate practicing on a black mat, preferring instead purple or green.

Maybe I am revealing too much about myself, but even my position in the yoga room seems to make a difference to my practice. I am not attached to an exact spot, but definitely an area. In the Purple Valley *shala*, where I have practiced for many years, I wanted to be somewhere in the front right section. I have a feeling it might have been slightly brighter. If I was somewhere in front of the door where I could feel the draft coming under it, I might just as well have gone home. I think I actually did one day.

I also remember on another occasion putting my mat on the exact spot where, moments before, superstar yogi Mark Robberts had been practicing, and I immediately thought with a smile, "Let's hope he left some of his energy behind." I think it was a good practice!

It might be useful at this stage to make a list of all the things that really help your own practice and those that are a hindrance. See if you can take this opportunity to remove a negative environmental influence.

Finally, it's worth reminding ourselves that bad things can also make you stronger. I remember having to practice for a time where the windy conditions made it hard to balance, that training made me much better when I then found myself in normal conditions. The same can happen with any negative influence. It can also be an opportunity to draw your focus inward.

Oh yes, don't forget the moon.

Lifestyle

There is no doubt that practicing yoga can have positive effects on our health and lifestyle, but what we do off the mat can also positively or adversely influence our body and hence the physical practice. One of the places we spend most of our time is at work, and it is easy to build up tensional patterns that will be highlighted by the yoga. The unwinding of these patterns through the yoga will no doubt be of benefit, but in the interim, they will also provide significant physical restrictions and potential sites for injury. We spend much more time off the mat than we do on the mat, so one of the first things we should do when we notice imbalance or tension is to explore our habits and working practices and try and change those that are detrimental.

A good example is students who have office jobs involving long periods at the computer. There is likely to be a significant shortening of structures on the front of the body, so when it comes to postures like backbending, there can be resistance from the front of the hip, shoulders, and chest. Conversely, if you have a profession that uses comparable skills with the yoga practice, you will probably enjoy some freedom in those same movements. As we mentioned earlier in the book, a person who plants rice all day is likely to be able to fold forward easily—whether they feel like going to yoga after all that is another thing altogether.

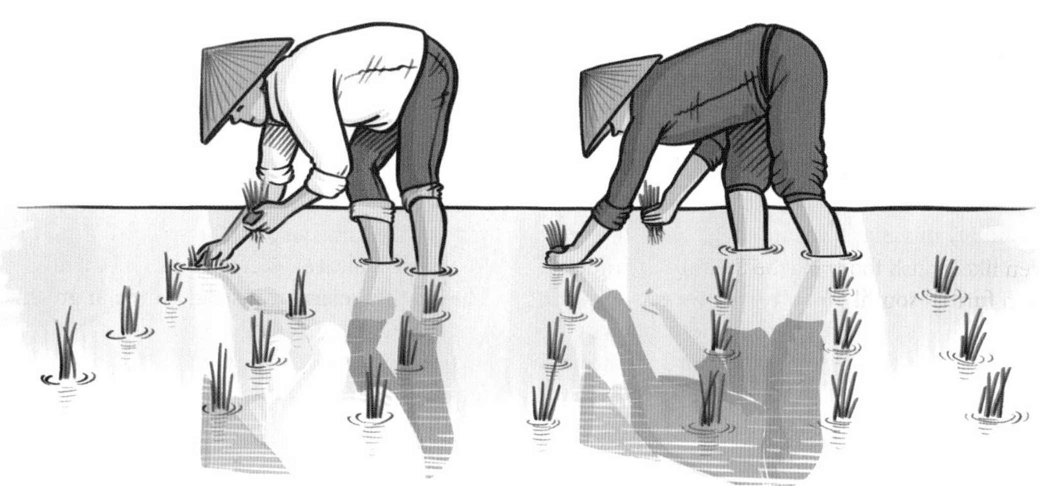

The pursuance of other sports is something that is often discouraged by yoga teachers for fear of them negatively influencing the ability to perform postures. Personally, I take the opposite view. From a health and fitness perspective, yoga does not address all aspects evenly or sufficiently. We have discussed the preponderance of pushing actions rather than pulling, external rotation of the hip as opposed to medial. There is also not the same workout for the cardiovascular system as there is in, say, running or cycling. As well as that, increasing ROM is generally given greater emphasis than creating the strength to control it.

The problem with addressing these types of issues by including too much conditioning into the practice is that there is a chance of it becoming less recognizable as yoga. I always advise students to keep doing other forms of exercise if they enjoy it, but also to take action to address any potentially detrimental side effects. Running is a good example. Some students feel that they need the buzz from running to deal with stress, or enjoy being out in nature, find it assists weight control, or gets them fitter. Repetitive movement below full ROM will shorten certain muscles, but this could easily be alleviated with a proper cool down and stretch after the run.

There is a much greater expectation of what we can do with our bodies nowadays, and many of what I call the new breed of teachers look outside of the practice to borrow techniques. The approach to Handstands is a good example, but also to make improvements in areas such as strength, control, and stability that can then help with the physical practice. One of my favorite alternative pursuits is calisthenics, but surfing would also complement yoga, because it has the paddling out that provides the pulling missing in yoga.

A popular saying is, "We are what we eat." We won't go into the whole nutrition thing here, but it is important to eat in a way that supports your level of calorie output and provides the nutrients for the body to repair and renew. As the body contains about 60 percent water, and the muscle tissue specifically about 75 percent, proper hydration is a good thing to ensure. Some people say that meat-eaters—besides smelling different—are also stiffer. I will wait for the research to come through on this one.

Looking back at *Flexibility* in Chapter 2, I suggested that some of the fundamental movements, such as squatting, can be incorporated easily into our lifestyle. Yoga is a lifestyle, and the more the physical practice can also merge with our time off the mat, the more significant impact it will have on our time on the mat.

Personal History

Everything that has gone before this moment in time has impacted us in some way. It can be positively or negatively, infinitesimally or massively, isolated or compounding. What is happening today is history tomorrow. We are not separated from our past, even though we are in the present. If we have experienced, trauma, injury, loss, extreme joy, exhaustion, or anything else, it will play out in the body now. We can live in the moment, but it doesn't mean we didn't also live the moments before.

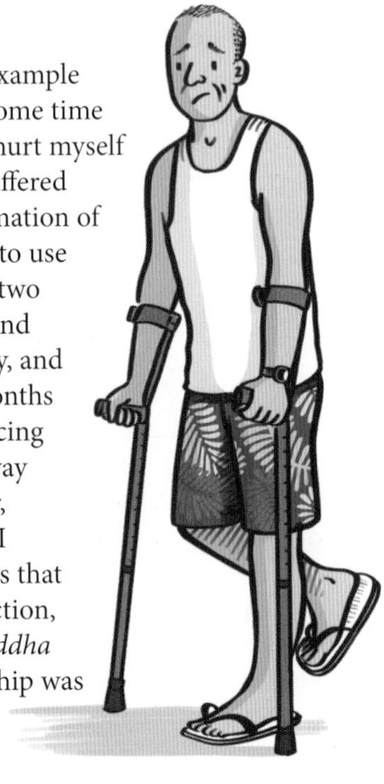

I will give you an example from my history. Some time ago, I managed to hurt myself pretty badly and suffered from acute inflammation of the right SIJ. I had to use crutches for about two months to get around during my recovery, and it was about six months before I was practicing yoga in the same way as before. However, I found that when I performed postures that involved hip abduction, for example, in *Baddha Konasana*, my left hip was considerably more restricted, with my left knee staying up in the air and the right side going down to the floor.

For a long time, I couldn't figure out how I now had some tension at the front on the left side of the pelvis, yet the injury had happened around the back on the right side of the pelvis. Then one day, my brain suddenly presented the solution—I think the problem must have been worked on in my subconscious, which is not that uncommon for me. During the time when I was using the crutches, I had almost no use of my right hip, so I would plant my left leg and drag my right side to it. That action involved the contraction of my left adductors, which had tightened up as a result of being overworked. Their tension was keeping my left knee in the air, as they were resisting hip abduction.

It is very common for imbalances caused by a previous injury to express themselves far from the original site of damage because of all the compensatory movements and adopted patterns initiated during recovery. I have also found that the timespan from the initial incident can be immense, probably because those same adaptations were never entirely let go. This was a physical example, but I have come across plenty of individuals limited by past psychological traumas. Of course, not all influences of the past have to be negative. We can definitely learn a lot about ourselves from the challenges we have faced, but also joyous times can give us an openness and willingness to explore.

Psychology

Psychology plays a significant role in everything we do, and yoga postures are no different. How do we approach the whole practice? Are we chilled out, ego-driven, or lazy, do we have trouble focusing or are we intense? Are we motivated and committed, or do we find it hard to keep a regular practice? Are we flexible in mind as well as body, or are we rigid and reluctant to change things? There are many other traits we could list, and in a way, these are just an extension of our personality and repeated in many different areas of life. One of the purposes of yoga is to provide an opportunity to work with these obstacles, but it is equally easy to avoid or ignore them. Yoga's sister science Ayurveda would direct us to look at our ayurvedic constitution (Vata, Pitta, Kapha) to help determine what we need from our yoga practice.

Although we won't go into much detail here as it is not one of my strong points, many people get clarity about themselves and why they do particular things by viewing them from an ayurvedic perspective. I would urge you to read much more about this topic if it catches your interest.

From my rudimentary understanding, the basic tenet is that your constitution will be a combination of the three doshas, Vata, Pitta, and Kapha, in different degrees (prakriti). For the most part, either one or two of the doshas are the primary influencers. With dual prakriti, the most influential contributor is expressed first, for example, Vata-Kapha, Vata-Pitta, or Pitta-Kapha. Any imbalance in the doshas will heavily influence the way you practice, which, in turn, is affected by your constitution. However, anyone can experience an imbalance in any of the doshas.

If you want to try and balance your doshas, it might be best to practice in a way that goes against your natural inclination. In other words, if you are feeling quite Kapha, you could be calm and grounded, but your practice is likely to be somewhat slow in tempo, maybe heavy and sluggish. You could decide to inject a bit of zip into it. If you are primarily Vata or your Vata is off, you might find it hard to concentrate, tend to rush through your practice, and be a little anxious. It might help in this case to slow things down, focus on the breath, and firmly ground through your feet and legs. You may also decide to do specific sequences designed to work with particular doshas.

It is not uncommon for students to have a fear of inversions or a reluctance to try something if they have had previous bad experiences. As a teacher, you may even feel your student has all the other elements in place. It could be just their mind that is stopping them from being able to do a specific posture. In my own experience, when I first tried a freestanding Handstand with other students on their mats right next to me, there was a spike in the fear factor in case I fell on someone (Figure 5.1). That could be enough to scupper your attempts even though you have done it loads of times in a different situation.

Fear might also be related to what other people might think, not wanting to hurt oneself, trying something new, insecurity, failing, and I'm sure many other things. From my lay perspective, I see psychological inhibitors, such as fears and phobias, as not based on logical thought processes. That doesn't make them any less real for the individual but means that it is harder to get a letting-go of that inhibitor through logical reasoning. Lateral thinking and stepped progressions are often the way to go.

Previous injuries also result in us wanting to protect an area (see *Personal History*). Although sensible at the start, those feelings may last well after the injury has healed. This could set us up with abnormal movement patterns that will need addressing. A desire to please or be recognized may lead us to try too hard or risk things that we are not ready for. There may also be psychological traumas associated with some regions of the body. It may be

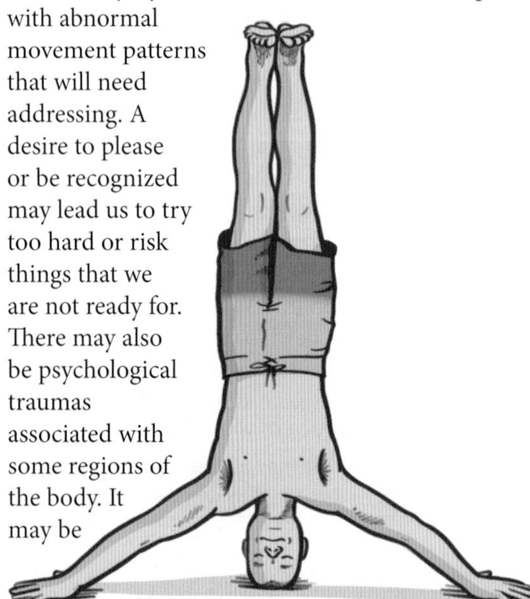

Figure 5.1 With all your foundations in one plane, this posture can play with the mind. I know it did for me.

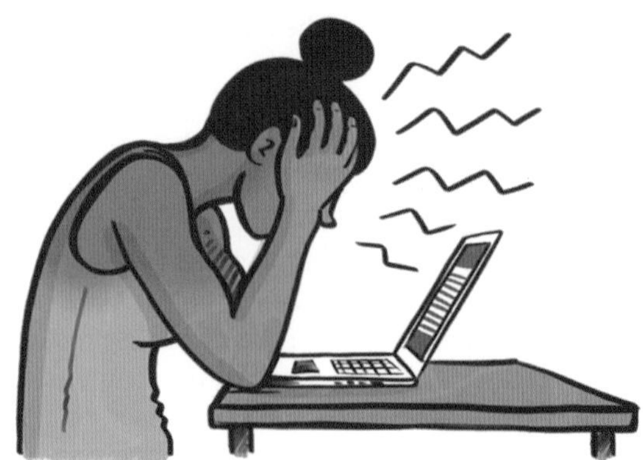

Figure 5.2 What did I spend that money on? Yoga classes?

easy to hypothesize that work and financial stresses might reside around the neck and shoulders (Figure 5.2), sexual abuse around the hips and pelvis, fear or insecurity in the chest and abdomen. I am not a trained psychologist, so don't take this as fact. There could well then be a reluctance to move freely in those areas, a dislike for particular postures because of the feelings they evoke, or even an outpouring of emotions after a deep posture. I recently met a student who got intense feelings of anger while doing powerful shoulder openers.

There is also a somewhat natural tendency to do more of what we feel we are good at and less of what we find hard. The trouble is that in yoga, this often relates to openness or strength in particular areas. Accordingly, we should be trying to do the opposite, as those are most likely the areas we need to work on to create balance in the body.

So, I suppose what we can get from *Psychology* is that we should enquire within ourselves as to why we practice the way we do and compare that with what we feel the body and mind need most. The individual yoga poses are chances to work with fears, obstacles, ego, lethargy, and, of course, many other aspects of our psyche. If we are not doing this, we are missing out on an ideal opportunity to take learning experiences from the mat to the real world.

I think, sometimes, we also need to consider what it is that is driving us to want to master particular postures, especially those that require extreme ROMs. I'm constantly amazed at some bubbling desire in myself to do *Eka Pada Sirsasana*, even though I'm incredibly dubious about any potential health benefits, and risk analysis would say forget it. So, I continue to work toward the posture, albeit slowly and vigilantly, maybe reassured by the fact that as an old git, I'm unlikely to succeed at this late stage in the game.

As homework, identify something about the way you practice. Decide to change or work with it for the next weeks to see where it leads.

Risk Factors

I remember when I started getting into yoga, my mum said to me, "Make sure you don't start going weird." By that, she meant becoming vegetarian, chanting, dressing funny, and taking on an unusual name.

So, of course, there is the risk with yoga that you may change in some way that others don't understand, but here I am referring to the risk of potential injury rather than anything else. We are not even talking about slips, trips, and the like. Accidents can happen somewhat independent of what we are doing (not entirely correct, but for now it will suffice). How we position our body—either intentionally or otherwise—is our concern, because making shapes is our business.

Because yoga is enveloped in its mystical healing bubble, a lot of the time people have the assumption that whatever they are asked to do in a yoga class must be good for them.

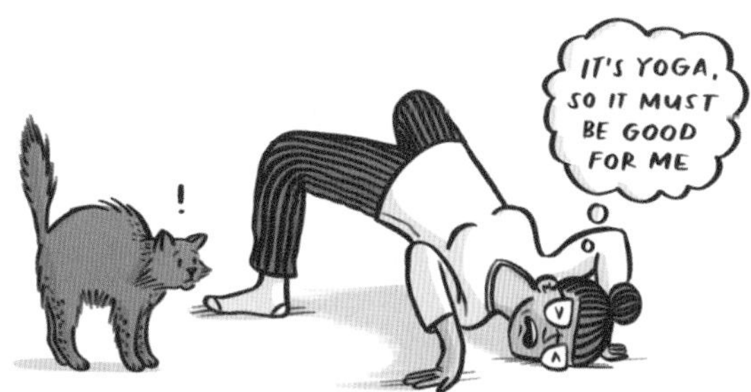

Of course, this is not the case, and I think that although the motivations behind much of the media attention this topic has received in recent years might be questionable, the outcome of greater public awareness of the potential for injury has been a good thing. Many moons ago, when I was doing a personal trainer certification, we used to have to list all the health and safety points for a particular exercise. I remember at the time being utterly bored with that aspect because many were the same, and in your youth, you feel invincible and don't necessarily relate to things going wrong. However, as time goes by, if you are lucky, you become wiser. I think that same type of critical eye that I was reluctant to cast back then could be put to good use when considering yoga postures.

It is easy to see that some of the intricate and more extreme postures, where we are testing the

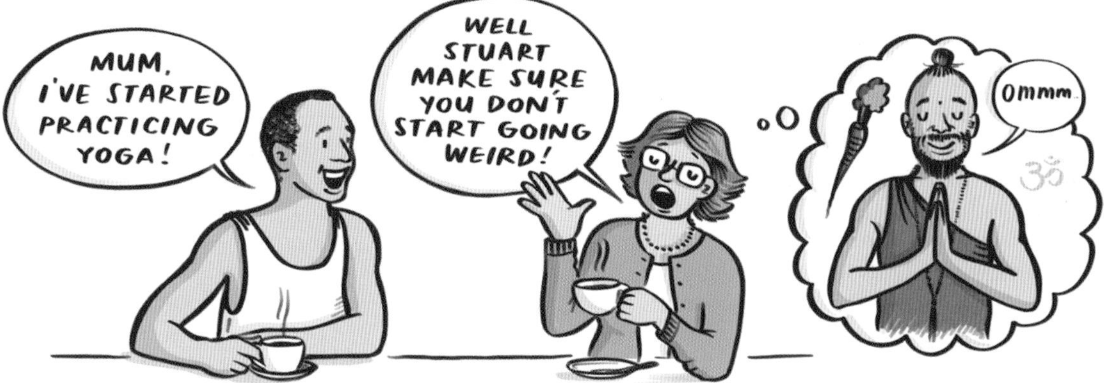

limits of strength and ROM, have the potential to place stress on bodily structures. However, a pose doesn't have to be complicated to cause problems for some people, even something as seemingly straightforward as *Paschimottanasana* can place stress on the low back if done incorrectly. Yoga is not a team sport, we are not moving at speed, and we don't have people ready to jump on us (apart from the odd overzealous adjuster), so the variables for risk potential are small. They are limited to the posture itself, the practitioner, and external forces.

Let's deal with external forces first. I consider these come in two forms: the adjuster and gravity. The purpose of an adjustment is a whole discussion in itself, so for the moment, we will just say that adjustments serve many uses and can be performed with a variety of intentions.

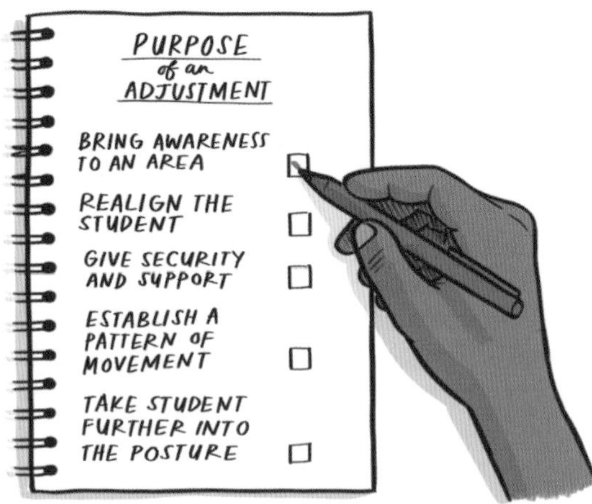

The following are some examples: bringing awareness to an area, realigning the student, giving security and support, establishing a pattern of movement, and taking the student further into the posture. Most of these situations carry minimal risk but fair to say, negative things can happen when being taken deeper into postures. Unfortunately, through my bodywork, I meet many individuals that attribute their current issue to being taken too far by an adjuster. That is not to say that it was the adjusters' fault because there is a high percentage of personal responsibility necessary. Many students give their teachers way too much credit for their ability to assess how far they can go.

Some postures lend themselves to over adjustment because of the leverage available, *Prasarita Padottanasana C* and the shoulders is a good case in point (Figure 5.3). Enough on this for the moment because it is not really part of the posture itself.

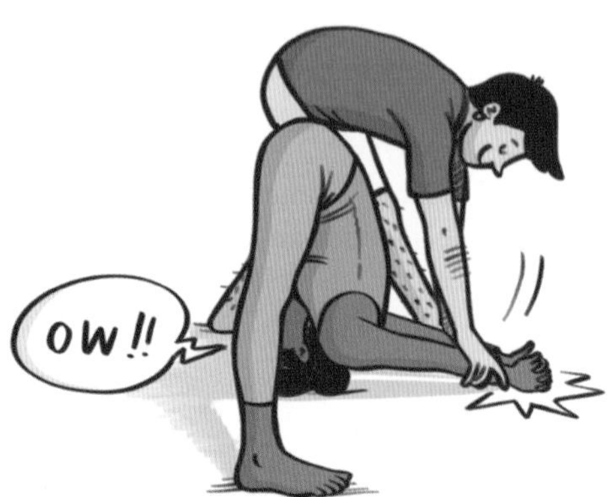

Figure 5.3 Long levers are just too tempting for some people.

Gravity, on the other hand, even though an external force, can play a role in our undoing, depending on the way the posture has called for us to be oriented in space. We looked at the role of gravity in balancing poses, and I have definitely fallen out of things with a thud before, which vigorous rubbing failed to appease. We might want to question whether that is gravity's fault, unrealistic expectations, or unpreparedness on behalf of the student. It is perhaps the more insidious effects of gravity that is of interest to us. Gravity is a downward force, and as such, will add to the stresses experienced at joints. If we are doing a Handstand, for example, the wrists may be placed under strain; in *Sirsasana*, the neck and postures such as *Virabhadrasana B*, the medial aspect of the knee are under strain. The detrimental effects can mostly be avoided through the correct activation, but we need to know how to be working.

The role of the practitioner is a good one. We can, for sure, be a risk to ourselves through pushing too much, ignoring instructions, failing to be in tune with the body, and having unrealistic or goal-oriented expectations. All those things sort of tie into psychology, but a practitioner also brings with them the baggage of restrictions, strength imbalances, or deficiencies, and previous or existing injuries. We are coming with our stuff, and some postures will be more or less accommodating to it. So, the risk factors of a posture can be highly practitioner dependent. If you have some existing condition or known weakness, you may need to heavily modify a pose to avoid further aggravation.

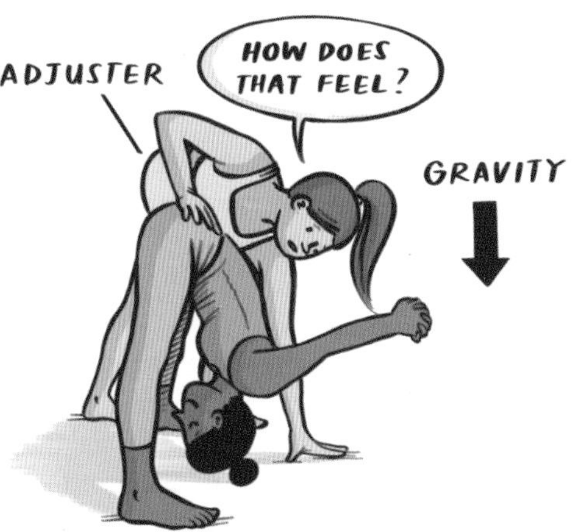

Restrictions in ROM can cause another area to have to take up the slack, often to its detriment. If we are an experienced practitioner who is familiar with a posture and has built the appropriate strength and ROM necessary over some time, then that posture might be considered quite safe even though it may, for many people, present numerous risks. This is one of the concerns about multi-level classes. So, in one way, the posture is the posture, and it is how we perform it that adds to the risk, but that is not the whole story.

How risky is the posture itself because of what it is asking us to do? In many poses, we can do things that, in the long run, won't benefit the body. Hyperextending knees or elbows, flexing the neck too strongly, taking too much weight on the head, and hinging the back are cases in point. Still, in a way, these issues are related to correct technique and not specifically the fault of the posture itself. Some poses contain a higher level of risk because to perform them, we must position ourselves in such a way that parts of the body are more vulnerable. Of course, this ties in somewhat with the previous section relating to the individual's readiness for a posture and the bodily health and safety mentioned in Chapter 1, *Alignment*. Let me give some examples, and you will see what I am getting at.

Performing the posture *Bakasana* requires the shoulders to move in front of the wrists. If you want to perform the posture with straight arms, you will have to go further forward, and if you wish your butt not to be pointing in the air too much, even further forward. All of this must happen to balance your COG easily. Maybe the more strength you have, the more you can temper this. Should your weight distribution be a bit butt heavy, then this will also make you have to go further in front of the wrists. This forward position of shoulders relative to wrists calls for a lot of wrist extension, which, in itself, can be detrimental for the wrists in this weight-bearing position (Figure 5.4).

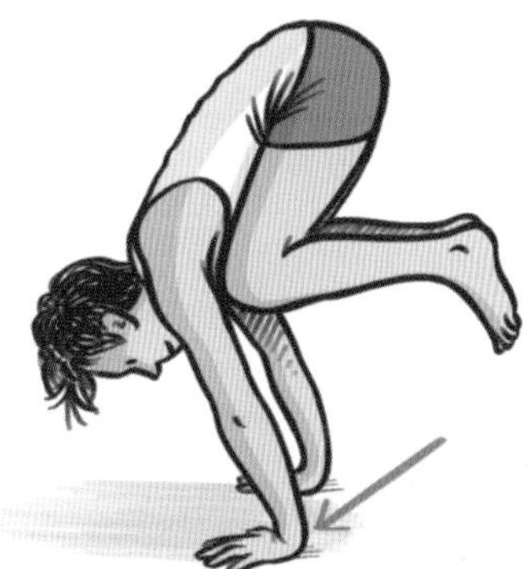

Figure 5.4 A lot of wrist extension may be too much for some practitioners.

Here are some more examples:

- Stressing the cervical spine in Shoulderstand through excessive neck flexion if the shoulders are not raised on blankets (Figure 5.5).
- Loading the lumbar spine when coming forward to meet the leg in *Utthita Hasta Padangusthasana*, when less than about 120 degrees of flexion in the hip of the raised leg is available.
- Torquing forces around the sacrum in *Parivrtta Parshvakonasana* (Figure 5.6), if performed with the back leg sole of the foot placed on

the floor, when sufficient external rotation of the hip is not available. Same sort of thing with *Virabhadrasana A*.

- Holding the ankles in a standing backbend. You can see how easy it is to hinge more in a specific area of the spine when performing intense backbends (Figure 5.7).
- Torquing forces at the knee in *Janu Sirsasana C* if the external rotation of the lower leg relative to the upper leg is not controlled and limited (Figure 5.8).
- Compressive forces being placed on the cervical spine in *Sirsasana* when the head is on the floor (Figure 5.9). More so as the arms and hands come away from the head, such as in *Mukta Hasta Sirsasana A, B, and C.*

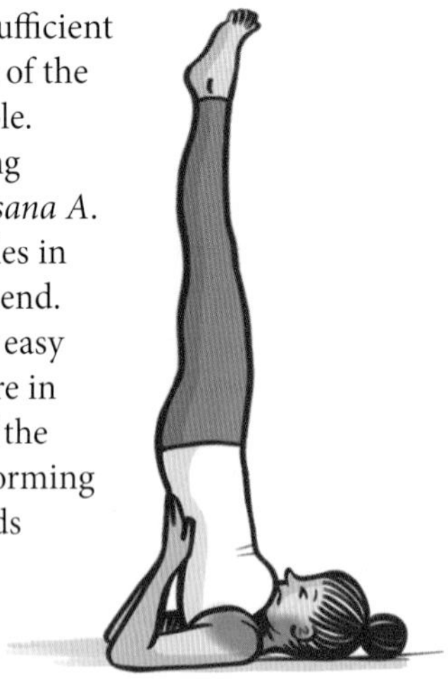

Figure 5.5 The cervical spine can be vulnerable.

Of course, with those examples above, the factors of strength, ROM, technique, and familiarity will play significant roles in diluting the risk. There are also many postures whose compromised form is somewhat the accepted norm unless you are studying with the most alignment-based teachers.

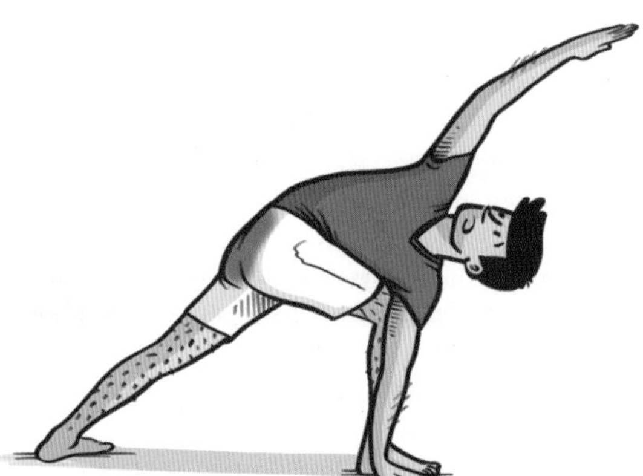

Figure 5.6 With the foot turned out, it can lock the pelvis in place.

Marichyasana D would be one such posture where there is an accepted version that is less than perfect. With one hip raised, the pelvis is uneven, and the spine laterally flexed. Then there is the adding of a twist and the potential floating knee of the leg in *Padmasana* (either one or both often visible).

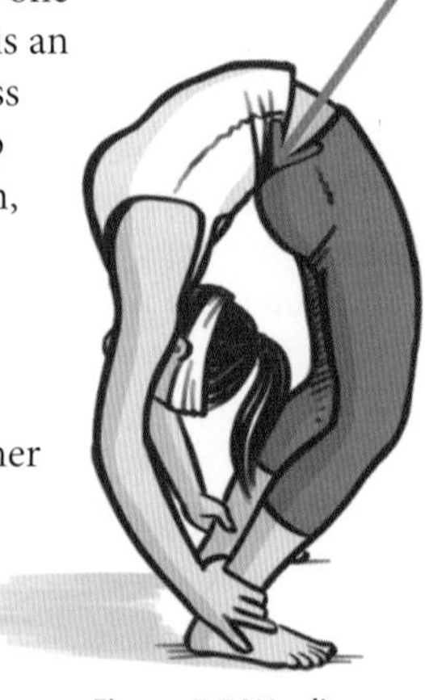

Figure 5.7 We discuss hinging in the Backbends *chapter.*

In my eyes, *Marichyasana D* is an excellent example of where—for the majority of students—posture risk and student technique don't sync up. If performed with both hips grounded and the knee of the leg in *Padmasana* on the floor, with no sickling of the ankle, and minimal flexing of the spine, then it could be said the posture is not risky (Figure 5.10A) because, positioned like this, it is not asking for joint alignment and weight-bearing that is undesirable, unlike the example of *Bakasana* previously. However, the widely accepted norm for the posture, which is with one hip way up and quite often a knee too, does have risks, even if the idea is that you will work one or both down over time.

The posture calls for one leg to be in *Ardha Padmasana* and then to add a bound twist. For those students with insufficient external rotation in the *Ardha Padmasana* hip, bringing that knee down further will lift the opposite hip, making the

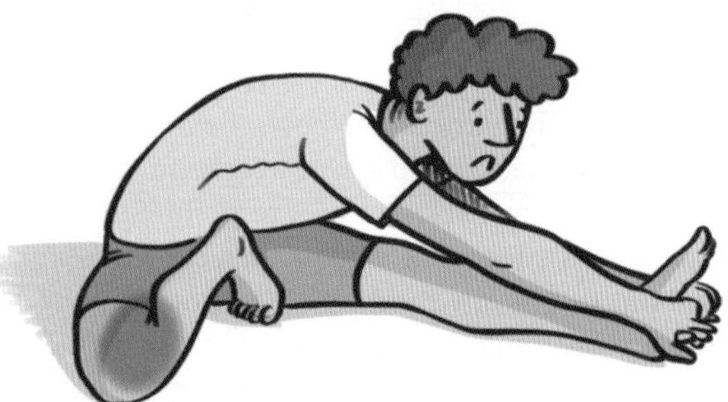

Figure 5.8 Janu Sirsasana C, *one of my least favorite postures for its potential to create torquing forces.*

pelvis more unlevel. From that position, if the upper body is then moved toward the side of the raised hip to grab or bind the leg, the spine will have to side bend and flex (even more so if the student is in the habit of leaning way forward to wrap the arm). From this bent position, a twist to the spine is added as the knee is passed and the bind taken (Figure 5.10B). Because the arm is in contact with the leg, it is possible to add some force into the equation (sometimes a lot if this posture is not freely available and the student is determined).

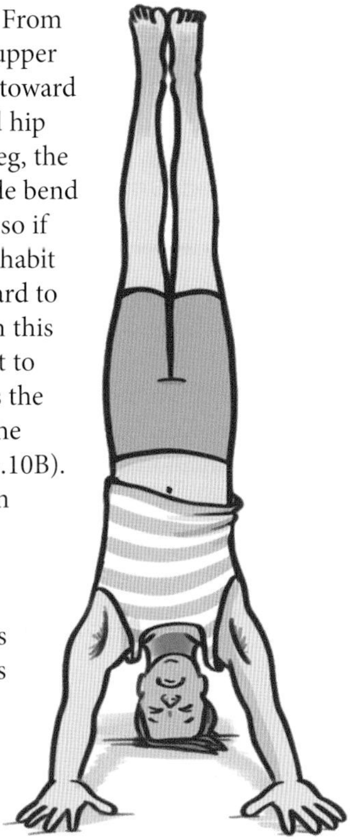

Figure 5.9 In Sirsasana *variations like these, there is no way to take weight out of the cervical spine.*

One of the most common ways people hurt their backs in everyday life is with a flexed spine that is rotated and loaded. An example would be taking something heavy out of the boot of the car and then twisting and flexing the spine to place it down on the floor

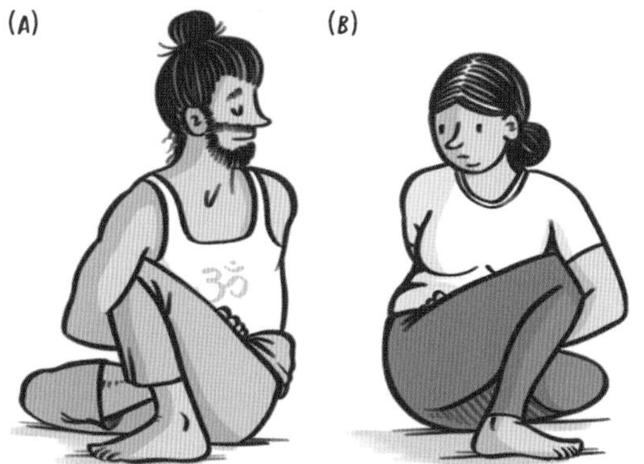

Figure 5.10 (A) Zane is properly positioned, (B) Wendy has her hip way too high, and her spine has had to flex laterally.

beside them. So, you can see how easy it is to create negative forces in this posture. We can also add to this equation the fact that often the knee of the leg in *Padmasana* is up in the air, which again makes it vulnerable. Because of the inaccessibility of safer positioning—for most students—a compromised form is widely accepted.

In reality, it is only those students with a specific proportional relationship between their upper and lower legs that will be able to keep their same side sit bone on the floor as the bent leg foot is placed down near the hip. However, a highly tilted pelvis should be avoided. We will revisit this pose in Part III, *Posture Groups*.

Other postures where I have observed a high incidence of sloppiness are *Eka Pada Sirsasana*, Drop Backs, and *Supta Kurmasana*. I'm sure if you start to think, you will come up with loads of others. It comes down to what degree the form should be compromised to make a pose more accessible.

Other factors that might make a posture more or less risky are:

- **Sequencing**: Have we opened up the correct areas prior to the more complicated postures? Where are we transitioning from to get into the pose? It might be, for example, that we are already loading a joint and then adding load by rotating on that to get into the next posture, for example, going from *Virabhadrasana C* to *Ardha Chandrasana*, where the standing hip might be vulnerable. How you transition into rock star or wild thing (if you do those postures)? We might even add in here regard for how you set yourself up to do the pose.
- **Heat and lack of**: Are you physically cold and less pliable because you have not warmed up properly. On the other hand, are you in a hot environment that makes you more flexible than usual and likely to go too deep if you are not accustomed to it?
- **Age**: Are you past your prime and should be watching TV and drinking tea (no, not really!)? With age, soft tissue becomes less elastic, and

structures can get more fragile. In particular, the vertebral discs tend to compress, making those individuals even more compromised in weight-bearing on the head. Also, along with age comes often more baggage from the affront of life on the physical body. On the bright side, occasionally there is more wisdom.

- **Joint instability**: Due to a previous injury, lack of strength, or excessive mobility.
- The **time** that you spend in the posture.
- **Suitability of surface**: The quickest way to hurt your wrists is to practice Handstand on the beach because the soft sand provides an unstable base and doesn't allow for the even/proper distribution of weight.
- **Motor skills and coordination**: For example, have you learned how to balance in Handstand before you start trying to do other fancy stuff in it. Are you just a clumsy person? We must all know someone who is always getting injured.
- And of course, all the other elements we have mentioned in the other topics (e.g., **alignment**, **strength**, **psychology**, etc.).

At the end of the day, what I want to instill, is that a posture itself can hold more or less risk but that we can also reduce or increase that risk by our actions, preparedness, psychology, awareness, etc. Additionally, each individual will react differently to a given situation depending on their restrictions, previous injuries, proportions, etc.

Our environment will influence the whole gamut.

PART II

BODY BITS

"Although it is handy to break the body down into bits, it is integrated at every level, nothing exists in isolation, and everything is far from simple."

Introduction

In the following chapters, we will be discussing the body based around the significant joints, foot and ankle, knee, hip, spine, shoulder, and wrist and elbow. As we move here to create the shapes of particular posture groups, there is a crossover between this section and the next. With that in mind, I will, along with joint construction and muscle actions, focus more on the ways in which we might position ourselves that could negatively impact the joint.

When you read about where muscles go to and from in a regular anatomy book, they will give precise detail about the origin and insertion (where the muscle attaches). This specificity is perfect if you can make use of it, but for our purposes, it is sufficient to know the rough location, front, side, top, bottom, etc., to allow us to apply our "Key Concepts." Occasionally, there may be a well-known landmark that is worth using—otherwise, I will try and keep the terminology simple.

You might think that considering which muscles move a particular joint would be relatively straightforward, but although we will present it in this way, in reality, this is not the case. Muscles have a depth and size. This might mean that particular groups of fibers within the same muscle have different directions of pull. Therefore, these areas are responsible for different actions.

Take the large trapezius muscle that spans the back from the base of the skull to the lowest thoracic vertebra and across to the shoulders. The fibers change direction so completely within different parts of the muscle that they can have opposite actions, for example, scapula elevation and depression. With other muscles, if you wanted to be very specific, you would find that sometimes there would be a change of action between superior and inferior fibers or deep and superficial. If you look in detail at the actions of gluteus medius (Gmed), the anterior fibers medially rotate the hip and the posterior fibers externally rotate the hip.

Even muscles that are grouped because of the primary action they perform may have different secondary actions, for example, the deep external rotators of the hip, where some of the six muscles in that group also abduct the hip while others adduct the hip instead. To add even more detail, some of those that perform adduction alternatively perform abduction if the hip is flexed.

If your brain has just started to curdle at the thought of all the possibilities, don't worry, for our purposes, we are going to keep it simple and stick with the main actions. I want you to appreciate that, as with most things relating to the human body, simplicity doesn't exist in reality. One point that is worth remembering is that the actions a muscle can perform depend on the direction of pull of the fibers. As we move a joint through a ROM, that direction of pull will change, and so too will the muscles that are most efficient at creating a particular movement.

I suggest you do this short practical to make some sense of what I have just covered. We are just going to move the leg out to the side and make changes to the hip position so you can feel how the muscles working alter slightly. At any time you need to rest, come down, recover, and go back up. You will be able to feel more easily what is working if you put some effort into lifting the leg as high as possible.

We are going to start close to a wall with one shoulder resting on it to help isolate the movements and prevent you from leaning sideways. Take the weight into the leg closest to the wall and then:

- Lift the other leg out to the side without turning it or taking it out of line with the body. This movement is straightforward hip abduction.
- Stay there, turn the foot toward the floor.
- Turn the foot toward the ceiling.
- Bend forward 90 degrees at the hip and repeat the previous three moves.

While in each position, have a feel of the butt and hip area on that side to establish which muscles are working hardest—you will probably sense it too. It is not necessary to know what muscle is which, just investigate the whole area from the side of the hip to the sacrum at the back. Notice also if anything is working deeper down.

You might even have felt that you don't typically work those muscles much. I know I did when I was running through this practical. Maybe you also noticed it was easier to lift the leg with a particular rotation, or the hip flexion. Hopefully, what you gained from this little experiment was an appreciation that, in yoga poses we are not in anatomical position, so the ways the muscles work and interact will not be cut and dried.

We have already talked about the fact that we live in an integrated body where there is considerable interaction and accommodation by adjacent and more distant areas. Muscles may cross multiple joints, and the position of one joint will influence another's capabilities. Furthermore, any given posture may have several variations and nuances. Breaking up the body into bits certainly makes learning more manageable, as we can think about one area at a time. However, the complication is when to talk about a particular point of interest involved in a multi-segmental movement. For the most part, in these circumstances, I have placed the material within the chapter for the joint influenced most by the body's placement. When it makes more sense, I have, on occasion, introduced an idea in one chapter and then expanded further in another.

CHAPTER 6

Foot and Ankle

The foot is a fantastic construction of 26 bones, 32 joints, and more than 100 ligaments that allows us to accommodate and balance on uneven surfaces as well as transmit forces for locomotion. They are excellent barometers of our body awareness during asana as well. Like flags at the end of sticks, they wave at us hanging limp, sickling, or unforgivingly dropping out when we are not, for example, engaging our legs in seated postures. They may even give us clues that we are over engaging specific muscles or trying to escape restrictions, such as when the feet turn out when doing Dropbacks or *Urdhva Dhanurasana*. Their orientation will be affected by those structures above them and, conversely, how and where we place the feet will not only affect the ankle but also everything else above them.

Take a look at people walking by, and you will be staggered at the variation in what we might consider an almost subconscious task. Some feet are turned out, others in, a few even straight. Now look at their knees and hips. One person's knees may be pointing straight ahead with the feet turned out, the rotation coming from the ankle or knee. Someone else may have the knees pointing out like the feet with the rotation seemingly coming from the hips. Even the way the hips move can be different, with some looking jammed up, others loose and rhythmic. Build on that and look at people running, and you will see more pronounced differences. Some feet make loops as they move forward, maybe striking the ground with one edge or other. The gait can be heavy and lead-like, or light and floaty—there may even be marked differences between the way each side is working.

These individuals will bring their movement patterns onto the yoga mat and watching what happens to their feet will lead you down many paths of discovery. Next time you get the chance to view a class in *Shavasana*, look at their feet and ask yourself some questions as to what might be going on with their bodies (Figure 6.1).

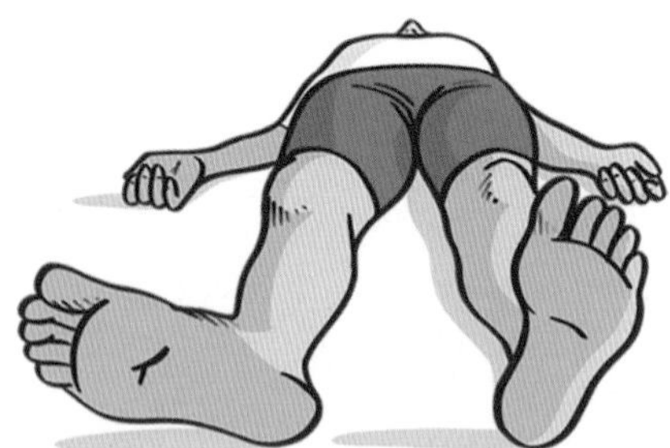

Figure 6.1 It is very common to observe uneven legs.

Construction of the Foot and Ankle

The bones in the foot come in all sorts of shapes and sizes. In what we might call the forefoot, they are long and slender. The bones that make up the toes are called phalanges, and just behind them, the metatarsals. In the midfoot are the tarsals, which resemble irregular cubes, and as you move further back to the hindfoot they are pretty substantial lumps. The largest of all is the calcaneus, your heel (Figure 6.2).

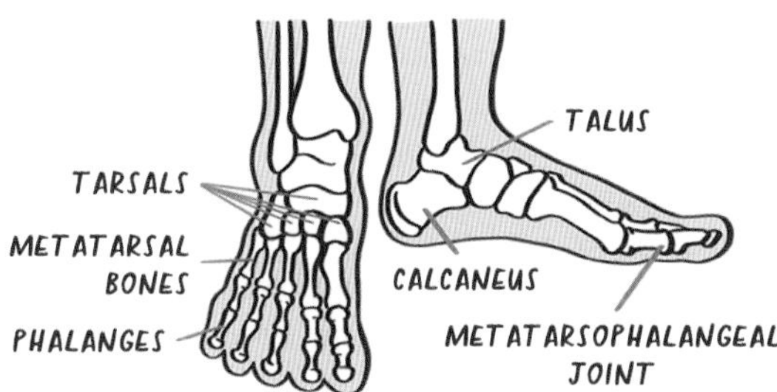

Figure 6.2 Construction of the foot and ankle.

The two bones of the lower leg—the tibia and fibula—form an articulation with the most superior tarsal bone, the talus. About 60 percent of body weight is distributed from the talus into the calcaneus, with the remaining 40 percent toward the ball of the foot by way of the other tarsal bones. You can feel your tibia as that sharp ridge running down the front of the lower leg, often referred to as the shin.

The fibula is a much smaller bone and hardly carries any of the body weight (less than 15 percent), but its distal end (further from the body) helps form the ankle joint. The fibula is the more lateral of the two bones, and remembering this makes it easy to determine which leg you are looking at in a photo (as long as you know if you are looking from the front or the back). The many bones of the foot help it to adapt to different and uneven surfaces and to maintain the characteristic shape.

We can scrunch our foot up and spread our toes (what my wife calls fleece your toes), press through the ball of our foot, etc., but the gross movements of the foot happen at the ankle.

What we commonly refer to as the ankle is, in fact, two different joints (Figure 6.3). The ankle joint itself is where the ends of the fibula (lateral malleolus) and tibia (medial malleolus) meet the talus, forming a mortice-type joint that allows only for dorsiflexion (foot drawing back toward the shin) and plantar flexion (foot pointing). Take a feel of your ankle now; those two prominences just above the foot that we often call the ankle bones are the malleoli. Then just below is the subtalar joint, where the talus sits on top of the navicular and calcaneus bones. Here we have the movements of eversion (the sole turning toward the outside of the body) and inversion (the sole turning toward the midline of the body).

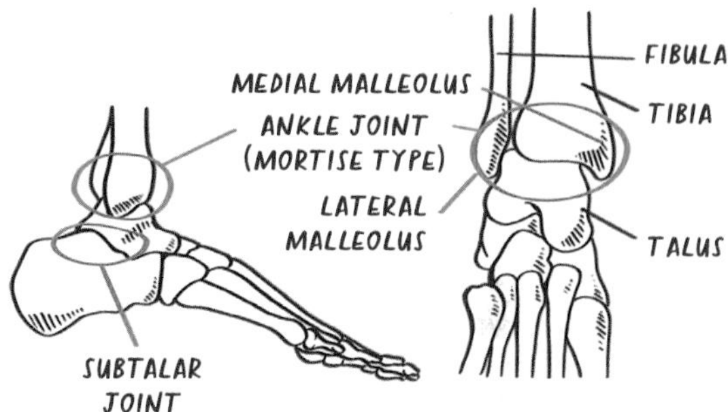

Figure 6.3 Construction of the ankle.

The talus bone is such an integral part of so many movements that 70 percent of it is covered in hyaline cartilage. The construction of this joint and the oblique angle of a stabilizing ligament result in us having a greater ROM in inversion than eversion. So don't expect it to be even; we are not built for that.

The idea here is not to get bogged down in detail but to appreciate that the ankle is more complicated than we might have thought, with many muscles having to create the necessary movements. In my mind, wherever there is complexity, there is a high chance for adaptability but also greater instability. Think how easy it is to sprain your ankle. We need to take that vulnerability into account when performing the less-than-straightforward asanas.

That said, there is one specific detail about the ankle joint that I think is useful to know to help prevent injury through repeated stressing of the ligaments.

The talus bone itself is not entirely symmetrical. The trochlear surface (the part that articulates with the distal end of the tibia) is wider at the front than the back. The consequence of this is that as you plantar flex (point) your foot, the fit of the talus within the mortise is a bit looser than when the foot is dorsiflexed. This extra play results in less stability and more strain being taken up by the ligaments. The least stable position is when the foot is inverted and plantar flexed. This is precisely the position the foot can land up in when we place it into *Ardha Padmasana* or *Padmasana* if we do not have enough external rotation in the hip to position it correctly. We will come back to this in Chapter 8, *Hip*.

Ligaments are connective tissue and go from one bone to another to increase joint stability and resist undesirable movements. Therefore, we don't want to overstretch ligaments because it will introduce instability. After about a 6 percent stretch, damage is likely to occur, called a sprain or tear. In people termed hypermobile, the ligaments can be stretchier and allow for more significant joint movement, but along with this can also come pain and a higher likelihood of dislocation. Building muscular strength would be one of the priorities of hypermobile yoga practitioners so that they can enjoy their freedom while also protecting their body.

For every practitioner, being active in postures is more likely to protect the ligaments than being passive and hanging in the joints. Ligaments are quite good at resisting sudden forces, but with prolonged forces, they tend to weaken and lengthen. As ligaments help support the arches of the foot, the repeated and extended periods of weight-bearing experienced by people that have to stand a lot as part of their job can result in their arches flattening. You can often observe the same flattening arches in hypermobile students because of their potentially weaker and more flexible ligaments.

Muscles that Move the Foot and Ankle

Often, the arrangement of muscles in the body is such that they are positioned in the adjacent body part to the one they move or stabilize. For instance, the soleus, whose job it is to plantar flex, is on the back of the lower leg. With the foot and ankle, we have muscles that reside in the foot (intrinsic) and others that are in the lower leg (extrinsic), Figure 6.4. We won't single out the intrinsic muscles, but as a group, they have an essential role in supporting the arches of the foot, distributing forces during gait, and moving the toes individually. Exercises such as grabbing a towel with your toes and lifting individual toes can help strengthen these muscles and, in turn, help toward supporting a falling arch.

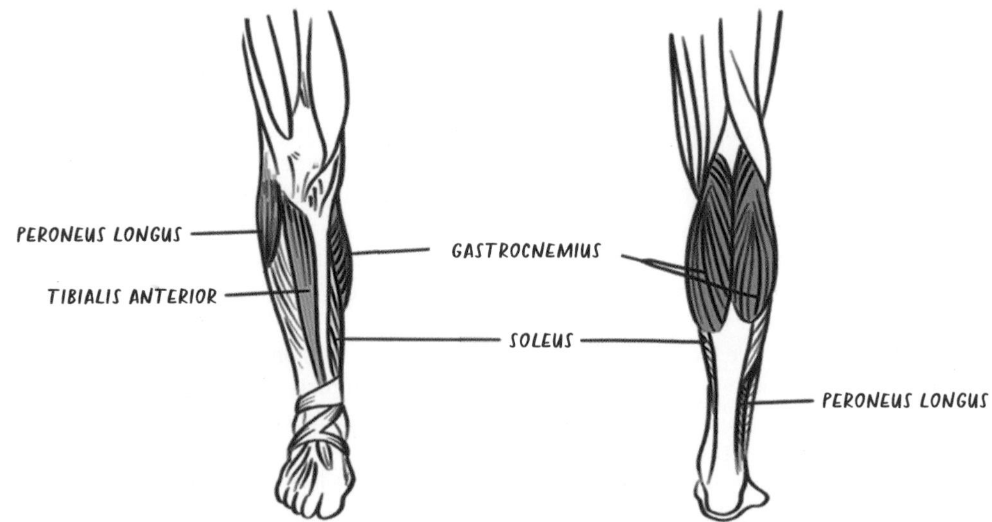

Figure 6.4 Muscles that move the foot and ankle.

The gross movements of the foot and ankle happen due to the extrinsic muscles located on the posterior, anterior, and lateral aspects of the lower leg. For our purposes, the most important of these are tibialis anterior, gastrocnemius, soleus, and peroneus longus, as they produce the movements of plantar flexion, dorsiflexion, inversion, and eversion.

Tibialis Anterior

Tibialis anterior is found on the front of the lower leg (tibia), but because of the wedge shape of the tibia, it is on its lateral aspect. Interestingly, it crosses over the front of the ankle and attaches under the medial arch of the foot. Because of this oblique pulling angle, it not only dorsiflexes the foot but also inverts it (Figure 6.5).

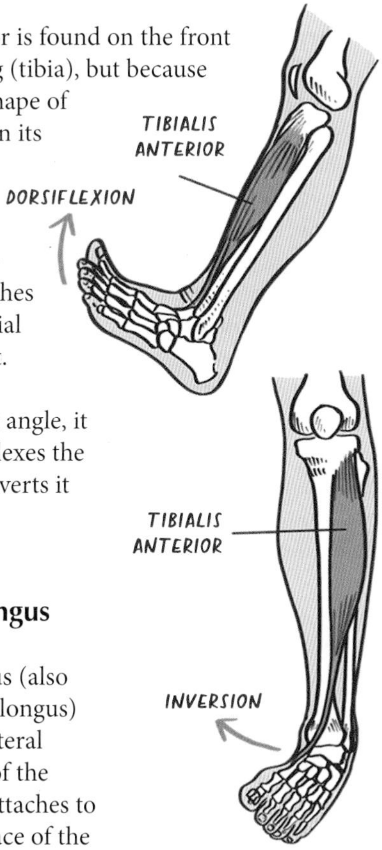

Figure 6.5 The actions of tibialis anterior: dorsiflexion and inversion.

Peroneus Longus

Peroneus longus (also called fibularis longus) is part of the lateral compartment of the lower leg and attaches to the lateral surface of the fibula (Figure 6.6). Its tendon passes behind the lateral malleolus and under the foot to connect to the medial arch in near enough the same place as tibialis anterior. So, this muscle will dorsiflex the foot the same as tibialis anterior but then also evert because it has crossed under the foot.

Tibialis anterior and peroneus longus act together to form a stirrup that helps support the arches of the foot. These muscles will also help with side-to-side balancing, such as when you are standing on one leg.

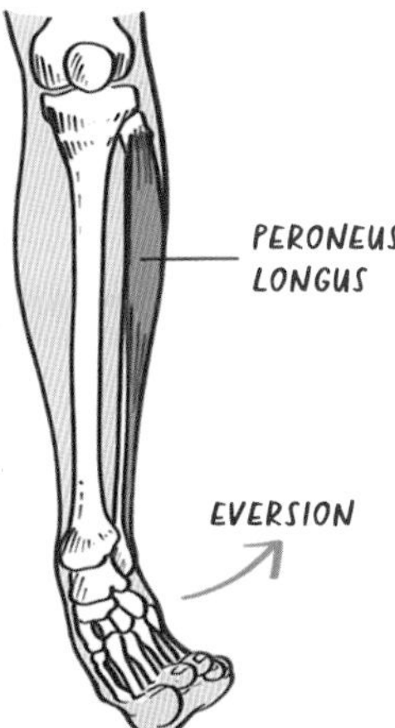

Figure 6.6 Peroneus (fibularis) longus.

Gastrocnemius

Gastrocnemius is a polyarticular muscle and has two bellies, which, at the upper end, cross the knee and attach to the back of the upper leg bone (femur) close to the knee joint (Figure 6.5). The hamstrings pass on their outside on the way to attach to the lower leg. The lower end of the muscle connects to the calcaneus via the Achilles tendon. When it contracts, it causes both plantar flexion and knee flexion, but will resist dorsiflexion. It might resist knee extension if the ankle was already strongly dorsiflexed.

Soleus

The soleus doesn't cross the knee but instead attaches to the back of the lower leg bones (tibia and fibula), Figure 6.7. Then, like the gastrocnemius, it

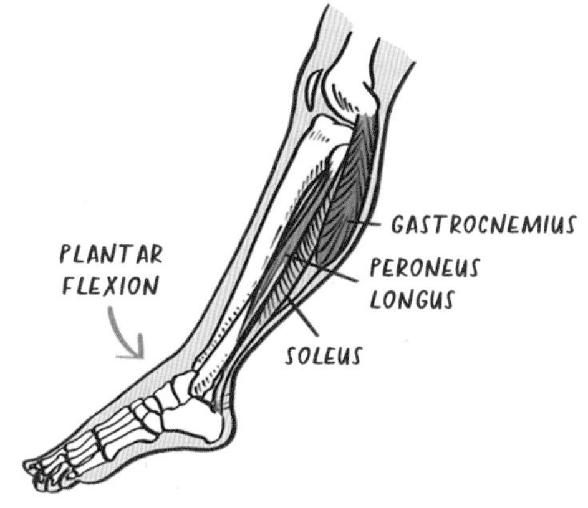

Figure 6.7 Gastrocnemius and soleus both plantar flex the foot.

connects to the calcaneus via the Achilles tendon. Because it doesn't cross the knee, it only plantar flexes and will resist dorsiflexion.

Quick Reference Muscle Action Tables

Plantar Flexion	Dorsiflexion
Gastrocnemius	Tibialis anterior
Soleus	Peroneus brevis and longus
Tibialis posterior	Extensor digitorum longus
Peroneus brevis and longus	Extensor hallucis longus
Flexor hallucis longus	Peroneus tertius
Flexor digitorum longus	

Inversion	Eversion
Tibialis anterior	Peroneus brevis and longus
Extensor hallucis longus	Peroneus tertius
Tibialis posterior	Extensor digitorum longus
Flexor hallucis longus	
Flexor digitorum longus	

You will notice that there are more muscles listed in the tables than we have introduced. To keep things simple, we are focusing on the main muscles that do specific actions, and they are listed first in the tables. However, often there will be other muscles that can help or perform the same actions. We have included these in the tables for those who are interested but don't feel you need to know this level of detail. The same applies for all muscle action tables in this section of the book.

Arches of the Foot

The feet have three arches, two longitudinal (medial and lateral) and one transverse (Figure 6.8). They help distribute the body weight across the foot, create leverage when walking and running, and act like shock absorbers similar to the curvatures of the spine. The arches themselves are maintained by the shape of the bones, ligaments, muscle activity, and muscle tendons (acting somewhat like ligaments). If they weren't supported in this way, the weight of the body would flatten the arches.

You can see from the images that some bones are considered to be part of more than one arch. In some ways, the division is somewhat

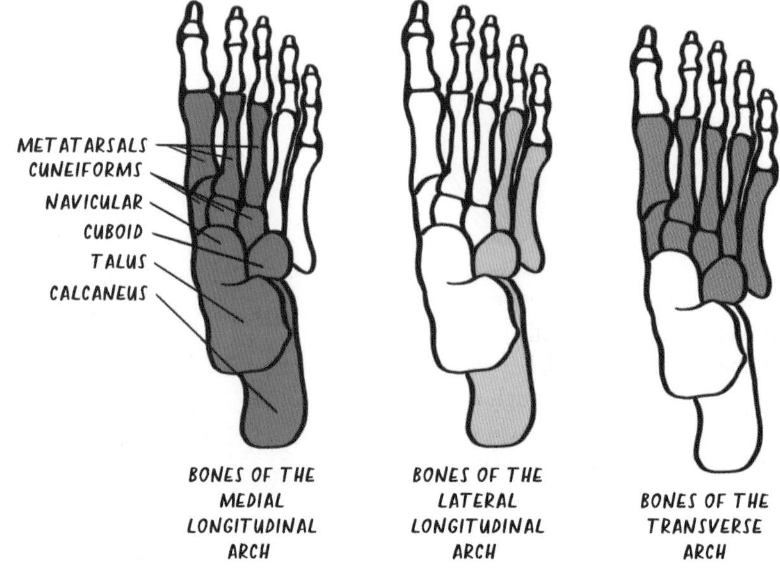

Figure 6.8 The three arches of the foot.

arbitrary—you might consider there to be one three-dimensional arch spanning the whole rear and midsections of the foot (Figure 6.9).

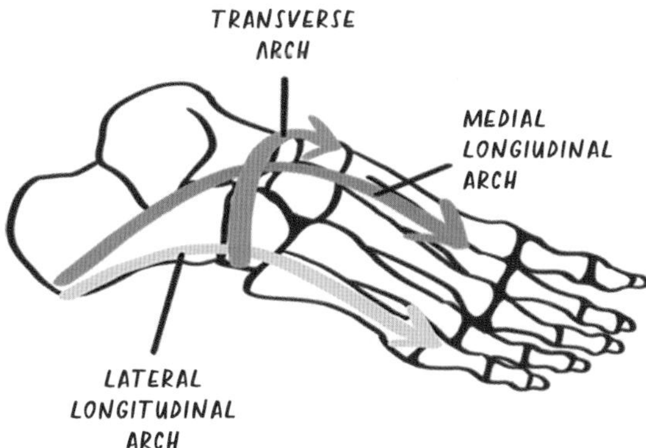

Figure 6.9 There are three arches in the foot, but they all blend into one three-dimensional structure.

When the medial longitudinal arch is not being appropriately supported and decreases in height, the condition is known as pes planus (flat feet or fallen arches). Often flat feet are congenital, but they may also be acquired by placing repeated stress on the supporting structures by, for instance, jobs that require standing stationary for long periods and chronic tension in the gastrocnemius and soleus muscles. If you are considered hypermobile, then you might also be prone to flat feet. Those same more pliable ligaments that allow for excessive movements around other joints will also be problematic in the feet as the ligaments play a crucial role in supporting the arch.

The causes are varied, but in many circumstances, much can be done to bring some life back into the arches. Working the muscles that support the arch, actively seeking to align the foot in a better way, avoiding long periods of standing still, and generally using the feet more actively will go a long way to halting the progression and, hopefully, reversing the decline.

One of the frequent consequences of the arch flattening is for the foot to turn out (abduct) and evert as more pressure comes onto the medial part of the foot. This is likely to be combined with a mild increase in dorsiflexion. Those three movements in combination constitute pronation. In circumstances when this is excessive, it would be called overpronation, characterized by an inward collapsing of the heel. This places stress on the ligaments on the medial aspect of the ankle and can cause some impingement of soft tissue on the lateral aspect of the ankle. Yoga offers an ideal opportunity to work on addressing this issue. Still, it will need constant awareness by the practitioner because the natural inclination will be to keep collapsing the medial side of the foot. Particular attention will need to be paid to single-leg balancing postures as the ankle is carrying more weight. It will be noticeable in all standing poses, apparent in some more than others. The main thing is to try and create a new pattern of supporting the medial side of the foot and ankle in many varied positions.

One very good way of trying to establish some lift of the medial arch is to make use of one of the structures already there and designed to do the job. The plantar fascia is a band of thick fascia (well, actually an aponeurosis, but let's not get pedantic) that, at one end, attaches to the calcaneus (heel bone) and at the other to the base of the toes (Figure 6.10). By connecting to both ends of the arch, it provides support and resists the arch dropping. I think of it as much like the cross beam of an A-frame or easel. It is different from that example, of course, by the fact that it can stretch, which allows it to act as a shock absorber and can

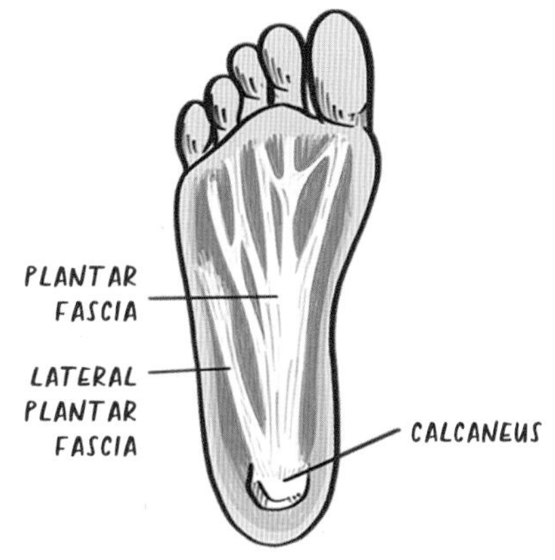

Figure 6.10 The plantar fascia spans the sole of the foot.

return energy in phases of the gait cycle. If the toes are dorsiflexed, then this tensions the plantar fascia further, causing a rise in the arch.

So, if we have that collapsing tendency after trying to align the foot, we can raise the toes and get some lift to the arch (Figure 6.11). This immediately reduces how much the ankle drops in and the willingness of the foot to turn out. The tricky bit now is to feel the muscles that were engaged in this process and keep some activation in them as you lower the toes back to the floor. With practice, you will then be able to recreate the action without lifting the toes first.

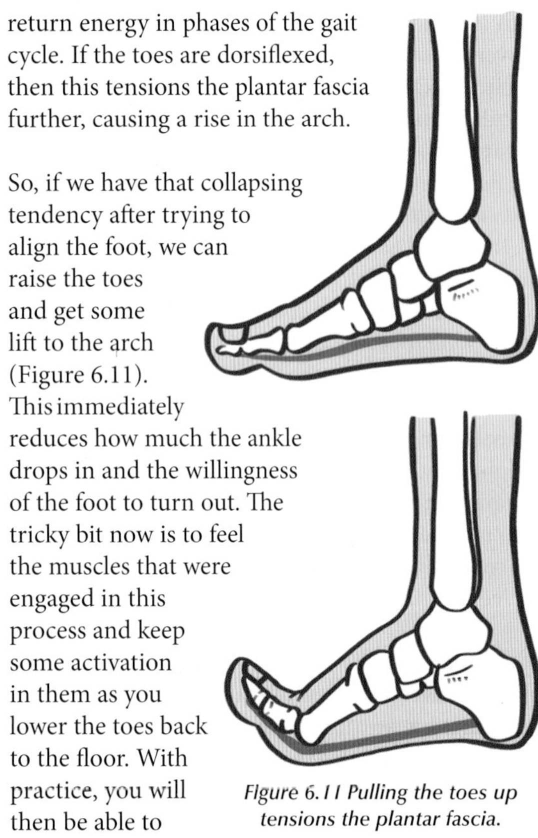

Figure 6.11 Pulling the toes up tensions the plantar fascia.

There are also many people who take the weight more to the outside edge of the feet—that inversion, plantar flexion, and adduction combination accounts for supination and can also present itself in excess (over supination). It is not as easy to spot as over supination (unless you are watching someone running), but in balancing postures, you may begin to see the medial side of the foot lifting.

These students will need to actively encourage eversion to help bring the foot and ankle back toward neutral. A cue like pressing through the base of the big toe into the floor might go some way to help. It wouldn't be at all surprising to observe the same students' feet in inversions, twisting and parting with the soles moving toward each other. Giving the instruction to bring together the knees, ankle bones, and big toe joints, while at the same time reaching away with the ball of the feet, will help straighten things out. As a teacher, you often find yourself viewing the student from the front, as you can see from the image below when it comes to ankle alignment—a view from behind speaks volumes (Figure 6.12).

As I mentioned at the beginning of this chapter, the positioning of the feet will have a consequence on other body parts, in particular, the knee as it is the closest articulation (more in Chapter 7, *Knee*). The asana practice is a great time to be working on strengthening the muscles of the legs that support the arches. Awareness built up now

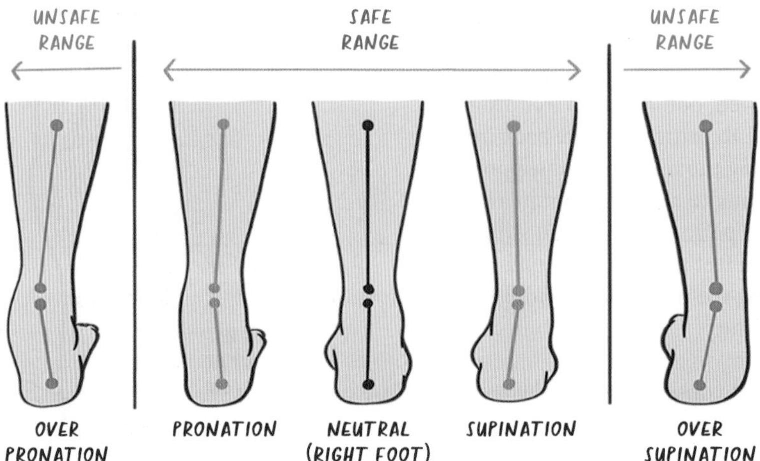

Figure 6.12 It is much easier to see the ankle dropping inward or outward from the back.

will help you carry this alignment into daily life. If you are a teacher, you will need to keep reminding your students as we all happily fall back into our ingrained patterns.

Foot Alignment

The longitudinal alignment of the foot is through the second metatarsal (the toe next to the big toe), and the center of the heel. The toes themselves are the phalanges, so we are talking about the area of the foot just behind that toe, but you get the idea. This means that when you are aligning your feet in, say *Tadasana* you may have to have the sides of your big toes touching and your heels slightly apart (Figure 6.13A). Check it out on yourself. Bear this in mind when you are setting up for your standing postures. Get your foot aligned first and work up from there (Figure 6.13B).

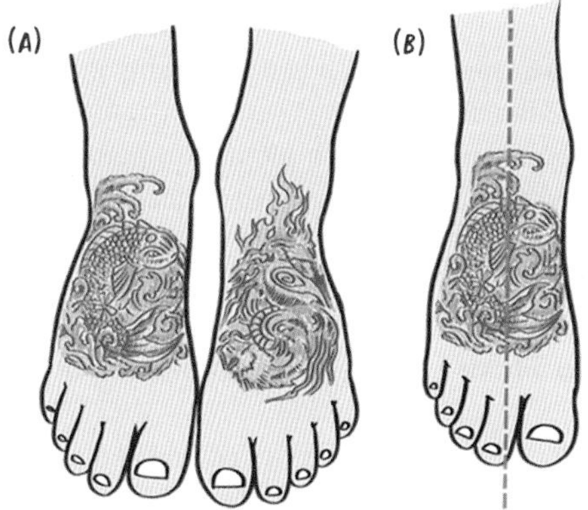

Figure 6.13 The feet in Tadasana *(A) toes touching and heels slightly apart, (B) foot aligned.*

Down Dog is another good posture to check out your alignment as it is easy to see your feet (Figure 6.14). If you have flat feet and overpronate, the chances are that as your ankle drops in, your heels will move toward the center line of the mat. Keep an eye out for this and encourage them back to neutral. It may be exaggerated if the heels are not down—we might also notice that if our feet point outward and we straighten our feet up without incorporating other actions, it may have the undesirable result of the knees pointing in. Think about which of the examples we might be referring to?

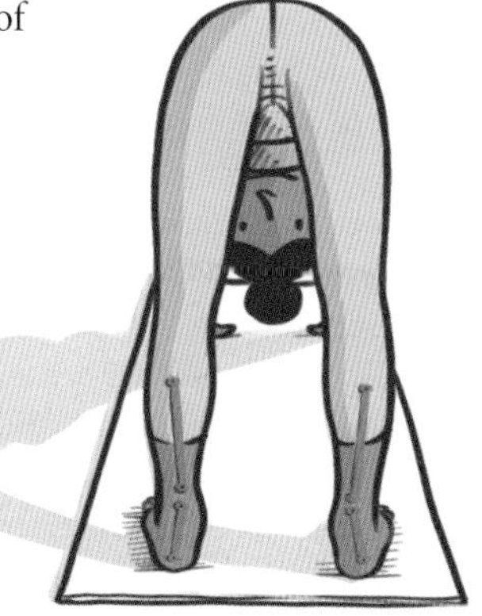

Figure 6.14 Down Dog is an ideal pose to look out for wayward ankles.

The knees moving too far toward the center when the feet are moved to align them is problematic. It is most likely to happen if the reason for the feet pointing out in the first place is to do with either collapsing of the arch, or tensional patterns causing the lower leg to be laterally rotated relative to the upper leg. In the normal stance, you will notice the knees and feet are not facing in the same direction. When the rotation is from the hip, the feet and knees tend to be facing the same way, and when you move the feet, the knees and feet keep that same orientation. Of course, I am sure that it is possible to have all of these occurring simultaneously.

If the arch is the problem, then when we align the feet, if we re-establish the arch by engaging muscles and lifting the toes, the knees will move back to the center. It won't stay there though if, as we focus on other things, we let the arch go again. If, however, the reason is the lateral rotation of the lower leg, then the alignment of the knee will not be as easy to correct. Here we have to decide what is more important—the knees facing forward but the feet out, or the feet aligned and the knees turned in. I would say that it is more important to have the knees facing forward as otherwise, the knees are vulnerable. You can see now it is not as easy as just getting someone to move their foot to a particular position.

So, let's say we have adjusted our alignment and then we do a vinyasa and jump or step back to standing, for most people, you will already be back to your usual pattern. So, attention is required before or as we come back up.

It is not just *Tadasana* but all postures—standing, seated, or inverted. The former gets more attention because we are in the ready-to-start position, but actually, I find once students start to move, they forget all about what they did when standing still. Inversions are a great time to observe and correct foot alignment because it is easy to follow a pattern through the body.

Balancing postures are another good time to bring attention to what is happening with the feet. There may be a tendency to take the weight to the inside or outside of the feet, as well as forward or backward. In yoga, we are trying to ground through the four corners of the feet (Figure 6.15).

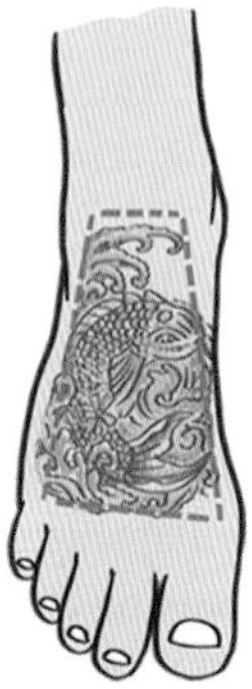

Figure 6.15 Grounding through the four corners of the feet.

If your weight is toward the outside, you will, as mentioned previously, need to press more firmly into the base of the big toe and think of everting your feet. If you are prone to flat feet or overpronation, you will more than likely drop your weight to the inside and see the foot turning out. Here, you can work on inverting the feet and spreading the weight more toward the outer side of the foot. You will be astonished by how much you can realign the foot by drawing up the medial arch. As the arch rises, it tends to reduce the amount of abduction that has occurred, bringing the foot back toward the center line and neutrality. Remember the tip to draw the toes off the floor, feeling the lift in the arch, and then trying to place the toes back down while maintaining that lift.

Even if you set up with your foot aligned, you may well turn it out once you are balancing, especially if there happens to be a little wobble. It is quite a good practice to check your feet periodically when exiting a pose to see what you may have done unconsciously while in it. With balance in general, it helps not to be too rigid and forceful. Instead, play with the edges of balance, softly shifting your weight and not overcorrecting.

Patterns of aberrant foot orientation will repeat themselves over many different and seeming unrelated postures. For example, we could consider the common problem of feet twisting in poses.

Let's say that in *Paschimottanasana* the soles of the feet, instead of facing away, turn toward the midline and the ankles start to separate. This is a pattern likely to repeat itself in many postures, not only those that fall within the same seated forward fold category, e.g., *Janu Sirsasana*. You may well experience the same actions in *Salabhasana*, *Sirsasana*, Shoulderstand, *Virabhadrasana C*, in fact, any posture where one or more legs are straight and not constrained by the friction of the floor.

Particularly problematic are postures where the feet are out of sight because we must rely on spatial awareness, which can invariably give us false feedback. Things feel square or inline, but if someone showed you a picture or, better yet, adjusted you, it would be hard to accept. It felt right, but such is the nature of patterns.

So How Do We Start Working on This?

If you notice that your feet twist one way or the other in the seated postures, then this is a good time to work with them because they are right in front of you. You could take your hand and physically turn the foot back to where it should be and then maintain its position there with continued contact. I feel this is a sensible starting place because it tells you if the foot will go to where you want it to or if something is physically stopping it. It may even make you have to release muscular engagement somewhere for you to move the foot. If it moves, then you can consider if it is tensional patterns pulling the foot out of place or if you are using muscles to do the posture in such a way that the side effect is distortion of the foot position.

So, we have started the ball rolling by physically moving the foot, but we are not adequately establishing new patterns. We need to begin engaging muscles in such a way as to keep the foot where we have put it. What we need to do is loosen our grip on the foot until it is the softest of touches and see if we can maintain the foot position there while we do the posture. The hand still in place will let us know if the foot starts to drift back. You can then build it up by removing the help from the hand but supported by visual feedback, and then begin to position the foot with the eyes closed. Now we are building up the motor skills to move and keep the foot where we want it and the spatial awareness to be able to do the same when we can't see the foot, e.g., in *Sirsasana*.

I see many students with their legs and feet not symmetrical in *Sirsasana*, and if you look very closely, the chances are their whole body is a bit off-angle. Working with the alignment of the legs and feet can start to straighten out the body and add more stability. Depending on how your legs are shaped, different parts will not come in contact. For example, if your legs are a little bowed, the knees won't touch. The main thing is to sense the same body bits on both sides in contact with the same pressure and positioning. If structure allows, aim to feel the inside of the thighs, inside of the knees, medial malleoli (ankle bones), and medial bases of the big toes, all touching evenly. Don't be happy with just them contacting, bring your focus onto the exact same points of each area.

Here's an exercise you can try out. Arrange a little helper to take some photos. Do your *Sirsasana* with your usual level of awareness and ask your friend to take some images from behind. Then with their vocal cuing, tune into your body and make sure everything is touching in exactly the same way as described previously (inner thighs, inner knees, medial malleoli, and medial surface of the big toe joint). Then, keeping all this the same, really reach toward the ceiling, either with the bases of your toes (if you plantar flex the feet) or the whole sole of the feet (if you dorsiflex the feet).

When you compare, don't just focus on the legs but also look at the entire body. Did it also make you feel more secure? While the camera is out, you might as well have them also take some pics of you doing postures such as *Virabhadrasana C*, *Ardha Chandrasana*, and *Salabhasana*, so that you can see if your feet and legs are aligned the way you think you are.

In *Salabhasana*, many people allow the knees and ankles to come apart even if they keep the big toes touching. Has this been a conscious choice, and if so why, or is it just a lack of spatial awareness and focus? Another good time to do some work is in Shoulderstand because the leg position is similar to *Sirsasana*, but we can see the feet to correct their positioning. Again, you can try with the eyes closed and then look to see if they are where you think they are.

Putting Things into Context

Let's consider what we are asking of the ankle in certain poses, and when we might use some of these actions. Remember here the material we talked about in Chapter 3, *Opposing Muscles Restrict*, namely that the muscles that create movement in one direction can resist the movement in the opposite direction. Also, from Chapter 3, *Strength*, that by engaging muscles that cross a joint, we can create stability in that joint.

In *Baddha Konasana*, we are inverting the feet. The instruction is often, "Try and open your feet like a book." We can even use our hands to encourage this movement, but the intention is not to create more inversion at the ankle but to elicit a greater opening higher up the chain (external rotation and abduction of the hip), Figure 6.16.

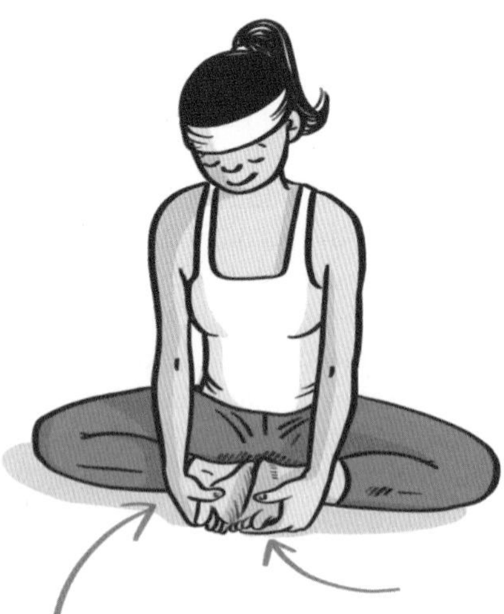

Figure 6.16 Inverting the feet hopefully helps access the hips.

We don't want to overdo it—once the hips hold fast, we shouldn't keep trying to invert the feet by using our hands because we will only place stress on the ankle or knee. The ankle is, however, in a much more stable position here than when in either *Padmasana* or *Ardha Padmasana* because the foot is dorsiflexed not plantar flexed, and the lateral aspect of the ankle is resting on the floor.

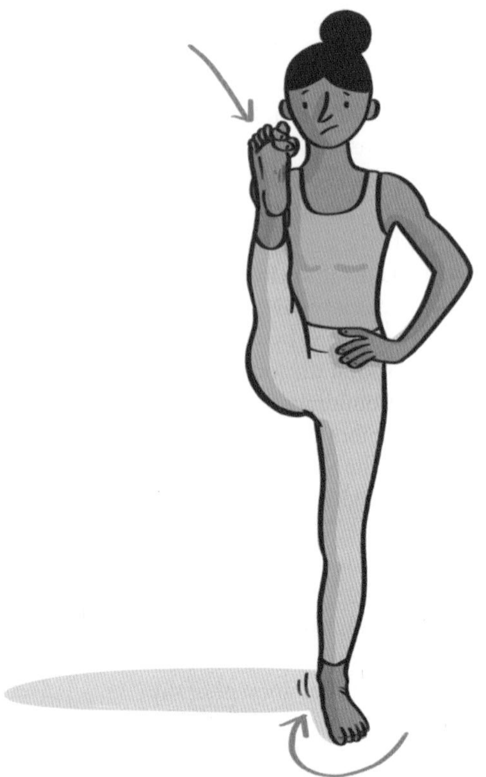

Figure 6.17 There is much work to do in Utthita Hasta Padangusthasana.

By grasping our big toe in postures like *Utthita Hasta Padangusthasana* (Figure 6.17) and *Paschimottanasana*, we may tend to pull the foot into inversion, counter this with actively everting the foot, and pushing away with the base of the big toe to level off the foot. In the same posture, if the arch of the standing leg is collapsing and the ankle rolling in, actively engage tibialis anterior (and its friends) on the front and lateral side of the shin to encourage inversion and a drawing up of the arch. You can also try lifting the toes to get the plantar fascia to help raise the arch. This idea can be repeated in any single-leg balancing posture.

Getting the heels down in *Pashasana* is often difficult for people not used to squatting (you can also think of sitting deep in *Utkatasana*). The ankle needs to be able to perform enough dorsiflexion for this to happen but may be restricted by tension in the soleus because it is a plantar flexor (Figure 6.18). Why not the gastrocnemius you ask, also being a plantar flexor of the ankle? Tension in the gastrocnemius will be reduced because it crosses the knee, and the knee is bent in this posture, bringing the lower and upper attachment points closer together. Therefore, to improve dorsiflexion with a bent knee, you need to focus on poses that also have a bent knee. Down Dog won't cut it.

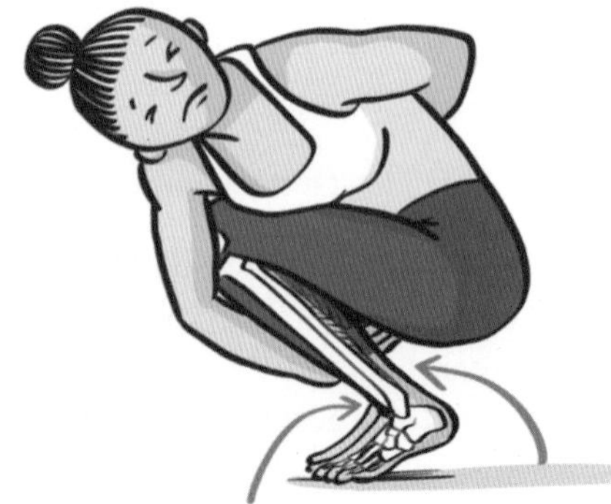

Figure 6.18 Soleus could well resist the ankle moving deeper into dorsiflexion.

There is a common perception that dorsiflexing the foot, e.g., in *Eka Pada Rajakapotasana*, will help stabilize and protect the knee. If you look at Figures 6.4–6.7, you will see that no muscles responsible for dorsiflexion cross the knee. Therefore, it is tenuous to say that the action in isolation would perform this function. However, it does seem to help, probably because as you are engaging muscles to dorsiflex the foot, at the same time, you are subconsciously engaging muscles to stabilize the rest of the leg (Figure 6.19). Although useful, depending on the orientation of the leg, it will not always be the best thing to do. I will explain more on this in Chapter 7.

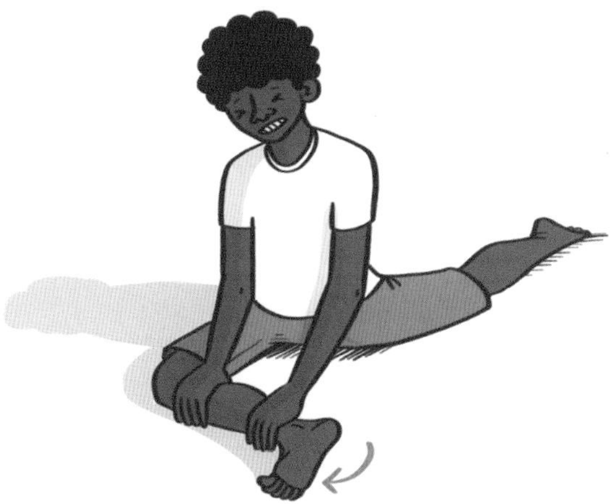

Figure 6.19 Aren would need to change the orientation of his foot if the front shin moves back toward the hip.

Check out the wear patterns of your feet on the mat. Are they even? If not, ask yourself, why not? Chances are that if you have a practice that involves jumping forward, you are either using more strength in one leg or are not square when you push off.

When we are rolling over the toes (or sliding our feet back) to go from *Chaturanga* to Up Dog, many students let their ankles drop out (even to a lesser extent going from Up Dog to Down Dog) rather than keeping the foot running straight (Figure 6.20). The reasons behind this may be

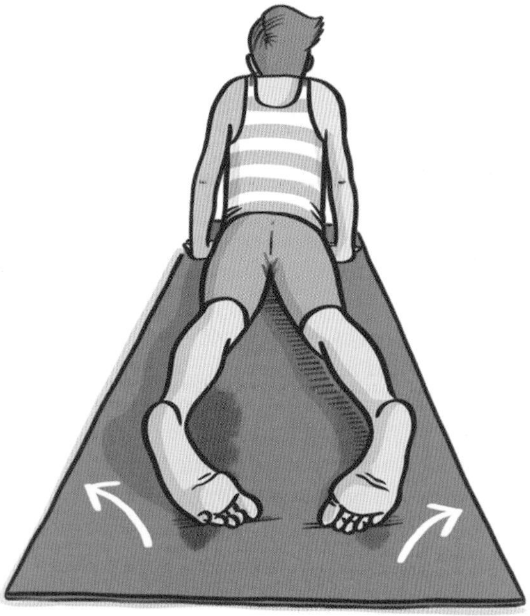

Figure 6.20 Ben really needs to control his ankles when transitioning.

anything from lack of awareness to stiff big toe joints, long big toes, and restrictions on the front of the ankle and shin. The result, however, is a less than perfect position in Up Dog because, more often than not, the feet will stay in that ankle rolled out position. This makes it hard to press evenly onto the top of the feet and tends to take the legs wider. This can all lead to more tension being placed into the low back as the pelvis drops toward the floor.

You may notice that a student looks high and uncomfortable in *Balasana*. Tightness in the Gmax and low back muscles may be one reason but also look to see if there is a gap between the front of the ankle and the floor. This would indicate a potential restriction in those muscles that perform dorsiflexion (e.g., tibialis anterior) as they will restrict plantar flexion, which is what needs to happen in this example (Figure 6.21). Consider also *Purvottanasana* and the soles of the feet not contacting the floor. Although, the reason in this last example is more often a weak core or restriction in the shoulders.

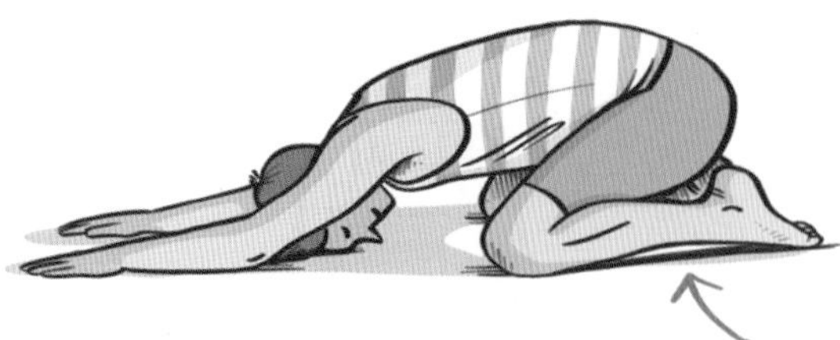

Figure 6.21 Tibialis anterior can resist the ankle plantar flexing sufficiently.

In postures such as *Parshvakonasana* and *Virabhadrasana B*, you may often notice more weight coming into the inside edge of the back foot or even the outside edge of the foot lifting off the floor. Actively inverting the foot is the action that will help even off the contact with the floor and reduce stress on the inside of the knee (Figure 6.22).

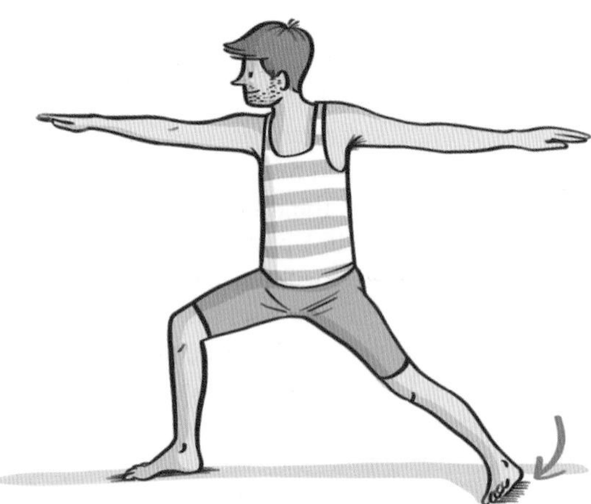

Figure 6.22 Actively inverting the back foot will help to keep it grounded.

When we look at the knee, we will consider why it is important to have the feet and knees pointing in the same direction in many postures, also, whether the knee needs always to stay behind or in line with the ankle.

We could go on, but you get the idea: the feet are very important. If you notice they are doing something that you did not want them to, ask yourself why. There will be a reason. In your practice during the next weeks, bring more attention to your feet and observe if you are doing any of the things brought up here or, indeed, something we haven't. Then play with trying to change things and if you can't, think about why it is difficult. Often, it is about creating a new pattern and sticking with it. If you are a teacher, start to notice if you see patterns of particular foot movements in your students and whereabouts in the practice—it might be easiest to begin addressing them.

CHAPTER 7

Knee

The knee is a critical joint in yoga and one where many students experience issues. Situated between the two longest bones in the body, the femur and tibia, there is great potential for the interplay of many forces. Muscular restriction around the knee itself and adjacent joints, alignment, or spatial placement of the knee relative to the foundation and body mass, are all factors that come into play. Due to the construction of the knee, it is particularly vulnerable to shearing and torquing forces. We will look at how the placement of the body can create this potential. The risks to the knee are very much related to hip freedom and the ability to move in the necessary amounts when creating postures. Another consideration is the movement patterns of many Western practitioners.

The knee is what we might call a modified hinge because, as well as the movements of flexion (bending) and extension (straightening), there is also both medial and external rotation, but only when the knee is bent. These extra movements allow the knee to be more adaptive, for example, to uneven surfaces. On average, there is almost twice as much external rotation available as there is internal.

Construction of the Knee Joint

Unlike the elbow that has a bony stop to prevent excessive extension, there is nothing in the shape of the bones at the knee joint that would limit movement in any particular direction. Thankfully, however, we know from experience that the knee is relatively stable when undamaged. This stability is primarily the responsibility of ligaments in and around the knee, and the multiple muscles crossing the knee joint.

The distal end of the femur finishes with two large rounded eminences, called condyles. Conversely, the end of the tibia is like a plateau with a ridge in the middle. There are several factors in the construction of the knee that help counter the potential instability. Between the two bones are horseshoe-shaped pieces of cartilage, the medial and lateral menisci (sing. meniscus), which also perform some shock absorption and distribution of forces. It is the ligaments, however, that provide the most stability (Figure 7.1).

On the lateral aspect of the knee is the lateral collateral ligament (LCL) and on the medial aspect, the medial collateral ligament (MCL). These ligaments stop any sideways movement of the two bones as well as resisting gaping. They also help protect the knee in the event of a hit from one side or the other.

Inside the knee are the cruciate ligaments, anterior (ACL) and posterior (PCL). These ligaments resist the forward or backward relative movement of the femur and tibia. The ACL tries to prevent the tibia

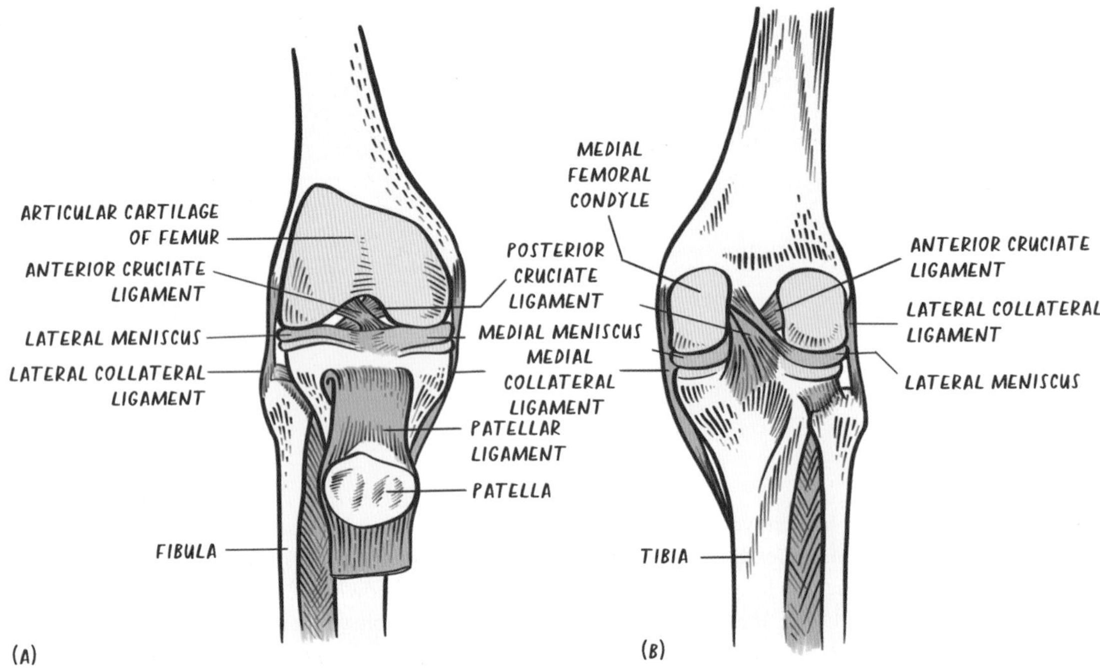

Figure 7.1 Construction of the right knee joint, (A) anterior view, (B) posterior view.

from moving anteriorly, and damage to it is one of the most common sports injuries, often involving the MCL as well. The most common mechanism of ACL injury is either an impact from the side or a pivot action where the femur and tibia rotate in opposite directions under full weight-bearing, likely including momentum as well. Luckily, the ACL is not something we tend to hurt in yoga, but we can cause damage to the collateral ligaments. More on that later.

One bone that we haven't mentioned yet is the patella or "knee cap." It sits within the quadriceps tendon helping to smooth the travel of the tendon across what would otherwise be an open space when the knee is flexed. It also increases the contraction force potential of the quadriceps by holding the tendon further forward than it would otherwise be (if you want to know how that works, you can look it up).

Muscles that Move the Knee

There are quite a few muscles that cross the knee, and as we mentioned earlier, not only do they move it but also play an essential role in stabilizing it (Figures 7.2 & 7.3).

Quadriceps

The quadriceps consist of vastus lateralis, vastus medialis, vastus intermedius, and rectus femoris, and they all perform knee extension. I can't foresee you needing to differentiate between the three vastus bellies of the quadriceps, which all attach to the upper femur. What is important is that rectus femoris passes the hip joint connecting to the AIIS, therefore, indicating that to stretch this belly efficiently, there would need to be hip extension as well as knee flexion. The quadriceps cross the knee attaching to the tibial tuberosity (just below the knee on the front of the tibia) via the patellar ligament. Strength in these muscles is an essential factor in providing stability of the knee.

Gastrocnemius

Gastrocnemius you met in the previous chapter because it also crosses the ankle where it performs

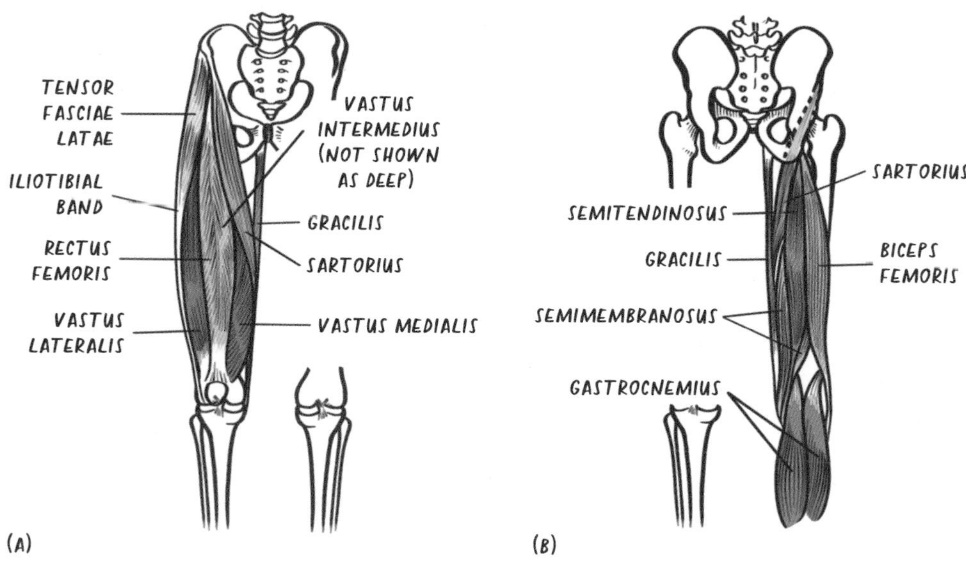

Figure 7.2 Muscles that move the knee, (A) anterior view, (B) posterior view.

plantar flexion. At the knee, it is one of the muscles responsible for knee flexion.

Other Muscles

The hamstrings are the strongest knee flexors but, sartorius, gracilis (an adductor), and popliteus (a small muscle behind the knee) all cross the knee and can help with knee flexion.

When the knee is straight, there is no rotation available at the knee but if the knee is flexed, the medial hamstrings (semimembranosus, semitendinosus), gracilis, sartorius, and popliteus, can all medially rotate the knee. The lateral hamstring (biceps femoris) can externally rotate the knee. We will cover these muscles in more detail in Chapter 7 because they also cross the hip (except for popliteus).

The lower tendons of sartorius, gracilis, and semitendinosus combine to create a three-pronged tendon called pes anserinus, meaning "goose foot" (Figure 7.4). Geese have three webbed toes in case you didn't realize. Because of the converging forces, it can be a site for overuse injuries, and it is not uncommon to find some tenderness on palpation (fancy word for having a feel). There is a bursa under the tendons that can become inflamed, and pain can also be referred to the medial aspect of the knee.

Quick Reference Muscle Action Tables

Flexion	Extension
Hamstrings: Semitendinosus, semimembranosus, biceps femoris	Rectus femoris
Gastrocnemius	Vastus lateralis
Sartorius	Vastus medialis
Gracilis	Vastus intermedius
Popliteus	
Plantaris (weak)	

Medial Rotation	Lateral Rotation
Semitendinosus, semimembranosus	Biceps femoris
Gracilis	
Sartorius	
Popliteus	

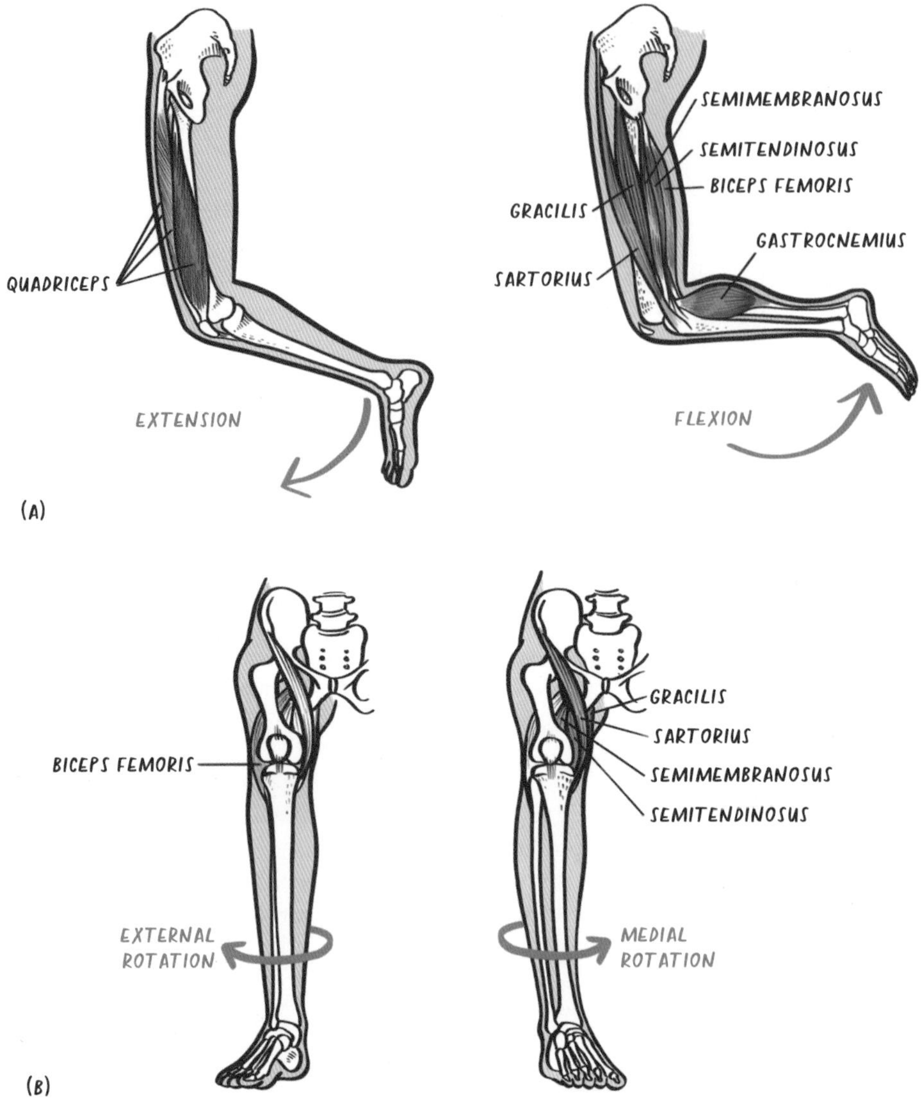

Figure 7.3 Movements of the knee, (A) flexion and extension (medial aspect of right leg), (B) rotation (bent knee, anterior view, right leg).

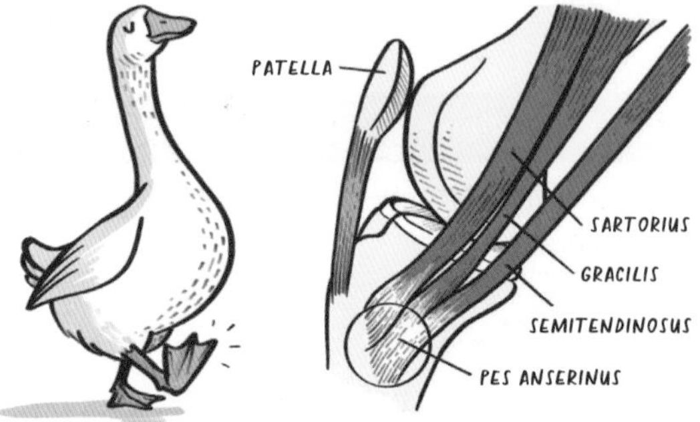

Figure 7.4 Pes anserinus, meaning "goose foot."

Putting Things into Context

Due to the limited number of large movements available at the knee, we could divide our interests into two main areas: postures that require knee flexion and vulnerabilities. Why not knee extension? Well, unless the knee is damaged, just straightening the leg is not a problem of the knee itself but rather the positioning of the body. What I mean by that is should we find ourselves in a position where we can't straighten our leg, it will be due to one of the polyarticular muscles that cross the knee. The most straightforward example to use would be when we have bent the knee to allow us to get as much hip flexion as possible. Remember, as the hamstrings cross the knee and hip, if we have some restrictions, we can bend the knee to allow a greater ROM at the hip. Once you have got that deeper hip flexion, if you maintain it and try and straighten your leg again, you may find that you can't because the hamstrings won't lengthen enough to allow the movement to happen.

Back in Chapter 1, *Fighting Own Restrictions*, we used the example of *Tittibhasana* to illustrate this point. I also don't think we need to work to increase the amount of rotation that is available at the knee—it is more of an accommodating movement than something that would stop you doing the vast majority of postures.

Many postures require us to fully close the knee joint to be able to place the foot in the desired spot or enable a level pelvis. *Padmasana* would be one such posture, which, to complete safely, requires the knee joint to be closed so that the lateral edge of the foot can be placed in the hip crease. Albeit that, certain conditions at the hip also need to be met. When sitting back on or between one or both heels, as in *Virasana*, *Balasana*, or *Triang Mukha Eka Pada Paschimottanasana*, failure to completely close the knee will result in the sit bones not grounding (Figure 7.5).

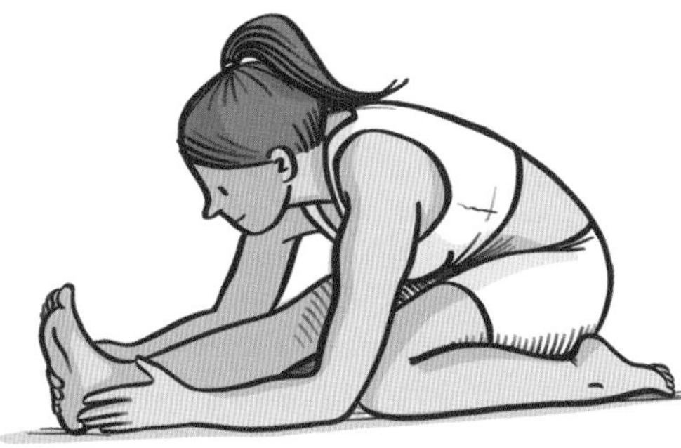

Figure 7.5 If you can't fully close the knee joint, then in some postures, the sit bone will lift.

The quick check for the necessary ROM is to lay on your belly and see if you can bring your heel to your butt. As a side issue, if when you are in that position, you find the heel is almost touching your butt even before you press it down, and it requires virtually no effort to make it touch, then it could well indicate weakness in the quadriceps. If that is the case, then you should seriously think about strengthening them.

When we are in a squat or a posture like *Utkatasana*, then the knees will be in front of the ankles. But in many poses, we will want to keep the knee in line with the ankle, both horizontally and laterally. Probably one of the most repeated cues is, "don't let the knee go forward of the ankle," but why, when it's clear that sometimes it does go in front. As with most things, it all depends. I think the key factors are how much weight is going forward into the knee and how strong are the leg muscles of the individual. The cue is aimed at protecting the knee from experiencing forces that may be too high. So, when in a pose such as *Virabhadrasana A*, it seems sensible to keep the knee over the ankle as it is in a more stable position there (Figure 7.6).

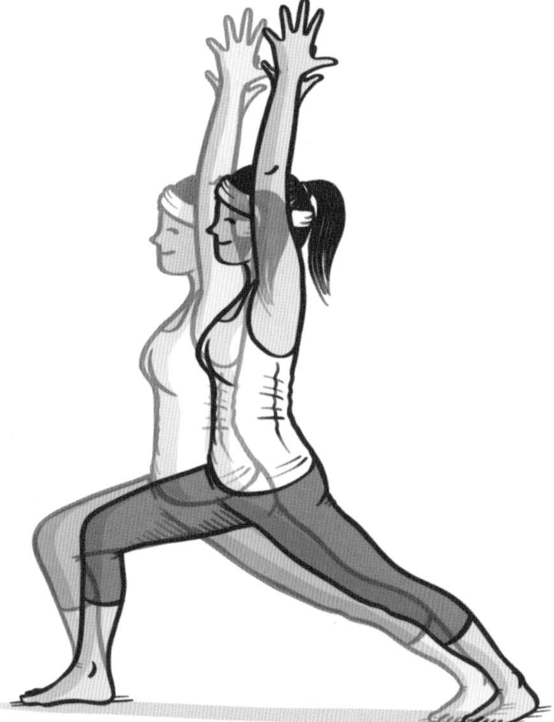

Figure 7.6 In Virabhadrasana A*, it makes sense to keep the knee in line with the ankle but that is not always the case.*

There are times when it is perfectly fine to take the knee well forward (Figure 7.7). I often perform a deep lunge with the shoulders flexed and the arms reaching behind to access the front of the body. In this example, most of the weight is going backward, meaning there is very little weight in the front knee.

So how about letting the knee drop in or out from the vertical line?

Well, again there will be times when this is fine and others when it's not. In lunge type postures, such as the previously mentioned *Virabhadrasana A*, or *Parshvakonasana*, I would agree that you should not let the knee drop in or out because it could place strain on the ligaments (Figure 7.8). Often, the front thigh is pulled out of position by restrictions in the back hip, repositioning the pelvis. If the knee is fully closed, it should be fine. Postures such as *Marichyasana C & D* are often shown with the knee taken across to the center line of the body (Figure 7.9).

When we are cueing in a class, we are generally trying to look after the vulnerable students, but there may be times as an individual when we decide to challenge our strength by purposefully taking the knee forward. As always, this sort of thing should be a conscious choice rather than poor positioning due to not being focused on what you are doing.

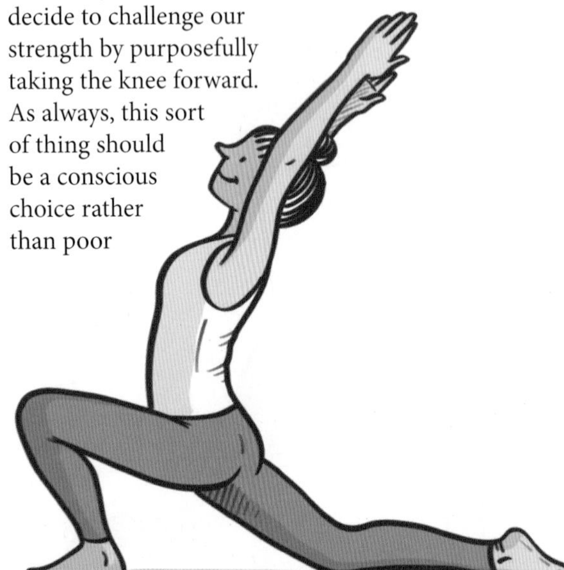

Figure 7.7 In this posture, the weight is going backward so it is perfectly fine to have the knee in front of the ankle.

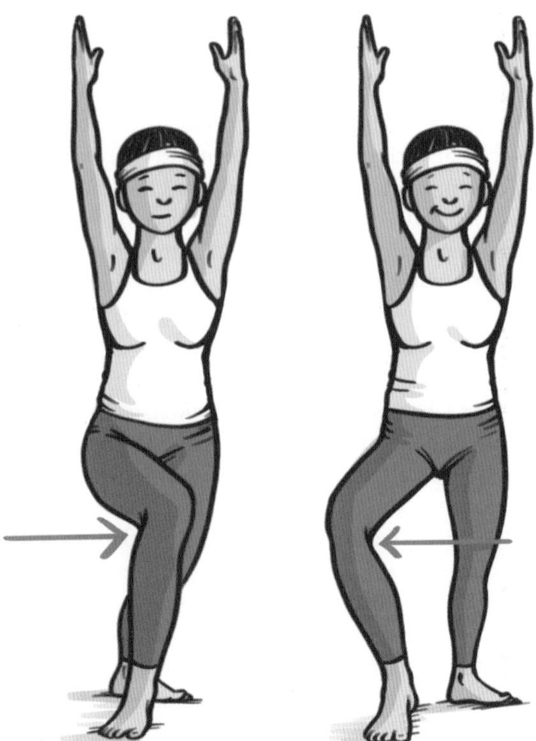

Figure 7.8 It is very common to see knees being allowed to drift sideways.

Probably one of the most troublesome positions for the knee is when the lower leg is levered sideways relative to the upper leg, either medially or laterally. One of the most common times this happens laterally is when the leg is folded back and the heel is taken to the outside of the hip.

In seated positions, students regularly move the flesh of the calf to the side. The more soft tissue there is to reposition, the higher will be the forces imposed on the knee, and I strongly advise against doing this movement (Figure 7.10). If you experience medial knee pain during this maneuver, you are probably putting pressure on the MCL. I would recommend instead taking the lower leg flesh down and away from the back of the knee.

Bhekasana must be one of the poses that makes me cringe the most when it comes to seeing what some

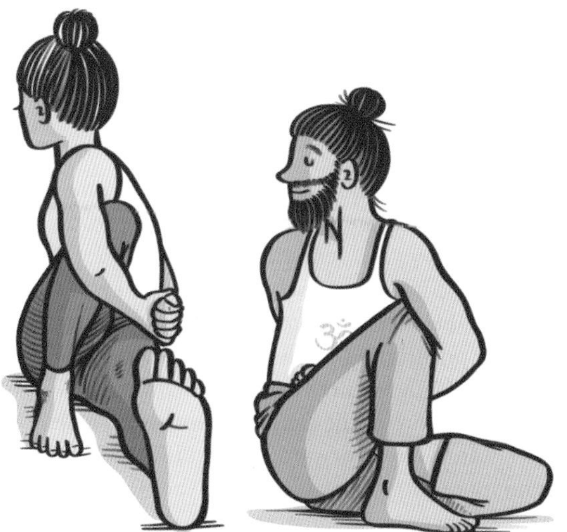

Figure 7.9 Taking the knee across the body in some postures allows for the twist to happen along the central axis.

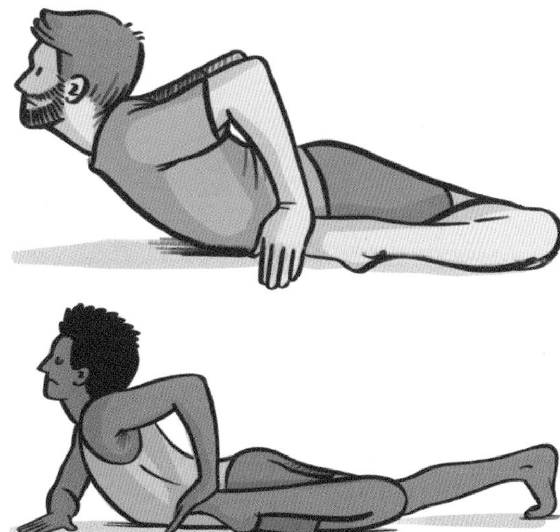

Figure 7.11 What the hell? How can this distortion of the knee joint ever be thought of as a good idea! Just don't do it like this!

practitioners do. I often observe students wanting to bring the feet to the floor, and in doing so, parting and rolling the thighs out—then with the lower leg in a nasty torqued placement, press the foot strongly to the floor (Figure 7.11).

I can't see anything beneficial happening to the body in this situation. It would be much better to be less enthusiastic about reaching the floor with the feet and instead press them back into the hands. At the same time, resist the thighs from parting too much and keep the heels close to the hips. Imagine an active prone (face down) *Supta Virasana*. With the positioning outlined, the knee is closed fully and in a much safer relationship between upper and lower leg (Figure 7.12).

A similar force can be introduced into the knee with *Ardha Padmasana* or *Padmasana* when the hips don't have enough external rotation. This time, the lower leg is levered medially with the potential of pinching the medial meniscus, especially if

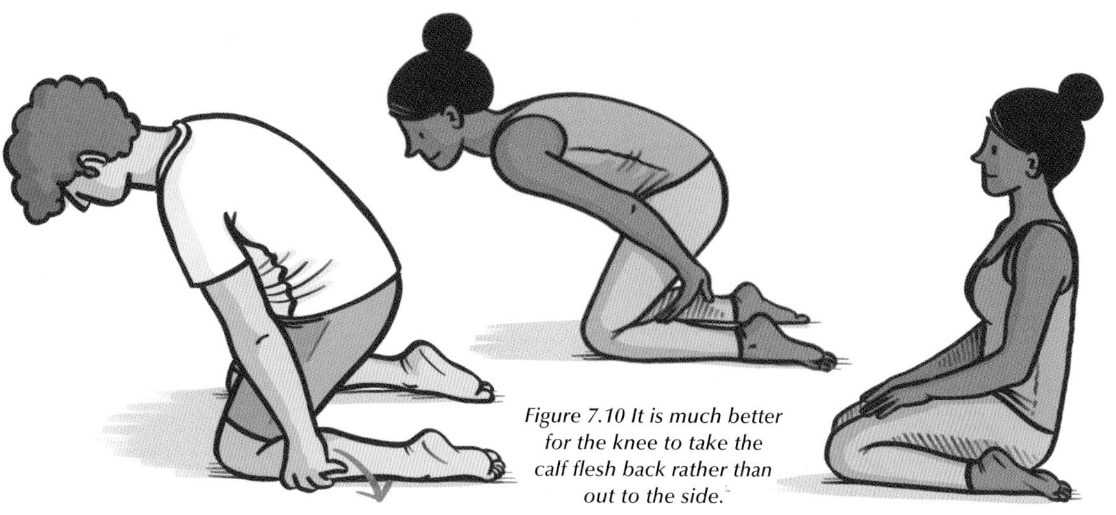

Figure 7.10 It is much better for the knee to take the calf flesh back rather than out to the side.

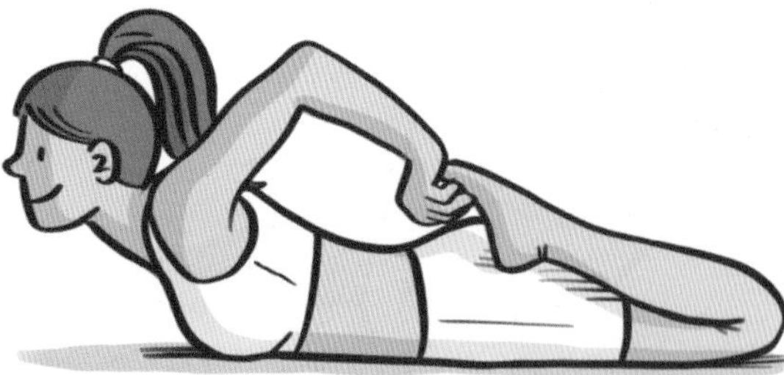

Figure 7.12 Victoria is happy to demonstrate a knee-friendly version.

the knee closure mentioned at the start of this chapter is absent. The body is forced to try and accommodate the missing external rotation by the lower leg moving sideways. This is particularly relevant to the second leg in *Padmasana*. The thigh of that leg is fixed by the other foot on top of it, making insensitive handling very risky.

Having been a manual therapist working exclusively with yogis for many years, it is incredibly depressing to have encountered a considerable number of students who have damaged their medial meniscus by this sort of repeated abuse. If you are super sloppy, you can have the double whammy of sickling ankle (Figure 7.13) and levered low leg. Open those hips in external rotation or don't do those postures that use *Ardha Padmasana* or *Padmasana*. I'll save some more discussion of *Padmasana* for Chapter 8.

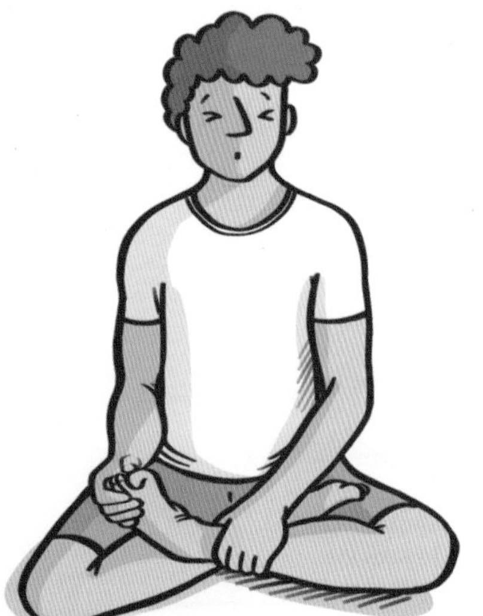

Figure 7.13 Doug is putting strain on his ankle.

The last body positioning I will cover here relates to when the foot can act as a rotational lever of the lower leg. We touched on this in the previous chapter, so now we will expand the idea.

With the foot dorsiflexed and up against something like the floor, it can prevent the lower leg from rotating. If you can remember in Chapter 2, *Relational Movement*, then hopefully you will recall we used the example of *Janu Sirsasana A* to explain that the positioning of the bent leg foot against the opposite thigh requires external rotation of the hip. Then more of the same movement is needed if we want to fold forward. As mentioned, if there is no more rotation available and the student pulls themselves forward, then the upper leg can rotate along with the pelvis. As it does so, it rotates medially relative to the lower leg because the dorsiflexed foot is preventing the lower leg from rotating along with the upper leg (Figure 7.14). The consequence can be that the student experiences medial knee pain due to the medial meniscus pinching.

A similar experience can happen in the lying variation of *Eka Pada Rajakapotasana* for the same reasons. This variation, sometimes called "Sleeping Pigeon," can be a very effective hip opener for external rotation, but is fraught with problems. As straightforward as the shape may look, I would consider the full expression an advanced posture for many reasons, which we will address in the next

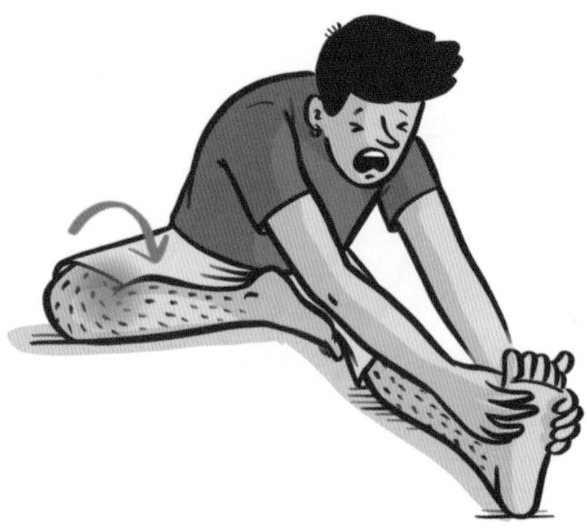

Figure 7.14 The upper leg is being medially rotated against the lower leg.

chapter. For the moment, we will discuss how the positioning of the foot will influence the knee.

If the shin of the front leg is parallel with the front of the mat, then the foot can be plantar flexed or dorsiflexed. Most often, the instruction is to dorsiflex the foot. I feel that this is based on the assumption that the action will introduce some knee stability, in much the same way as contracting the quadriceps in postures like *Trikonasana*. However, no muscles that dorsiflex the foot cross the knee. It probably means that it is the gastrocnemius being under a stretch from the dorsiflexion that is responsible for this sensation, as it does cross the knee. Hence if the hips have the ROM available to ground the whole upper leg, I suggest either foot position can be used with a parallel shin (Figure 7.15).

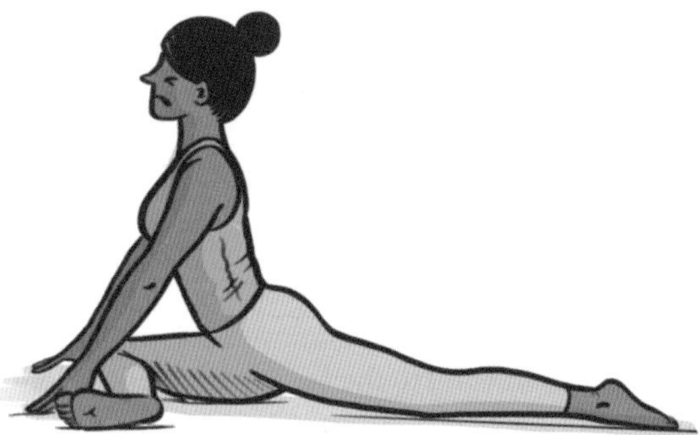

Figure 7.15 Myra has lifted up so that you can see the foot position more easily. The same principle of foot position goes whether up or down.

More important is what happens at the ankle as the foot moves away from a parallel position and toward the groin. The upper leg will want to rotate medially, especially if lying down. Now if the ankle is in dorsiflexion, it will fix the lower leg, as in the previous example, and the upper leg will rotate relative to it, potentially creating discomfort at the knee. For this reason, it is better to plantar flex the foot in any position other than parallel to the top of the mat (Figure 7.16). I would suggest that the same plantar flexed ankle placement should also be used in the full upright *Eka Pada Rajakapotasana* posture, even though you will see many images with the foot dorsiflexed. However, it is vital in the lying version because the upper leg can be pulled into rotation as the pelvis tilts forward.

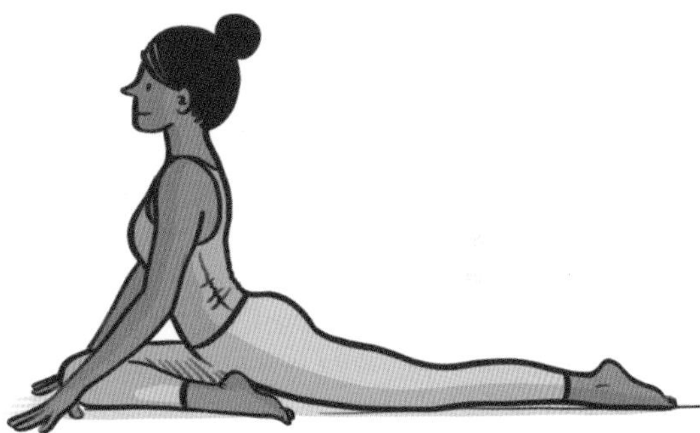

Figure 7.16 As the foot moves back toward the hip, the foot must be plantar flexed to protect the knee.

It is crucial to look after your knees in yoga because so many postures involve a bent leg. Once damaged, many practitioners land up having to stop the physical practice and even have trouble finding a comfortable seat for meditation or *pranayama*.

CHAPTER

8 Hip

What could be more straightforward than sitting on the floor with your legs out in front of you and folding forward to take your chest down onto your legs? There are no complicated shapes, testing binds, or tricky balances involved, but for many students, *Paschimottanasana* is anything but simple (Figure 8.1). Their weight can even be going backward rather than forward if they have less than 90 degrees of hip flexion available. How about even just sitting comfortably on the floor with your legs crossed, something many Asian cultures do, no matter their age.

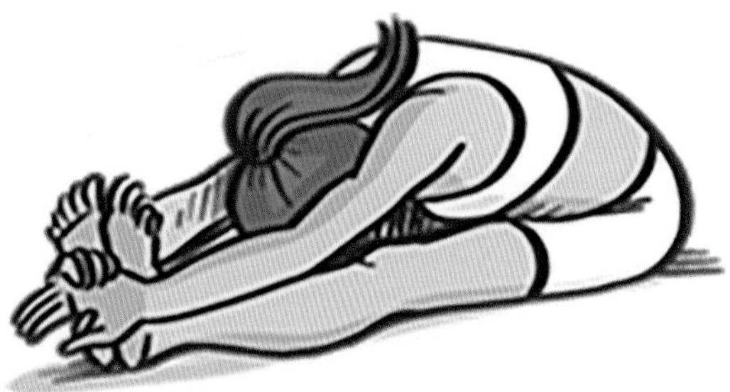

Figure 8.1 Paschimottanasana.

Open hips are essential for yoga. If that student sitting upright in *Paschimottanasana* has a one-pointed focus, they can be perceived as doing yoga more successfully than a student physically deeper in the posture, but with a wandering mind. Nevertheless, from an anatomical perspective, we are more concerned with why that upright person can't fold down onto their legs.

What do we mean when we say, "You need to open your hips?" Generally, people are thinking of the knees going down in *Baddha Konasana* or sitting comfortably in *Padmasana*. However, our hips can move through many more directions than just those needed to perform the types of poses mentioned. It's just that we associate the word "opening" with the imagery of opening a book, the two sides dropping out.

The diverse combination of movements available at the hips are integral to the accomplishment of the vast majority of yoga postures, and many students experience challenges in moving through the desired ROM in one or more directions.

The hip is a ball-and-socket joint that allows the movements of flexion, extension, abduction, adduction, horizontal abduction and adduction, circumduction, and medial and external rotation. What we should think when we refer to open hips is freedom of movement in every available direction. We are not necessarily designed to move to the same extent in each direction. Often, a posture requires a specific set of these movements, for example, when we bring the foot into an *Ardha Padmasana*. In this instance, we need hip flexion, abduction, and external rotation to place the foot nicely in the hip crease (we also need movements at the knee and ankle). If the hip doesn't move freely, then forces can easily be placed on the ankle, knee, spine, or SIJ. Each posture will need a combination of specific movements.

For each of those directions we want to move through at the hip, there will be muscles to take us there and others to bring us back. As you know by now, our general rule of thumb is that if a muscle's job is to move a joint in a particular direction, then tension in that muscle will resist movement in the opposite direction. What we experience is much more complicated than this, and we will find that many muscles can resist movements that are not directly related to their functions. For example, the rotational muscles of the hip can restrict flexion in many students.

We are hopefully getting the idea by now that the structural differences between individuals will influence our ability to do certain things with the body and no more so is it experienced at the hip (ok, and the shoulder). So pivotal is the hip to making pretty-looking postures, that many students are left grappling with discomfort and gravity as their body stubbornly rejects their attempted contortions.

As the hip joint is part of the pelvis, now is an excellent time to introduce some of the bony landmarks that are often referred to. As you know, I'm not a fan of knowing every nook and cranny of the body, but some are used so commonly that it is a lot easier to use them than try to explain the position with ordinary language. The pelvis is in two halves, separated at the front by the pubic symphysis and at the back by the sacrum. It is comprised of three fused bones: ilium, ischium, and pubis (Figure 8.2). You will notice the following bony landmarks often draw their name from the bone they are on.

The large flattish part of the pelvis (ilium) has a rounded top, the iliac crest. There are two bony projections (iliac spines) at the front, one higher than the other, and the same at the back. When naming these, first you say if it is at the front (anterior) or back (posterior), and then if it is higher (superior) or lower (inferior), for example, anterior superior iliac spine. Typically, the names are abbreviated to the acronyms ASIS, AIIS, PSIS, and PIIS. Don't be thrown, just think it through (see *List of Abbreviations*, page 9).

The sit bones are on the bottom of the pelvis, and because they are rounded prominences on the ischium, they are called the ischial tuberosities (the famous hamstrings attach here). Between them and the pubic symphysis is the pubic arch. In real basic terms, that space between the two halves of the pelvis is the pelvic inlet.

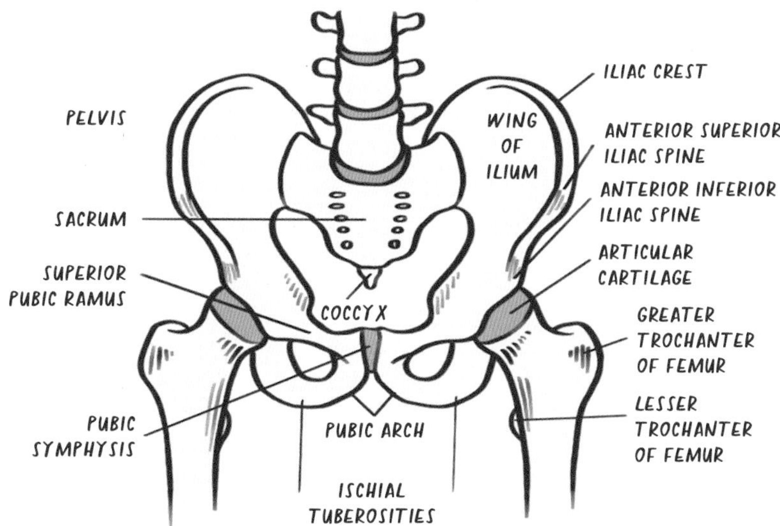

Figure 8.2 Bones of the pelvic girdle.

On the side of the pelvis is the hip socket, called the acetabulum, and around the back where the sacrum meets the ilium is the SIJ. Let's move over to the femur. There are so many muscles that attach to that big lump of bone at the top that it is worth knowing that the name of it is the greater trochanter. And as the yogi's favorite muscle, the psoas, attaches to the smaller lump around the corner; also remember the lesser trochanter.

Construction of the Hip Joint

As mentioned, the hip is a ball-and-socket joint, which allows for all those different movements (Figure 8.3). The socket sits on the side of the pelvis (its fancy name is the acetabulum). The ball bit is the femoral head (end of the upper leg bone). The depth of the socket will differ between individuals as well as its orientation. There is likely to be less stability the shallower it is, but there may be a reduced risk of compression, albeit also dependent on other factors. There is also a ring of cartilage in and around the acetabulum, called the labrum, which deepens the socket. It is this cartilage that can be prone to damage if we are levering into the socket in some of the yoga postures.

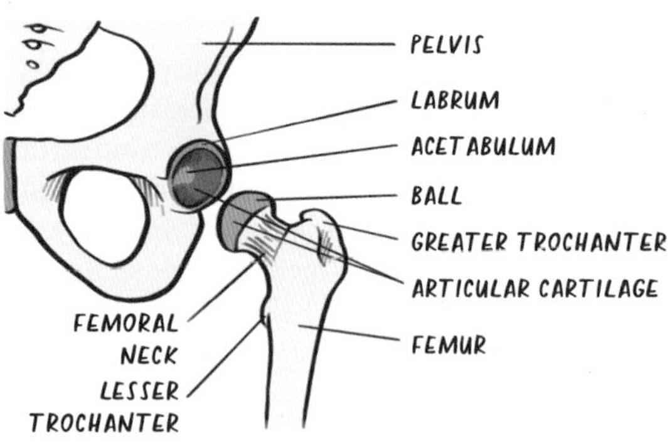

Figure 8.3 Construction of the hip joint.

We need to transmit the strong forces of locomotion from the legs to the body, so the hip is additionally stabilized by being heavily ligamentous. The direction most resisted is extension, and hence our accessible ROM in that direction is usually only 20 to 30 degrees. Most students find it difficult to comprehend that last point because they visualize people doing poses like the *Hanumanasana*, so we will clarify this a bit later.

It's funny because although there are so many movements possible at the hip, the stability offered by its design means that it is more difficult to injure than, for example, the knee. Of course, we can still strain a muscle or sprain one of the ligaments, but that can happen everywhere. Therefore, the emphasis in this chapter will be on appreciating those design differences that add to our individuality, rather than how we can damage it. I'm going to put the next few paragraphs in our anatomy geek sectioning

The primary hip variabilities center around the orientation of the acetabulum and the angulation of the femoral head. I'm not going to go into great detail because we wouldn't know what our hip joint looks like unless we had an X-ray. However, generally, men and women have a slightly different shaped pelvis because women need to give birth.

The female pelvis is characterized by being wider and shorter with more of an oval-shaped pelvic inlet. The angle of the pubic arch is also typically greater than 90 degrees. The consequence of this is that the acetabulum is usually more anteriorly facing than in males to bring the legs back under the body. A wider pelvis may also make the ischial tuberosities (sit bones) more rounded and hence more comfy on which to balance in postures such as *Navasana*. The angle across the face of the acetabulum can also vary, one of the elements that influence hip impingement (what we have been referring to as hard compression).

There is also some diversity in the shape and orientation of the femoral head. The angle at which the neck of the femur leaves the shaft (angle of inclination) is typically about 125 degrees but can be more or less. Think of this as how much the neck points up (Figure 8.4). If the angle is less than normal, the greater trochanter is likely to bang on the pelvis much sooner during hip abduction.

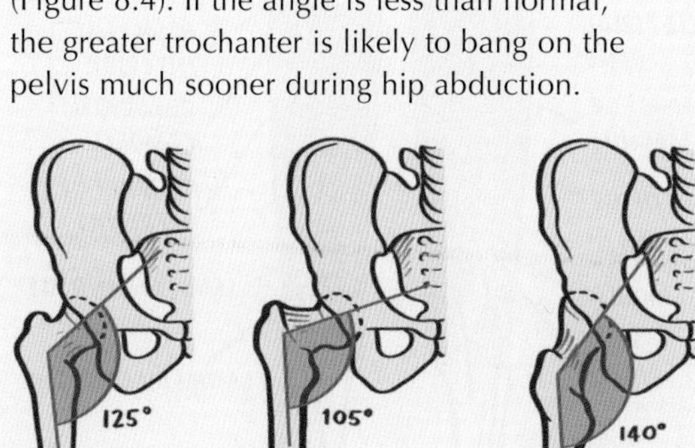

Figure 8.4 Angle of inclination.

It can also point more or less forward (femoral neck anteversion) (Figure 8.5). When the angle is less than normal, it is called retroversion. We haven't shown it here, but this variation can also be a factor in toe in and toe out gait.

As well as that, the femoral neck can be longer or shorter and the greater trochanter larger or smaller.

Therefore, with all these possibilities, and without making distinct comparisons, it is easy to appreciate how human variability will indicate that some students' shapes will facilitate more movement and others less, just by the underlying structure. It is beyond the scope of this book to draw specific conclusions, but if you fancy reading more about this topic, I can recommend *Your Body, Your Yoga* (Bernie Clark).

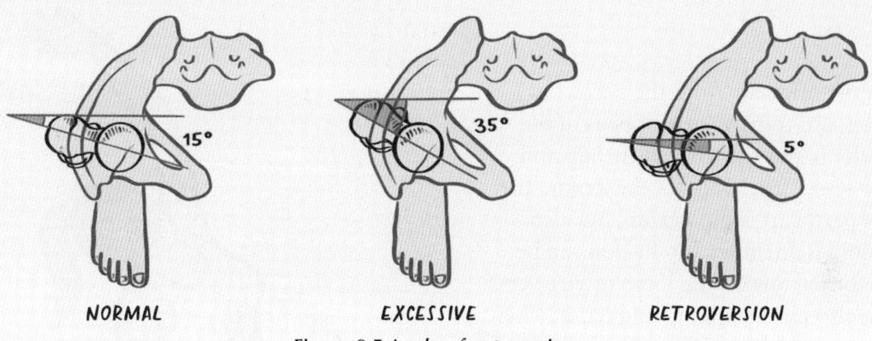

Figure 8.5 Angle of anteversion.

because, really, it is okay just to think that hip shapes can be slightly different and that this explains some of the increased vulnerabilities and ROM limitations between individuals not related to soft tissue (muscles, tendons, and ligaments) restrictions.

In Chapter 3, *Opposing Muscles Restrict*, we introduced the idea that the muscle that does one action will resist the opposite action. That still holds true for the hip, but it is worth recognizing that some students will have bone structure that allows for greater external rotation or abduction, others the opposite. Students with ligamentous laxity (stretchier ligaments) will be able to extend and probably externally rotate the hip further because the same strong ligament resists both movements.

Muscles that Move the Hip

All the movements available at the hip mean there are a whole load of muscles to take the leg through them and then others to bring it back. It looks like a bit of a nightmare when you see all the labels, but once you start grouping them together (e.g., quadriceps, hamstrings, adductors, deep external rotators) it's not so bad (Figures 8.6, 8.8, & 8.9).

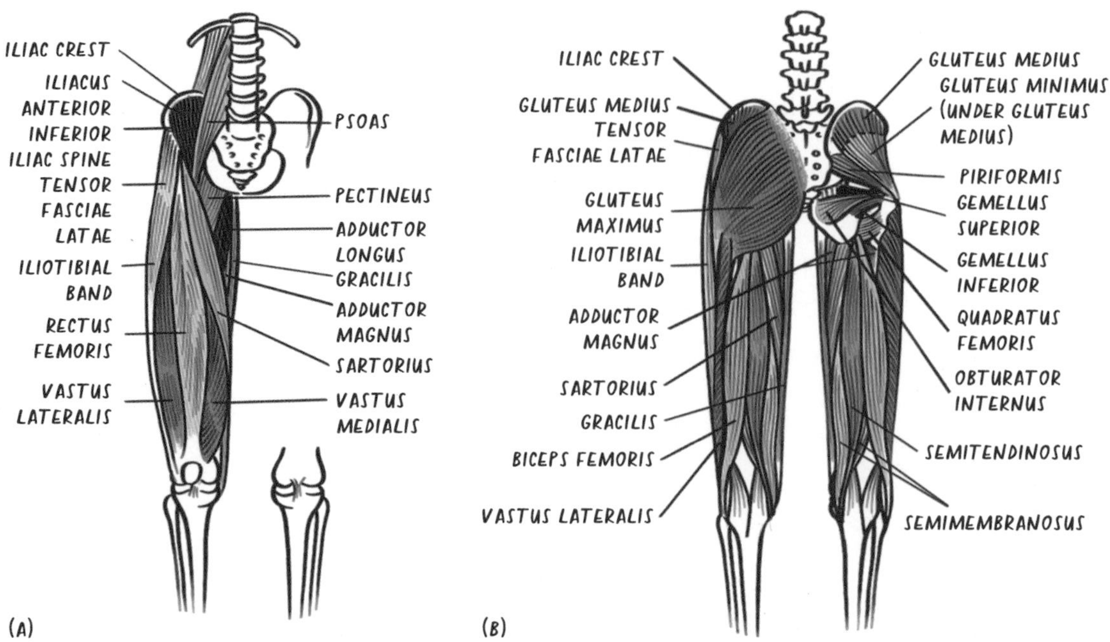

Figure 8.6 Muscles that move the hip, (A) anterior view, (B) posterior view.

Psoas

The psoas doesn't originate from the pelvis but from the bodies and transverse processes of the lumbar spine. It crosses the front of the hip and attaches to the lesser trochanter of the femur. The main action it performs is hip flexion, but also external rotation. Remember, hip flexion can be thought of as the leg toward the torso or vice versa. The psoas can also assist with hip adduction when the leg is in certain positions. Along with the back muscles, it will help stabilize the pelvis and torso. To stretch the psoas, you need to take the hip into extension, but it doesn't matter how much the knee is bent. As it crosses the spine, some practitioners like to add a lateral flexion to this positioning (Figure 8.7).

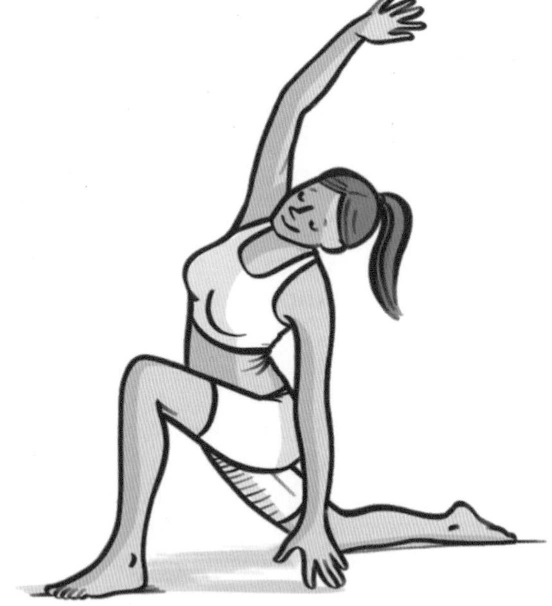

Figure 8.7 Adding a side bend can increase the stretch on the psoas as it attaches to the lumbar spine.

Iliacus

The lower end of iliacus has a common tendon with the psoas, attaching to the lesser trochanter, but at the top, it doesn't cross the spine. Instead, the iliacus attaches on the inner surface of the ilium (iliac fossa). Like the psoas, it flexes and externally rotates the hip, and may also help to adduct hip.

Rectus Femoris

Rectus femoris (a quadricep) is a polyarticular muscle, crossing the hip and knee, and we covered where it goes to and from in the previous chapter. At the hip, the action of rectus femoris is to help with hip flexion.

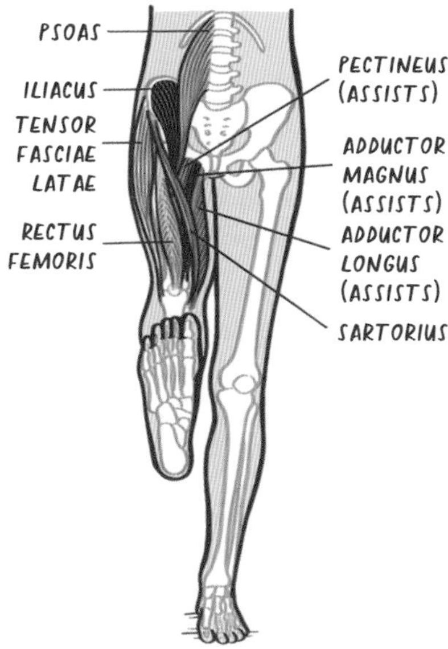

Figure 8.8 Hip flexion (anterior view).

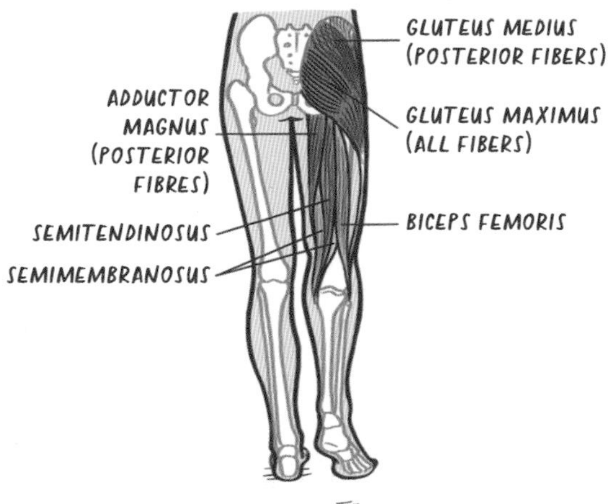

Figure 8.9 Hip extension (posterior view).

Gluteus Maximus (Gmax)

The most visible muscle on the pelvis is the Gmax. It goes from the posterior surface of the sacrum and iliac crest to the top of the femur and IT band. Its actions are hip extension, abduction, and external rotation.

Gluteus Medius (Gmed) and Minimus (Gmin)

The other two gluteal muscles, Gmed and Gmin, travel from the ilium to the greater trochanter of the femur. The main actions are hip abduction (Figure 8.10) and medial rotation (Figure 8.11), but they can also help flex the hip. We are going to leave it at that, but to be honest, it's not 100 percent correct because, as we've mentioned, different fibers within the same muscle can have alternative actions, and this is the case with these muscles.

Deep External Rotators

There are six deep external rotators, the most noteworthy being piriformis, which you will notice from Figure 8.12, attaches to the front of the sacrum. The others are gemellus superior and inferior, obturator internus and externus, and quadratus femoris. You don't need to remember all their names, but think of them as a group as they all externally rotate the hip. The muscles create a fan-like appearance attaching to various places around the inferior pelvis and then on to the greater trochanter of the femur. When the hip is flexed, the piriformis can also abduct the hip.

Hamstrings

The hamstrings are probably the most well-known muscles among yoga practitioners. They consist of three muscles, semitendinosus, semimembranosus,

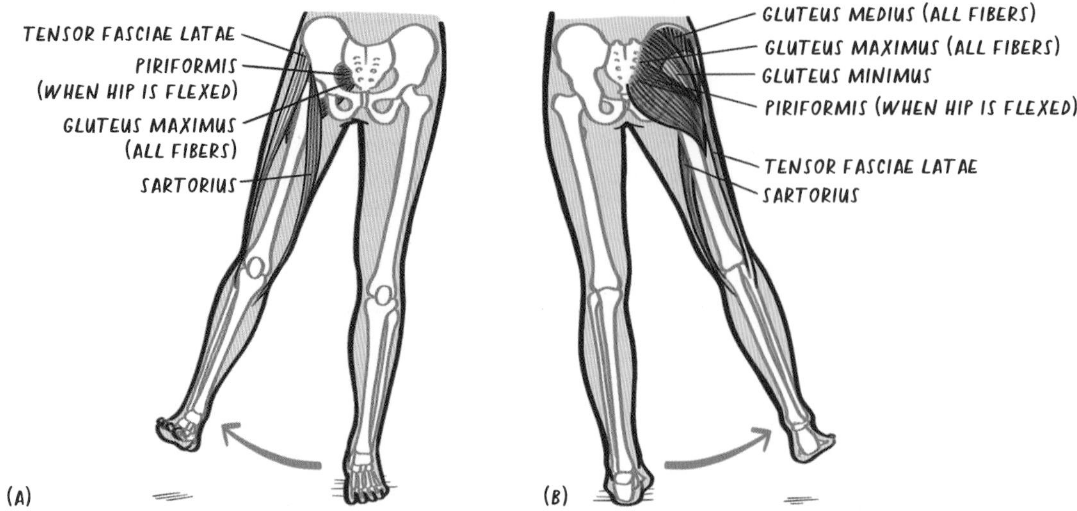

Figure 8.10 Hip abduction, (A) anterior view, (B) posterior view.

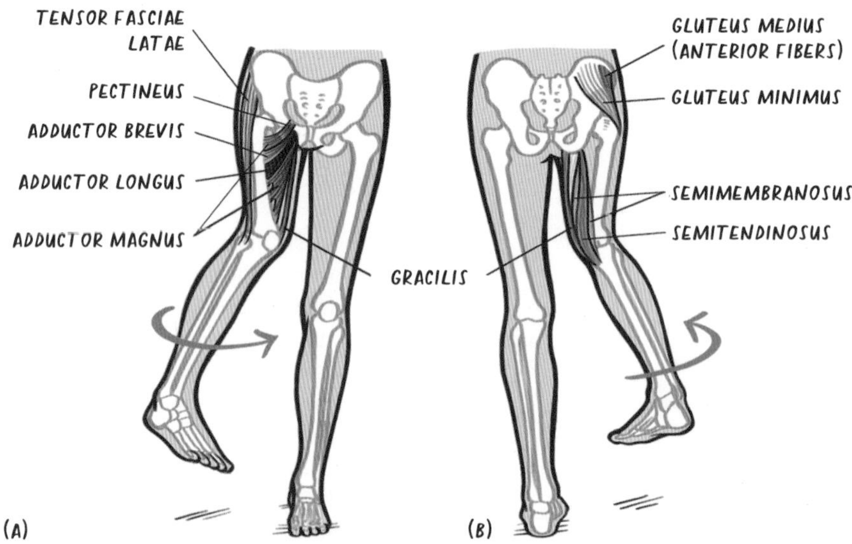

Figure 8.11 Medial hip rotation, (A) anterior view, (B) posterior view.

and biceps femoris. They are situated on the back of the upper leg and perform hip extension and knee flexion. Two hamstrings attach below the knee medially and one laterally. At the top, they all attach to the ischial tuberosity, although biceps femoris has two bellies, one of which connects to the femur. Besides hip extension and knee flexion, they can rotate the knee, but only when flexed. Also, they can posteriorly tilt the pelvis. You can see this in a posture like *Ustrasana*. Essentially, the action is still hip extension, but the pelvis is moving instead of the leg.

Sartorius

Sartorius is listed as the longest muscle in the body and is polyarticular, crossing the hip and knee.

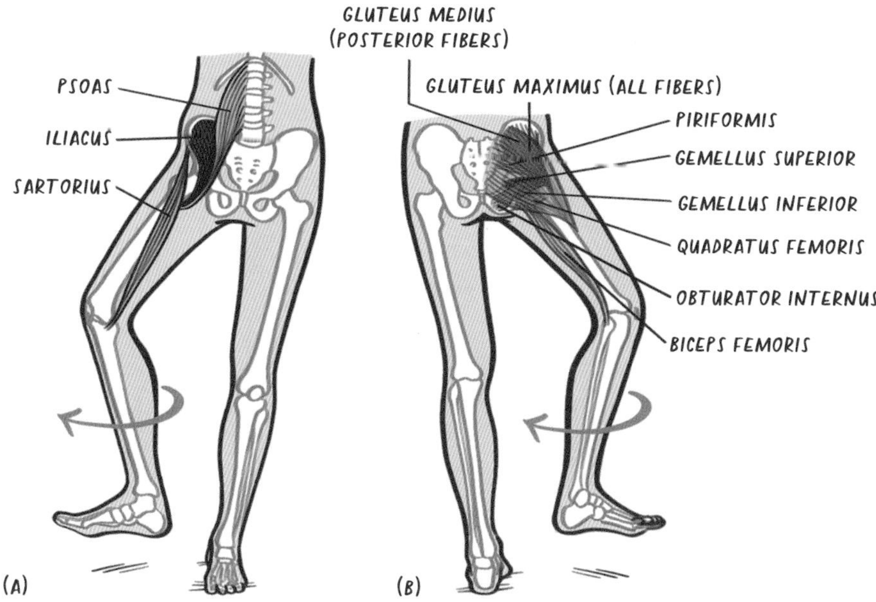

Figure 8.12 External hip rotation, (A) anterior view, (B) posterior view.

It goes from the ASIS to the medial aspect of the tibia just below the knee. For the most part, I think it is one of those muscles not talked about so much, which is not to say that there aren't any negative tensional patterns related to it. Still, I haven't heard anyone say, "I'm going to stretch out my sartorius."

Its name is thought to derive from the Latin word for tailor (*sartor*)—the tailor's muscle—because they spent all day sitting crossed-legged on the floor. In this position, the muscle is shortened, as its actions are to flex, externally rotate, and abduct the hip, as well as flex the knee. I would say that it is a synergist or helper in all these movements rather than the prime mover. As with all sustained aberrant positional patterns, it is likely to result in a shortening of muscles. Maybe this resulted in conditions linked to their profession and others that spent most of their days in a similar way. It would be interesting to investigate students who have attended one month or longer vipassanās.

Tensor Fasciae Latae (TFL)

TFL originates from the iliac crest (just above ASIS) and then like part of Gmax, merges into the ITB. Students will use the TFL, particularly when trying to stabilize the pelvis relative to the leg, such as in balancing poses.

Adductors

There are five adductors; brevis, longus, and magnus, plus pectineus and gracilis, and as their name suggests, their dominant action is hip adduction (Figure 8.13). You will notice that their superior attachments are different, with two attaching to the upper bony arch (superior pubic ramus) and two to the lower one (inferior pubic ramus). Adductor magnus connects to the ischial tuberosity, as do the hamstrings, just a little more medially. Their location will influence their direction of pull, but I can't imagine you will be targeting specific adductors based on these attachments other than adductor magnus. However, it helps to understand why they have different secondary actions.

Also notice that only one adductor (gracilis) crosses the knee and, because of this, it can also help with knee flexion. For the most part, the

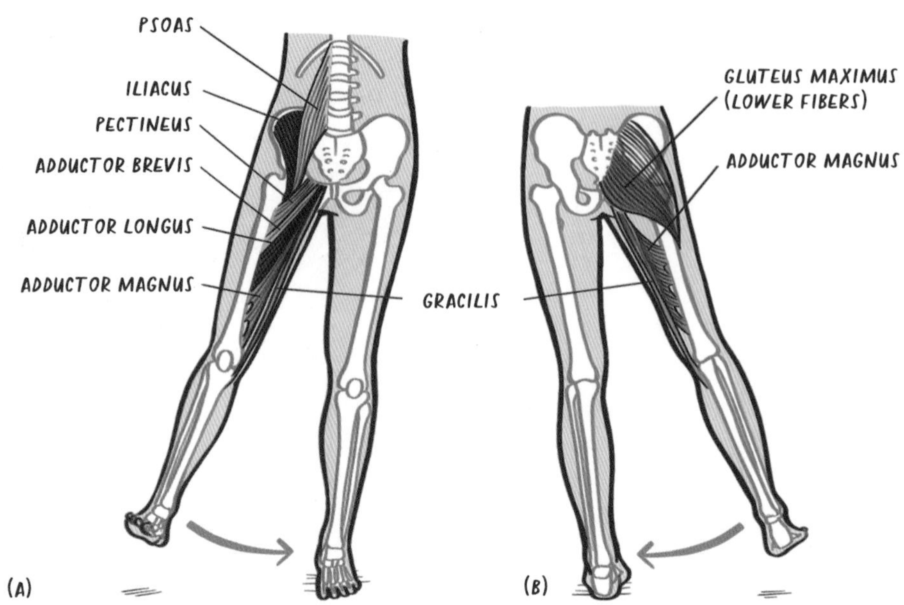

Figure 8.13 Hip adduction, (A) anterior view, (B) posterior view.

inferior attachments of the adductors are on the posterior aspect of the femur. This fact and the position of the pelvis relative to the femur will influence their ability to perform an additional action of either medial or external rotation. Unless you are otherwise inclined, just remember their names, which one crosses the knee and which one attaches to the ischial tuberosity.

Quick Reference Muscle Action Tables

Flexion	Extension
Psoas, iliacus	Hamstrings
Rectus femoris	Gmax
Sartorius	Gmed (posterior fibers)
TFL	Adductor magnus (posterior fibers)
Gmed (anterior fibers)	
Gmin	
Adductors: Magnus, brevis, longus, pectineus	

Medial Rotation	External Rotation
Gmed (anterior fibers)	Deep external rotators
Gmin	Gmax
Semitendinosus	Gmed (posterior fibers)
Semimembranosus	Adductor magnus (posterior fibers)
Adductors: Magnus, brevis, longus, pectineus, gracilis	Biceps femoris
TFL	

Abduction	Adduction
Gmed and Gmin	Adductors
Gmax	Psoas and Iliacus
TFL	Gmax (lower fibers)
Piriformis (when hip is flexed)	

Putting Things into Context

One of the most common cheats I see when students are trying to access the front of the hip to stretch the psoas and iliacus is letting the pelvis tilt forward (Figure 8.14A). It may seem like there is a more significant hip extension because you can lunge deeper but, in reality, there is less. Students with a bendy lumbar area can manage to keep the torso upright because they have used it to accommodate the anterior tilt of the pelvis. Instead, keep the pelvis neutral as you lunge forward (Figure 8.14B).

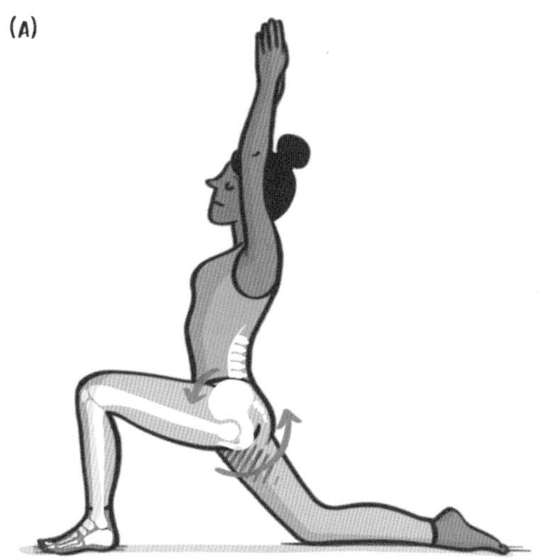

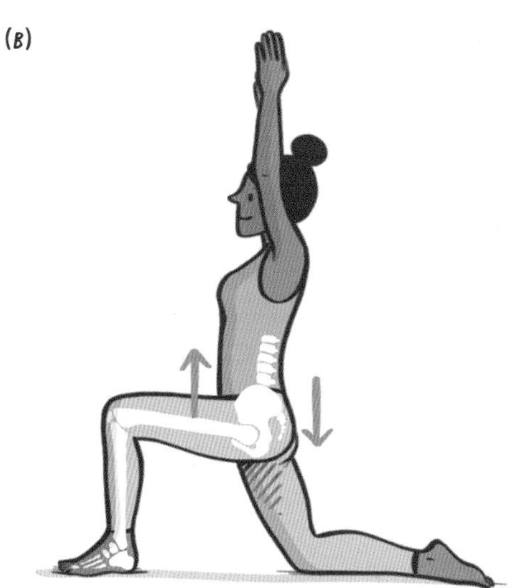

Figure 8.14 (A) Myra has allowed the pelvis to anteriorly tilt. The lunge is deeper but is a less effective stretch for the psoas and iliacus, (B) Myra is pulling up the pubic bone and down with the sacrum to keep the pelvis neutral and maintain a natural lumbar curve.

The same pattern will show up in many postures where one or more hips are in extension, such as *Virabhadrasana A* (Figure 8.15) and *Ustrasana*. Students that have this pattern often have trouble opening up across the front of the hip because they keep escaping from the work. When it comes to the deeper backbends, they are then likely to do precisely the same and increase the likelihood of using excessive movement from the spine, instead of spreading the load. More on that later when we look at backbends.

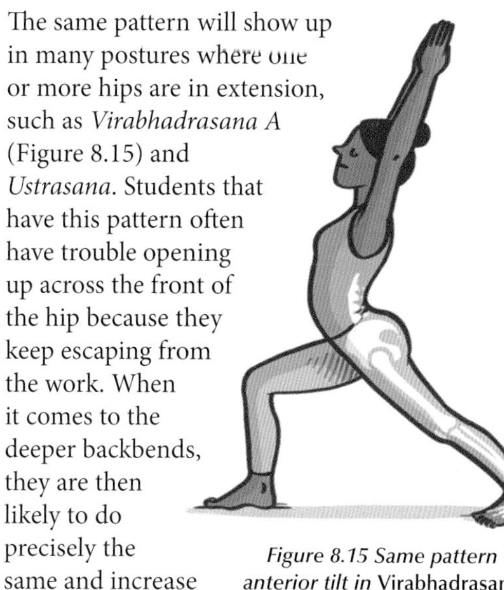

Figure 8.15 Same pattern of anterior tilt in Virabhadrasana A.

In Chapter 3, *Secondary Actions of Muscles*, we used the examples of *Hanumanasana* and a Dropback to illustrate the potential pull into external rotation by the stretched psoas and iliacus. This pattern of allowing the hips to roll out is also a common cheat to avoid the restriction on the front of the hip. The problem is it can tend to send stress toward the SIJ. Giveaway signs are thighs rolling out, feet turning out, and the space between the knees increasing (Figure 8.16). If the foundation is actively maintained and the thigh drift resisted, this pattern can be neutralized.

As you take the legs apart in postures such as *Upavistha Konasana*, the medial hamstrings will be put under more of a stretch than the lateral one. Depending on how far apart you take your legs, you might not sense much going on in the adductors until you start folding forward. We will go over forward folding in detail later, but basically, the pelvis will tip forward as you go down.

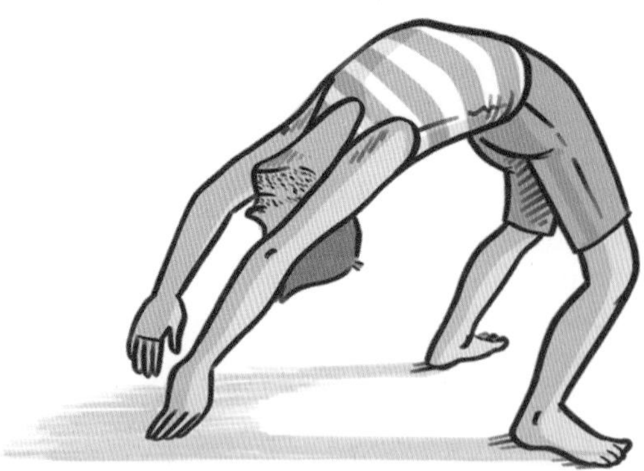

Figure 8.16 A very common pattern is letting the feet turn out to avoid some of the restriction from the hip flexors to hip extension. However, it is much more likely that this will create some tension in the low back and SIJ.

This sends the pubic bone and ischial tuberosities backward and away from the adductor muscles' distal attachments. In particular, the ischial tuberosities will travel further. Adductor magnus, which attaches there, will be put under a double stretch because the legs are also apart (Figure 8.17). It acts like an adductor and a hamstring, and some people even refer to it as the fourth hamstring. For this reason, it is not advisable to push someone forward in this posture as adductor magnus is vulnerable.

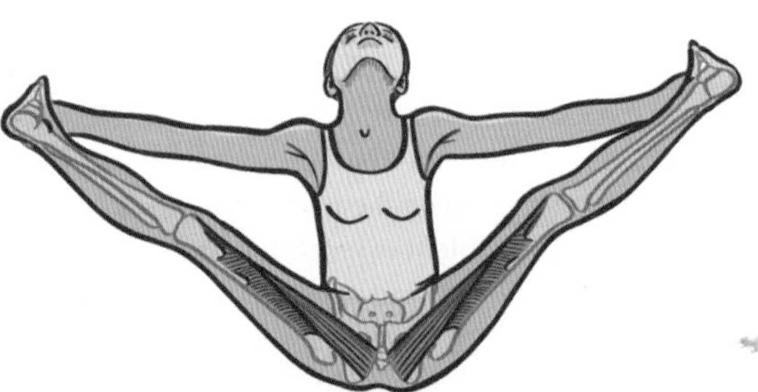

Figure 8.17 Upavistha Konasana *viewed from below, showing adductor magnus*

Weakness in the Gmed muscle has been associated with low backache. One of the tests to see if the Gmed is not strong enough can be done from a standing position. If the individual takes one foot off the floor and can't maintain a level pelvis, then the Gmed is likely to be too weak (Figure 8.18). Holding postures such as *Utthita Hasta Padangusthasana* and Peeing Dog with good pelvic alignment would be ideal options for improvement.

On the other hand, students who also run a lot or participate in associated sports may have tightness in the TFL and the connected ITB, which can lend itself to lateral knee pain. Focusing on some postures that include hip adduction, for example *Supta Padangusthasana C*, could help encourage some release. This is often a movement overlooked in many yoga sequences.

As the hamstrings cross the knee, it is essential to keep the legs straight when flexing at the hip if you want to elicit a change in flexibility. In single-legged hip flexion postures like *Utthita Hasta Padangusthasana* and *Supta Padangusthasana*, it is quite common to see the opposite leg to the one being stretched unintentionally bending. This indicates that the stretch has been taken too deep, pulling the pelvis out of position and along with it the opposite leg.

If we take the standing version as our example, enthusiastic students will keep trying to pull the raised leg higher even though hip flexion has really stopped. The result is that the hamstring attachments pulling on the ischial tuberosities will start to move the pelvis into a posterior tilt. As this happens, the knee of the standing leg will bend to facilitate it. Fix: don't let the standing leg bend or you are escaping the work (Figure 8.19).

The same can be seen when you are lying down in *Supta Padangusthasana*, the knee bending even if the student manages to keep the heel down (Figure 8.20). My instruction is to feel the calf on the floor as well as the heel. In this way, the leg must be kept straight.

Let's revisit Chapter 3, *Opposing Muscles Restrict*, with respect to the rotational muscles of the hips. Many students are fine with the logic when

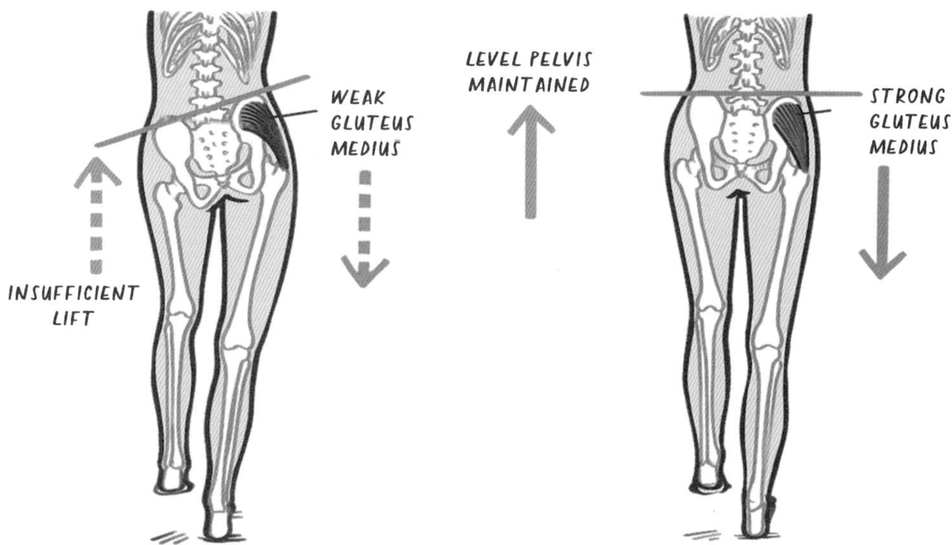

Figure 8.18 If Gmed is weak, the pelvis won't stay level as the leg is lifted.

thinking of hip flexion and extension but start to get a little confused when it comes to rotation.

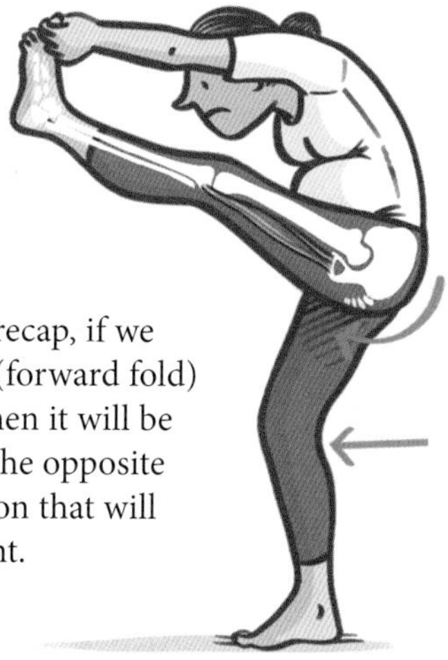

As a little simplistic recap, if we want to flex our hip (forward fold) with a straight leg, then it will be the muscles that do the opposite action of hip extension that will restrict the movement. This is primarily hamstrings and maybe Gmax. Applying the same thought process to hip rotation, the medial rotators will resist external rotation and the deep external rotators (piriformis and friends) will resist medial rotation.

Figure 8.19 Hmm. Wendy has pulled that leg high but can only do so because bending the knee has allowed the pelvis to tip back.

I think the confusion comes when we start talking about postures and the phrases we use. For example, *Padmasana*, requires us to take the hip into external rotation. If we can't get comfortable, we need to work on more external rotation, not the external rotators. We must endeavor to gain more flexibility in Gmed and Gmin (medial rotators) by using accessible postures that also use external rotation.

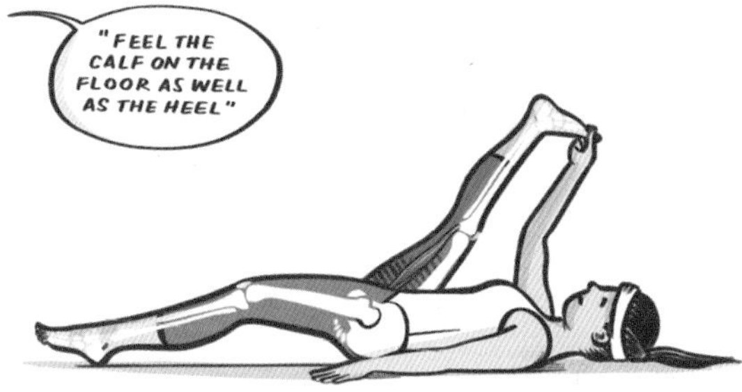

Figure 8.20 The calf coming off the floor is another cheat that gives the illusion of greater hip flexion.

The hip movements are central to so many yoga postures that we will be covering a lot more postures and "Key Concept" examples in the next section of the book.

CHAPTER

9 Spine

The spine is the center of our being, axial rotation, and inner strength. Rigid at times, pliable and undulating at others, resilient but also vulnerable. In this chapter, we will look in detail at this fantastic and sometimes frustrating area of the body. You only need to hurt your back to appreciate how much it is involved in everything we do, from allowing the mobility to twist and bend, to providing a central inner foundation from which we can stabilize and move the extremities. Often, there is an emphasis in yoga to create flourishing deep backbends, but a lot of students would probably do better to spend more time working on strength and stability. In many classes, it is easy to spot a sagging *Chaturanga*, a sinking *Navasana*, and wobbly inversions. Creating body integrity at the same time as flexibility is key to a healthy practice.

Construction of the Spine

When we look at the spine from the front or the back, it is a straight line, unless there is scoliosis (a condition resulting in the spine curving sideways). However, when looking from the side, the characteristic double S-shape is evident. Because it has these curves, it is much more adaptable to shock and more easily distributes body weight and loading.

The spine is divided into five sections, cervical, thoracic, lumbar, sacral (sacrum), and coccygeal (coccyx), with cervical and lumbar having lordotic curves (bending toward the front) and the thoracic, sacral, and coccygeal having kyphotic curves (bending toward the back). Individuals naturally have accentuated or diminished curves as part of human variability, but they may also be exaggerated by posture, sport, working practices, psychology, etc. If there is too much additional curvature, then the term hyperkyphotic or hyperlordotic is used. Changes in bone shape and density, as well as soft tissue tensional patterns, can be responsible for the increase in the curvature.

There are medical conditions that can be the cause of spinal abnormalities, but the most common non-exercise-related reason for hyperlordosis is disproportionate weight distribution in front of the spine, such as with pregnancy and obesity (Figure 9.1). Another common cause is that the muscular strength and flexibility

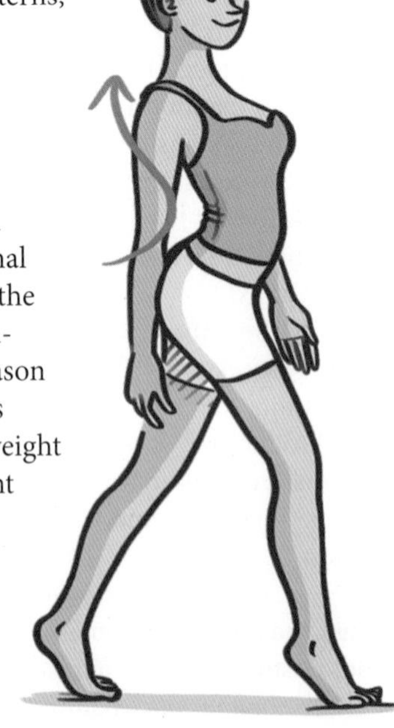

Figure 9.1 Hyperlordosis caused by, for example, pregnancy or obesity.

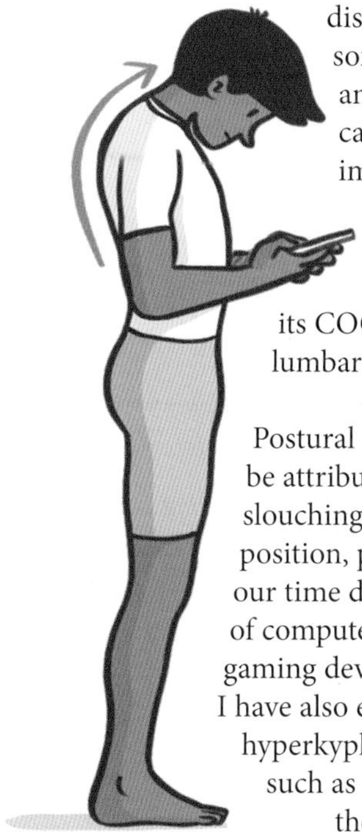

disparities present in some sports (e.g., dance and gymnastics) and can cause tensional imbalances that result in the pelvis tilting anteriorly. The body will have to maintain its COG by increasing the lumbar curve.

Postural hyperkyphosis can be attributed mostly to slouching and the head forward position, predominant of our time due to excessive use of computers, phones, and gaming devices, etc. (Figure 9.2). I have also encountered marked hyperkyphosis in sport fighters, such as Thai boxers, due to the rounded upper back protective stance. The good thing about curvature changes due to posture and muscular imbalance is that they should be correctable with the prescription of the right exercises.

Figure 9.2 Hyperkyphosis caused by, for example, excessive computer or phone usage.

Each section of the spine has a certain number of vertebrae—cervical (7), thoracic (12), lumbar (5), sacral (5 fused), coccygeal (4 fused)—but anyone can have one more or less (Figure 9.3). When identifying a particular vertebra, we give it the letter from the name of the section and a number counting from the top. So, the top cervical vertebra is C1 and the last C7. If talking about a particular part of the spine where movement is taking place, the two adjacent vertebrae are referenced, as in T12/L1, the bottom thoracic and top lumbar vertebra.

The spine gets its incredible mobility through the number of movable segments, 24 sites in total if we include the L5–S1 junction. I think you can see in Figures 9.3 and 9.4 that the vertebrae are quite small in the cervical area and then increasingly larger as you move down toward the sacrum (Figure 9.4).

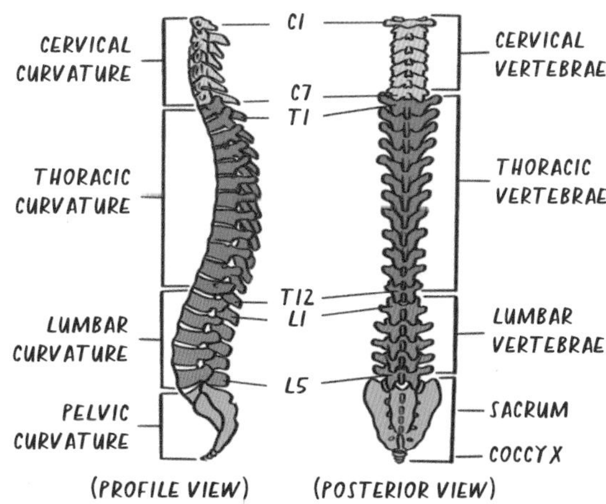

Figure 9.3 Construction of the spine.

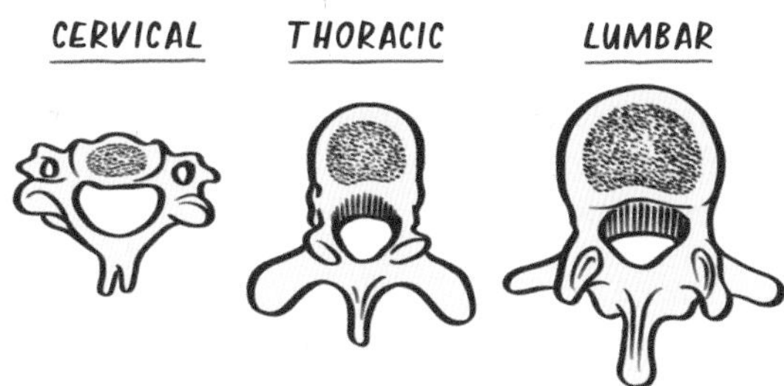

Figure 9.4 The size of the vertebrae vary considerably as you go down the spine.

A vertebra can be divided into a front part, which is basically an oval lump of bone (vertebral body), and a back part which consists of several bony projections (processes) (Figure 9.5). Between each vertebral body is an intervertebral disc. These cartilaginous joints are classified as slightly movable, hence the importance of the number of opportunities for movement (articulation). The discs are vulnerable to damage, such as bulging and herniation (rupturing), but are not in themselves the limiter to directional movement—that happens due to the rear section of the vertebra.

Right behind the vertebral body is the oval-ish space (vertebral foramen) through which the spinal cord travels, and then we have the processes. The ones that stick out sideways are called the transverse processes, and although muscles and ligaments attach to them, they are not of that much

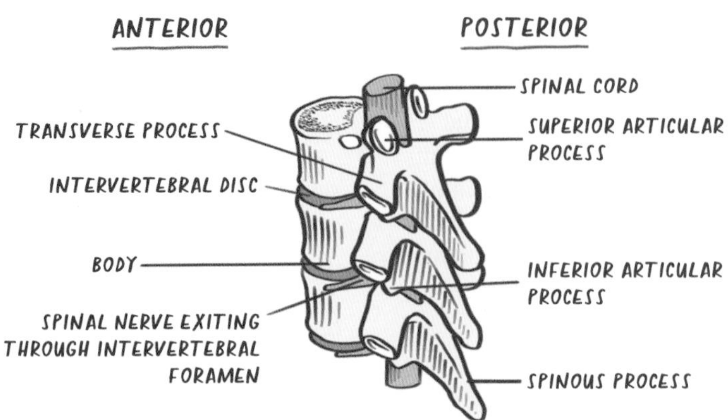

Figure 9.5 You might consider the front section of a vertebra as weight-bearing and the rear as restricting and allowing movement through muscle attachments and process shape.

interest to us as they provide no bony restriction to what we can do with the spine. Pointing backward are the spinous processes, and they vary significantly and consequentially between the different sections.

In the thoracic area, the spinous processes are the longest and project downward, roughly 40 to 60 degrees (it changes throughout the section) and therefore almost lay down on the one below (Figure 9.6). If you remember from Chapter 2, *Compression*, when bone meets bone, there is no more movement in that direction. In this area of the spine, there is then an absolute limiting bony restriction to extension. Although it may look like you are getting a significant curve when you look at the ribcage, you are not.

Look at the X-ray reproduction of a contortionist doing a backbend with the butt sitting on the head (Figure 9.7). Even though it is much deeper than we would do in yoga, you can see there is almost no extension in the thoracic spine. To go this deep, you literally have to hinge in several places.

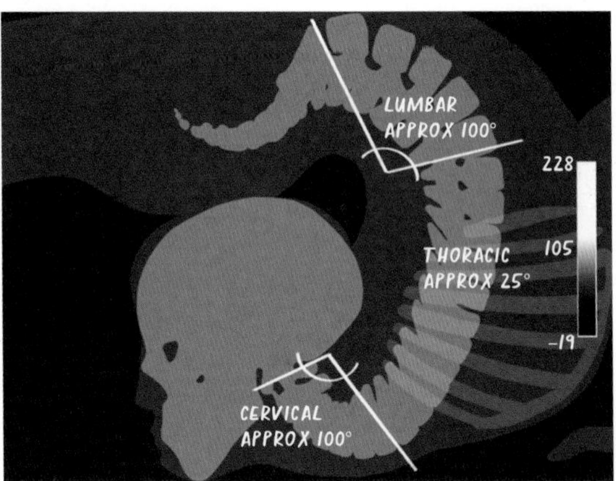

Figure 9.7 The curve of the ribcage is not representative of the curve in the thoracic spine.

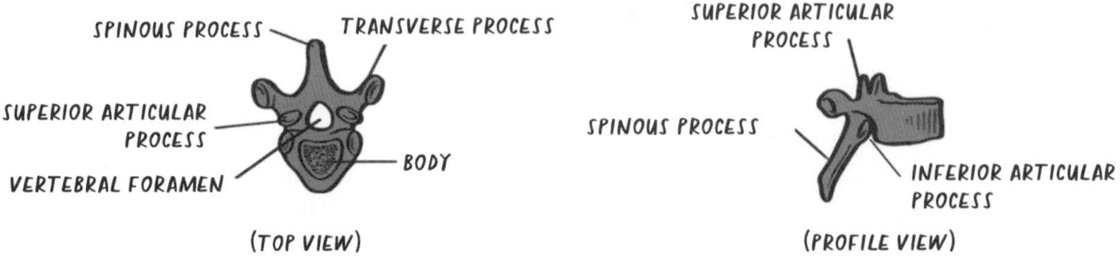

Figure 9.6 Thoracic vertebrae: Pay particular attention to the angle of the spinous processes in the thoracic vertebrae.

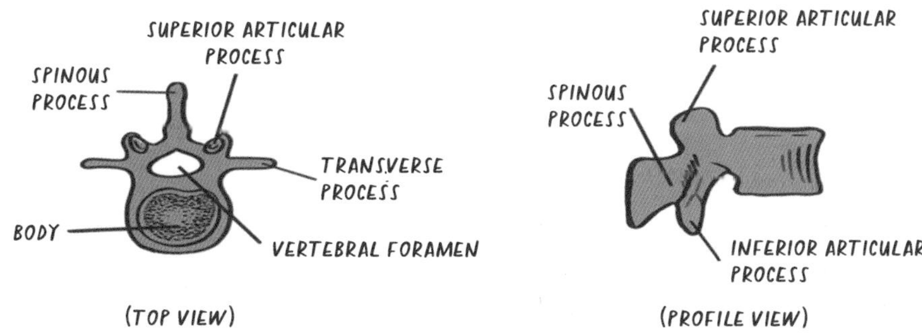

Figure 9.8 Lumbar vertebrae: Here the spinous processes are relatively straight but wider.

When we reach the lumbar area, the spinous processes are pretty straight but wider (Figure 9.8). The space between them will vary among individuals and can often reduce with age due to a thickening of the spinous processes themselves or a narrowing of the intervertebral disc. Again, we have the potential for hard compression stopping further backbending, but this area is definitely designed to allow some to happen.

The spinous processes in the cervical area are generally shorter but do increase in length in the lower ones (Figure 9.9). C7 is often prominent when you look at the back of someone's neck because it is one of the longest spinous processes in the cervical area, and the angle at which it leaves the vertebral body is a bit straighter. Apparently, about 50 percent of the generous amount of flexion and extension we have available in the cervical spine happens between the skull and C1. Almost 50 percent of rotation happens one joint down between C1 (Atlas) and C2 (Axis).

We have talked about the bits that stick out sideways and backward, so now let's cover the most important from our perspective. It is the small facet joints between each pair of vertebrae that ultimately determine what movements are readily available as their orientation differs as we travel the length of the spine (Figure 9.10). These facet joints are created by articulating processes that point superiorly (up) and inferiorly (down) on both sides of the vertebrae. If, for example, we consider T9, the two superior articulating processes meet with the two inferior processes of T8, and the two inferior articulating processes of T9 meet with the two superior articulating processes of T10.

These articulating processes in the thoracic spine are oriented in the frontal plane, which means they will happily allow rotation but resist flexion and especially extension. In the lumbar area, they are oriented in the sagittal plane accommodating flexion and extension but resisting rotation. In the cervical region, the ROM that we can happily demonstrate is due to the facet joints being oriented approximately 30 to 40 degrees anteriorly from the frontal plane (Figure 9.11).

Let's consider some other factors that may limit ROM. One of the main functions of the

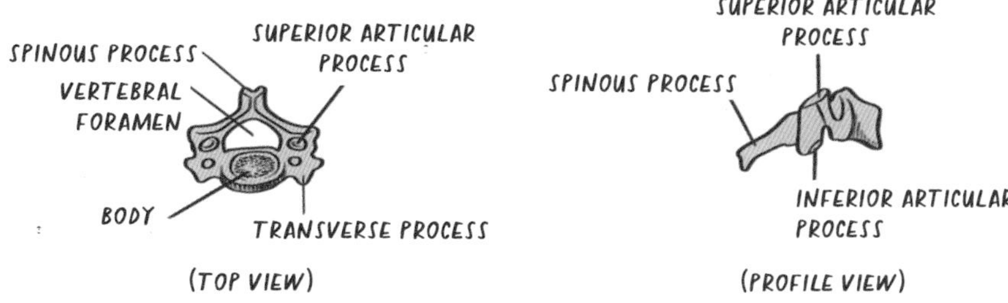

Figure 9.9 Cervical vertebrae: Here the spinous processes are generally shorter.

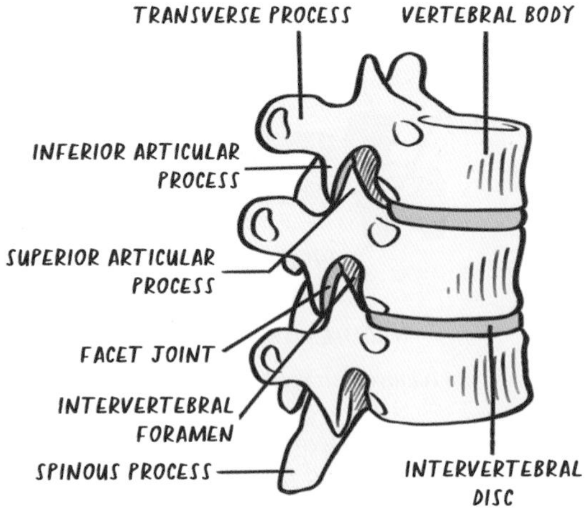

Figure 9.10 The articulating processes determine the movements available in the spine.

thoracic area is to provide protection for our vital internal organs. One of the ways this is achieved is by having the ribcage around them. You can appreciate that if you have a protective container, you won't want it to deform much otherwise the stuff inside would get squished. So, in delivering its functional requirements, the ribcage severely restricts flexion and, even more so, extension in this area of the spine. A pair of ribs attach to each thoracic vertebra at what is called the costal facets (that doesn't mean near the sea but referring to the ribs).

Because the spine curves, there is also a change in the center of rotation for each vertebra (Figure 9.12). In the lumbar region, it is at the

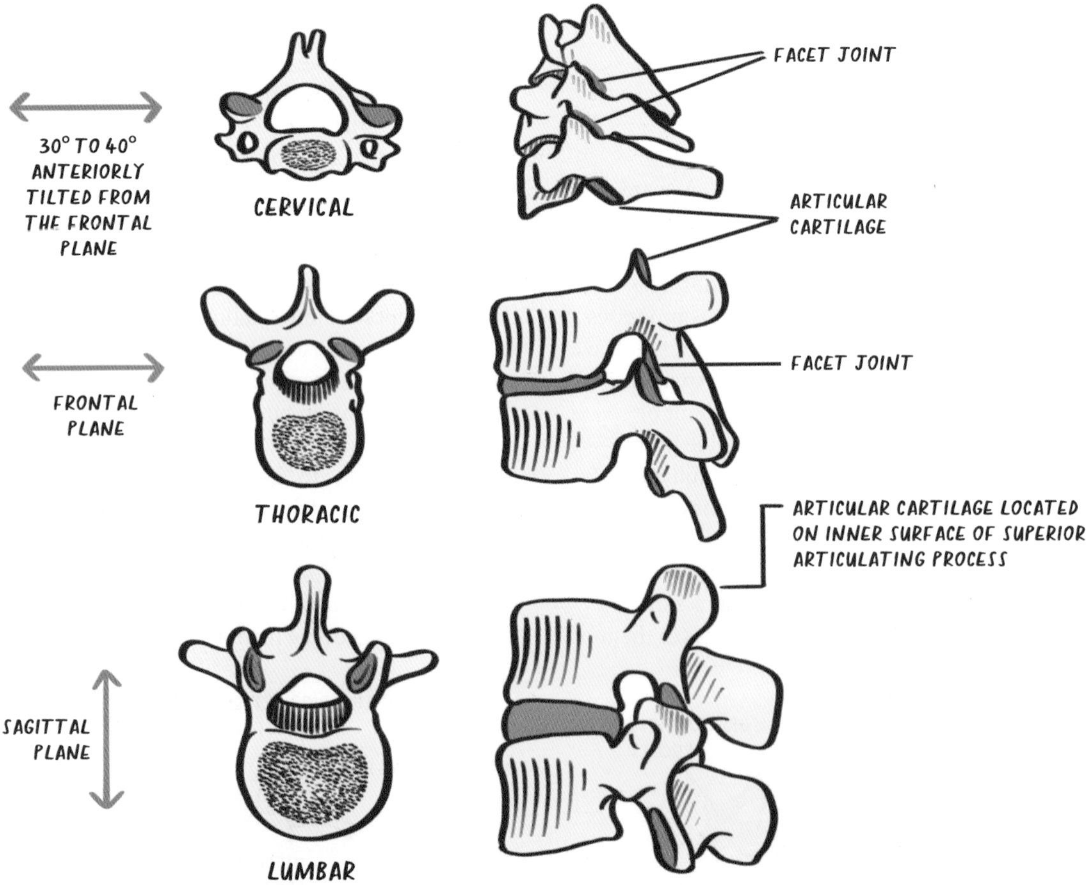

Figure 9.11 The directionality of the articulating processes changes along the length of the spine.

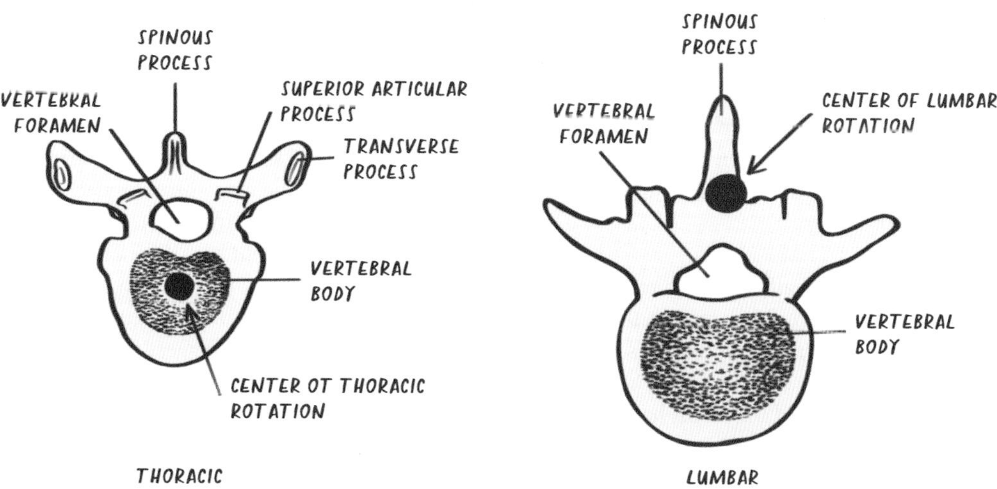

Figure 9.12 The center of rotation is in a different place for the thoracic and lumbar vertebrae.

bottom of the spinous process, while in the thoracic area, it is the center of the vertebral body. This, again, assists the thoracic region in its role of providing the rotational movement.

It is useful for us as yoga practitioners to understand the structural differences between the three movable regions of the spine (cervical, thoracic, and lumbar) and the subsequent implications for where we should try and focus specific movements. This amounts to a thoracic area designed to twist but flex poorly and resist extension, a lumbar area designed to flex and extend but resist twisting, and a cervical area that can accommodate most movements.

We are now going to think about general stability in the spine (Figure 9.13). Two long ligaments run all the way up the spine, just in front and behind the vertebral bodies. Up the front is the anterior longitudinal ligament (ALL), and at the back is the posterior longitudinal ligament (PLL). The ALL resists spinal extension, the PLL flexion, and they both help support the intervertebral discs. The ALL is stronger and thicker than the PLL, which might indicate that the body sees excessive extension as more dangerous. We will come back to this in Chapter 14, *Backbends*.

Where there is a transition between one area and another, for example, thoracic to lumbar or lumbar to sacral, the facet joints are more liberal in their orientation and incorporate a degree of movement from the adjoining section. This leads to a certain amount of instability and, hence an increased risk of injury. By far, the most common sites of

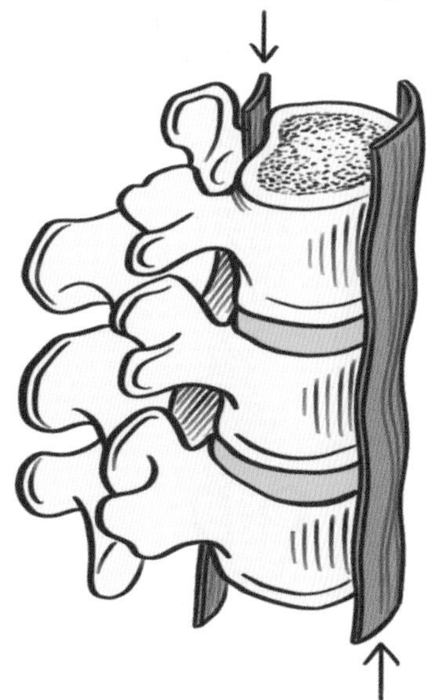

Figure 9.13 General stability in the spine: ALL and PLL.

injury are between L4/L5 and L5/S1 (between 90 to 95 percent of herniations) with the junctions between C6/C7, C7/T1, and T12/L1 also showing a greater incidence of injury. These are also the areas you can observe some students moving in, predominantly when doing deep backbends. I refer to this excessive localized movement as "hinging." The money question is whether this is detrimental to spine health or not.

As a starting point, we really have limited functional requirement to interact with the world behind us without turning around. That's not to say that we don't need to be able to extend our spine, but we have no need to fold in half apart from entertaining punters at a circus. Most of us spend too much of our time on computers and interacting with the world in flexion, so it definitely seems sensible to unwind some of this pattern by going backward. But how far is enough? Research also seems to suggest that what we require most from this region of the body is stability and strength rather than instability. If students regularly move into those already fewer stable areas, the most likely outcome is that those areas will become increasingly mobile. At the same time, the adjacent sites of articulation will remain the same. There is often an association made with the incidence of back pain and lack of stability.

An argument could be made that, with enough abdominal and back strength, the spine can be protected even in the extreme extended positions. I might concede that in the short term this may be valid, but what about as we age and become weaker and those same places of instability are no longer able to be supported equivalently? In addition, I would like to suggest that postural yoga lives within the health and wellness sphere, not the entertainment arena, so what positive purpose are intense backbends providing?

Scoliosis

When the spine has a postural pattern that includes a lateral flexion, it is called scoliosis. There can be one curve (C-shaped) or sometimes two (S-shaped), with the second curve trying to bring the head back over the COG (Figure 9.14).

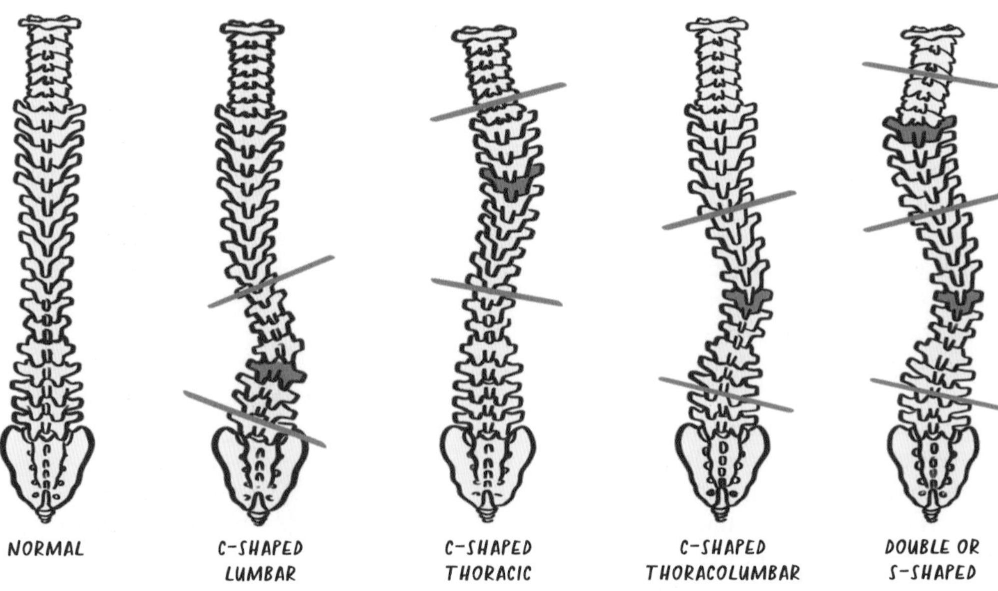

Figure 9.14 Types of scoliotic curve (the apex of the curve is in orange).

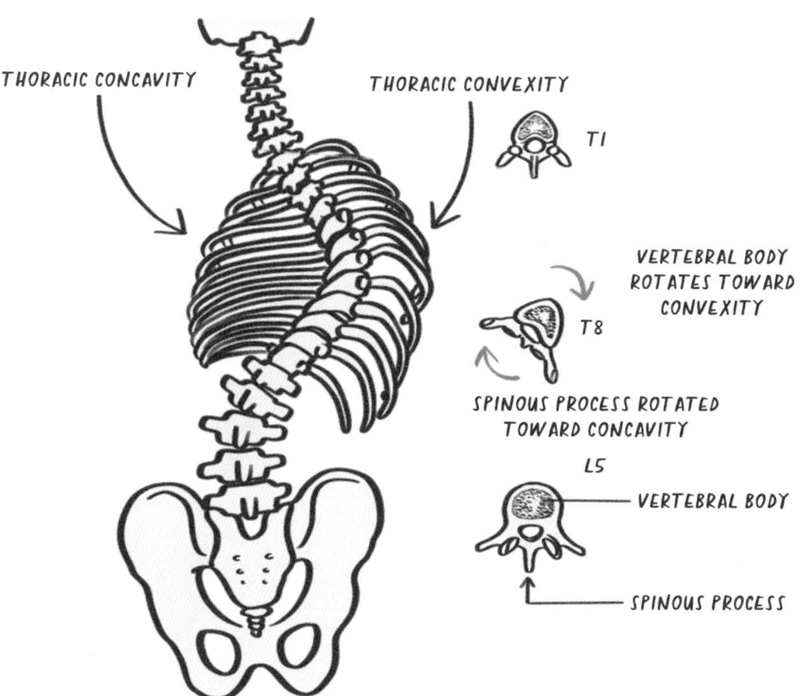

Figure 9.15 A scoliotic spine will often rotate toward the convexity of the curve.

The apex of the curve can be in any region of the spine, and regularly there will be a rotational element as well. The outer side of the curve is called the convexity, and the spine will rotate toward this direction (Figure 9.15).

You can see then that scoliosis is a three-dimensional adaptation, and as such, is a complex issue to address. Scoliosis can be structural, where there have been changes to the vertebrae, or functional, where often the spine itself is fine but is held in a laterally curved position by muscular tension or due to uneven leg length. Many people can have mild scoliosis and not even know because quite often there is no associated pain (Figure 9.16).

Several factors might highlight possible scoliosis, both visually and experientially (Figure 9.17). A student may stand with one shoulder higher and forward, place the hands unevenly on the mat in Down Dog, have a crease under the ribcage on one side, or a scapula (shoulder blade) and underlying ribcage that look more raised from the back. Additionally, their pelvis may not look square, or they may seem to rotate along the spine when in forward folding postures (Figure 9.18).

I have found that it is postures like *Balasana*, Cat, Down Dog, *Uttanasana*, and *Paschimottanasana* that bring attention to scoliosis, with what appears like more muscular bulk in one erector spinae group. In reality, there is often no muscular hypertrophy (increased muscle bulk), but it presents as such because the underlying vertebrae are rotating and their transverse processes are pushing the musculature up from underneath.

The individual with scoliosis may notice that they twist or side bend more easily to one direction or look slightly rotated or curved in inversions (e.g., Handstand, *Sirsasana*, and Shoulderstand). If the scoliosis is more pronounced, then it can influence other bodily functions, such as breathing and digestion, or involve a degree of pain. As mentioned earlier, setting out to address scoliosis itself, or indeed any associated symptoms, is less than straightforward and should be done under the guidance of a trained professional.

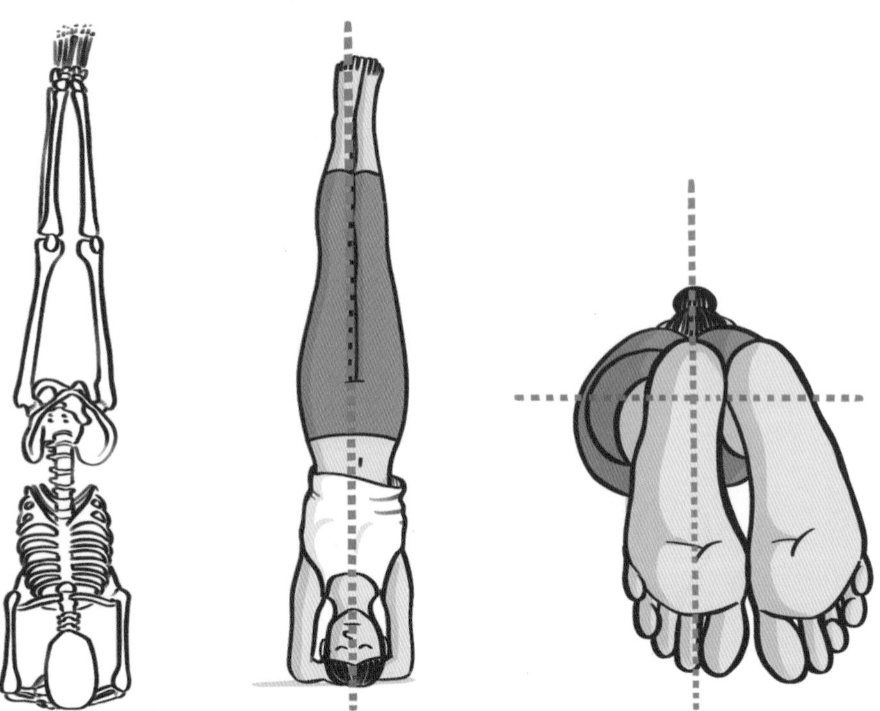

Figure 9.16 Many students have a mild scoliosis that they are not even aware of as it generates no discomfort and has minimal visual cues. A keen eye can sometimes notice slight rotations or dissymmetry in postures like Sirsasana.

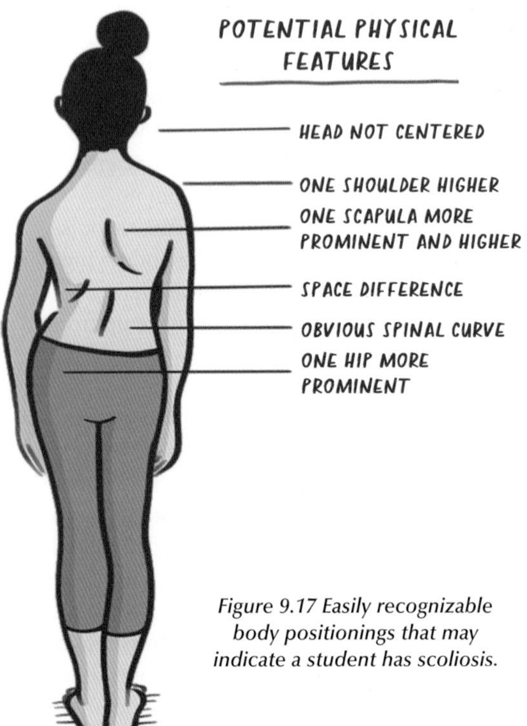

Figure 9.17 Easily recognizable body positionings that may indicate a student has scoliosis.

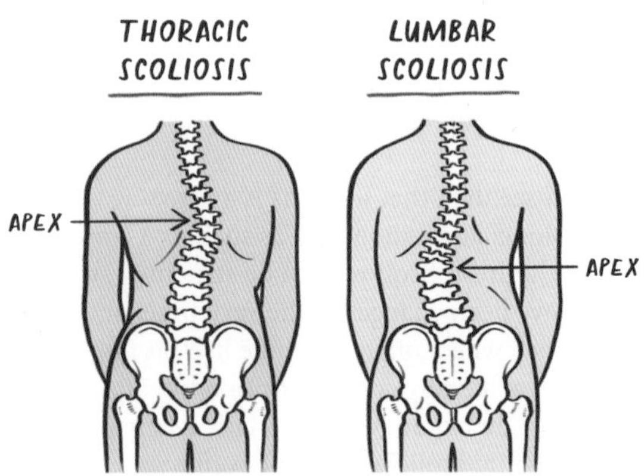

Figure 9.18 The apex of a scoliotic curve can be in different places in the spine.

Intervertebral Discs

This is not a yoga therapy book so we won't be discussing intervention related to disc issues, but what follows is an overview of what can happen to them and some subsequent possible contraindications.

Between every vertebral body and its adjacent neighbors is an intervertebral disc, which has a soft inner core (nucleus pulposus) and a tougher outside (anulus fibrosus) that act as a spacer and shock absorber. Owing to the effects of gravity on our body, the discs tend to compress during the day and plump up again overnight while we are non-weight-bearing. During our lifetime, they can undergo a degree of degradation, much like the rest of us, including thinning, drying out, and cracking (degeneration) (Figure 9.19). Damage to them can be gradual as in age-related changes, trauma, disease-induced, or as a result of wear and tear (osteoarthritis).

Two common conditions are disc bulges and herniated discs. A disc bulge can be diffuse, where there is a relatively symmetrical outward expansion of the disc, or focal, where the disc has bulged more in one area than another. In both cases, however,

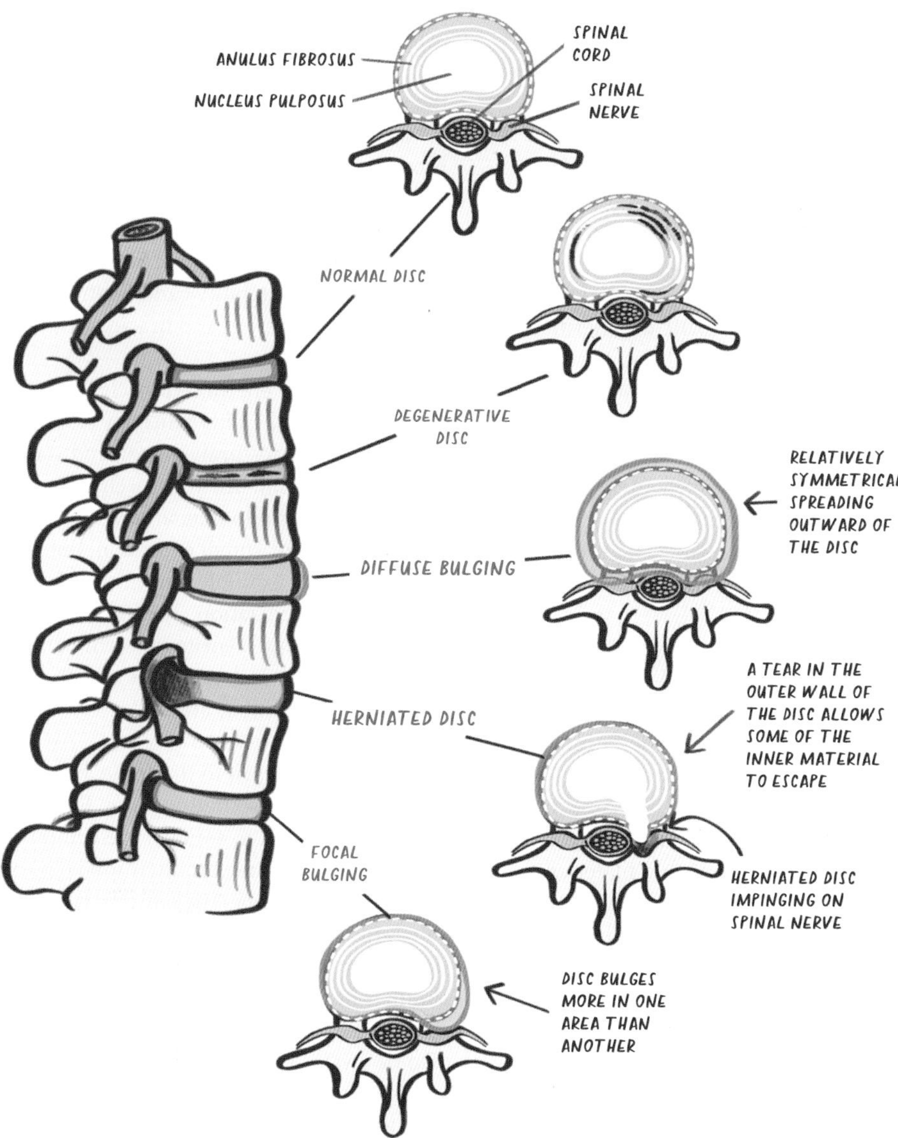

Figure 9.19 If disc material presses on a spinal nerve, pain and dysfunction may well be likely.

none of the nucleus has come out. There can still be associated pain and muscle tension, but many people will have bulging discs and be completely oblivious.

Alternatively, when herniated (also called prolapsed), a tear in the outer wall of the disc has allowed some of the inner material to escape. Depending on the direction of herniation, there is a strong likelihood of ensuing pain due to the disc material pressing on a nerve route. There will also be local inflammation and responsive muscle spasm. Apparently, it is also possible to have a herniated disc and be in no pain, but I imagine this could only be the case if there is no nerve route involvement.

Most of the pain associated with herniated discs resolves with conservative care within six weeks. Mindful movement seems to be the best course of action rather than complete rest unless movement is out of the equation, as is the case sometimes. The usual mechanism of traumatic disc herniation, not involving impact, is due to a flexed overloaded spine, sometimes also including a twisting element, such as when taking something heavy from the boot of the car. It is fair to say that injuries rarely happen in isolation—there is likely to be a history of bad posture, repetitive stressing, or just aging, that causes deterioration over time and sets the scene for the more severe injury.

Nearly all herniations happen at the bottom of the lumbar spine, segments L4/L5 and L5/S1. Due to flexed posture and the PLL supporting the back of the vertebral column, the direction of most herniations is posterolateral (toward the back and to the side). Unfortunately, that is the same location where the spinal nerves leave the intervertebral foramen. Consequently, the escaped material is likely to press on the nerve root and cause pain. It follows then that with posterolateral herniations, forward folding postures would be contraindicated because they can involve the same flexed spine position. Should the herniation be anterior, then backbending would be contraindicated. Deep twisting would also be ill-advised for any of these situations as this movement tends to compress the spine and increase the pressure on the nerve root.

Muscles that Move the Spine

There are a lot of muscles that move the spine, but we won't single out most of them because in yoga, you are not going to target them individually. I think it's more helpful to start by dividing them into two groups. Firstly, there are muscles involved with the gross movement of the ribcage and upper limbs, only some of which attach directly to the spine itself but will certainly greatly influence its position.

None of the four layers of abdominal muscles—transversus abdominis, the obliques (internal and external), and rectus abdominis—attach to the spine but instead to the ribcage and pelvis. As the ribs are connected to each vertebra of the thoracic spine, movements such as spinal flexion, rotation, and lateral flexion can be achieved by the contraction of these abdominal muscles moving the ribcage and hence the spine. Similarly, a significant degree of spinal stability can be introduced by their isometric contraction and bracing of the torso.

The other group are those muscles that attach to the spine itself and are directly responsible for movement, postural control, and stability of the spinal column. The most well-known is the erector spinae group that, among other actions, is responsible for spinal extension, but there are also others, for example, multifidus and rotatores involved in stabilization. The quadratus lumborum (QL) is one of my favorites, attaching to the spine, ribcage, and pelvis, laterally flexing the spine, and stabilizing the lumbar area.

Some muscles attach to the spine, but their primary action is to move something else. For example, rhomboids attach to some of the spinous processes of the thoracic spine, but their job is to move and stabilize the scapula. The famous psoas attaches to the lumbar vertebrae, and although if the legs are stabilized relative to the pelvis it can assist with lumbar flexion, its primary role is as a hip flexor.

Do be aware that there are other more sophisticated ways of grouping and dividing the muscles that influence spinal position and movement. Still, I reckon this is good enough for our purposes.

Erector Spinae Group

The erector spinae group of muscles run up either side of the spine from the sacrum to the skull and are easily visible on many individuals (Figure 9.20). It consists of three subgroups, iliocostalis, longissimus, and spinalis. These subgroups themselves have parts in the cervical, thoracic, and lumbar regions. Their combined action is to extend the spine if both sides contract together (bilateral action) or to laterally flex the spine when each side contracts independently (unilateral action).

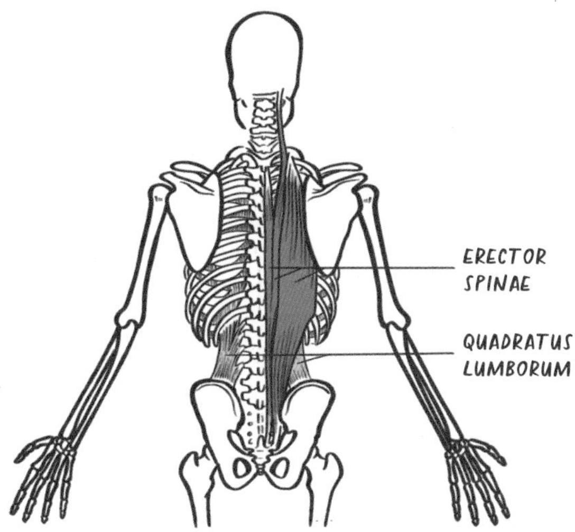

Figure 9.20 Erector spinae and QL.

Quadratus Lumborum

Spanning the gap between the bottom rib, the iliac crest, and the lumbar spine is the QL muscle (Figure 9.20). Again, there is a unilateral and bilateral action, lateral flexion, and stabilization of the lumbar spine, respectively. They can also assist in spinal extension.

Remember the idea that when a muscle contracts, area A can move toward area B or vice versa? Well, the same goes here. The QL can draw the ribcage to the iliac crest or the iliac crest toward the ribcage. Both scenarios result in a shortening of the side body, but with a stable pelvis, the movement is a side bend, and with the pelvis moving, the action is a hip hike. If there is a unilateral spasm of a QL, then the resulting hip hike can emulate a shorter leg and trigger a compensatory tensional pattern. The QLs often spring into action to immobilize the lumbar region if it has been overstressed. Their bilateral contraction will stiffen the low back, often preventing bending forward, and usually the individual experiences an aching across the whole low back. I have encountered many students with this type of protective spasming after attending enthusiastic backbending workshops.

Abdominal Muscles

The abdominals consist of four layers (Figure 9.21). Starting from the deepest and working toward the surface: transversus abdominis, internal obliques, external obliques, and the "six-pack" rectus abdominis. The transversus abdominis provides thoraco-pelvic stability and compression of the abdominal viscera by drawing the abdominal wall inward. It wraps around the body spanning the gap between the ribcage and the iliac crests. Around the back of the body, it merges into the thick fascia of the low back (thoracolumbar fascia), and attaches to the inner surface of the ribcage (lower six ribs).

Rectus abdominis, rather than coming around the sides, runs down the center of the abdomen, from the xiphoid process and ribcage to the pubic crest and pubic symphysis. A concentric contraction will cause flexion of the lumbar spine, while isometric contraction will brace the abdomen. Forceful

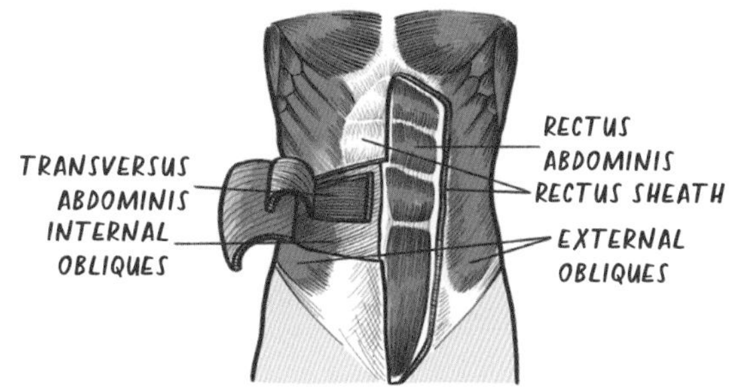

Figure 9.21 Abdominal muscles.

expiration is facilitated by this muscle, creating a powerful drawing in of the belly area.

The obliques again connect to the ribs and iliac crest but in slightly different ways, resulting in muscle fibers that run perpendicular to each other, and consequently, opposing muscle actions (Figure 9.22). If you visualize the shoulder moving as the ribcage and spine rotate, then we can say that the internal oblique draws the same side shoulder backward and the external oblique draws the same side shoulder forward. So, they work in pairs when we twist, external on one side and internal on the other. If the obliques contract on one side, then they will produce lateral flexion of the spine. All together they assist spinal flexion, as well as being accessory muscles of respiration.

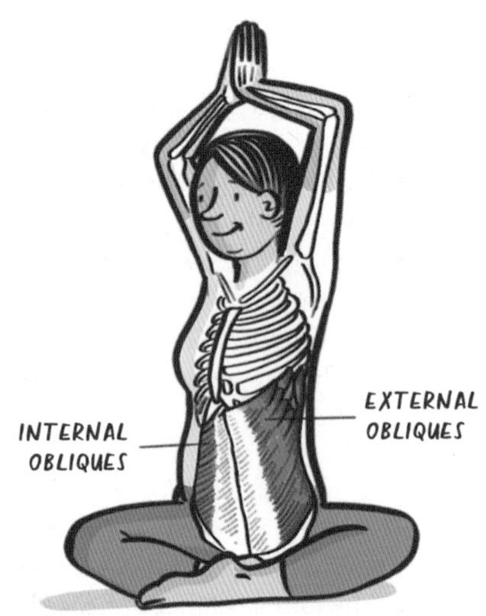

Figure 9.22 Obliques.

Quick Reference Muscle Action Tables

Flexion	Extension
Rectus abdominis	Erector spinae group
External obliques (bilateral contraction)	Quadratus lumborum (bilateral contraction)
Internal obliques (bilateral contraction)	

Lateral Flexion	Rotation
Quadratus lumborum	Obliques in opposing pairs
Erector spinae (unilateral contraction)	

Putting Things into Context

In Part III, we will have chapters on backbends and twists so, in the following paragraphs, we will focus on how the information detailed above informs us about likely movement patterns and injury risks.

A student who is hyperkyphotic will likely feel comfortable rounding the spine and have difficulty extending the spine. Therefore, there is a higher chance of them falling into that rounded pattern doing postures such as forward folds and twists. When it comes to poses that involve a rounded spine, for example, *Baddha Konasana B* or *Karnapidasana*, the student may well excel. However, it would be my recommendation that they avoid these postures as they will be encouraging their existing pattern. Although the thoracic spine does not typically extend much, the hyperkyphotic spine will, at best, still be in a level of kyphosis when attempting to backbend, the consequence of which is that other areas will try and compensate for the lack of movement there.

I would say that there will be a high risk of the student hinging in the lower spine. The deeper the backbend, the more the other areas will have to accommodate the movement. In my opinion, students exhibiting hyperkyphosis and an inclination to hinge should restrict themselves to the more shallow and controllable backbends, such as *Bhujangasana* and *Ustrasana*.

Setu Bandhasana, performed in the Ashtanga style, is a posture that I feel nearly everyone should avoid (Figure 9.23). The most fragile part of the spine, the cervical area (neck), is in an extended position and loaded. Worse still is that instruction is often given

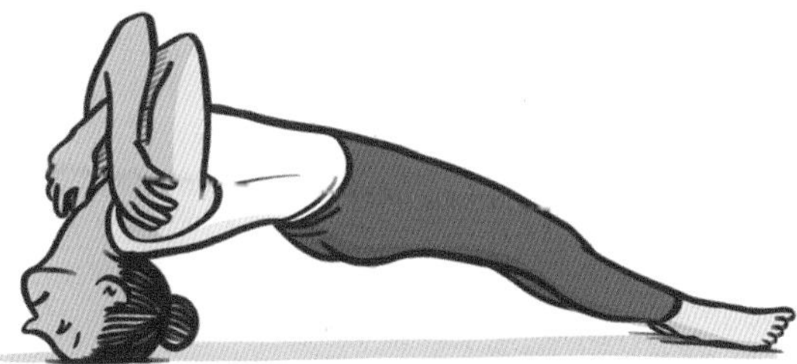

Figure 9.23 I feel that taking the neck into this much extension in Setu Bandhasana *is inadvisable for most students, and especially for those with existing neck issues.*

to take the forehead toward the floor, which further increases the neck extension. This movement is nearly always an exaggerated hinge because of the minimal thoracic extension combined with many students not having the strength to lift the hips very high.

Following on from the part on hyperkyphotic students, this for them is a "don't even think of it" posture, as they would hinge even more. The pose is often touted as a necessary neck strengthener, particularly with a view to placing the leg behind the head, for example, *Eka Pada Sirsasana*.

My view on that point is to choose a less complicated way to strengthen your neck and don't do a posture like the one just mentioned in a way that it will put such a strain on it (Figure 9.24).

Let's stick with neck vulnerability for the moment and consider *Sirsasana*. The size differential between the cervical and lumbar vertebrae, and in particular the vertebral bodies, suggests that the weight-bearing capabilities increase as we travel down the spine. This makes sense as there is more and more of us above each vertebra as we descend. In *Sirsasana*, all our body weight, apart from the head, is now above the cervical spine. Although the instruction is generally given to reduce the pressure by actively using your forearms and shoulders to press the floor away, this really does very little unless you can lift your head clear of the floor. Think for a moment how quickly you would tire if I asked you to hold *Chaturanga* (and that is not even all your body weight because the feet are on the floor).

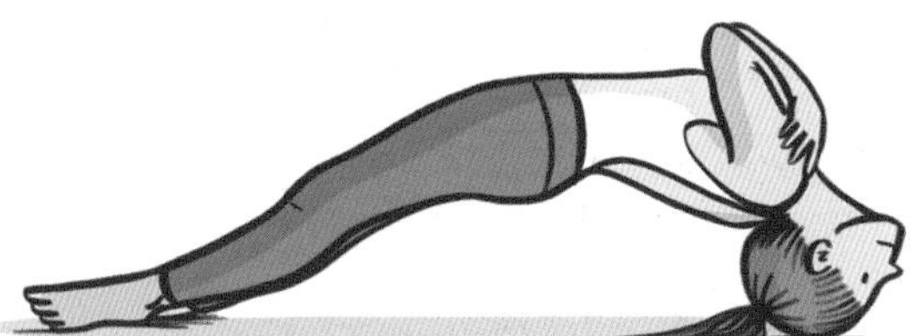

Figure 9.24 This is a healthier alignment because the hips and chest are higher and the cervical spine is in neutral. But I would still be happier if students didn't do the posture.

Continuing with *Sirsasana*, I am going to single out our hyperkyphotic student again. I can't see the possibility of them achieving a neutral spine, so I would say it is ill advisable for them to do this posture without the use of a prop, such as a headstand stool. Along with them, I will add anyone with a head forward posture or who suffers from neck pain or tension. From my point of view, I would prefer to see all students attempting this version of *Sirsasana* to do so by lifting their head clear of the floor.

I'm sorry, but I'm still not ready to leave this topic yet. The entry and exit into *Sirsasana* are the times when the neck is most vulnerable because of the potential for instability and being in a position that is not neutral when loading occurs. Subsequently, no hopping or jumping in is advisable. Entry and exit need to be controlled, and the best way is by using a straight leg raise.

The classic *Sirsasana* is the only variation that either allows the head to be lifted clear of the floor or at least allows attempting to reduce the weight-bearing. *Mukta Hasta Sirsansana A* is a popular variation where you have no choice but to spread the weight throughout your head. It is a very useful posture for entry into arm balances and other challenging sequences, but I would recommend that if you are going to use this pose and similar variations, you limit your time in them. Make sure you are stable and be highly aware of your spinal positioning.

In the main text, we mentioned that students coming from certain sporting or exercise backgrounds, for example, dance and gymnastics, may have hyperlordotic lumbar spines. Because of the dominance of hip flexion and a need for strong hip flexors and quadriceps, the chances are that the hamstrings are flexible but weak. This then leads on to an anteriorly tilted pelvis and increased lumbar lordosis. There may have also been some influence over the standing posture promoted, as the butt and chest pushed out with deep lordotic curve has often been thought to be aesthetically pleasing in these disciplines. Strengthening the core to decrease the space between the ribcage and pubic bone as well as strengthening the hamstrings themselves may go some way toward changing the postural pattern. As it is a pattern, bringing constant awareness to how one stands—and also yoga postures that reinforce it—will again allow the student to sense their positioning more easily.

Hyperlordotic students will usually find backbending easy because the spine is already heading that way in the area designed for extension, but they may also suffer from back issues or sensitivity because of over-accentuating the use of this area. Whenever there is a posture that involves both hip and back extension to make the shape, these students should emphasize a firming of the belly to reduce the availability of excessive movement in the lumbar area and focus on accessing the front of the hip more.

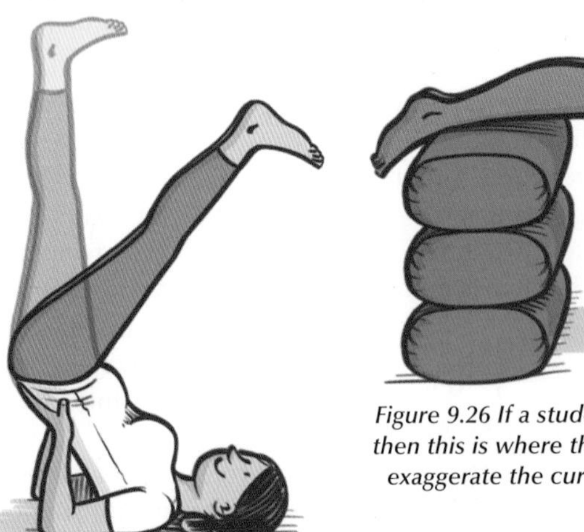

Figure 9.25 A 90 degree angle change is a lot to ask of the cervical spine in Shoulderstand. It is preferable to use a block of blankets or adjust your hip position, and care for your neck.

When it comes to Shoulderstands, I'm sure you already know that the weight should be in the shoulders, not the back of the neck. Even so, for most students, I feel that taking the body perpendicular to the floor without the use of a block or blankets to raise the shoulders and allow for a kinder angle in the cervical spine, is not sensible (Figure 9.25). The other option is to keep the hips further back and raise the legs perpendicular from there.

Following on from Shoulderstand in many sequences is *Halasana*. To take the feet to the floor requires a good helping of straight-leg hip flexion. Those students without it will be tempted to take too much strain into the neck to get the feet down. Leaving them hanging in the air is also not desirable because gravity will gradually drag them down. Having a bolster or blocks on which the student can rest their feet is a safer option (Figure 9.26). With hyperkyphotic students, as with *Karnapidasana*, I would advise not to do it as the lever of the legs will reinforce the rounding pattern in the thoracic spine.

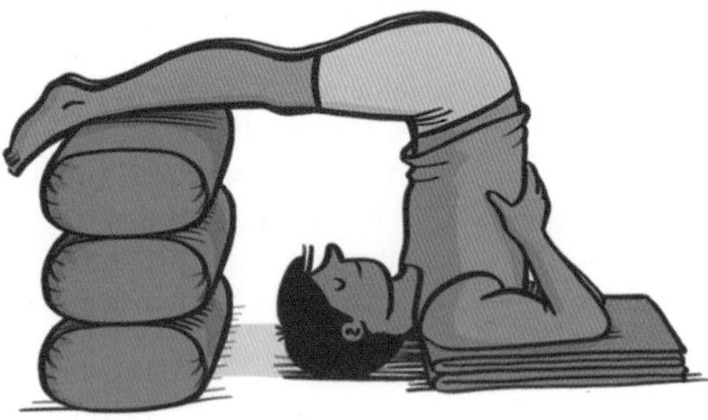

Figure 9.26 If a student has only 90 degrees of hip flexion, then this is where the legs should be. Otherwise, they will exaggerate the curving of the spine to try and bring the legs down.

CHAPTER 10

Sacroiliac Joint

Construction of the Sacroiliac Joint

Where the sacrum meets the ilium bones (ilia), we have the SIJs, one on each side. Looking from the back, they would run about 15 degrees from horizontal. They are slightly boomerang-shaped joints containing both fibrous and hyaline cartilage (Figure 10.1). The joint becomes more fibrous and restricted as we age, and even in our teens, there are only a few degrees of movement available.

The sacrum can tilt forward relative to the ilia (nutation), and backward relative to the ilia (counternutation) (Figure 10.2). Each half of the pelvis can also tilt anteriorly or posteriorly relative to the sacrum. Again, this movement is minimal and happens primarily in motions like the gait cycle, helping to transfer locomotive forces up into the spine. In this example, each half of the pelvis is going in different directions.

Both anterior and posterior sacral surfaces are heavily ligamentous, and this, along with the shape of the articulation, maintains the joint stability (Figure 10.3). Although some muscles attach to the sacrum (including multifidus, piriformis, and Gmax), it moves relative to the ilia, not due to muscular action but because of the positioning of the body. For this reason, as well as the incredibly strong ligaments and the few available degrees of motion, I don't think it is sensible to try and work toward increasing movement here. Instead, in the paragraphs on putting things into context, I will

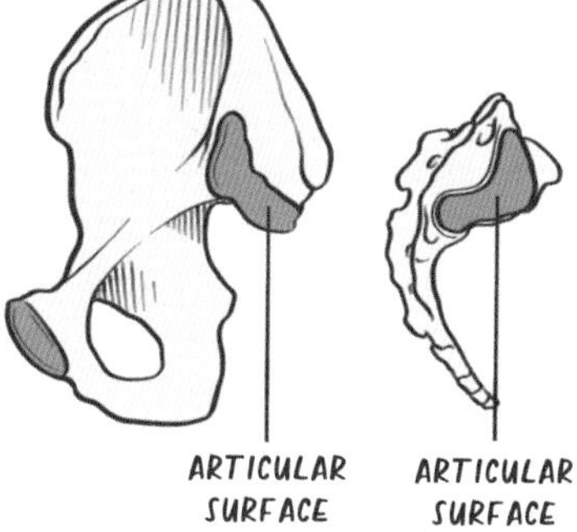

Figure 10.1 The right half of the pelvis (innominate bone) with the sacrum rotated on the vertical axis 180 degrees so that the corresponding articulating surfaces can be seen.

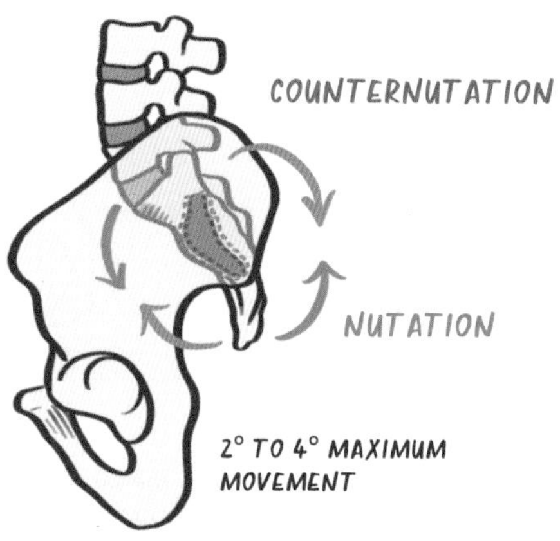

Figure 10.2 Dotted line shows potential movement.

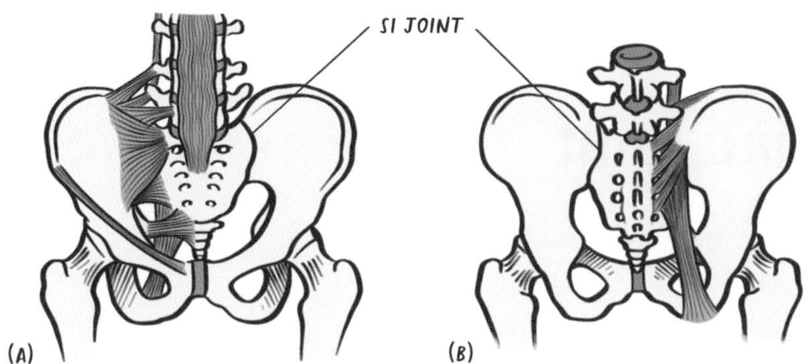

Figure 10.3 The SIJ is heavily ligamentous on both the anterior (A) and posterior (B) surfaces.

focus on protecting the SIJ from the sort of torquing forces we can generate in postural yoga.

Below the sacrum is the coccyx (tailbone), and along with the sacrum, this can be more or less curved across the spectrum of individuals. If the arrangement is on the straighter side, the student may find it uncomfortable to roll around and balance on their tailbone.

Muscles that Move the Sacrum

The piriformis is the only muscle that attaches fully to the sacrum—the others only attach with some fibers that are part of a broader connection to the pelvis—and then attaches to another bone other than the pelvis (Figure 10.4). The piriformis originates from the anterior sacral surface but skips over the pelvis and connects to the greater trochanter of the femur. So, I am going to stick with the idea that no muscles directly move the sacrum. Many muscles may have a role to play in the SIJ moving, but indirectly by changing the positioning of the body.

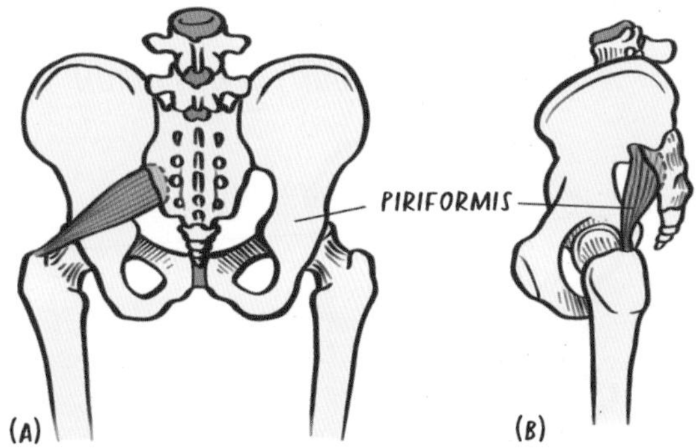

Figure 10.4 The piriformis attaches to the sacrum but not the pelvis, (A) posterior view, (B) profile view.

We have talked before about the problems involved in segmenting the body to try and discuss joint actions, stability, and movements. The SIJ is a prime example of an area that is influenced not only by adjacent bones but by far-reaching fascial connections, muscle chains, global positioning, and regional stabilization.

If you have stretched the ligaments around the SIJ, then you are going to have trouble stabilizing it again because of precisely this lack of direct muscular involvement. Usually in these situations, the instruction is given to strengthen all the surrounding muscles, especially those that travel transversely.

Typically, SIJ pain is felt directly over the SIJ itself, often seeming to emanate from a specific location rather than the whole length of the joint (Figure 10.5). But it may also refer pain into the buttocks, low back, back of the thigh, or even the groin, particularly if you are getting protective muscle spasm. The pain itself is regularly experienced as a dull ache, but can also be sharp, stabbing, or unimaginably painful. What you experience will be dependent on the issue, for example, ligament sprain, joint inflammation, instability, or misalignment.

To give you an idea, I have come across numerous students who have reported their symptoms as a dull ache that lasted over between a couple of months and several years. I was not so lucky when I caused acute inflammation of the SIJ. The pain I experienced was so intense that within several hours of the first onset of discomfort, I needed pethidine injections (extremely strong opioid-based pain medication). All sorts of muscles went into a protective spasm, and the recuperation involved several months on crutches.

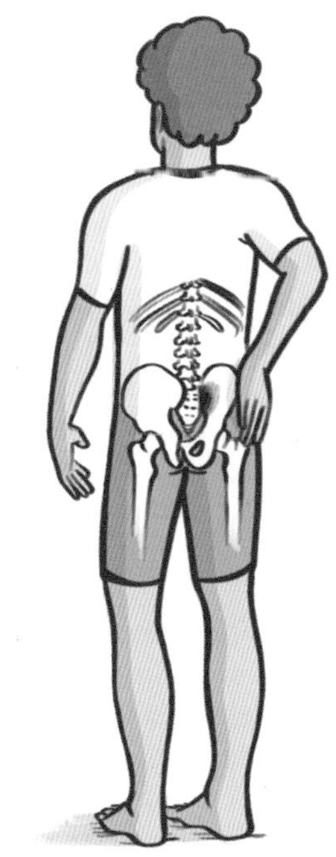

Figure 10.5 SIJ pain is typically felt directly over the joint itself.

The important thing is that SIJ pain is not something to be ignored. Take action by exploring what you are doing to aggravate the area. Some misinformed students feel that pain and discomfort are part of the journey to a more open body. That is never the case and even more so in this area because we are not looking to gain increased ROM at this joint. The good news is that not everything that presents as SIJ pain is actually that, and in many cases, it can be trigger points in Gmed or Gmin referring pain to that area.

Putting Things into Context

It is possible to hurt or misalign the SIJ through accidents such as sporting collisions, falls, and car crashes, which may involve tearing or spraining the ligaments. Luckily yoga involves controlled movement, so it is unlikely that students will suffer a traumatic injury. We are much more likely to stretch or sprain a ligament by introducing torquing forces repeatedly into the area. Many yoga students can land up with nagging SIJ pain or worse. It's handy then to know some of the ways we can stress these supporting ligaments.

I consider there to be three main types of movements that may pose significant problems: passive twisting, asymmetric postures, and using the leg as a lever. They collectively relate to the introduction of a force that is, in effect, trying to move the sacrum within the ilia, or vice versa, against the protective resistance of the ligaments.

With active twists, you are going to move in the right places because you are only using your rotational muscles to do the job. However, if there is assistance by way of gravity or a lever (passive twist), then when the thoracic area stops rotating, that rotational force can move into the lumbar or sacral area. Should the pelvis not be free to move with the spine, then that twisting action can place strain on the SIJ. Examples of a lever could be an elbow or arm to increase the depth of the twist, a strong adjustment, or using a bind.

The posture we will use to explore this idea is *Parivrtta Parsvakonasana*. If this pose is done with the foot turned out to the side, it effectively locks the pelvis in position. Should the student then use the arm or elbow on the outside of the front knee to increase the twist, there is nowhere for this force to escape, and the energy can easily be taken into the lumbar or sacral area (Figure 10.6). If the student is instead on the ball of the foot and applies too much effort, then the pelvis will start to rotate with the spine. We will continue with a more in-depth look at *Twists* in Chapter 16.

Postures that involve having asymmetric hips can impose forces trying to take each half of the pelvis in different directions. The gait cycle is an example of this as a natural movement that a healthy SIJ can comfortably accommodate. However, when you are fixing legs in position and then adding force, there can be a vulnerability.

Hanumanasana is an excellent example. In this posture, the front hip is flexed, and the back hip

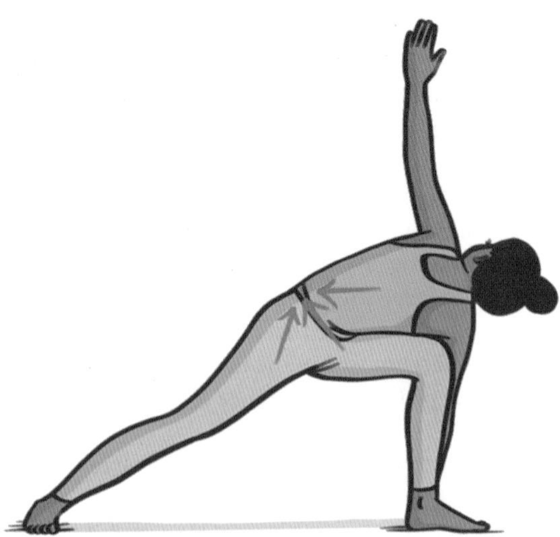

Figure 10.6 If the arm is used on the outside of the leg as a lever to increase the twist, there is the potential to take stress into the SIJ.

is extended. If both upper legs are grounded easily, then there is enough ROM at the hip joints. On the other hand, if there is space under the upper legs, then the downward force of gravity will be challenging the available ROM at the hips. If the muscles resist any further ROM, the ilia can be pulled by the legs in opposite directions. This can again place stress on the supporting ligaments around the SIJ (Figure 10.7). What do you think I would say about bouncing in this position?

The legs don't always have to be in opposite positions to have a similar effect. The previous example had one hip flexed and the other extended, but something like the popular pose, *Kapotasana*, can easily present problems. In this posture, if the shin is parallel to the front of the mat, the hip is externally rotated deeply, as well as being flexed. This position is extremely challenging for many students, and what you might observe is that the thigh and hip of the front leg are not grounded. As well as putting pressure on the outside of the knee (LCL), this positioning will also cause the pelvis to twist, again making the SIJ susceptible to gravitational forces (Figure 10.8). For these reasons, I consider *Kapotasana* with the shin in this position an advanced posture and not something to be placed in a beginner's sequence.

Both the previous examples of asymmetric postures could also be included in the group of "using the leg as a lever." Still, many poses where the legs are doing different things can place stress on the SIJ, especially if the SIJ is already irritated or the ligaments are lax.

We previously talked about the posture *Janu Sirsasana A* concerning the potential for placing pressure on the knee. It is also possible that restriction in that bent leg hip will hold the pelvis in place as the student tries to move forward. If they are rounding their spine and pulling themselves forward, it is possible to place additional stress on the SIJ of the bent leg side. Incidentally, this same idea applies to all forward folds where the spine has been rounded. If the stress doesn't go into the low back, it will go into the SIJ instead.

The last group I mentioned was to do with using the leg as a lever. A typical time for Ashtanga practitioners to start experiencing SIJ pain is when they embark on the leg behind head postures in the intermediate series. Unless adequate external

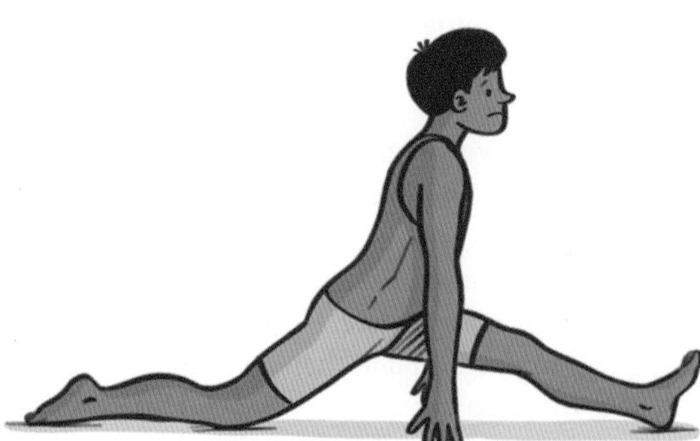

Figure 10.7 Weight-bearing asymmetric postures can place stress on the SIJ.

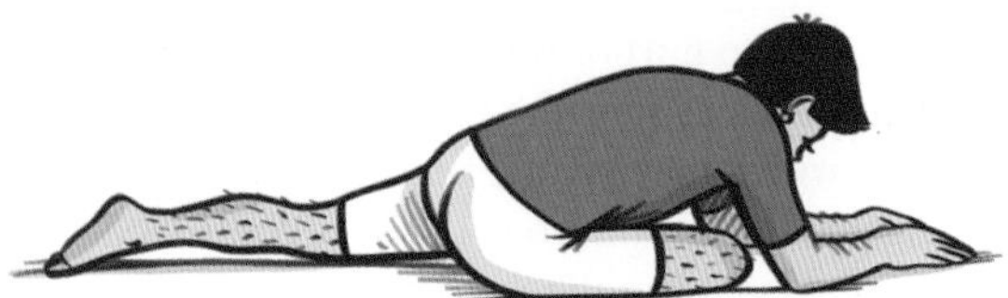

Figure 10.8 Here, Dave has taken the shin forward, but his restriction has caused the pelvis to twist.

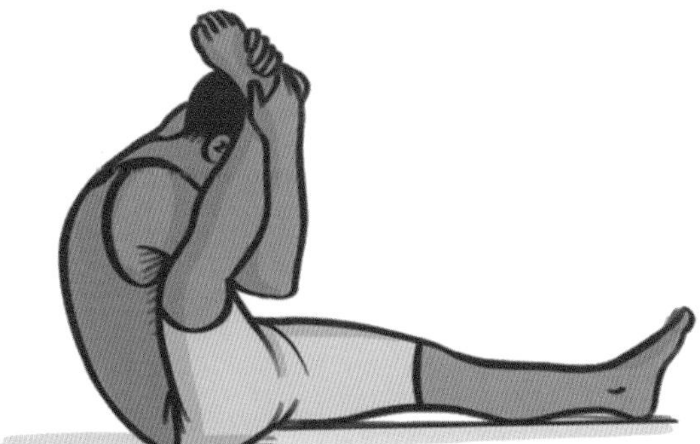

Figure 10.9 I cringe every time I see this type of body distortion. And I have to cringe a lot!

rotation and hip flexion are available, the student will round the back excessively, with the foot probably placed on the back of their neck. If that is not bad enough for the cervical and lumbar spine, to make matters even worse, they may have lifted the hip off the floor (single-leg seated version) as they raised their leg, making the pelvis uneven in the process. Then, in trying to sit up straighter, they use the back of their neck to lever the leg, which, in turn, levers the pelvis on the sacrum (Figure 10.9). This can generate a very powerful force on all accommodating areas involved but notably the SIJ.

This time, instead of thinking about taking the two halves of the pelvis in different directions, we will consider the legs going out to the sides. In poses such as *Baddha Konasana* and *Samakonasana*, the legs can act as levers on the pelvis, pulling the ilia apart from the sacrum. Of course, this will be resisted by the ligaments, but the legs are long and can be heavy.

As ligaments play such a fundamental role in providing the stability of the SIJ, anything that influences their pliability will affect the integrity of the joint. Students who are considered hypermobile need to take extra care of this area, because their ligaments already have a tendency of laxity. One of the other special interest groups would be pregnant students, as their body will release the hormone relaxin to prepare the pelvis for birthing. Some students may experience that their body feels less integrated into the second half of their menstrual cycle, also because of relaxin release.

The way I go on, it may seem like it is safer to sit in a chair and have a cup of tea instead of doing yoga. Most of the time, most students can practice safely. The purpose of this chapter is to bring your attention to the fact that things can go wrong, and it's usually due to a lack of awareness. If you or your student is experiencing discomfort in the SIJ region, then it is time to take a close look at the postures being performed.

CHAPTER 11

Shoulder

Much like the relationship between the hip-knee-ankle-foot chain, there is a lot of interaction between the elements of the upper body combination of shoulder-elbow-wrist-hand. In the yoga setting, we generally start questioning what's going on with the shoulder when we find we have trouble binding or doing Reverse Prayer, can't stop the elbows sticking out, or if we can't straighten the arms in some poses. We do have to support ourselves on our hands or forearms in some yoga postures, and I think many more students notice that they are weaker or less stable in the upper body than the lower body.

The bone and joint configuration of the arm and leg are somewhat similar. Working outward there is a ball-and-socket joint, then a modified hinge, and lastly a joint combo. This arrangement of lots of movements, followed by fewer movements, and then lots of movements again, enables superb functionality and adaptability while also providing greater control of the limbs. With the bones themselves, we have one in the upper arm and leg, two in the lower (one thick, one thin), and then a load in the wrists, hands, ankles, and feet (Figure 11.1).

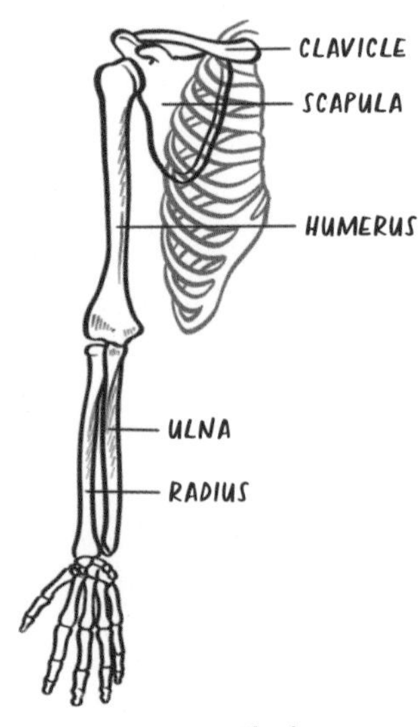

Figure 11.1 The bones of the upper limb.

Construction of the Shoulder Complex

Unlike the hip joint that is built for weight-bearing and is somewhat robust due to strong stabilizing ligaments, the shoulder joint is designed for interaction with our environment. We want to be able to reach up high, scratch our backs, and position our hand with precision and agility. The shoulder joint construction reflects these functional requirements with a shallow socket and much lighter ligaments than those of the hip. However, this need for mobility comes at a cost. The compromise is a reduction in stability and hence an increased risk of injury.

When we say, "shoulder joint," generally we are talking about where the humerus (upper arm bone) articulates, but really this is called the glenohumeral joint (GHJ) because the name of the socket is the glenoid fossa, situated on the scapula (shoulder blade). The shoulder is more complicated than the hip because the scapula is part of the shoulder girdle, which itself articulates with the axial skeleton (skull, vertebral column, ribcage, and sternum). The other bone that comprises the

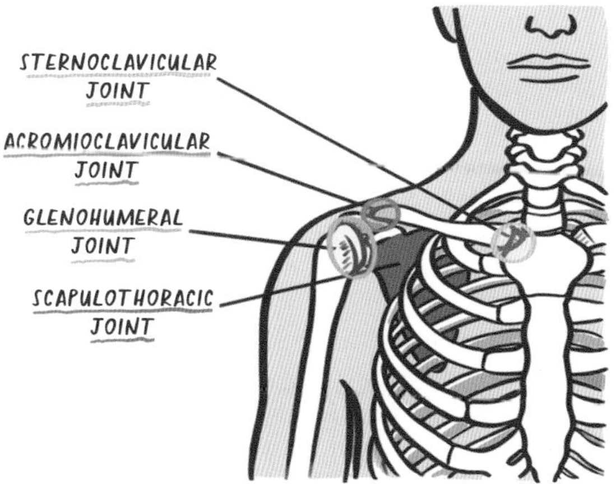

Figure 11.2 Shoulder complex joints.

shoulder girdle is the clavicle (collar bone), so we also have a joint at both ends of the clavicle. Where it joins the sternum is the sternoclavicular joint (SCJ), and where it connects to the acromion process of the scapula, the acromioclavicular joint (ACJ). Lastly, the scapula articulates with the ribcage, the scapulothoracic joint (STJ). This is not a joint in the same way as the others because there is no joint capsule or synovial fluid (Figure 11.2). The scapula just fits nicely on the back of the ribcage and is held there by muscles. We can refer to the combination of these four articulations as the shoulder complex.

A big difference between the pelvis-leg relationship and that of the arm-scapula is that the scapula can move around on the back. In conjunction with the shoulder girdle arrangement, it can slide backward around the ribcage and toward the spine (retraction), forward and laterally (protraction), up (elevation), and down (depression). The scapula can also rotate up and down, which changes the angle of the glenoid fossa and, consequently, how far up we can take our arm. I don't want you to blow a gasket, but the scapula can also tip forward and backward, and rotate externally and medially about its vertical axis. We might notice this last movement in a student when the inside edge of their scapula (medial border) pops away from their back when lowering in *Chaturanga*. We tend to refer to this appearance as "winging scapula," although this is not the same as the medical condition by the same name.

Don't get bogged down, just appreciate that by the scapula moving we can accentuate some of the movements available to the arm, but that we may also need to stabilize the scapula on the back (Figure 11.3). When the scapula is moving, there will also be articulation at the ACJ and SCJ.

The scapula has three projections, the acromion process that comes across the top of the shoulder, the coracoid process that pokes through to the chest just below the clavicle, and a ridge across the back called the spine. The spine of the scapula is a handy landmark, but it is knowing more about the acromion process that is useful for us as yogis.

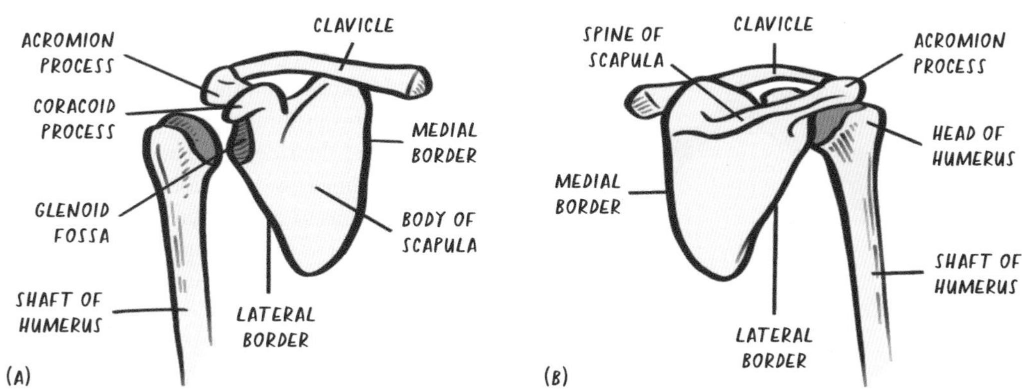

Figure 11.3 As with the pelvis, it is handy to know the landmarks of the shoulder girdle, (A) anterior view, (B) posterior view.

There are three classified shapes of the acromion process: flat (type I), curved (type II), and hooked (type III) (Figure 11.4). I'm sure when we take into account human skeletal variability, it is also possible to combine different length acromion processes, ones that overhang more laterally, as well as slight differences in the shape, angle, and depth of the glenoid fossa. With a person who has a hooked acromion process or another variation that means more bone overhangs, the humerus will likely bang on the acromion process (hard compression) before the full range of shoulder flexion is completed. This translates into the same person who in Down Dog was not able to get a straight line between their torso and wrists. Any posture, e.g., Handstands, *Virabhadrasana A*, or *Utkatasana*, where the shoulders are fully flexed would be the same.

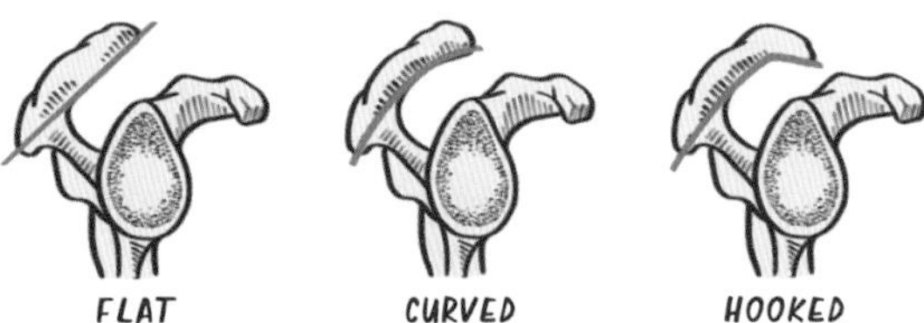

Figure 11.4 Different shape acromion processes. There is actually a fourth that curves the other way.

Most people have type II, but as with all underlying bone structures, you wouldn't know unless you had an X-ray. What is important to appreciate is that this skeletal structure can be one of the impediments to shoulder flexion (Figure 11.5).

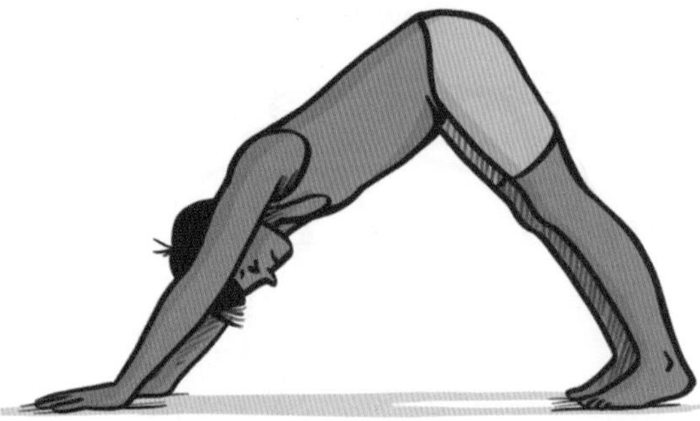

Figure 11.5 Hard compression of the humerus bone on the acromion process can prevent the full range of shoulder flexion being achieved.

The same compression rules would apply: don't force against the bone, and discomfort would be felt in front of the direction of travel. The only thing that might influence the situation is if the scapula is not moving on the back as it should. As a side point of interest, a much higher percentage of people that get rotator cuff tears have type III shaped acromion process.

Movement available at the SCJ and ACJ is there to facilitate the scapula moving on the thoracic cage as the shoulder girdle is elevated, depressed, protracted, or retracted. As with the SIJ, there are no muscles whose job it is to specifically move these joints. Therefore, if the ligaments maintaining their skeletal relationship are damaged, it is hard to recreate stability. Later, we will look at how we can put these two joints under stress in yoga.

Muscles that Move the Shoulder Complex

There are many muscles around the shoulder (Figure 11.6). We will start with the shoulder girdle and then move to the shoulder joint (glenoid fossa joint). The movements possible with the shoulder girdle are elevation, depression, protraction, and retraction.

Serratus Anterior

Serratus anterior is that fantastic looking bunch of fingers wrapping around the torso, so easily visible in boxers. It comes from the medial border of the scapula, but travels underneath the scapula and reaches around the side of the body to attach to the first eight or nine ribs. Its action is to protract the scapula as well as to rotate it upward when flexing or abducting the shoulder (Figures 11.6, 11.7, & 11.8). I also think of it as sucking the scapula to the ribcage. When we see a winging scapula, it is a good indication that the serratus anterior is weak, maybe also the next muscle as well, the rhomboids.

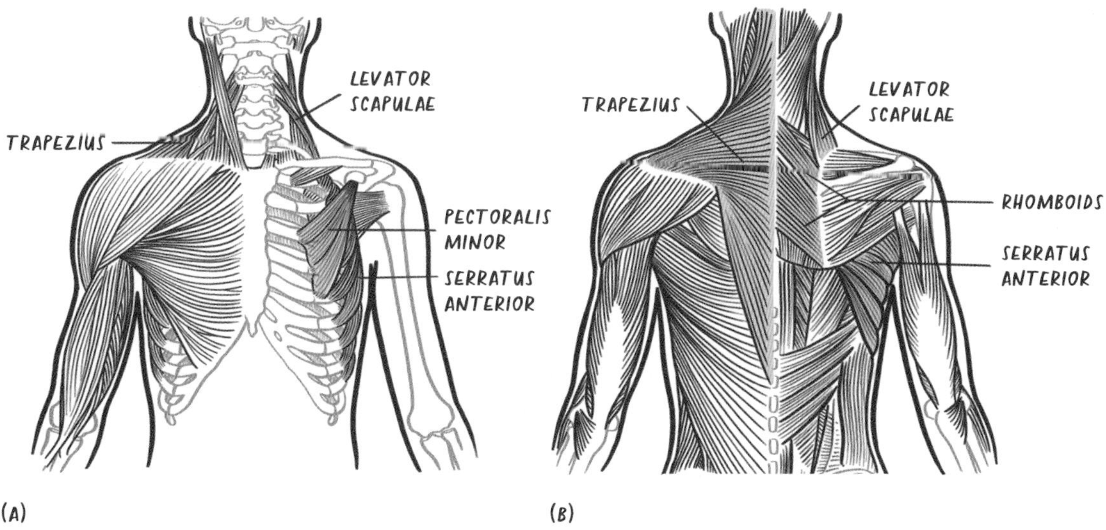

Figure 11.6 Muscles that move the shoulder complex, (A) anterior view, (B) posterior view.

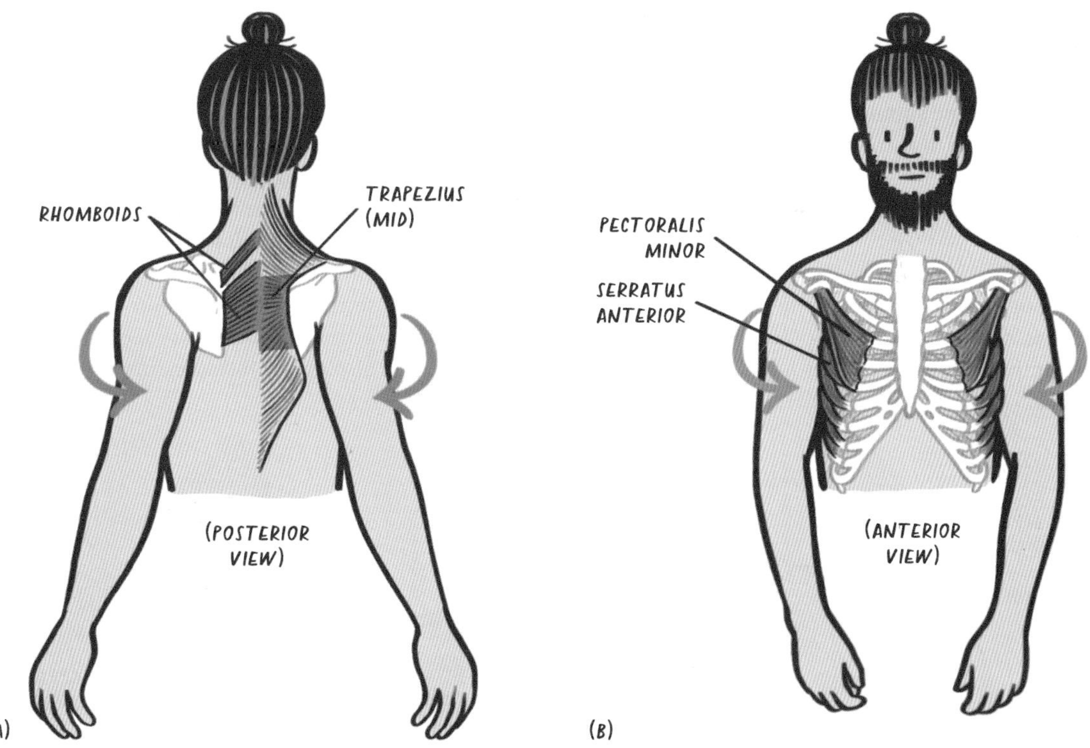

Figure 11.7 Serratus anterior is like the new psoas, everyone wants to talk about it, and to be fair, it does play an essential role in stabilizing the shoulder girdle. But the rhomboids and trapezius also work in conjunction to balance retraction (A) and protraction (B).

Rhomboids

Lying between the spine and the medial border of the scapula are the rhomboids. There is a major and minor, but they do the same actions, which is to retract and elevate the scapula as well as assist with its downward rotation (Figures 11.6, 11.7, & 11.8). Working with serratus anterior, they help stabilize the scapula on the back, so we can use the arms without the shoulder girdle moving as well.

Levator Scapulae

This muscle does what it says on the box, scapular elevation (Figures 11.6, 11.7, & 11.8). It attaches to the top medial corner of the scapula and then to the transverse processes of the upper four cervical vertebrae. So, like the rhomboids, that upward pull on the medial side can help to downwardly rotate the scapula. If you are trying to visualize when you would use that movement, think of lifting for an L-sit—as the shoulder girdle is depressed, the scapula would also rotate downward.

Trapezius

The huge diamond-shaped muscle that spans the neck, mid-back, and shoulders is called the trapezius. Not only does it attach to the spinous processes from C7 to T12 but also to the ligamentum nuchae that runs up the back of the neck, the lateral clavicle, the spine and acromion process of the scapula, and the base of the skull. Because of its size, it has fibers running in different directions, and hence the three main parts have dissimilar actions.

The upper part elevates the scapula, the middle retracts, and the lower depresses. Upper and lower parts also help retract the scapula and can work together to rotate the scapula when raising the arm (Figures 11.6, 11.7, & 11.8). The trapezius is a very powerful muscle and is one of the main muscles stabilizing the scapula in place on the back when moving the arm independently of the shoulder girdle.

Pectoralis Minor

There are two pectoral muscles, major and minor, but only pectoralis minor moves the shoulder girdle because it attaches to the coracoid process of the scapula, and major attaches to the humerus. The other end of the muscle originates from the third to fifth ribs. It protracts the scapula and rotates it downward (Figures 11.6, 11.7, & 11.8). So, if it works together with serratus anterior (an upward rotator), protraction without rotation can be achieved. It is also one of the accessory muscles of

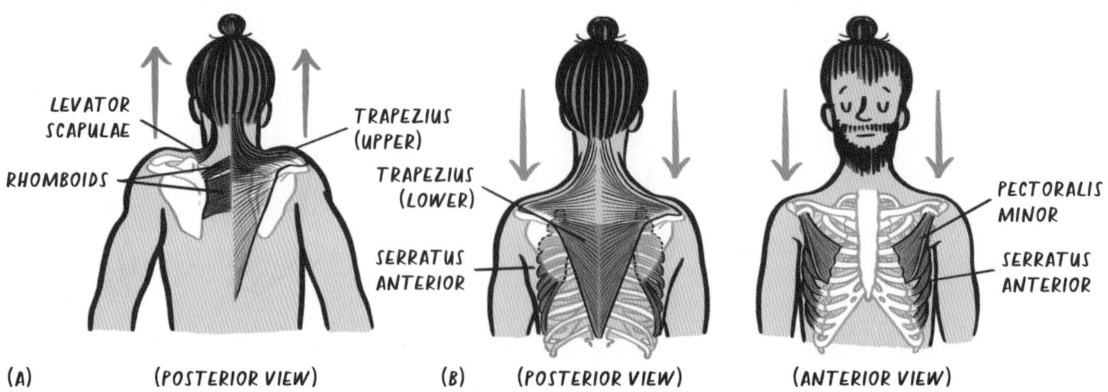

Figure 11.8 Muscles involved with shoulder elevation (A) and depression (B).

breathing, pulling the ribcage up to create greater volume.

Now let's think of the muscles that move the shoulder joint (Figures 11.9 & 11.11). When I speak to students, I find they are a bit confused about which muscles move the shoulder joint. Simply put, we are talking about the movement of the humerus, so the muscles that are going to create the actions must attach to it. Some of the muscles we have just covered attach to the scapula, the bone that the shoulder socket is on (glenoid fossa), but came from somewhere other than the humerus.

Now we have muscles, some of which originate on the scapula, but all of which will attach to somewhere on the humerus. It is a good time to remind yourself about the direction of pull and the Chapter 3 topic, *Secondary Action of Muscles*, as it will help you visualize why muscles create the actions they do around the shoulder. The movements we have at the shoulder joint are medial and external rotation, flexion and extension, abduction and adduction, and horizontal abduction and adduction.

Rotator Cuff Muscles

We are going to start with a group of four muscles collectively referred to as the rotator cuff because their tendons merge with the joint capsule of the shoulder and help to stabilize the head of the humerus in the shallow socket (Figure 11.9). As well as providing this crucial role, they are also responsible for many movements (Figure 11.10). This duality of purpose means that they are susceptible to injury, particularly from repetitive overhead actions or loading.

Supraspinatus

Supraspinatus sits above the spine of the scapula and then traveling under the acromion process attaches to the top of the humerus. It helps the deltoid with shoulder abduction. Incidentally, it is the most likely muscle tendon to be damaged in a rotator cuff tear. If you get pain when you raise your arm up the front or out to the side that is not going, it is worth seeking advice and guidance, as doing nothing may result in a cycle of further deterioration.

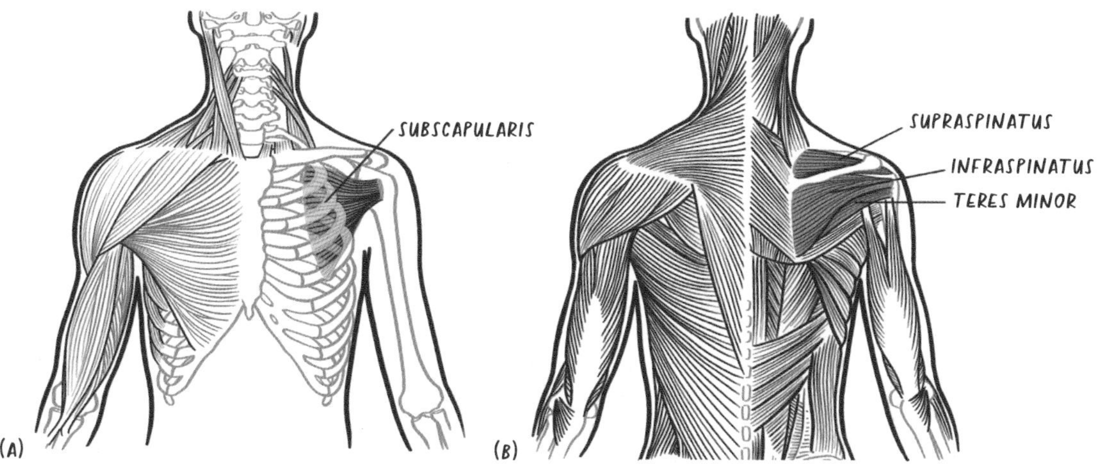

Figure 11.9 Rotator cuff muscles, (A) anterior view, (B) posterior view.

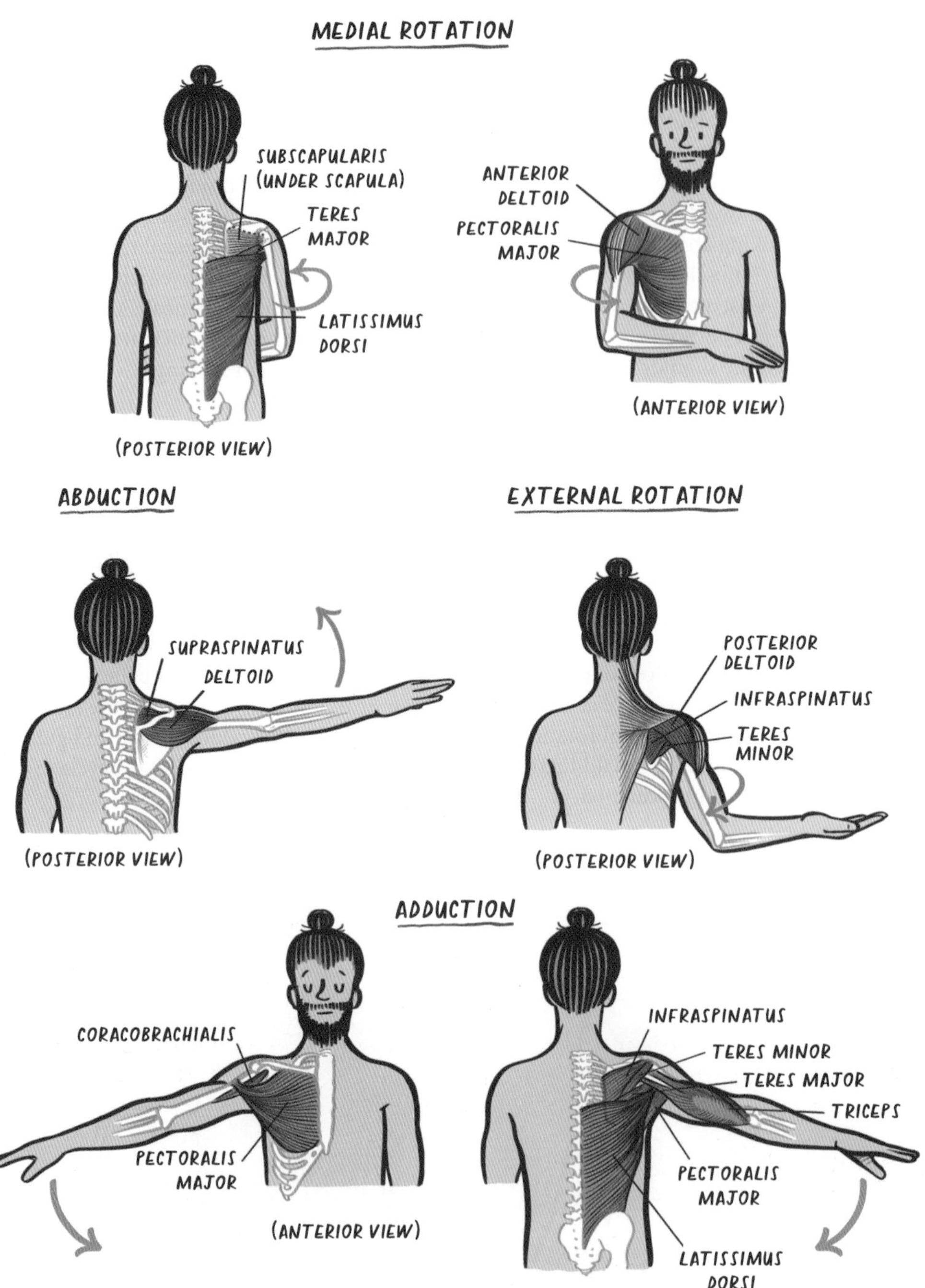

Figure 11.10 (Continued)

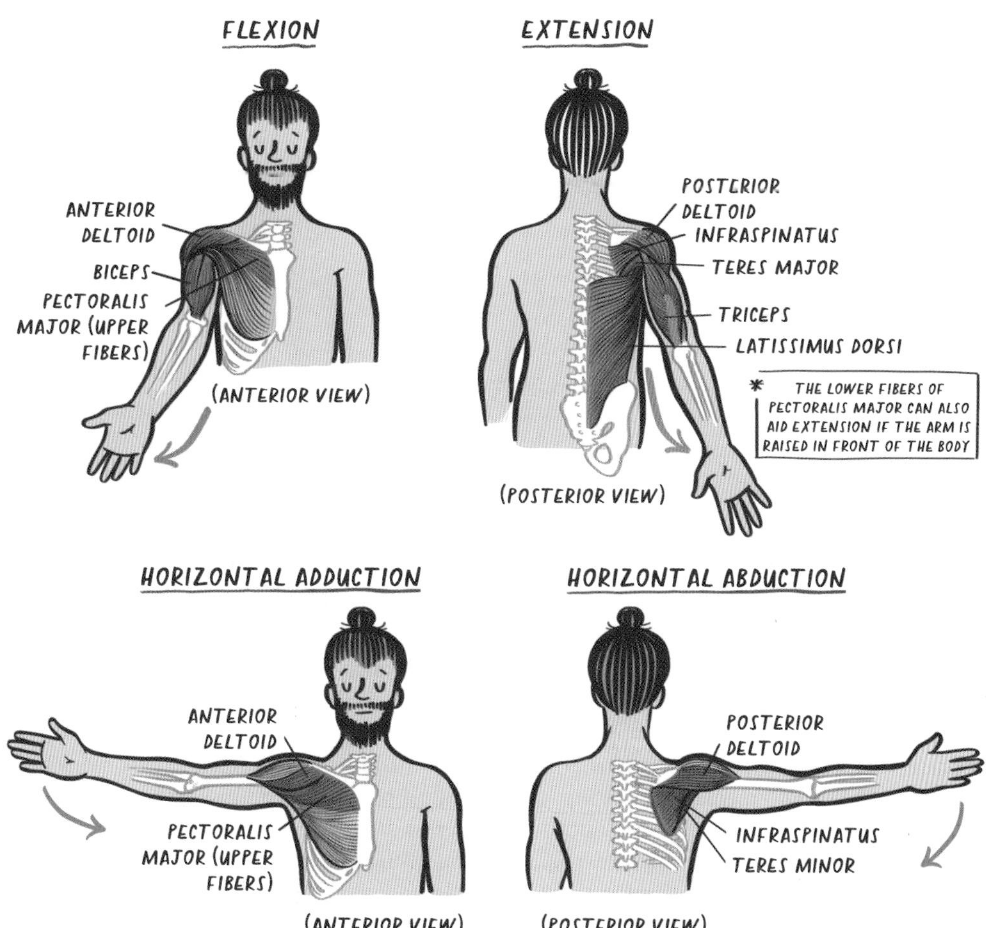

Figure 11.10 The many movements of the shoulder joint.

Infraspinatus

Infraspinatus is the main external rotator and, as such, is prone to trigger points due to overworking against the many powerful medial rotators. It can also assist with horizontal abduction and extension. The infraspinatus is the largest of the rotator cuff muscles occupying the entire area below the spine of the scapula and attaching to the posterolateral (back/side) aspect of the humerus.

Teres Minor

Teres minor goes from the lateral border of the scapula to the posterior aspect of the humerus and performs external rotation as well helping with adduction.

Subscapularis

Subscapularis runs from under the scapula (anterior surface) to the front of the humerus and therefore does medial rotation. It can also assist with adduction and extension.

Other Muscles that Move the Shoulder Joint

Pectoralis Major

Pectoralis major lays on the front of the upper chest, completely covering pectoralis minor. It attaches to the sternum and clavicle and cartilage of the first six ribs and then on the anterolateral aspect (front/outerside) of the humerus. Because it

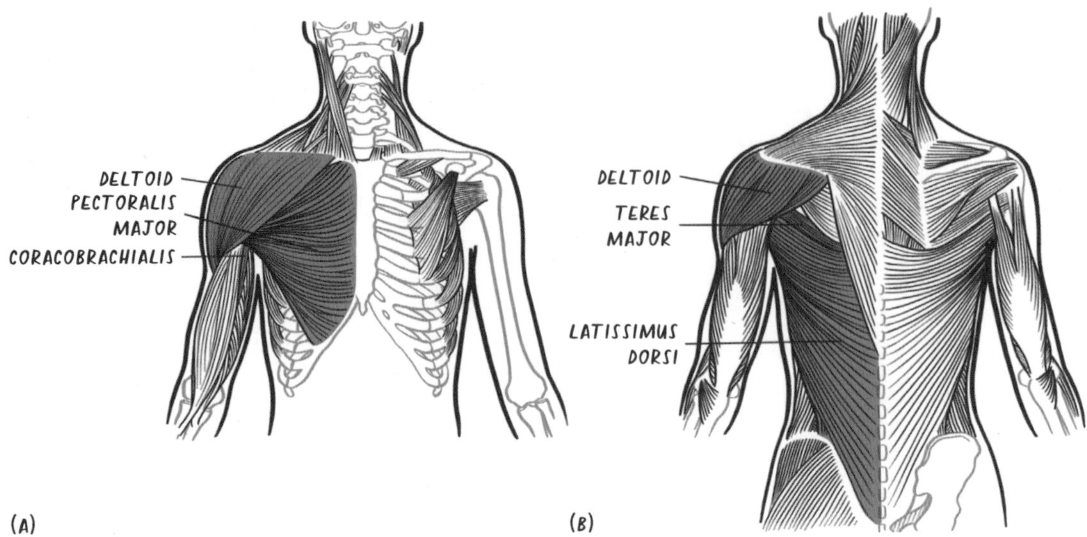

Figure 11.11 Other muscles that move the shoulder joint, (A) anterior view, (B) posterior view.

is large and powerful, again the fiber directionality produces different actions for the various parts, some pulling from high or low and others straight across. It is divided into three sections: upper (clavicular), middle (sternal), and lower (costal). All sections can adduct and medially rotate the shoulder. The upper fibers can flex the shoulder and horizontally adduct it, and the lower fibers can do the opposing action of extension. You can see that it is a pretty useful muscle. As the direction of pull is changing continuously, some of these actions will be better at certain stages of the arc.

Latissimus Dorsi

The latissimus dorsi covers almost the whole mid- and lower back. Being the largest muscle of the upper body, it has attachments all over the place, including all the spinous processes from T7 to the sacrum, the thoracolumbar fascia, iliac crest, and the bottom four ribs. At the other end, it goes under the arm to attach to the medial aspect of the humerus. When it concentrically contracts, its actions are extension and medial rotation.

It has the potential to be a huge and very powerful muscle, and if developed, it can give that classic "V" shape from narrow waist to wide shoulders. I think of it as the swimmer's muscle, having watched plenty of Olympic competitions, growing up. Then in my gym days, there was a bodybuilding pose called the "Lat Spread," which, from the back made someone look like a turtle, and from the front, an insect (Figure 11.12). I digress, but there is a purpose to my reminiscing. You wouldn't see much muscle tone in the latissimus dorsi of yoga practitioners because we do no pulling movements, and that is its job, shoulder extension.

It can pull your arms back from flexion or your body to your arms. Also, remember from Chapter 3, *Strength*, that if your arms are overhead, unless there is some resistance, gravity will be the force that brings them down, not a contraction of the latissimus dorsi. If you don't believe me about the lack of pulling movements, try and think of some now. For example, *Sirsasana*, Handstand,

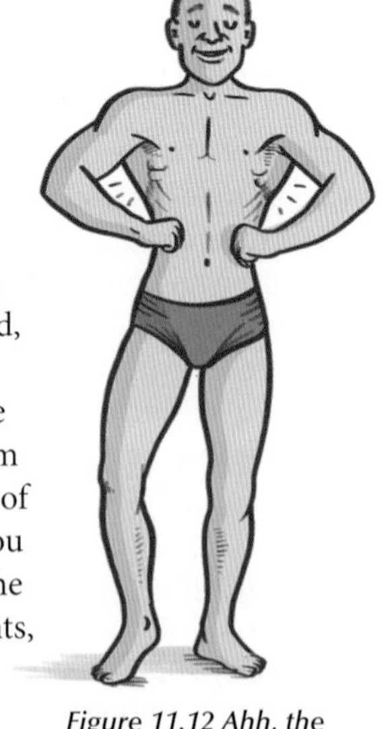

Figure 11.12 Ahh, the "Lat Spread."

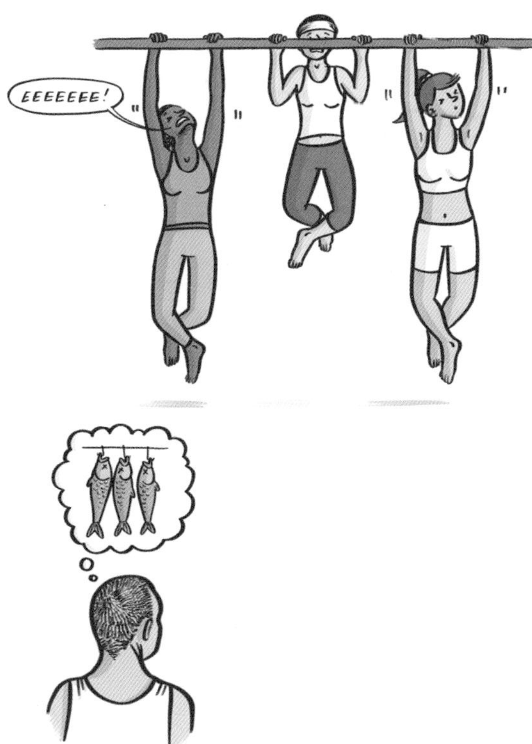

Figure 11.13 See if you can pull yourself up on a bar!

Shoulderstand, Down Dog, and *Chaturanga* are all pushing movements.

Sometimes for a bit of fun with a group, if there is a handy bar around, I'll lift students up so they can grab it and then see if they can pull themselves up (Figure 11.13). All, but the very few, dangle in place like a salted fish drying in the sun. Therefore, if we want to create a balance between the pulling and pushing muscles, we will have to find some other way of strengthening the pulling muscles of the upper body. This includes the biceps brachii as well.

Teres Major

Teres major is the brother (or sister) of teres minor coming from a similar place on the lateral side of the scapula. However, the other end dips under the arm to attach like the latissimus dorsi to the medial aspect of the humerus. Consequently, it has the opposite action to its sibling, medial rotation, the same as subscapularis. Teres major is not one of the rotator cuff muscles despite the similar name. My Latin is not brilliant, but apparently, teres means rounded. Coming from the back of the body to the front, it can also assist with adduction and extension.

Deltoid

Deltoid is named after its characteristic triangular shape, like the Greek letter delta Δ, although up the other way. That's probably the end of the highbrow stuff, so don't worry. The top of the muscle wraps around the shoulder, tracing a line along the spine of the scapula, the acromion process, and then the clavicle. It has, in effect, doubled back on itself, so even though all fibers have the same attachment on the lateral aspect of the humerus, there are three distinct sections, with one shared action and several different actions. The parts are generally referred to by their position, anterior, lateral (sometimes middle), and posterior. All three sections of the muscle can perform shoulder abduction, although the lateral fibers will work the hardest. The anterior and posterior parts then have additional opposite actions, flexion and medial rotation, and extension and external rotation, respectively.

Coracobrachialis

I must admit this is a muscle I have never actually referred to. But having looked at its actions, it is one of the muscles responsible for bringing the arms across the body in *Garudasana*, as it does shoulder flexion and adduction. It attaches to the coracoid process of the scapula like pectoralis minor, and then connects to the medial aspect of the humerus. It also helps hold the humeral head in the shoulder socket.

The biceps brachii and triceps brachii do cross the shoulder joint, but their actions are weak compared with the other muscles. The biceps can help with flexion and the triceps with extension. We will expand on them more in Chapter 11.

Quick Reference Muscle Action Tables

Elevation	Depression
Trapezius (upper fibers)	Trapezius (lower fibers)
Rhomboids	Serratus anterior
Levator scapulae	Pectoralis minor

Retraction	Protraction
Trapezius (middle fibers)	Serratus anterior
Rhomboids	Pectoralis minor

Horizontal Abduction	Horizontal Adduction
Posterior deltoid	Anterior deltoid
Teres minor	Pectoralis major (upper fibers)
Infraspinatus	

Flexion	Extension
Anterior deltoid	Posterior deltoid
Pectoralis major (upper fibers)	Latissimus dorsi
Biceps brachii	Teres major and minor
Coracobrachialis	Infraspinatus
	Pectoralis major (lower fibers)

Abduction	Adduction
Deltoid (all fibers)	Latissimus dorsi
Supraspinatus	Teres major and minor
	Infraspinatus
	Pectoralis major (all fibers)
	Triceps brachii (long head)
	Coracobrachialis

Lateral Rotation	Medial Rotation
Posterior deltoid	Anterior deltoid
Infraspinatus	Pectoralis major
Teres minor	Latissimus dorsi
	Teres major
	Subscapularis

Putting Things into Context

We need to be particularly careful not to stress the SCJ and ACJ because they will be hard to stabilize if we damage the ligaments. So, in what types of postures might this occur?

Starting with the ACJ, I think it can happen when the shoulder is in extension and movement at the shoulder joint stops, but there is an effort to still take the arm further behind the body. What I have determined is that as the shoulder joint is on the scapula, at the end of its ROM, muscular tension can cause the scapula to move with the humerus, resulting in perhaps excessive rotational movement at the ACJ.

As the arm is long, it can act as a strong lever. I'll give two examples, one with the arms moving relative to the torso, the other with the torso relative to the arms—in *Prasarita Padottanasana C*, if the arms are pushed down by an assistant too forcefully (Figure 11.14), and in *Purvottanasana*, if the hips are pressed or lifted too high (Figure 11.15).

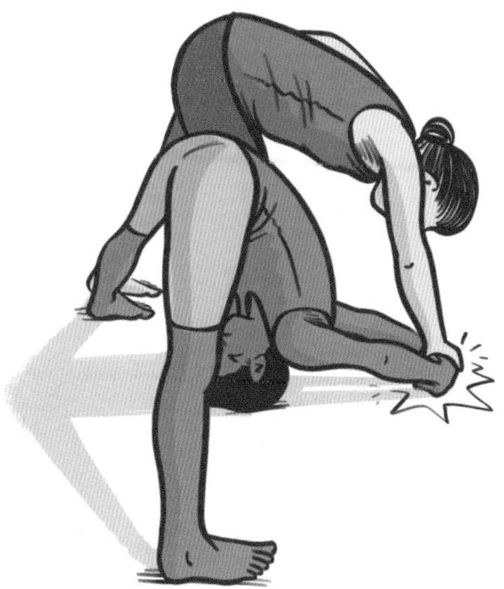

Figure 11.14 Nope, this is not necessary!

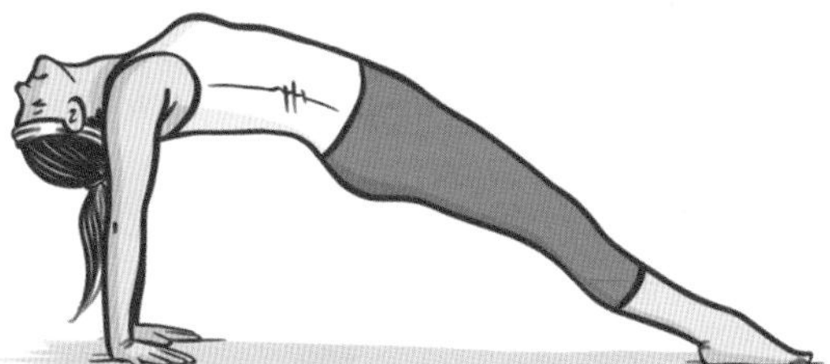

Figure 11.15 The adjustment for this posture can be to lift the hips for the student. If this is done too enthusiastically, it is possible to stress the ACJ.

The SCJ is vulnerable to the clavicle being levered on the sternum. This can happen in postures such as *Kurmasana* where the student does not have enough hip flexion and rounds the back excessively, shortening the space across the chest (Figure 11.16). With the weight of the legs on the arms, stress can be taken into the SCJ, as the clavicle is forced forward or backward depending on how much retraction of the shoulder girdle is going on. I think, for some students, *Supta Kurmasana* can raise the same problem.

Because the tendons of supraspinatus and the long head of the biceps travel between the top of the humerus and the acromion process, there is the potential for them to get squished between the two bones. This, repeated over time, can cause fraying or inflammation of the tendons. The movement that highlights this vulnerability is when the

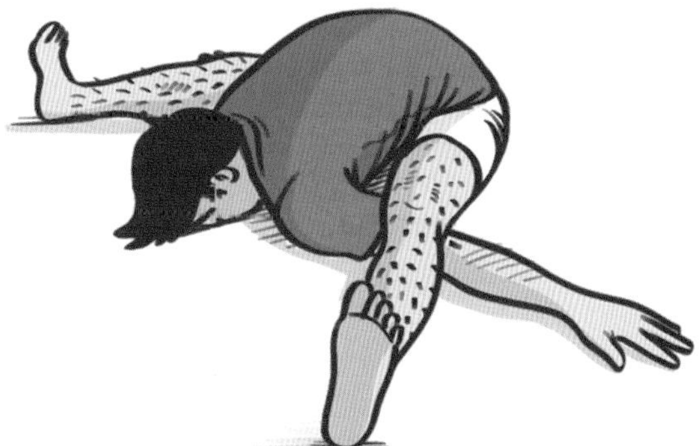

Figure 11.16 The SCJ is vulnerable in this posture if the spine is rounded too much.

arms are taken above the head, particularly when traveling in the abducted arc. Precisely this action is what can happen when doing a Sun Salutation, and many students landing up feeling some discomfort during this movement.

There are two useful adaptations to remove potential stress. The first is just as the arms leave the side, externally rotate the shoulders to bring the palms to face up. The second action is to bring the arms forward of the body slightly, so they are at an angle of about 45 degrees. These two actions put the tendons in a position where they are much less likely to become impinged.

Another thing that can happen when the arms are taken overhead is that the elbows can go out when we don't want them to. Common postures this can happen in include, the backbend *Kapotasana*, *Urdhva Dhanurasana*, *Virabhadrasana A* (Figure 11.17), and *Ardha Pincha Mayurasana*. It doesn't matter if the elbows are bent or straight because the restriction that causes the phenomenon is at the shoulder. It is just easier to spot if the arms are bent.

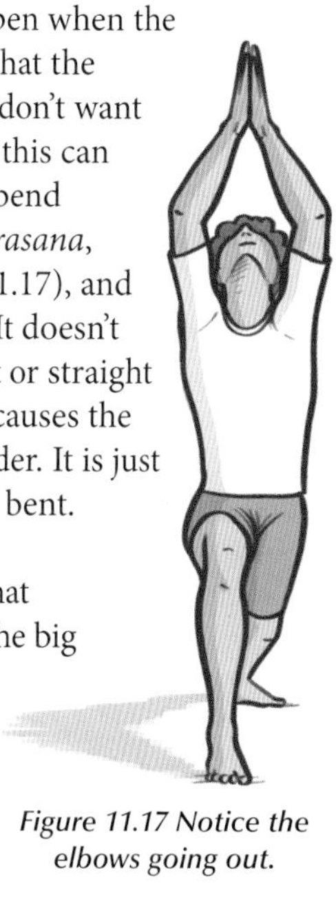

Figure 11.17 Notice the elbows going out.

If you think of the muscles that extend the shoulder, two of the big ones, pectoralis major and latissimus dorsi, have a secondary action of medial rotation. I'm sure you remember Chapter 3,

Secondary Action of Muscles, so we can apply that idea here. When the arms go up the front in shoulder flexion, it will be the opposing muscles that restrict the movement. As they are stretched, the line of pull of the muscle fibers can cause the secondary action to happen, in this case, medial rotation. As the arm rotates inward, the elbows will point outward.

If you are on the ball, you will already be thinking of other muscles that might be to blame, if the restriction is not in those two. Teres major and subscapularis both medially rotate the shoulder, so again, as they are stretched with the arms going overhead, they could also be responsible for the wayward elbows.

So how do we know which it might be? As a rule of thumb, what I do is to stretch out each of the muscles separately and retest the original position to see if there is an improvement. When we come to the *Posture Groups* (Part III), I'll show you how we can do that. Once you have found the right muscle/s, you can choose other yoga postures to work them effectively.

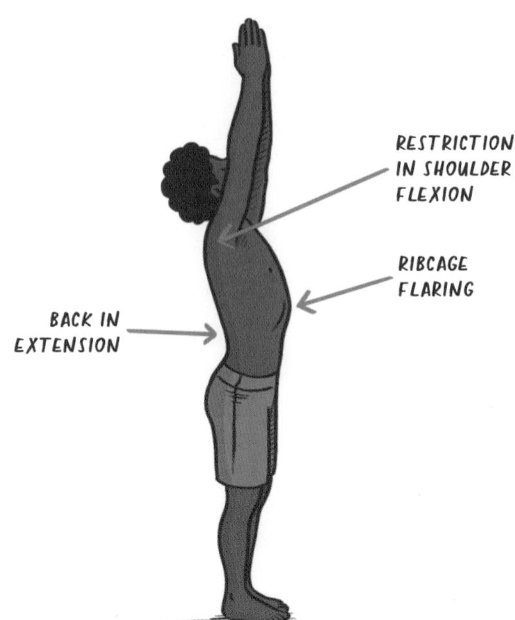

Figure 11.18 Restriction in shoulder flexion can cause the ribcage to flare and the low back to arch.

The elbow going out is not the only adaptation that can happen when we flex the shoulders, sometimes the chest gets pulled out. Coming back to our Sun Salutation example, most students have it in their heads that they will take the arms to point to the ceiling. If the shoulders have reached their limit of flexion before that movement has been completed, then the body will happily accommodate for you by arching the back (Figure 11.18). Now, I don't think this amount of lumbar extension will cause a problem even if repeated every time you do a Sun Salutation, but the student is missing out on the opportunity to work on shoulder mobility.

By maintaining an isometric contraction of the rectus abdominis, think ribcage to pubic bone connection, the lumbar extension will be prevented (Figure 11.19). Now, on reaching the restriction in shoulder flexion, the student can work the movement actively. If necessary, the belly can now be gradually relaxed to continue the progress upward. Even if you prefer to go into a backbend in the first stage of your Sun Salutation, the same principle can be applied. Work the range at the shoulder first and then start into the spine extension.

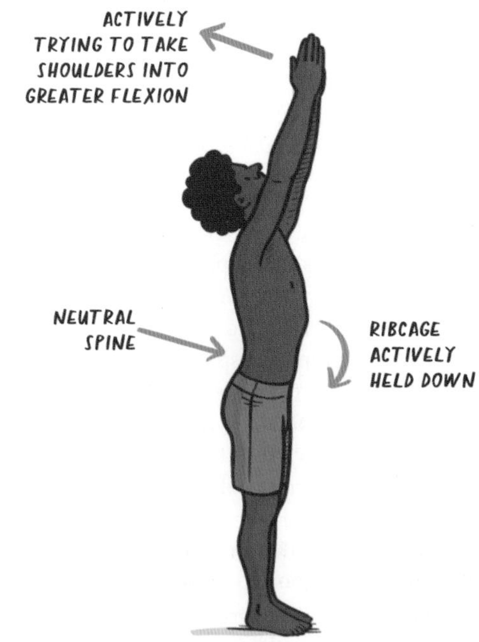

Figure 11.19 Maintaining the connection between the ribcage and pubic bone allows the student to address their restriction and work on active shoulder flexion.

We'll think of the shoulder girdle movements now, elevation, depression, protraction, and retraction. When we are supporting ourselves with our arms, we want the scapula to be nice and snug on the ribcage. In the fully protracted position, I think the back rounds too much and can also cause a narrowing across the chest. It is better to find that balance between protraction and retraction and use the interplay between the serratus anterior (protractor), and the rhomboids and trapezius (retractors), to encourage more dynamic stability. Holding a High Plank is a good place to train the positioning. Some students also drop their head toward the floor in this posture, which, again, causes unnecessary rounding of the thoracic and cervical spine. It is better to keep the head and neck neutral (Figure 11.20).

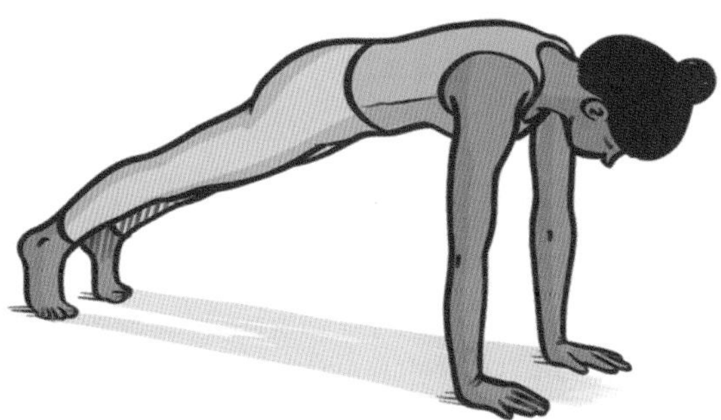

Figure 11.20 It would be better for Myra to draw her head away from the floor for a more neutral position.

When the shoulder girdle is retracted, it gives space across the front of the chest and helps to counter rounding of the upper back. In postures such as *Utthita Hasta Padangusthasana*, many students find the shoulder being pulled forward by the weight and restriction of the lifted leg. This is an ideal time to recruit the rhomboids and trapezius to pull the scapula back toward the spine.

Another great time to focus on retraction of the shoulder girdle is in bound twists like *Baddha Parsvakonasana* or *Marichyasana C*. The shoulder of the arm wrapping around the leg will get pulled forward, but I still think it is good to work on pulling it back (Figure 11.21). The free shoulder is easier to control, and retraction on this side will allow you to open up across the chest,

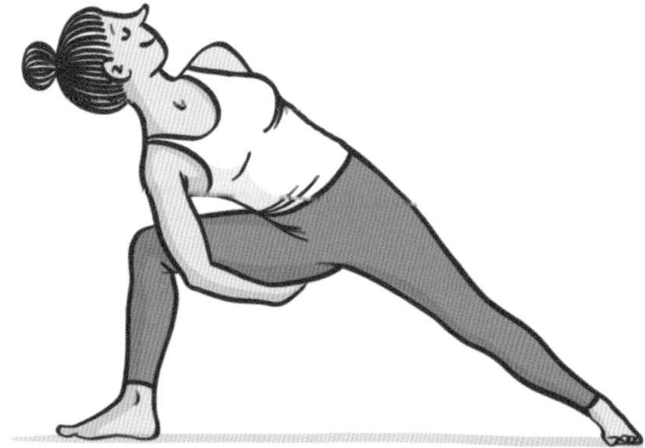

Figure 11.21 Sasha is working hard to keep open across the chest by retracting the shoulder girdle.

lengthen the spine, and increase the twist in the thoracic area.

Depression of the shoulder girdle is a good counter to the shoulders drifting up toward the ears, in anything from *Tadasana* to *Virabhadrasana B*. In any lifting postures such as the L-sit or *Utplutih*, it has the effect of making the arms longer, giving more clearance with the ground, or even allowing lift-off (Figure 11.22). Do be aware that when the arms are taken over the head, the scapula must rotate up. So, in postures like Down Dog, although we generally like to see some space between the arms and the head, the idea is more to release possible neck tension. The shoulder girdle doesn't need to be pulled down too far. The oft-used cue, "shoulder blades back and down" may be appropriate in postures like *Tadasana* but is not

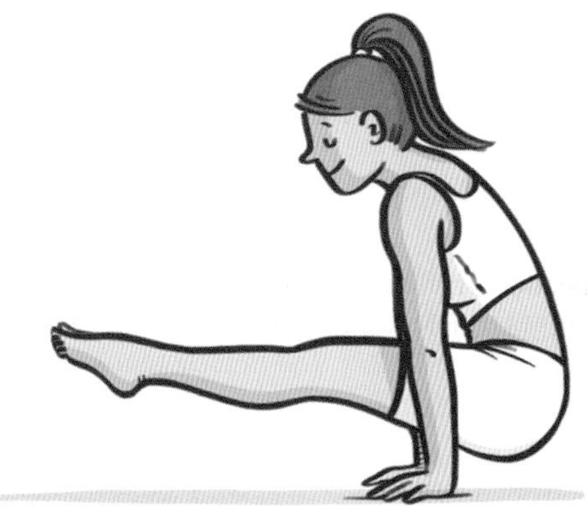

Figure 11.22 L-sits are great for working on strength and in particular shoulder girdle depression.

universal. In fact, in the modern Handstand, the movement of shoulder girdle elevation and arms touching the ears is actively encouraged.

One of the things that I question about the shoulder is how much shoulder extension do we need? On average, people have about 45 to 60 degrees, and that amount is undoubtedly sufficient to do things like scratching your back, swinging your arm, and reaching for something on the back seat of the car. It's not so easy to think of a functional requirement that would benefit from having more. Place that idea on top of an appreciation of the instability inherent in the shoulder joint and its propensity for dislocation, and striving toward 90 degrees or more extension capability seems misguided. For those students who are already overly mobile at this joint, something very common among hypermobile individuals, they should definitely work diligently on creating more strength around this area. As a teacher, when it comes to shoulder flexibility postures within your sequence, it is worth having strength options ready for these individuals.

A Bit About Moving the Head

This seemed the most logical place to add something about the head movements. We don't need to say anything about construction because we already looked at the cervical spine in Chapter 9. There are lots of muscles involved in moving the head and neck, but I'll just introduce another couple and then revisit some we have mentioned already.

Sternocleidomastoid (SCM)

SCM has such a bonkers name from the bones it attaches to, the sternum, clavicle, and mastoid process (Figure 11.23). The muscle tends to be easily visible when the head is rotated, and it reminds me of puppet strings. It laterally flexes the neck, drawing the ear to the same side shoulder or rotates the head to face the opposite shoulder.

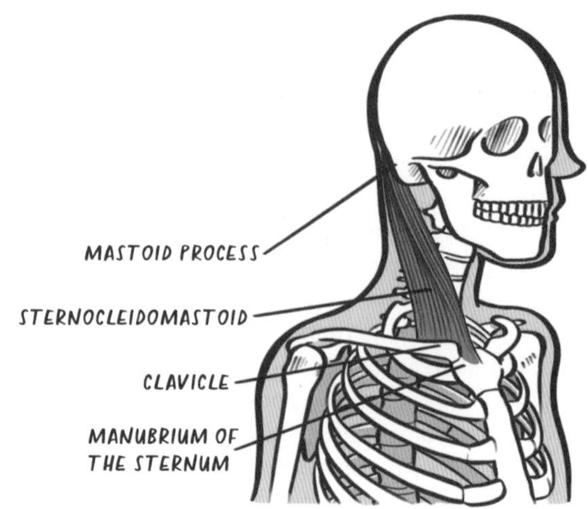

Figure 11.23 Sternocleidomastoid.

If both sides contract (bilateral), it flexes the neck. SCM also acts as an accessory muscle of breathing by elevating the ribcage.

Trapezius and Levator Scapulae

Both the trapezius (upper fibers) and levator scapulae muscles can assist with neck extension, lateral flexion, and rotation (trapezius to the opposite side, levator scapulae to the same side).

Putting Things into Context

What can be done with the neck is not a limiting factor of poses unless the neck is particularly stiff and preventing flexion, which is required for floor-based postures where the legs are over the head. We want to encourage natural movement in the cervical spine without creating stress. Turning the head last in twisting postures rather than leading with the head makes it less likely to create excessive tension in the neck muscles. In some postures, we can look with the eyes without exaggerating the head movement. I have already mentioned that taking into account the high incidence of head forward position, many students should avoid weight-bearing on the head altogether, the others should keep it to a minimum.

I think the two positions that need the most care are instability when the neck is loaded, for example, wobbling around in *Mukta Hasta Sirsasana A* and hinging the neck back in extension. It is always better in the latter case to imagine you are curving the spine over something the size of a tennis ball, rather than just tipping it back. If taking the neck back causes pain, cease the movement until you have had it checked out.

Many students arrive at yoga with existing neck tension, often due to their working practices or stress. It can be helpful to use some of the simple inverted non-weight-bearing positions to find some space and relaxation for the neck. Postures like *Uttanasana* can allow the weight of the head to give gentle traction. When using this pose to release the neck, it is fine to bend the knees as much as necessary to achieve a more vertical position of the upper body without overstressing the hamstrings or low back.

I've noticed that in standing postures like *Trikonasana,* where the gaze is at the raised hand, lots of students drop the head back to try and get a greater rotation in the neck (Figure 11.24). This can put a strain on the front of the neck due to the weight of the head. It is better to keep the chin slightly tucked and only turn as far as is comfortable. Eye movement can make up the difference.

In the previous chapter, I have already voiced my concerns over *Setu Bandhasana* (Ashtanga version). In case you skipped that, my advice is simple. "**Don't Do It**." I do remember being in a class a good few years ago now, and the teacher saying to me, "At least give it a go." Don't be afraid to say, "No thanks," it's your neck not theirs after all!

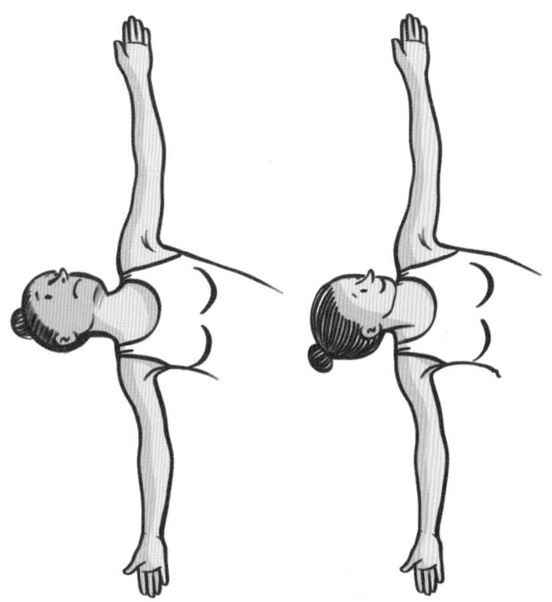

Figure 11.24 Some students drop the head back as it seems to allow for more rotation if there is restriction in the neck muscles. But it is healthier for the neck to keep the chin slightly tucked and turn the head not so far.

There is one more posture used in Ashtanga that has featured highly with students coming to me with neck issues—the backward roll transition called *Chakrasana*. It is not so problematic in itself, but student strength and technique are often lacking, causing them either to flick with the head to take them over, or laterally flex it to try and get it out of the way. I hope you are cringing with me. My advice on this one is that if there are any existing neck issues, leave it out completely, and if you are going to do it, make sure you understand and can perform the technique properly.

CHAPTER 12

Elbow and Wrist

The elbow isn't one of those joints where there's a need to increase flexibility, but it is certainly a useful one to understand (Figure 12.1). Mostly, we notice if it looks in a funky position or if we can't straighten the arm when we want to. The wrist is much the same with most students taking it for granted unless it starts to hurt.

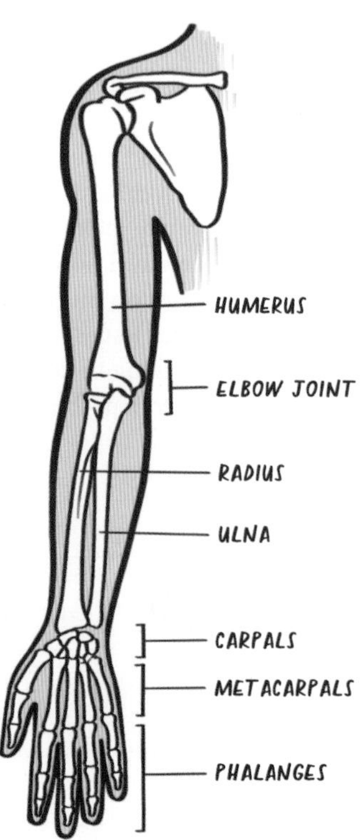

Figure 12.1 The upper limb.

Construction of the Elbow

The elbow joint is different from the knee in that both the bones of the lower arm articulate with the upper arm. The humerus-ulna joint (humeroulnar) is a simple hinge joint with a bony stop called the olecranon process, and the humerus-radius (humeroradial) joint is a pivot joint (Figure 12.2). This combination adds dramatically to the rotation available, with the radius crossing over the ulna when you go from palm up (supinated) to palm face down (pronated).

The olecranon process physically restricts how much extension is available at the elbow. Students who can hyperextend their elbow will usually have a greater available range before the olecranon process meets the olecranon fossa, the shallow depression on the humerus that makes the other part of the joint. Other factors that influence the

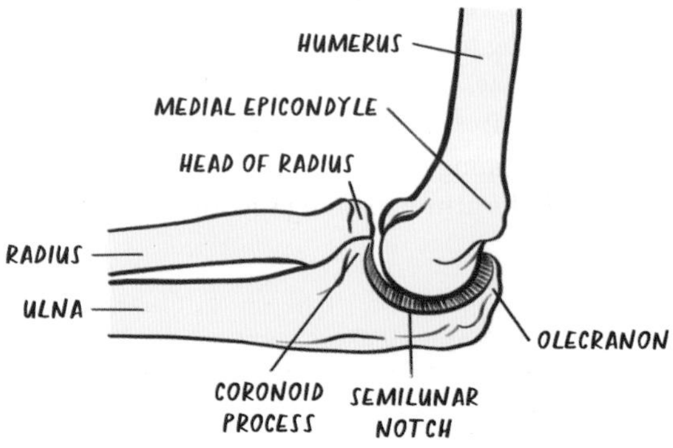

Figure 12.2 Construction of the elbow.

degree of extension at the elbow are ligament laxity, muscular tension in the elbow flexors, and joint capsule restriction.

The bone on bone compression is the definitive range limiter for hyperextension; on top of that, the other factors will play a role (Figure 12.3). We will use four students as examples to explore this phenomenon, with the extremes of hyperextension and staying flexed at both ends of the spectrum.

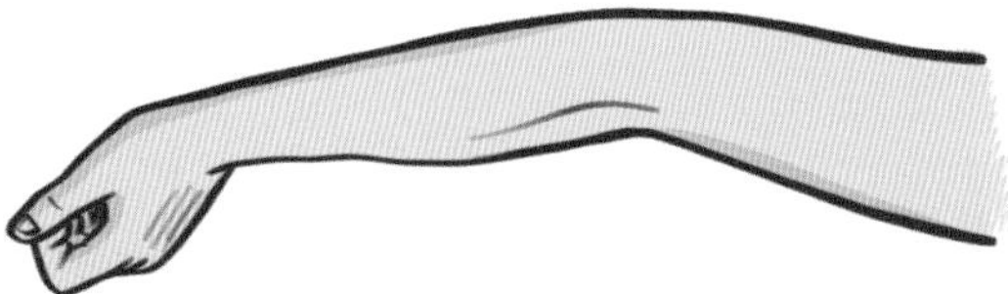

Figure 12.3 Hyperextending is not an unusual sight in a yoga room.

Student 1 has a range greater than the straight line of 180 degrees before the bones make contact but will not be able to go further than compression time irrespective of whether the soft tissue (ligaments, muscle, tendon, joint capsule) would allow.

Student 2 is at the other end of the scale and can't straighten the arm fully because the bones come into contact before reaching 180 degrees. I have come across several students like this over the years. Again, soft tissue changes are inconsequential. For this student, bone on bone has stopped the joint moving through the full range.

Student 3 has bones that would allow for greater than 180 degrees of extension, but muscular tension in the elbow flexors is preventing them from moving into hyperextension.

Student 4 has a bony arrangement that allows for the arm to straighten to 180 degrees, but muscular tension is stopping it short from the available range, with the arm remaining slightly flexed.

Hopefully you understood that compression will be the absolute limit, but soft tissue tension can be used to reduce the range if desirable and may also prevent the full range being available. In line with our *Compression* topic in Chapter 2, hard compression would be felt at the back of the elbow and soft tissue restriction in front. We will come back to whether elbow hyperextension is desirable as well as to how we can make use of the plentiful rotation later.

> Hold your straight arm out in front of you with the palm facing the ceiling. Now, look at the lower arm. Does it change direction at the elbow and head off toward thumb side (laterally) or does the whole arm look like it's in a straight line?

Do something for me now as you are sitting there (tinted box above). Whatever you see, don't worry, you're normal. This change of direction is called the "carrying angle" and is entirely separate to hyperextension (Figure 12.4). Some people have none or minimal deviation, and others have much more. The idea behind this design trait is to allow the arms to swing past the hips without banging on them. Even though women usually have narrower shoulders and wider hips than men, from what I've observed, the angle change seems to be inconsistent between the sexes and loosely tied to proportions.

The main concept to appreciate is that unlike hyperextension, which can be consciously controlled, the carrying angle can't be changed. It is regularly mistaken for hyperextension in postures, and speaking to students with large carrying angles, they report often being the target of confusion in poses like Down Dog. It is possible to have both

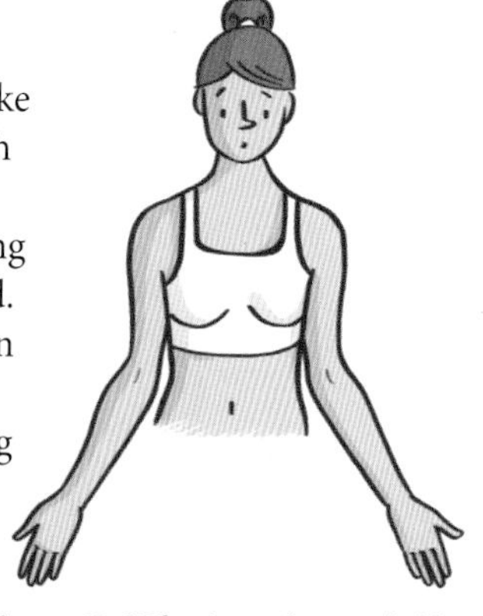

Figure 12.4 The "carrying angle" is not the same as hyperextension. You can have both a large carrying angle and hyperextension, just one or the other, or neither.

hyperextension and a large carrying angle, or only one or the other, or neither.

Muscles that Move the Elbow

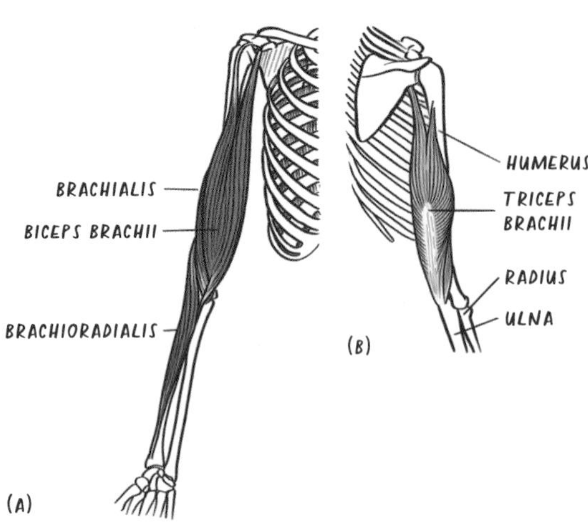

Figure 12.5 Muscles that move the elbow, (A) anterior view, (B) posterior view.

Biceps Brachii

I don't think anyone uses the last bit of biceps brachii, but it does differentiate it from the two bellied hamstring, biceps femoris. One point, if you guessed, is that brachii is Latin for arm.

At the top of the muscle, both heads attach to the scapula, but in different places. The long head attaches just above the glenoid fossa almost at the base of the coracoid process, and the short head attaches to the end of the coracoid process. At the far end of the muscle, it connects to the radius, making it a powerful forearm supinator and elbow flexor. It also assists with shoulder flexion (Figure 12.6).

Triceps Brachii

On the back of the upper arm is the triceps brachii (Figure 12.7). It has three heads, long, medial, and lateral, with the long head attaching to the scapula, therefore being able to assist with shoulder extension. The other two heads attach to the back of the humerus.

At the distal end, the triceps connects to the olecranon process of the ulna, making it a strong elbow extensor. Unlike the biceps, many yoga practitioners have strong triceps because it is a key factor in

Try this fun little exercise.

Fully flex your elbow with the forearm pronated (palm facing the floor) and have a squeeze of your little biceps (1). I say little because, as I mentioned earlier, we don't do much pulling in yoga.

Now fully supinate your forearm while keeping the elbow flexion going (2) and feel the muscle under your fingers grow and firm (3).

You are now using both primary actions of the biceps.

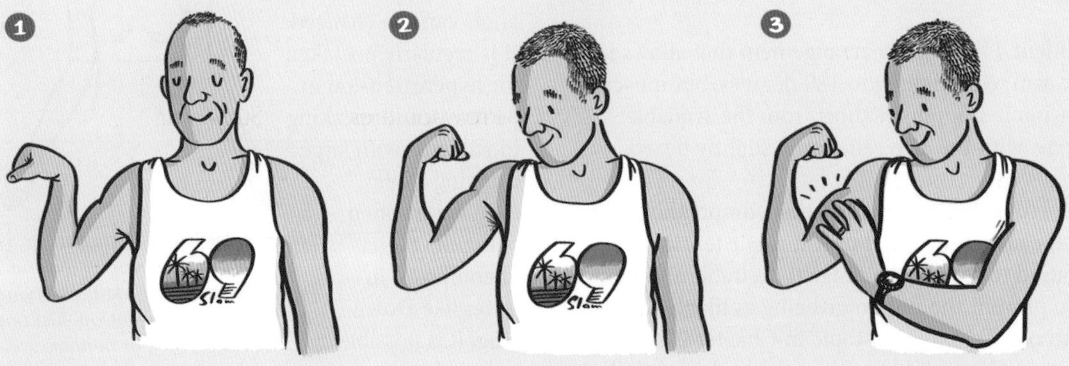

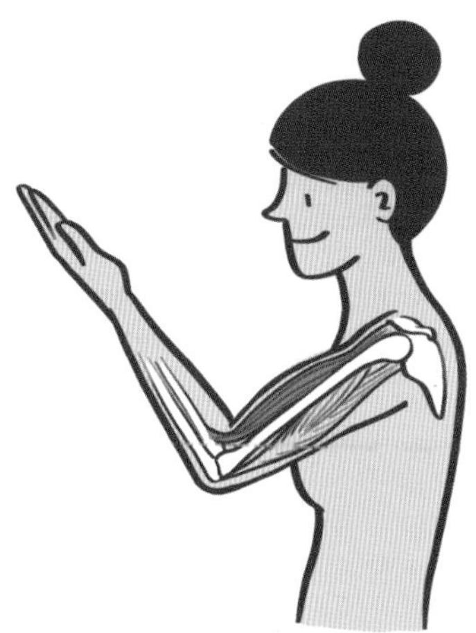

Figure 12.6 Shoulder and elbow flexion: The biceps are elbow flexors and weak shoulder flexors (profile view).

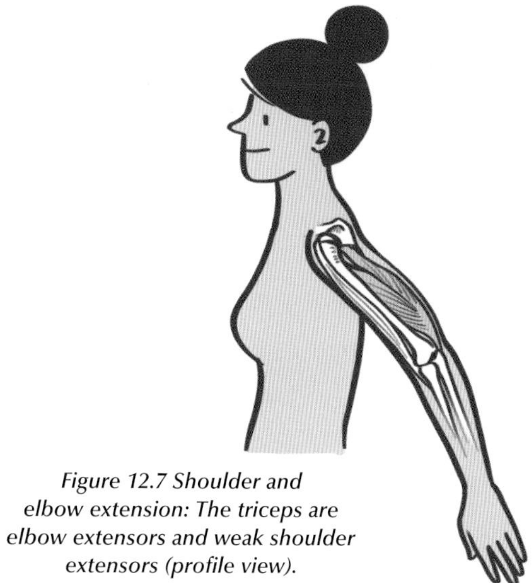

Figure 12.7 Shoulder and elbow extension: The triceps are elbow extensors and weak shoulder extensors (profile view).

bent-arm strength, holding us away from the floor in poses such as arm balances. Of course, it all depends though on what you do in your yoga practice.

Other Muscles that Move the Elbow

There are quite a few other muscles that cross the elbow and can help with flexion, pronation, or supination, but I think we have enough to work with (Figure 12.8). We always want to keep an eye on our focus, and that is to understand the body within the context of postural yoga. I can't think of any postures where we might say the limiting factor was pronation or supination of the forearm.

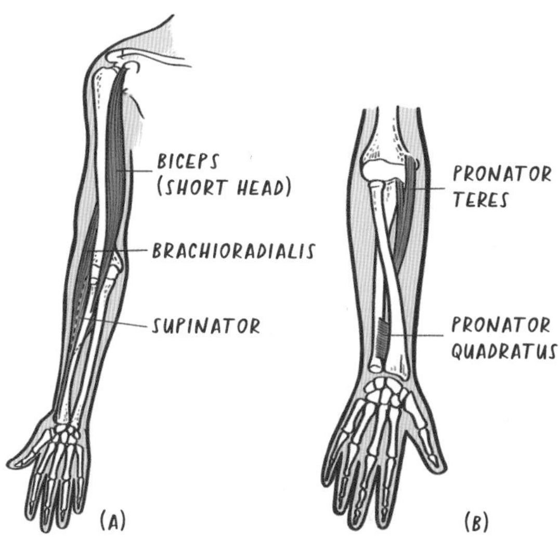

Figure 12.8 I really don't think you will need to remember the muscles that perform supination (A) and pronation (B), but they are here for completeness. Mind you, there are a couple of clues in the names of these.

Quick Reference Muscle Action Tables

Flexion	Extension
Biceps brachii	Triceps brachii
Brachialis	
Brachioradialis and a few others	

Pronation	Supination
Pronator teres	Supinator
Pronator quadratus	Biceps brachii (short head)
	Brachioradialis

Putting Things into Context

When we take the arm behind us to bind or go in to Reverse Prayer, often the cue that is given emphasizes the need to rotate the shoulder medially. I have experimented with this a lot, and I think this creates unnecessary stress in the anterior shoulder, with some students experiencing pain. If more use is made of the rotation available at the elbow, then less is required at the shoulder, which brings comfort to many. For the moment, think for yourselves how you might go about actioning this movement, and I will expand the idea in Part III, *Posture Groups*.

In the last chapter, I discussed the elbows going out in postures. I'm going to come back to the topic, but this time in *Chaturanga*. Here, the cause is not muscular restriction but rather weakness. When the arms are kept close to the sides on the lower down, it is the triceps working eccentrically that slow the elbow flexion and the anterior deltoid that primarily slows the shoulder extension, with a little help from the upper fibers of the pectoralis major. As the elbows drift out, the pectoralis major can help more (Figure 12.9). Hence students with weak triceps subconsciously try and avoid the work there by recruiting the larger pectoralis major.

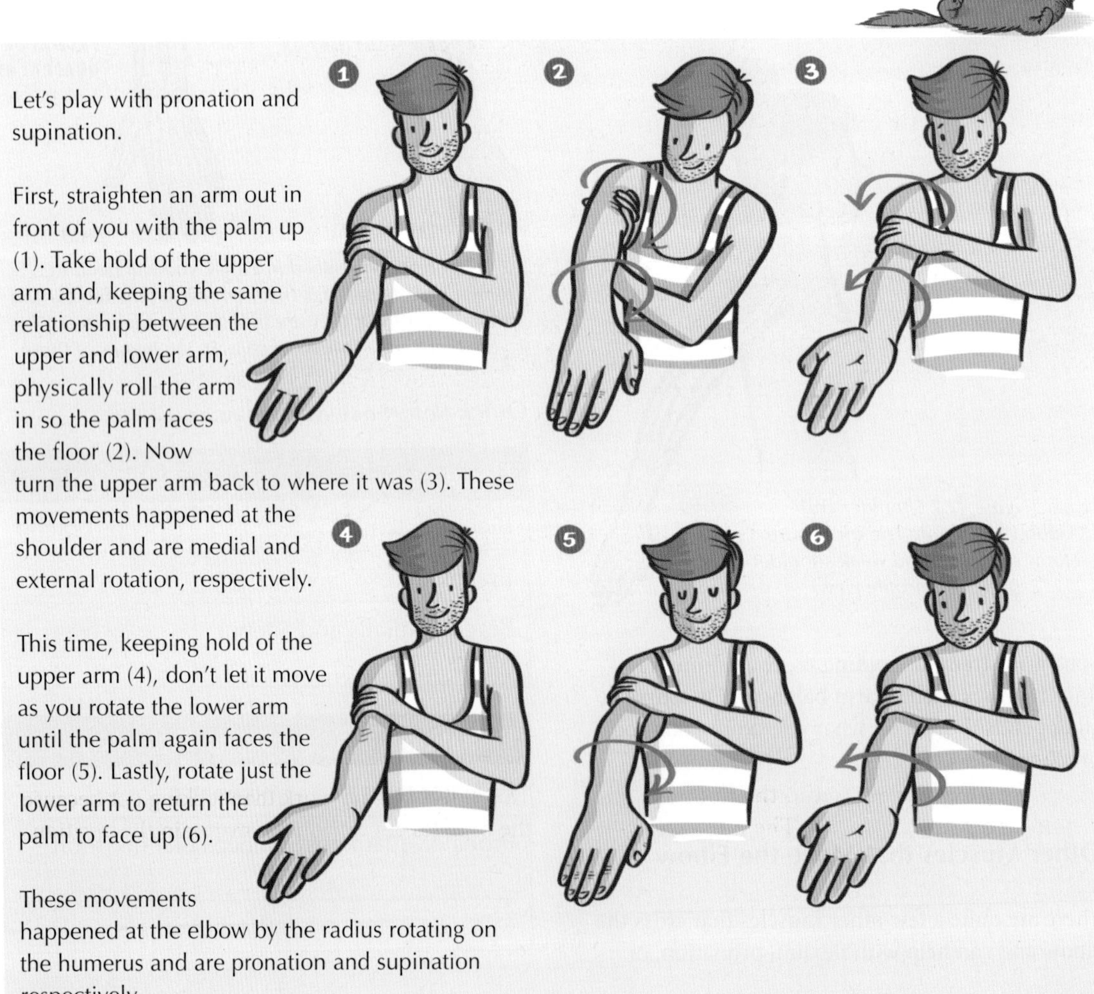

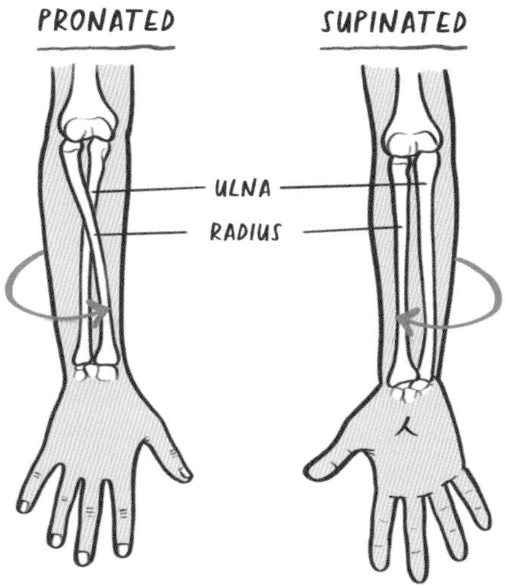

Figure 12.9 The pivot joint between the radius and humerus allows the radius to cross over the ulna when the forearm is pronated.

The first problem this pattern causes is that it will take longer for the triceps to become stronger. The second is that as there is probably already an imbalance between the pulling (latissimus dorsi) and pushing muscles of the torso, this will further increase the difference. This sort of imbalance can feed into a shoulder's rounded forward postural pattern.

Another posture I mentioned in the previous chapter was *Kurmasana*. This pose can also be a hazard for those students with hyperextending elbows if hip flexion is not available. As we would expect from our understanding of *Multi-Segmental Movement* (Chapter 2), what tends to happen when the shoulders are off the ground is that the weight of the legs pushing down on the arms causes the area of least resistance to give. With this type of student, that tends to be the elbow, from where they move into hyperextension. I have observed students where the forearms are flat to the floor, but the shoulders are still in the air. The movement we are looking for needs to come from the hips, by way of hip flexion. This compromise just places undue stress on the elbows.

It's time for us to consider if hyperextension of the elbow is problematic or not. The first thing we could say is that if a student's joint is designed to allow the elbow to extend greater than 180 degrees, then in a non-weight-bearing situation, it won't cause damage. The critical detail there is *non-weight-bearing*. When we think about the difference in a weight-bearing position, we now can have a substantial load being transmitted down the arm. The lower the number of foundational elements, the greater the force. If bones are lined up, there may be some compressive force, but the joint and ligaments are in a stable position. If the elbow is in a hyperextended position, then some of the force will be pressing the elbow back toward further hyperextension. The olecranon process will stop the movement, but you are levering against the joint structure. So, my verdict, at the moment, is the arm should be kept straight by using muscular engagement. There are so many postures where this is the case, for example, *Ustrasana*, *Purvottanasana*, *Setu Bandha Sarvangasana*, *Bakasana*, and of course, Handstands.

So, what to do then in those non-weight-bearing positions? This is where I think we can draw on the idea of encouraging new patterns. If the student just lets the elbow hyperextend in postures like *Virabhadrasana B* and *Ardha Matsyendrasana*, then that is the established pattern, and it will feel the most natural. In times of reduced attention, this pattern will just be repeated. My advice is to microbend the arm even when not weight-bearing, as well as to strengthen the elbow flexors (biceps) so they provide more tensional resistance to extension.

Working to maintain straight arms when there is a potential of hyperextension takes a lot of awareness. Simple guidelines are to start from a flexed position and then use the eccentric action of the flexor muscles of that joint to resist how far you take the joint. Stopping with a microbend is useful. This will be harder work than locking out because the muscles are working to maintain the position, but I feel it is healthier for the joint.

So how about another perspective to give a balanced overview. Many professional hand balancers and circus artists perform handstands with locked out hyperextended elbows as if that is what their elbows can do naturally. The reasoning behind this is that it uses far less energy to be locked out rather than maintain a position through muscular effort. From what I have read, there seems to a higher incidence of muscle tendon injuries from hyperextending in this group from trying to maintain a microbend than ligament or other injuries.

I think now you have to decide where you stand. If hyperextending in weight-bearing positions causes you elbow pain, then definitely don't do it. If you are pain-free, then you have more choice, but I will finish by saying that as yoga practitioners we don't have to be concerned so much with energy conservation because we are not holding postures or inversions for very long. With that in mind, I still think microbending is the right thing to do for yoga practitioners.

I have been asked by yogis before about the safety of Handstanding if you have a large carrying angle. Again, the same holds true as for hyperextending. Forces will find the change in direction on their journey down the arm and place stress into the elbow. Any negative impact is likely to be influenced by the degree of angle change as well as the robustness of the individual's skeletal framework. In this situation, I think it is best to proceed cautiously, gradually building up the time under load.

The chain of joints we have in the arm means that, like the knee, if the areas above and below do not have adequate ROM, then the one in the middle often has to compromise. One of the keys to elbow safety is having the required movement ranges at the shoulder, especially when it comes to flexion, because it is in this position that we are likely to introduce the greatest loading. Shoulder strength is also a major component when it comes to elbow safety because, unlike the leg, we are not used to taking the whole body weight on our hands. Any compromising of shoulder positioning due to lack of strength will have to be taken up by the joints below.

Construction of the Wrist

We went into quite a lot of detail in covering the ankle and foot, but when it comes to the hand and wrist, I am going to keep things simpler. The reason for this is that what we ask from it in the yoga practice is relatively straightforward. For example, we want to be able to grasp things, weight-bear, and place our hands in prayer position. There are lots of small accommodating movements that will be going on, but these are no different from those used in our everyday interactions with the world around us. The movement we need the most of, and which may present an issue for some students, is wrist extension. This is not to say that students don't get wrist issues, but these are mostly due to weight-bearing.

The two lower arm bones, the radius and ulna, articulate with each other at the wrist, but only the radius articulates with the proximal row of carpal bones (with three of the four) (Figure 12.10). It is called the radiocarpal joint, and this is where wrist extension, flexion, adduction, and abduction are available, and in combination, circumduction. Following on down, we have another row of four carpals, then in the hand, the metacarpals, and finally the phalanges (fingers).

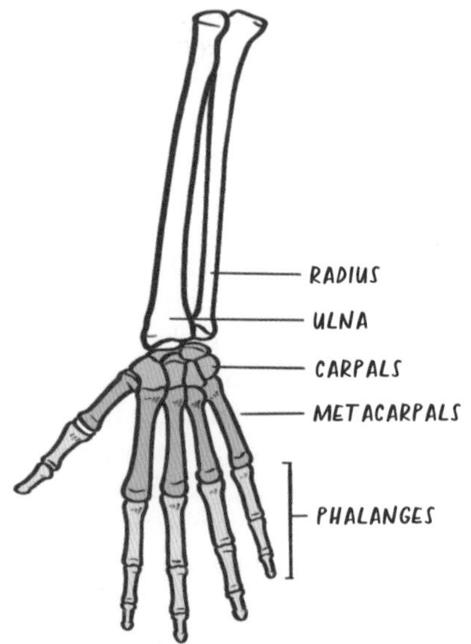

Figure 12.10 Construction of the wrist.

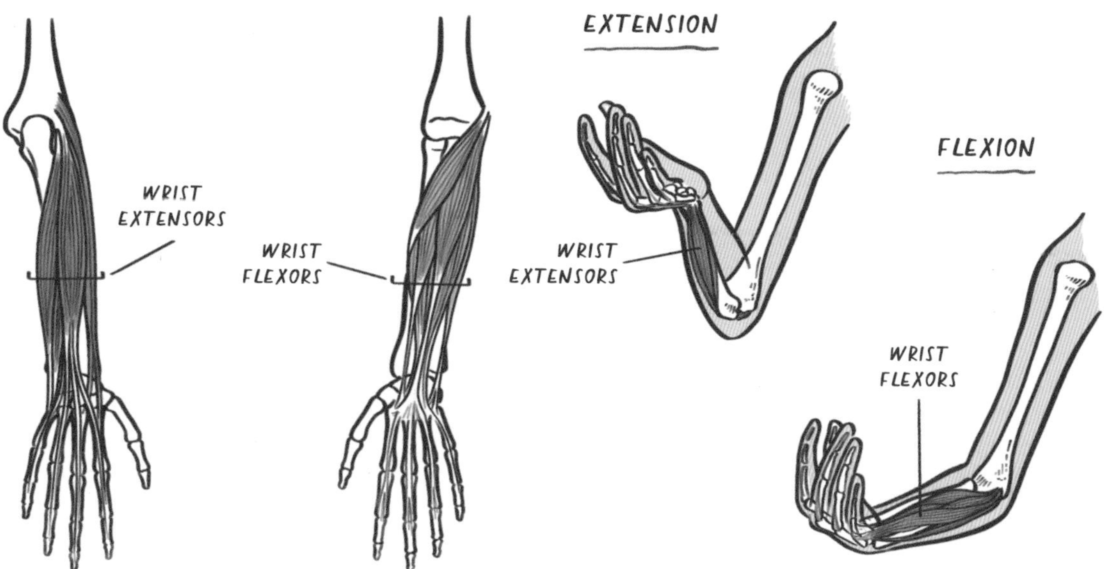

Figure 12.11 Muscles that move the wrist.

Muscles that Move the Wrist

There are four muscles that do wrist extension, and five that do wrist flexion (Figure 12.11). We are just going to lump them together and say the wrist extensors are on the back of the forearm and the flexors are on the front. Think anatomical position if you are wondering which is front and back. Combinations of them do wrist abduction and adduction. Students often get confused as to which movement is flexion, and which is extension. If you are in Down Dog, Plank, Handstand, or *Bakasana*, your wrist is extended to various amounts. See what I mean when I say that extension is an important movement.

Putting Things into Context

There is a relatively high incidence of wrist pain in yoga practitioners, particularly among new students. Our feet and ankles are designed in a more rugged way than the wrist and hand because we spend our time on our legs. One of the primary elements contributing to wrist pain can be too much too soon. It takes time for the muscles, tendons, and even bones, to get stronger and be ready to take a greater proportion of our body weight, so build up the amount of weight-bearing over several months.

Another key element is the existing wrist ROM. Working practices, such as high-volume computer use, can make the wrists more inflexible. If this is the case, the area may already be sensitive and more easily aggravated. Extra care needs to be taken in postures such as arm balances, where greater ROM is often necessary and more weight is taken into the wrists. Sometimes it is better to use wedges under the hands.

The last element I will mention is dynamic loading, for example, jumping backward and forward, especially to seated. When the body is in motion, it is much harder to control the ROM moved through, as momentum can take us further than we are ready for. Dynamic stabilization can place extra stress on the ligaments and tendons. It is especially important to carefully assess the impact these transitions are having if you are on the heavier side or have to jiggle around to get through the arms.

This point is just as relevant to the shoulders because once you are in the air, you are at the will of gravity to bring you back down. As our arms

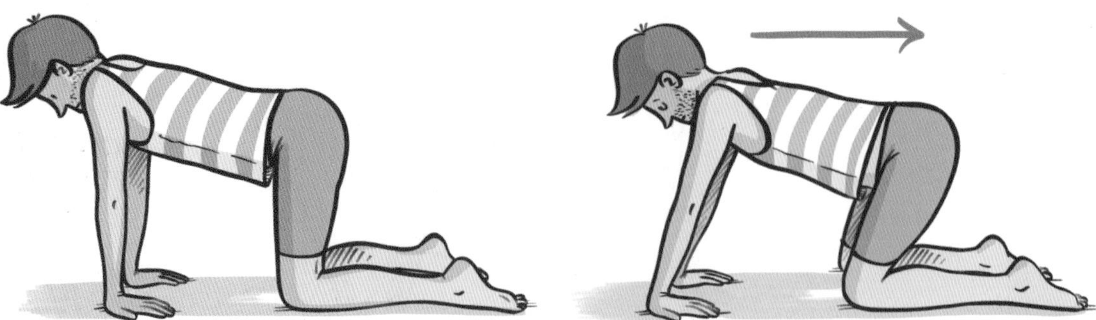

Figure 12.12 Keep the heels of the hands grounded as the body is gently taken back.

don't account for much of our overall body weight (approximately 5 to 6 percent), nearly all our weight has to be controlled down by the relatively small muscles of the shoulder, and they can easily fail under this load. Again, the key to maintaining healthy wrists and shoulders is to build up slowly the number of dynamic transitions you do.

Sticking with pain for a moment, some students report experiencing wrist discomfort in postures like a Reverse Prayer. It is my experience that these students don't require greater wrist mobility, but greater *shoulder* mobility. I haven't encountered any of these students that, when asked to do a prayer position in front of them, report the same discomfort. If your shoulders allow, you can recreate exactly the same relationship behind you as in front, between the forearm and hand. We can deduce then, that restriction in the shoulders is causing the alignment to have to change at the wrist, and it is this compromised positioning that aggravates the wrists.

If you are going to do some serious weight-bearing on your wrists and shoulders, like, for example, a Handstand segment, taking some extra time to do a specific wrist and shoulder warm-up is advised. I'll share with you my favorite wrist flexor stretch.

The basic starting position is a shortened Tabletop with the hands shoulder-width apart and reversed, the fingertips pointing toward the knees. Keeping the heel of the hands firmly grounded, slowly bring the weight back toward the heels by bending the knees (Figure 12.12). This will increase the amount of wrist extension and place the flexors under a stretch. You can alternate between periods of stillness and rotating in small circles clockwise and anticlockwise. It is very easy for those students who hyperextend to stop moving at the wrist and instead bend at the elbow. To avoid this, it is better to start with bent arms and keep them like that until the full range of wrist extension has been reached. Only then begin to straighten the arms, stopping when the microbend is achieved.

Although as I have mentioned wrist extension is the most useful movement at the wrist, there is a point when enough is enough. If you can move through even 110 degrees of extension, I would say that is plenty. There is no need to try and get more, instead work on the strength.

PART III

POSTURE GROUPS

"A single posture can be considered to be in many groups, including classifications not used here, such as standing, seated, restorative, balancing, and so forth. Maybe what is more important is the purpose or intention behind why it is being performed."

CHAPTER 13

Forward Bends

Forward bends are postures where the most significant hip movement is flexion. Under this umbrella, I include both straight-leg and bent-leg variations. It may be that a pose also contains a hip rotation or abduction and could be symmetrical or asymmetrical. I would say that the intention of the poses in this category would be to move forward past 90 degrees of hip flexion or that this movement is the only one going on at the hip (Figure 13.1).

For example, in *Marichyasana C*, both hips are flexed to varying degrees, but the essence of the posture is a twist. That's not to say that inability to flex the hips sufficiently won't influence the pose.

Some postures, of course, are in more than one group, so are placed where the discussion makes the most sense. For example, *Janu Sirsasana* has one leg in hip flexion and the other is rotated and abducted. When the torso is taken in the direction of the straight leg, the pose is made more intense by increasing hip flexion and opposite hip rotation. Therefore, this posture is an asymmetric forward bend, but it makes more sense to be in Chapter 14, *Hip Rotations*, because of what happens at the bent leg hip. The straight leg is the same as all the other adducted straight-leg forward bends.

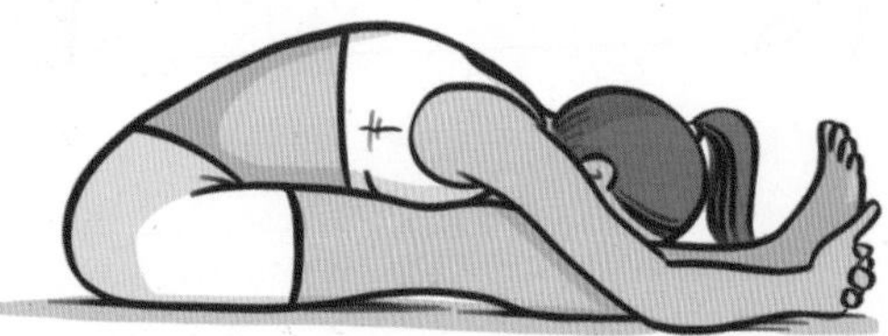

Figure 13.1 Forward bend.

Bent Leg or Straight Leg

The first major difference in forward bends is whether the leg is straight or bent, and by bent, I mean 90 degrees or more knee flexion. The change in the knee joint position completely alters which muscles will create the restriction to hip flexion. A small knee bend is often used as a modification for a straight-legged forward bend to allow a restricted student some forward movement of the pelvis, and a stretch will still be experienced in the hamstrings. However, because their distal attachments are below the knee, a large bend will effectively remove them as a restriction, and any significant limitation will come from Gmax. For example, one of the necessary actions for a comfortable squat is deep hip flexion with a bent knee.

As we will see when we broaden the discussion in a bit, there are quite a few muscles that influence the ability to move deeply into a forward bend, but the significant restrictions will be the hamstrings when the leg is straight, and Gmax when the knees are well flexed. The gluteal muscles may influence the ROM of a straight or bent leg forward bend, but the hamstrings will only restrict one with a straight leg.

Assessing Hip Flexion Capability

One of the old fitness test components was could you touch your toes either seated or standing, and you can still go to any park and see runners and other exercisers having a go. But of course, by now, I'm sure you realize that it's too easy to cheat by rounding the spine when the pelvis stops moving. For example, although *Paschimottanasana* would seem like an easy go-to test, we need something that keeps the back out of it. *Supta Padangushtasana* is perfect for isolating the straight-legged hip flexion movement. The leg in the air needs to be kept absolutely straight and the calf of the lower leg needs to maintain contact with the floor, otherwise it indicates that the pelvis has been pulled toward the face along with the leg (Figure 13.2).

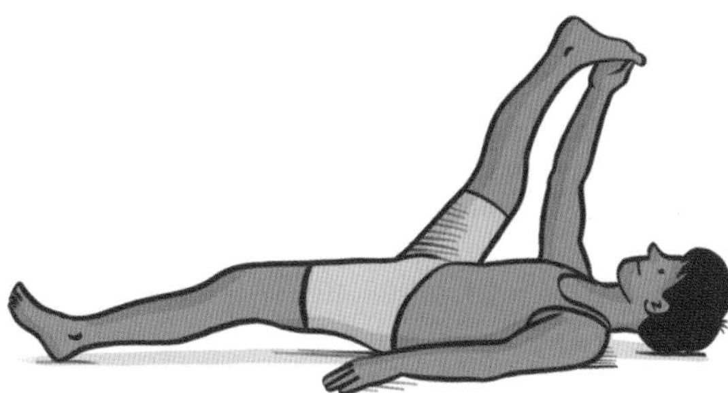

Figure 13.2 If the knee in the air or on the floor bends, it is not giving a true evaluation of straight-legged hip flexion.

This test gives the realistic position of the leg relative to the pelvis that can be expected in many other postures.

If there is a significant difference, it's a heads-up to look for where the adaptation is happening. If we are keeping it strict and the leg only points to the ceiling in *Supta Padangushtasana*, then that is 90 degrees of hip flexion. In *Paschimottanasana* that equates to sitting upright, in *UHP* the leg parallel to the floor and not coming forward toward the leg, and in a Standing Forward Bend, the torso parallel to the floor (Figure 13.3).

The position I like for assessing bent-legged hip flexion is Happy Baby (Figure 13.4). For a clean technique, the lower leg wants to be kept perpendicular to the floor, and the feet should not be twisted but positioned as if you were standing on the ceiling. It doesn't matter if the hands grasp the inside or outside edge of the feet. The thighs are kept relatively close to the sides of the ribcage.

As was mentioned in Chapter 2, *Compression*, some students may experience medium compression in this posture. If removing the flesh makes no difference to comfort, then they should not try to go deeper. The first giveaway for restriction will be that the student can't reach their feet and the

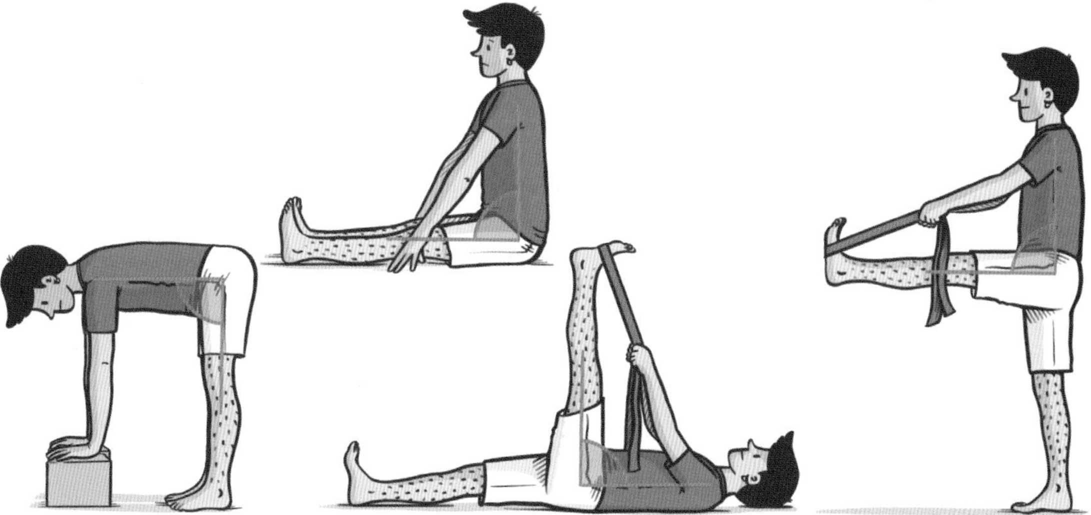

Figure 13.3 Essentially, the movement at the hip is the same irrespective of orientation. The only difference will be the effect of gravity.

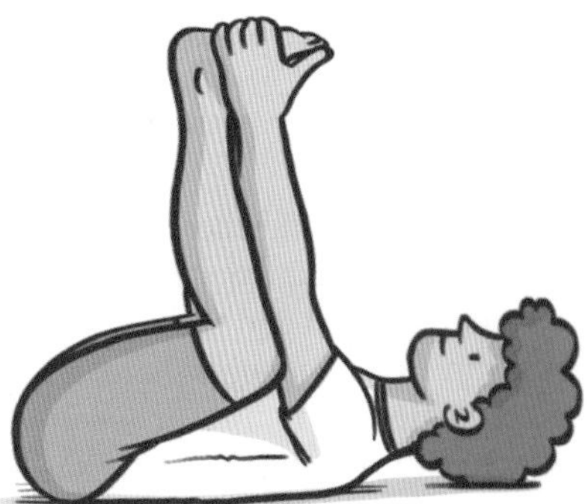

Figure 13.4 Happy Baby is one of my go-to postures for assessment, but also as homework.

knees are probably higher than their ribcage. In these instances, the student should use a belt so that their shoulders are not pulled off the floor. If the knees come down to the outside of their ribcage, that shows quite a good ROM, and if they come to the floor, then (a) they have a pelvis shape that will allow that, and (b) they shouldn't have any problem with postures that call for bent-legged hip flexion.

Rounding the Spine in Forward Bending

If you were at the physiotherapist and they asked you to reach down to your toes from standing, I don't think they would expect to see a hip hinge, but instead, for your pelvis to tilt forward and your back round as you went down. Usually, they would be looking to see if the spine curves evenly as well as having hip flexion. In general, we want a back chain of the body that works together to achieve a flexion movement and that there aren't areas that are inflexible relative to their neighbors. That doesn't mean we would necessarily pick something up like that, bent knees and neutral spine are still advisable.

However, there are even strengthening movements such as the Jefferson Curl (like a Standing Forward Bend holding a weight), which uses a controlled forward flexion, rounding the spine from cervical to lumbar, and finally hips on the way down (eccentric) and the reverse on the way up (concentric). Although not suitable for those individuals with segmental instability or mobility issues, it goes to show that rounding the spine is not always thought to be a bad thing.

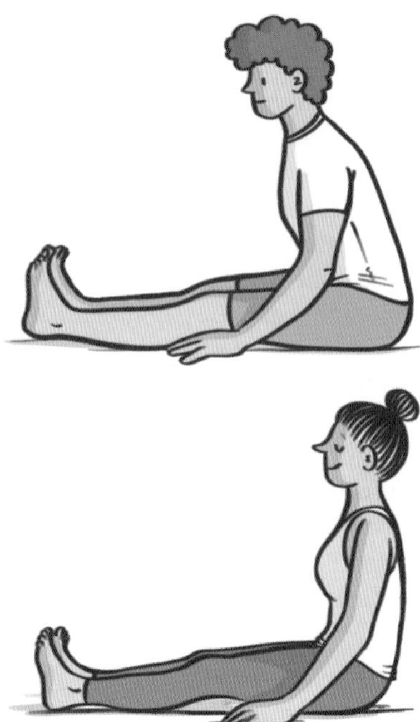

Figure 13.5 Unless the pelvis can move into an anterior tilt from Dandasana, *any seated fold will be compromised before it even starts.*

However, in a yoga setting, we are looking to emphasize the flexion at the hip in most poses (Figure 13.5). This focus will help protect the lumbar spine, bring awareness to where the flexion movement is coming from, and start to prepare the body for postures that will require a large ROM in hip flexion, such as *Kurmasana* and *Tittibhasana*.

Initiating forward movement with the pelvis, which tilts anteriorly, allows the spine to maintain its neutral curve for as long as possible. Inevitably in the deeper postures, the spine won't stay in that shape and will round, particularly once the ribcage touches the thighs (Figure 13.6). Students' backs will look rounded to varying degrees even when they are up against their legs, just because of their individual shape. When there is less straight-leg hip

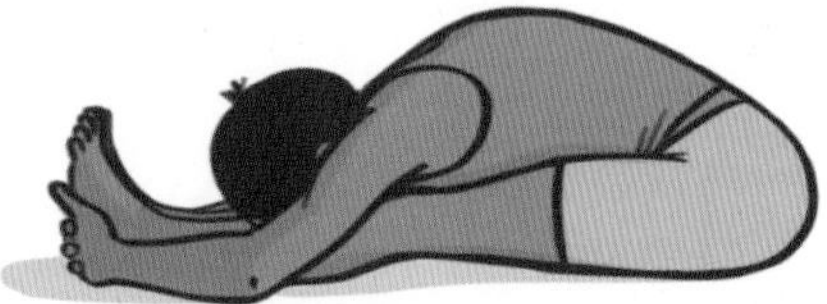

Figure 13.6 Once the ribs touch the legs, the spine will round as the head comes down.

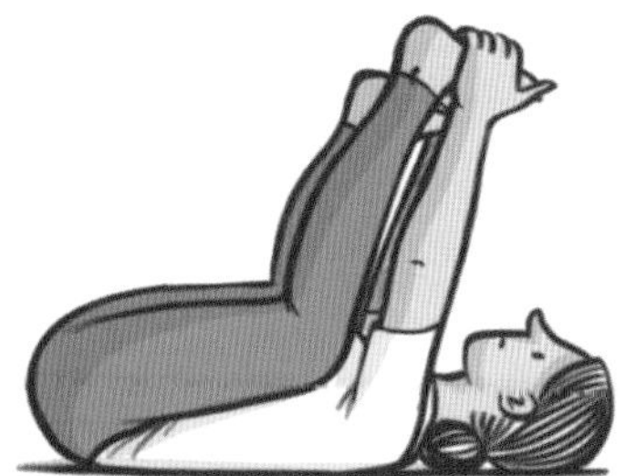

Figure 13.7 Keep the sacrum on the floor.

flexibility available, the student should try and not let the spine round and instead use a strap if they need to reach their feet. This is when it is good to refer to our strict ROM test, as it gives a realistic positioning to adopt.

With the bent-legged forward bends, there is often the same issue with trying to separate what is happening at the hip from the spine. In Happy Baby, for example, the knees come closer to the ground if the lumbar spine is allowed to flex. If this is our test, again it would give a false idea of ROM at the hip. In this posture, the cue is to keep the sacrum on the floor (Figure 13.7). In the squat, the rounding of the back can be reduced by not bringing the chest too far forward through the legs and emphasizing sitting up tall.

Gravitational Influence

Gravity is, of course, bearing down in all postures that we do, but I feel it is easier to discern its effect in forward bends and backbends. On the one hand, we can make use of this force, and on the other, it can be something to overcome. If we think of a forward bend as taking the upper and lower halves of the body toward each other, we can have both halves moving, just the top half, or only the lower half. All variations lead to an increase in hip flexion. Let's first consider some of the common orientations we can have and how that might influence students with different levels of flexibility.

From a standing position, if the torso is taken in the direction of the legs, then gravity will be assisting that movement (Figure 13.8). In fact, to control the descent, the muscles that are lengthening will also be contracting (eccentric contraction). Whether you find forward bending easy or difficult, gravity will be lending a hand. However, if instead you start to raise a leg when standing (Figure 13.9), then gravity will be pulling it back toward the floor. The more resistance you have to hip flexion, the harder you will have to work, with gravity added on top of that.

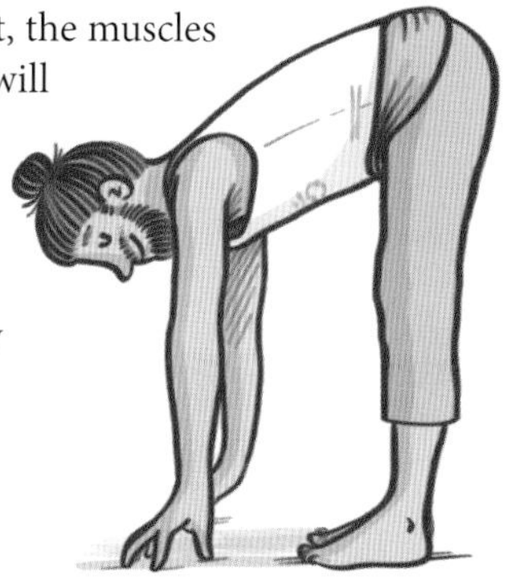

Figure 13.8 In this orientation, gravity will be assisting Zane to flex his hips.

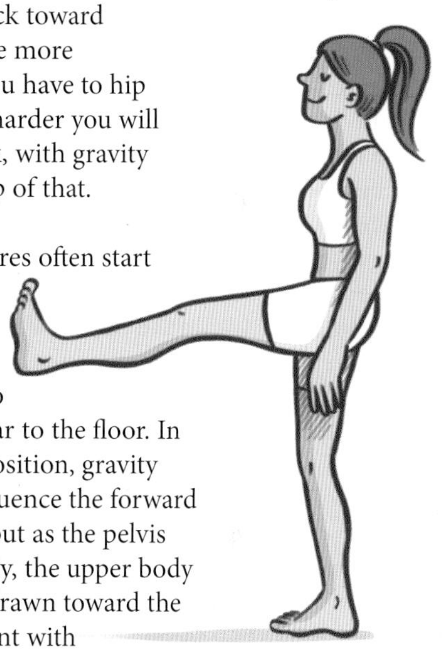

Seated postures often start with one or more legs outstretched and the torso perpendicular to the floor. In this initial position, gravity does not influence the forward movement, but as the pelvis tilts anteriorly, the upper body starts to be drawn toward the legs. A student with only 90 degrees of hip flexion will get no help as they are basically sitting in *Dandasana*. If they have less than 90 degrees, the pelvis is in a posterior tilt, and gravity will be taking them backward (Figure 13.10). As this positioning feels unnatural and is hard work to maintain, subconsciously these students will round the lower back to bring the mass of the upper body over the hips. The neutral spine is lost even before any attempt is made to move toward the legs.

Figure 13.9 Now gravity will provide a force to overcome.

It makes sense then to either bend the legs or place something under the butt to at least bring the

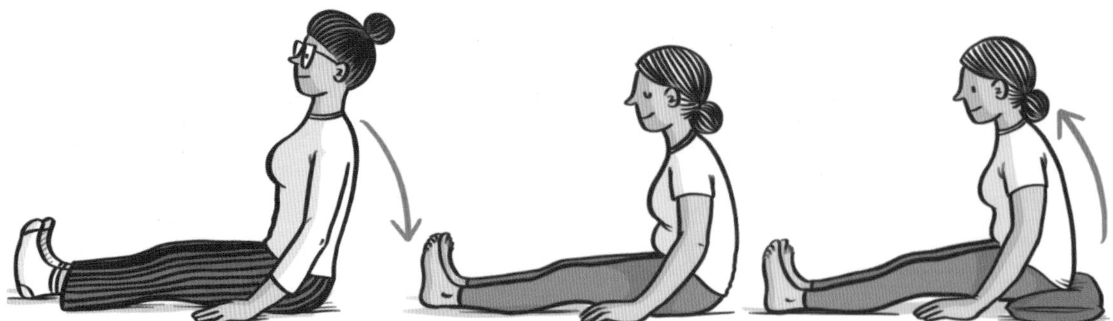

Figure 13.10 If the pelvis is in a posterior tilt, gravity is taking the torso backward and the student naturally rounds the back because it is less work.

pelvis into a slight anterior tilt. I would say that all students who can't initiate more than about a 15 degree anterior tilt of the pelvis would be better off using a strap around the feet to gently assist (Figure 13.11). The experience will be different for those individuals that can get a good tilt, as they will be able to relax and feel gravity aiding them on their way down.

In a reclined pose, such as *Supta Padangushtasana*, the leg is taken toward the torso. With the leg anywhere before 90 degrees, gravity is taking it back from where it came. Once you get past the halfway mark, you can start to feel the assistance of gravity, especially as the leg gets closer to the chest. The same goes here as with the seated postures—those students challenged in hip flexion would be better off using a strap to reach the foot, keeping the upper body on the floor, and cultivating that feeling of relaxed breathing. Working with active ROM, the restricted student will be fighting gravity and the tension in their soft tissues, whereas the freer student has an easier time because, for them, the leg wants to travel toward the body.

I think the time you feel the most assistance from gravity toward hip flexion is when you are inverted. In, for example, a *Sirsasana*, Shoulderstand, or Handstand, if the position of the pelvis is maintained as the lower limbs are taken toward the ground, the long lever of the leg under the influence of gravity creates a powerful action. This also makes it an ideal position to work on hip extension strength by controlling the movement up and down. Of course, we need to bear in mind the vulnerability of the neck in some of these positions (Figure 13.12).

Considering the above, I think restricted students will find working on hip flexion from a standing position more worthwhile. Poses like *Uttanasana*,

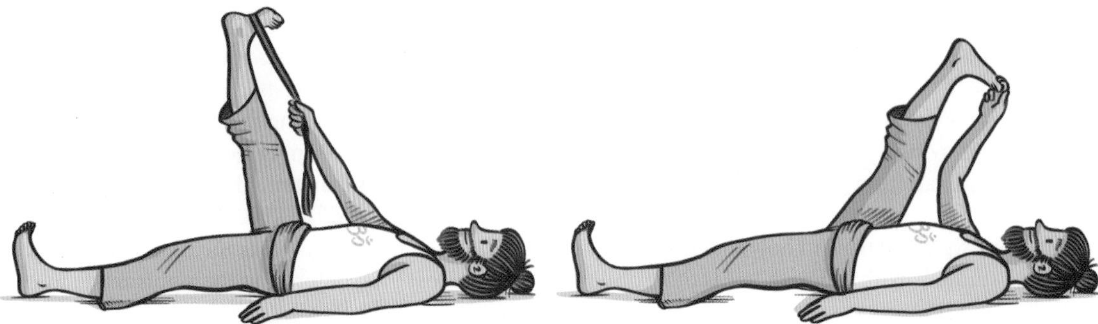

Figure 13.11 Flexible students have an easier time because gravity is also helping them flex the hip. Break out the strap to make life a little easier.

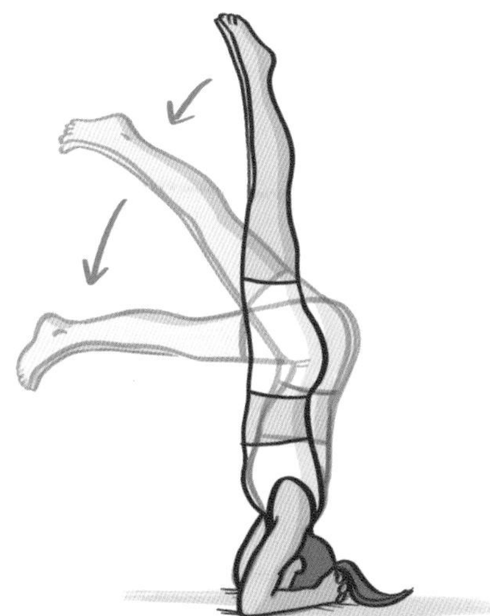

Figure 13.12 Controlling down, the hamstrings will be working eccentrically and concentrically on the way up.

Parsvottanasana, and *Prasarita Padottanasana* are excellent choices, because they are uncomplicated (that is not the same as easy).

However, the same gravitational assistance that is helping with hip flexion will also make rounding the spine more enticing. It is better to use blocks if the floor cannot be reached so that the neutral spine can be mindfully maintained. In addition, as the foundation of standing postures is considerably smaller than when seated, blocks will aid with balance (Figure 13.13). If the body feels like it will fall forward, then tension will be maintained in those muscles on the back of the body that need to let us go forward.

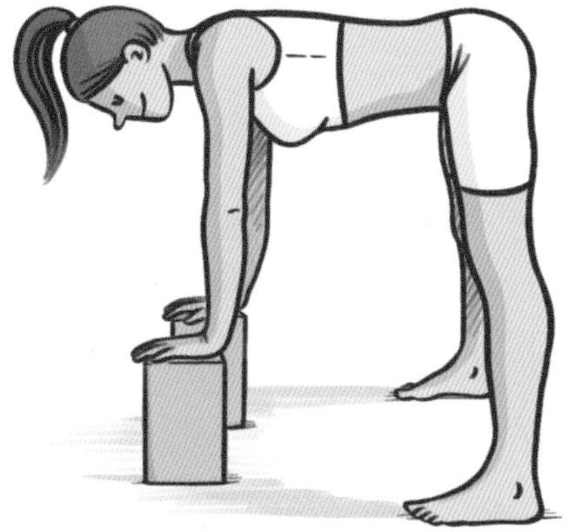

Figure 13.13 Make up any space between the hands and the floor with blocks rather than rounding.

This is not to say that we can't stretch a contracted muscle because, essentially, that is what is happening in an eccentric contraction. However, it will be challenging to go deeper from an unstable position. The reclined poses provide the best location as far as strictness, because the back is on the floor and rounding will be resisted. However, challenged students will get no help from gravity.

Hip Muscles that Affect Forward Bending

I will restrict this discussion to hip flexion with the legs in neutral alignment because what happens when the hips are rotated and flexed will be covered in another chapter. Sticking with our basic concept of opposing muscles restrict, the main inhibitors to hip flexion are those that perform hip extension, the hamstrings and Gmax. The story doesn't end there, however, because many other muscles can also play a role. When the legs are apart (abducted), the adductors will be placed under a stretch, and the forward tilting movement of the pelvis will increase this. The main culprit will be adductor magnus as it attaches to the sit bone (ischial tuberosity) similarly to the hamstrings, although in a slightly more medial position; because of this, it is even referred to as the fourth hamstring (Figure 13.14). The restriction the adductor muscles present will depend on their relative flexibility.

For example, a student who can easily abduct their hips will probably find they have minimal

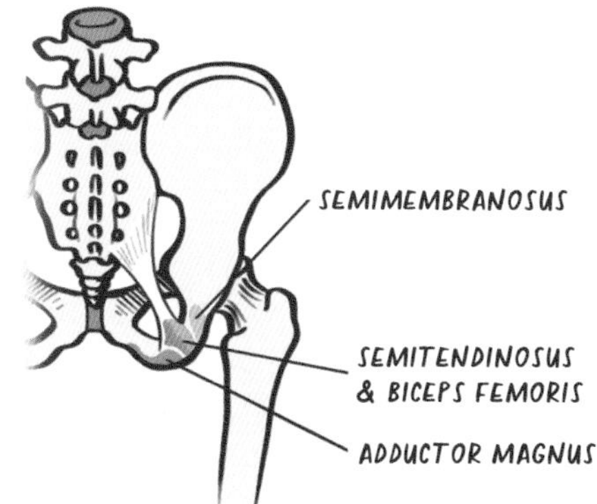

Figure 13.14 Adductor magnus attaches to the ischial tuberosity and acts similarly to a hamstring as well as an adductor.

resistance from the adductors when the legs are together, only feeling them come into play when the hips are well abducted, and then a flexion is added. On the other hand, a student who is more challenged with hip abduction may also be hampered by tightness in the adductors even when the legs are together. When the legs are taken a reasonable distance apart, as in *Upavistha Konasana*, the emphasis of the stretch will be lessened on the lateral hamstring (biceps femoris) because of the angle change in the leg relative to the pelvis, and increased on the medial hamstrings (semitendinosus and semimembranosus). For students who have significant restriction in the adductors as well as the hamstrings, taking the legs apart can easily send the pelvis into a posterior tilt. If so, modification by way of bending the knees or sitting on a block will be beneficial.

The same goes for the muscles that rotate the hip medially and externally, primarily Gmed and Gmin, and the deep external rotators. As they attach to the greater trochanter of the femur, they can also be placed under a stretch as the pelvis rotates around the femoral head in the forward bending movement (or vice versa). Again, students with easy hip rotation are only likely to experience minor resistance to hip flexion when the legs are neutral (i.e., seated forward bend). But students with limited rotational ability may notice quite an effect.

If you are in a straight-legged forward bend and you feel restriction to tilting the pelvis forward, it's most likely the hamstrings will be shouting the loudest, or as mentioned above, if the legs are apart, the adductors and medial hamstrings. But as we have said, that doesn't mean that other muscles are not also creating some resistance.

Then perform each of the following openers (or an alternative), below, repeating the original posture

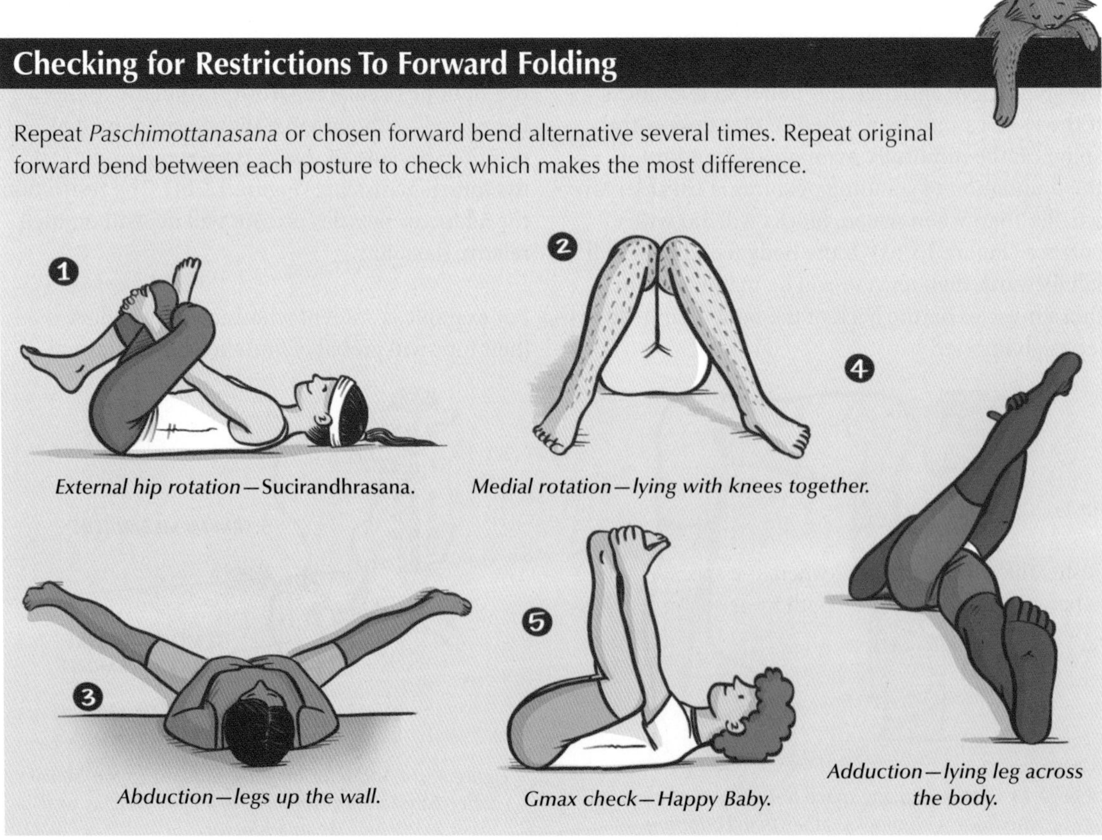

Checking for Restrictions To Forward Folding

Repeat *Paschimottanasana* or chosen forward bend alternative several times. Repeat original forward bend between each posture to check which makes the most difference.

1. *External hip rotation*—Sucirandhrasana.
2. *Medial rotation—lying with knees together.*
3. *Abduction—legs up the wall.*
4. *Adduction—lying leg across the body.*
5. *Gmax check—Happy Baby.*

after each. It is a good idea to test this out, as it is easy to get obsessed with seemingly uncooperative hamstrings. The way to do this is to warm up thoroughly and then perform several strict forward bends, such as *Paschimottanasana*. Repeat as many times as you need to feel that the current depth of posture is representative of your regular ability. Then perform each of the following openers (or an alternative) repeating the original posture after each. You will notice if there is a change in your ability to go into deeper hip flexion.

Once you have discovered if any other hip muscles are influencing your comfort in forward bends, you may then decide to sequence your yoga practice in such a way that you do some of the relevant types of postures first. Although we used what I termed "openers" in our little experiment, these can be replaced with poses that target the same muscles. On a larger scale, if teaching a group of students that you know to have a hard time forward bending, it makes sense to sequence postures in such a way as to address the other movements of the hips before introducing the forward bends.

Back Chain of the Body

We've suggested already that forward bending postures are mostly about accessing the movement of hip flexion, but as the postures get deeper, so too does the involvement of other areas besides from the hips. We can divide this topic into two parts: (1) those areas directly responsible for creating part of the shape, and (2) potential indirect influences.

When the ribcage touches the legs in the *Paschimottanasana* (Figure 13.15), the spine will round to bring the head down to the legs, which is part of the expected shape. The same is true of a deep posture like *Tittibhasana A*, where the shoulders need to be taken past the legs. In both these examples, the spinal flexion is creating part of the forward bend. Should there be resistance to this movement, then it will influence the final shape. In reality, I think the spinal flexion asked for in the type of forward bends we are referring to is comfortably within most students' normal range, unless there is something like injury creating back stiffness (Figure 13.16).

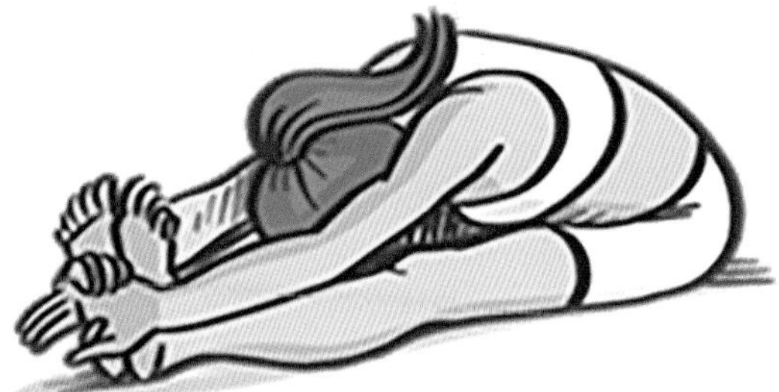

Figure 13.15 Paschimottanasana *is often referred to as a whole back of the body "opener."*

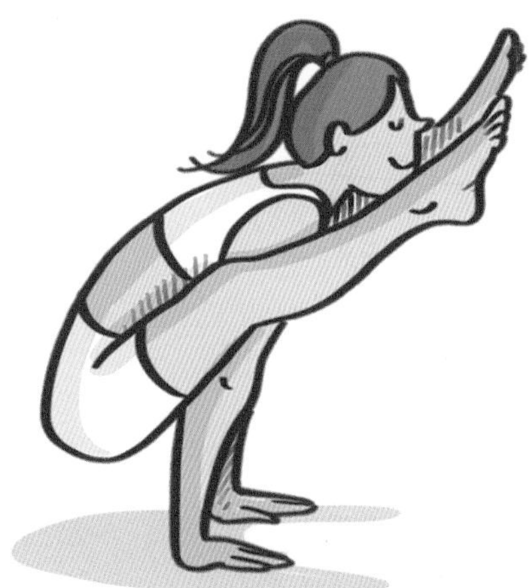

Figure 13.16 Tittibhasana *will have a natural rounding as it is such a deep forward bend.*

Of course, as with all postures, they can be exaggerated. I have seen pictures of students using so much spinal flexion in *Tittibhasana B* that they could comfortably inspect their own anus for piles (Figure 13.17).

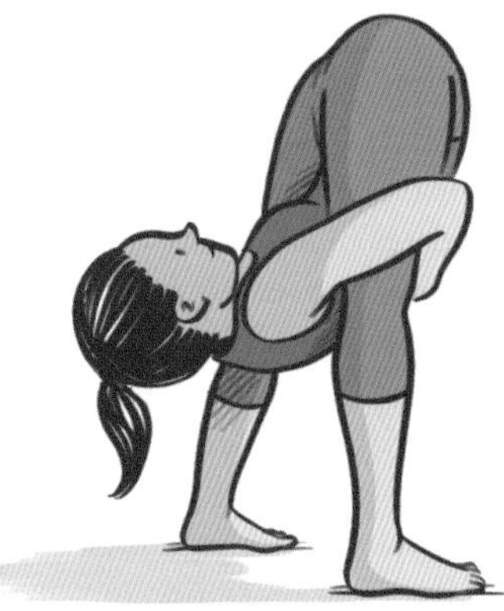

Figure 13.17 OMG, that's what I've got back there.

Experiment for Superficial Back Line

A very popular proof of concept for the Superficial Back Line is the experiment involving rolling your foot on a tennis ball and then retesting your forward bend. The proposed idea is that by releasing tension in the plantar fascia, which is what will be under the tennis ball, the Superficial Back Line will itself experience less resistance and allow for greater hip flexion (Figure 13.18).

Nearly everyone has a positive experience, folding deeper after the play with the tennis ball. The first thing is to have a go if you haven't done this before. A couple of minutes of rolling back and forth with moderate pressure should do the trick. The magic isn't in the tennis ball, by the way; it can be any rollable thingy—I've even used a fist before.

Now for phase two, best done at a separate time. Choose an area where you have less ROM than you would like and try out the movement several times until you feel you have got rid of the cobwebs. Now roll the sole of your foot with the tennis ball for several minutes as before and retest your original movement. Did you notice a difference? I often do.

My explanation for this phenomenon would again revolve around the systemic influence of the nervous system. Another plausible reason might be to do with the role the foot has in many other disciplines such as reflexology. If this sort of thing piques your curiosity, devise your own experiments to test out different scenarios of rolling and testing. You can always report your findings back to me.

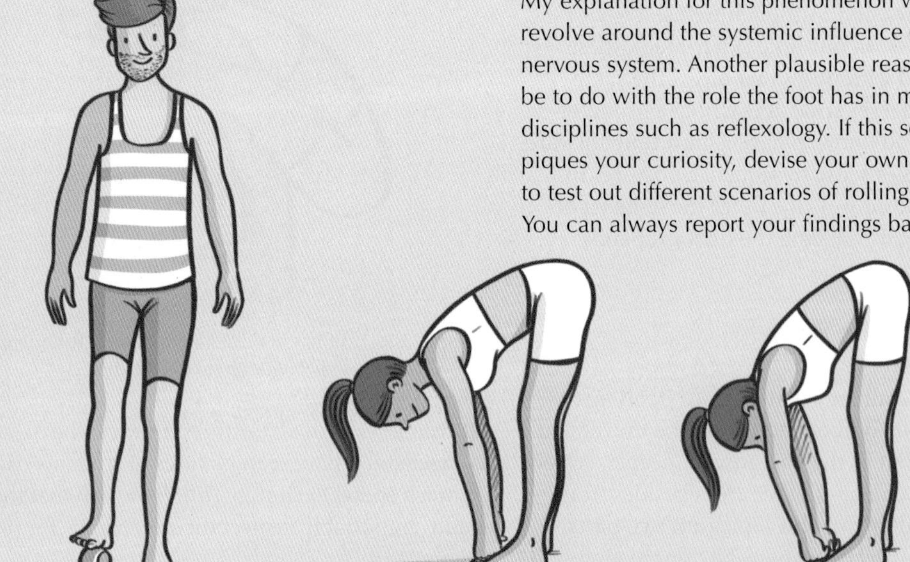

Figure 13.18 After rolling the sole of the foot, most students find a difference in their available hip flexion.

When it comes to indirect influences, I have found that all sorts of areas may be adding to the overall tensional resistance to hip flexion. This perspective relates most closely to envisaging a fascial connection between one area and another. Tom Myers has managed to dissect off from the body what appears to be a fascially-connected chain of muscles and connective tissue (Superficial Back Line) that goes from the front of the skull all the way to the plantar fascia on the sole of the foot. The suggestion is that tension in one area may be relayed to another in the chain. In myself, I have found that if I stretch out my neck, which is often tight because of all the computer work, it makes a difference to my hip flexion. I invite you to play for yourself, exploring the Superficial Back Line and see if anything contributes to a beneficial change.

As usual, I would like to offer some alternative perspectives to consider. I have experimented with stretching out areas unrelated to the Superficial Back Line, such as the forearm flexors, and still experienced differences in hip flexion. I wonder whether an explanation might be found again in the nervous system. Perhaps by addressing tension in one area, it is possible to alter tensional resistance on a systemic level. I would hypothesize that if the body feels vulnerable or overly sensitive in one area, it may well rein back the whole body just in case. Then as it begins to feel more comfortable with the protected area, it relaxes more globally. From this view, my easier hip flexion after neck stretching might be nothing to do with the existence of a "back line" but just coincidental, especially as I am probably stretching more trapezius than erector spinae. Here again, I invite you to test it out, both with your areas of tension and also the experiment on the previous page.

Foot Position

One other significant area on the Superficial Back Line is the lower leg. It is suggested that with the foot dorsiflexed, the tendons of gastrocnemius can push out against those of the hamstrings crossing the knee in the other direction to attach to the tibia, creating an increase in tension (Figure 13.19). Whether you go with the fascial connection scenario or the tendons, there does seem to be something in the positioning of the foot that influences ease in hip flexion. If you look, for example, at the deeper forward bending poses, a lot of them have a plantar flexed foot. Better still, you can try it out for yourself. In *Supta Padangushtasana*, bring the leg into your deepest hip flexion. keeping the knee straight. Now transition between a dorsiflexed and plantar flexed foot and see if you discern any difference.

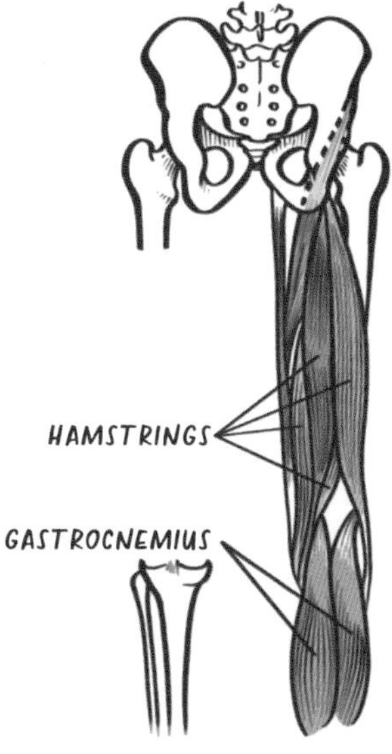

Figure 13.19 Gastrocnemius crosses the knee and passes on the inside of the hamstrings.

If you believe that the positioning of the foot changes the hip flexion in a positive way, even a little bit, then it is worth considering getting those students having trouble moving forward, to point their feet. I have also found that it can give some relief for those experiencing sit bone pain.

Counter Postures

Some students find doing the opposite hip movement first (i.e., hip extension) gives them space to move deeper into a forward bend. So, for example, you could try a low lunge then *Paschimottanasana*. I have never found this to be helpful myself but know many that do, so it is also worth exploring.

Asymmetric Postures

There are lots of yoga postures where one leg is straight in front and the other is doing something else. Both legs can be considered individually. In, for example, *Janu Sirsasana A*, the bent leg is externally rotated and abducted at the hip, and the other leg is pointing to the end of the mat (Figure 13.20).

What happens at the bent leg will be covered in the next chapter, but that may be the reason a student can't tip the pelvis forward, or it could be the hip flexion of the straight leg. It does seem to be that students who are challenged with hip flexion can find a little more forward movement when only one leg has to create that movement. As long as the other leg is not influencing the balance or quality of

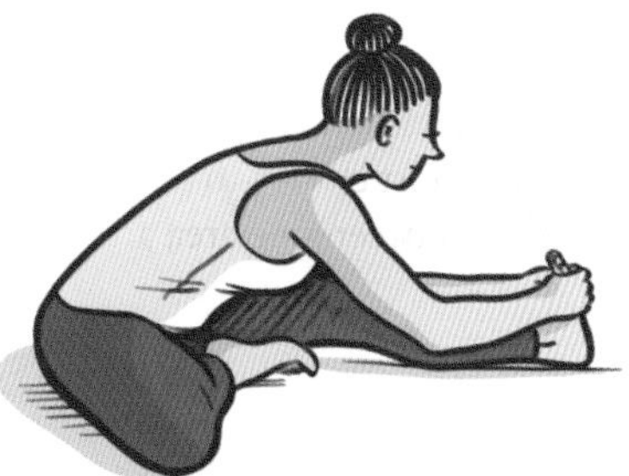

Figure 13.20 Hip flexion on the left side and external hip rotation on the right side.

the foundation, then the whole upper body weight can be used to address the resistance in just the one outstretched leg rather than two, as would be the case in *Paschimottanasana*.

Disguised Forward Bends

As you know by now, the shapes we create in yoga are made from the fundamental movements at the major joints. It doesn't matter if we are doing an inversion, arm balance, standing, or seated posture, if the neutral leg (not rotated) and torso have to move toward one another, then it includes the forward bending element. It is easy to overlook this simple issue when faced with different orientations and positionings. However, once you can recognize this, it makes unraveling any challenges more straightforward. The following examples will help illustrate what I mean.

Navasana is an uncomplicated shape, but it is associated with some balance and core work. When students can't create the sharp "V" shape called for by the pose, they presume they are not strong enough, but that is not the primary barrier for most people (Figure 13.21). The posture is a forward bend, just tilted, so that the balance point is the sit bones. If the legs are kept straight, the same limitations experienced in *Paschimottanasana* will be repeated here with the addition of gravity pulling the legs back to the floor.

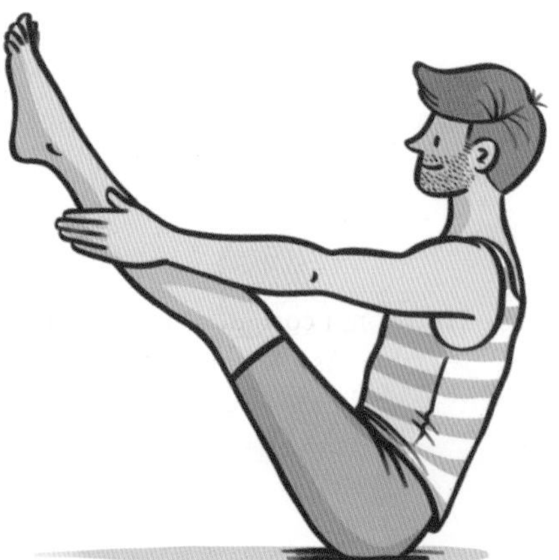

Figure 13.21 Lots of hip flexion available equates to a sharp boat.

If a student's forward bend is 90 degrees, then as with the seated posture, the distance between the torso and legs will not be able to be reduced without rounding the back. Kept strict, the result is a wider boat. If the student's forward bend is less than 90 degrees, then there will be an even greater tendency for the pelvis to tilt posteriorly, the back to round, and the speedboat hull will look more like a rowing boat (Figure 13.22).

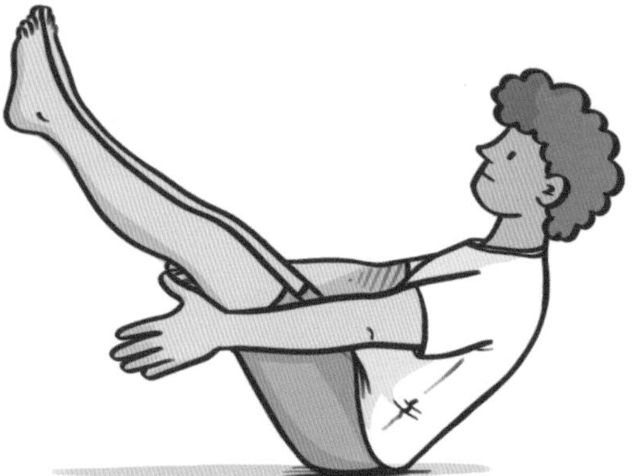

Figure 13.22 90 degrees or less hip flexion will result in a wide boat with more likelihood of rounding the spine.

You could do a thousand crunches a day, and the shape of the boat won't change because although the relationship of the ribcage to the pelvis needs to be maintained, the "V" comes from the movement of the legs relative to the pelvis (forward bend). The modification, therefore, is the same as with other forward bends: flex the knees as much as needed to allow the pelvis to tilt anteriorly (Figure 13.23).

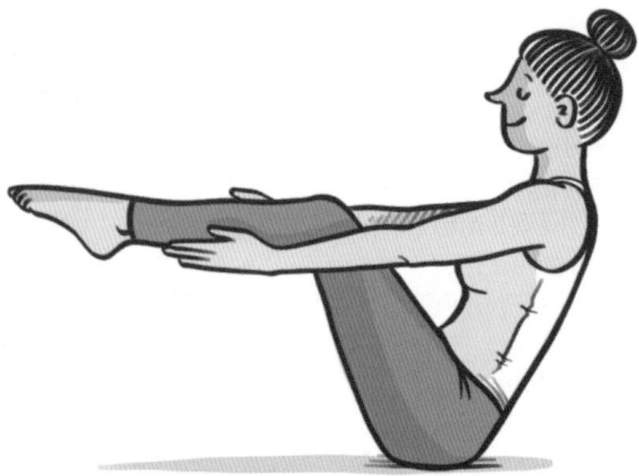

Figure 13.23 As with all forward bends, bend the knees to get more movement of the pelvis.

The legs can be straightened gradually as the student's forward bend improves.

Have you been in the situation where you want to do a straight leg raise to *Sirsasana*, but it feels like you are wearing diving boots, and there is no way the feet are leaving the ground (Figure 13.24)? You have probably guessed by now that the ability to perform this move doesn't involve strength, it's all about the forward bend. I bet you have never contemplated lifting both the feet off the floor in Down Dog (no jumping), but unless you can get your hips near enough over your shoulders in *Sirsasana*, it's a similar situation.

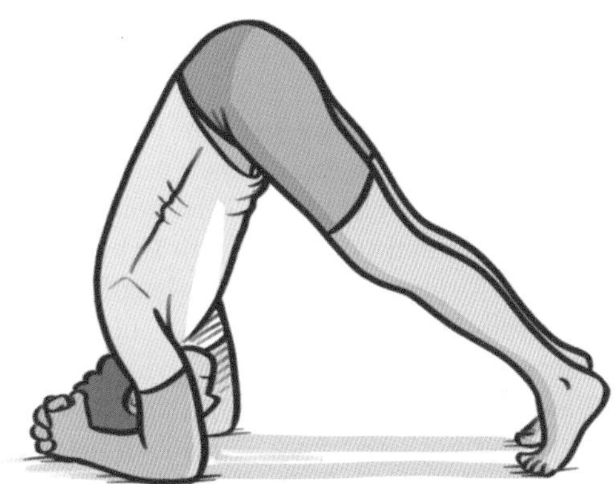

Figure 13.24 In this position, there will be too much weight in the feet to lift into Sirsasana *with straight legs.*

With the hips back from the BOS, there is too much weight in the feet for them to lift off. Hence the cue to walk the feet in until they feel light. But what happens for many students is that they just can't walk in far enough to get that lovely floaty feeling. And the reason they can't is that they don't have sufficient forward bending available. You need quite a bit more than 90 degrees hip flexion to be able to place the hips in the right position (Figure 13.25). Once there, everybody has the strength to lift their legs, although students may initially struggle to maintain a stable foundation or be stopped by fear.

We talked more about *Halasana* in Chapter 9, *Spine*, but the same concept applies here in bringing the feet to the floor. In the meantime, think it through for yourself and visualize why.

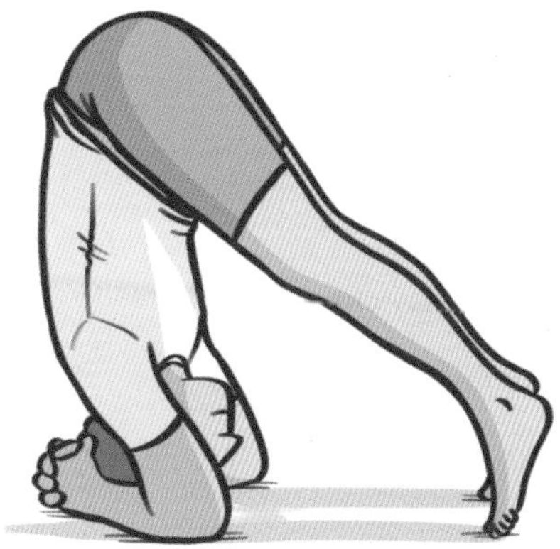

Figure 13.25 Now the hips are over the shoulders and the feet will float, but see how much more hip flexion is required.

We have also mentioned *Tittibhasana* a few times already, and the same is true here as with some other arm balances, good hip flexion is essential to be able to straighten the legs.

Active Forward Bends

Usually, the active hip flexion available is quite a bit less than passive, and although somewhat to do with hip flexor strength, I would say the overriding factor is tissue stiffness (Chapter 2, *Flexibility*). The stiffer you are—remember that is not the same as inflexible—the more hip flexor strength will be needed. It is often suggested that students should try and reduce the difference in ROM between active and passive movements. However, although students with compliant tissues may have good success in active control through the majority of available ROM, for stiffer students, a significant difference will probably remain. This will make postures that include gravity as an opposing force (e.g., *Navasana* and *UHP C*) particularly hard work for them.

Regarding hip flexion, I consider myself stiff but relatively flexible. As an example, in *Supta Padangushtasana* with assistance from the hand (passive), I can bring the leg through about 145 degrees of hip flexion, but my active range is only about 95 degrees (Figure 13.26). This difference shows itself up in postures. I can lay flat on my legs in *Paschimottanasana* with a bit of help from

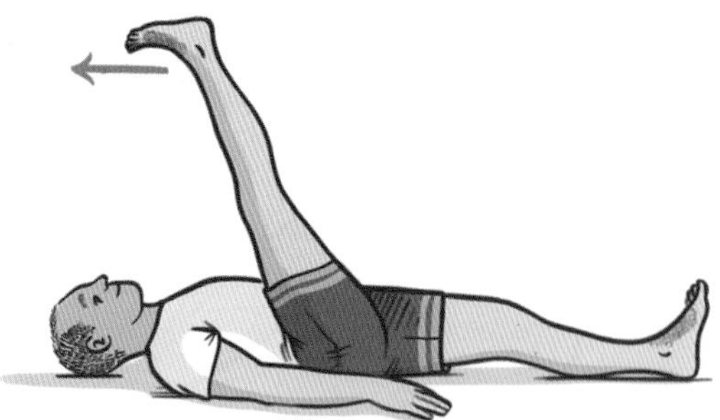

Figure 13.26 Keep both legs absolutely straight as you move through active ROM.

gravity and hands, but flip that orientation to *Navasana*, and it is a whole different story. In this position, I am stuck with my active range and the fight with gravity results in not as sharp a boat as I would like.

My wife, on the other hand, has good compliance and excellent active hip flexion of about 140 degrees, with only a little more available with help to bring her to about 150 degrees (passive). She can then, of course, lay comfortably on her legs in *Paschimottanasana*, and although her hip flexors are not as strong as mine, she breezes through *Navasana* with her sharp "V" shape. As I'm sure we have mentioned before, it is definitely desirable to be strong as well as flexible, but when it comes to making most yoga shapes that involve large ROMs, it is much more likely tissue resistance will be stopping you rather than lack of strength.

A useful way of including active ROM is to add it after passive work, or even before and after. In this way, the nervous system can be shown the usefulness of the newly achieved ROM, and I think it is more likely to be assimilated.

One of my favorite ways of doing this is in *Supta Padangushtasana*. First raise the leg, contracting the hip flexors for three or four breaths to see how far it is possible to bring the foot toward the head using only active ROM. Then grasp the big toe and bring the leg closer, relaxing the leg completely for a passive phase. This time hold for 5 to 10 breaths, gradually bringing the leg further as the nervous system gets used to the stretch. The third stage is to draw the leg closer using a combination of

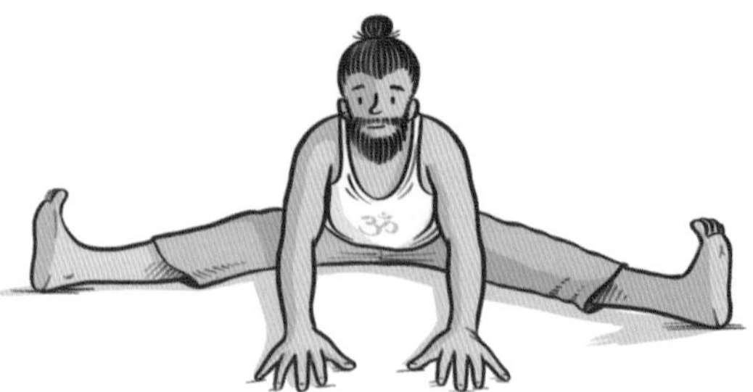

Figure 13.27 Hold the deepest position with neutral spine for 5 to 10 breaths.

active hip flexion and help from the hand on the foot. Lastly, release the hand and try to keep the leg where it is for three or four breaths using just the hip flexor engagement. In this manner, you are trying to use the increased ROM.

Another combination I like, this time for working in *Upavistha Konasana*, is to combine a passive gravity-assisted hold with a block push. After holding the deepest position available for 5 to 10 breaths (Figure 13.27), place a block at arms-length so that the fingertips just touch. Now contract the hip flexors to draw you lower at the same time trying to push the block further away (Figure 13.28). Spend another 5 to 10 breaths in active work, remembering to move from the hip, rather than rounding the spine.

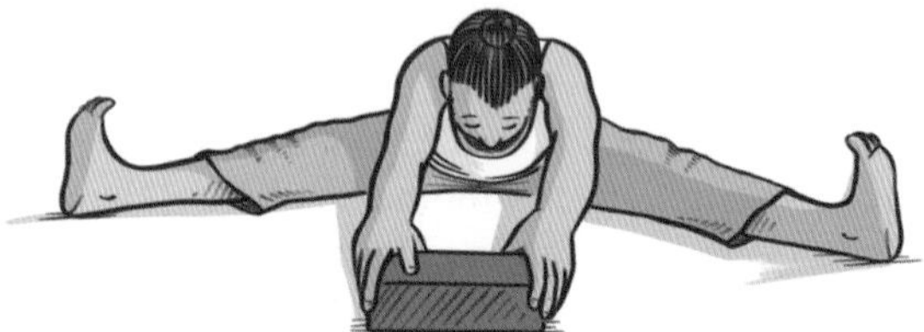

Figure 13.28 Use an active contraction to keep pushing the block away as far as possible. Knees stay facing the ceiling.

An alternative way to do the same sort of thing is to follow a predominantly passive posture with one that uses active ROM. An example would be to follow *Upavistha Konasana* with straddle leg lifts instead.

Activation at End Range

Hopefully, one of the key tenets coming through this book is that the nervous system is primarily responsible for regulating the available ROM. The more secure the body feels that you will be able to control your limbs through extended ranges, the more likely it will allow you to travel through them. It's a little bit like not taking off the training wheels on a kid's bike until you know they have a fair chance of not landing up flat on their face. Having strength and stability throughout a movement, but particularly at end range, are the best ways of building this control. A simple yet effective strategy is to engage the muscles being stretched once you have spent time in the posture. It will be easier to do this in some postures than in others just because of body positioning.

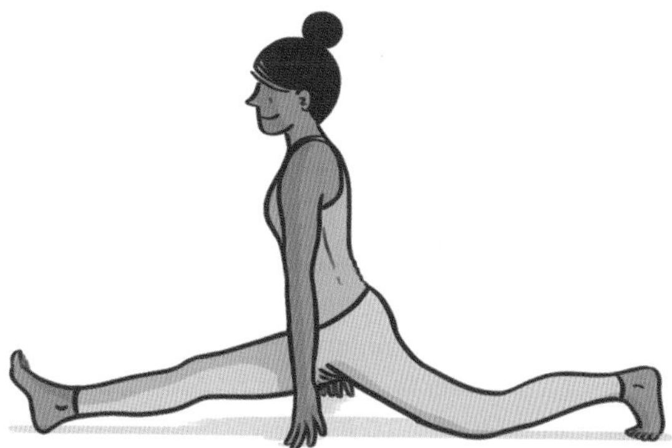

Figure 13.30 Over time, reduce the support from the hands so that the hip flexors of the back leg and hip extensors of the front leg are keeping you up.

For example, before coming out of *Parsvottanasana*, the front leg could be drawn backward against the friction of the floor. The leg doesn't need to move, just use the floor as resistance. When a muscle is at full stretch, it is more vulnerable to injury, so the amount of contraction needs to be built up gradually. In this example, it is easy to meter the amount of force exerted because we are not trying to hold up the whole body weight (Figure 13.29).

There are other postures such as *Hanumanasana* (Figure 13.30) where excellent work can be done, but more care needs to be taken. It is advisable to start much higher than the available ROM, engaging the hamstrings and gluteal muscles on the front leg and hip flexors on the back leg, to support the body weight for a number of breaths.

As muscular strength increases, the hold time can be extended. The hands can be used, on blocks, if necessary, to provide additional control of the amount of load placed on the muscles. Over subsequent yoga practices, the aim would be to work at deeper depths, moving slowly closer to the end ROM. Eventually, it may be possible to lower oneself into a full split, controlling the descent with eccentric muscle action rather than support of the hands. For the individual that is already quite strong, they will probably feel comfortable initially working much closer to their end ROM, but it would still be sensible to try out different depths rather than go straight for the maximum.

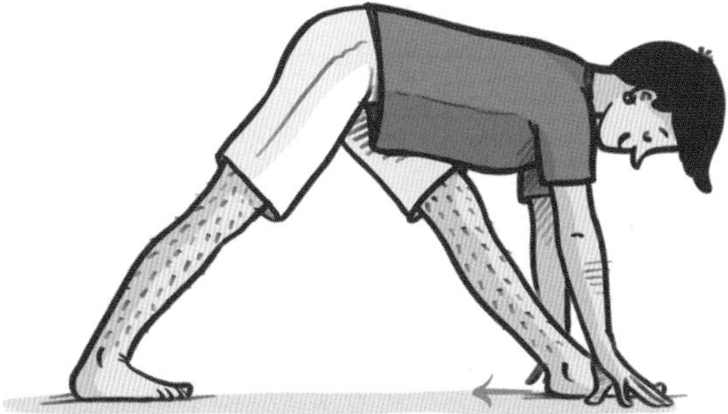

Figure 13.29 Engage the hamstrings and Gmax to draw the leg back. But it is an isometric contraction as the leg stays where it is.

Helping the Challenged Student

If we consider all the above points, we can come up with some ideas on what is going to be most pleasurable and productive for the more challenged students. The first thing is that it will be better to work with one leg at a time as there is less resistance to overcome. Another key point is that so many other muscles influence forward bending, it makes sense to sequence the practice in such a way that the hips and back of the body have been accessed before arriving at strict forward bends. The cheat of rounding the back will be very enticing for all but the most vigilant students, so it is better to remove that option by selecting postures where the likelihood is reduced. More straightforward postures will allow for the focus to be forward bending and not be diluted by other restrictions. Making use of props allows the body to be positioned in a way that is more conducive to relaxation. Finally, make use of gravity where possible and add in active work to reinforce the gain in ROM.

A suitable example would be *Parsvottanasana*, which we just used for active work. The posture is both asymmetrical and gravity-assisted. The front foot is more toward plantar flexion, and it is easy to use blocks under the hands to provide support and eliminate rounding. It is also straightforward and relatively easy to balance in because of the wide BOS provided by the scissored legs. Finally, active hip flexion can be effectively included to deepen the posture.

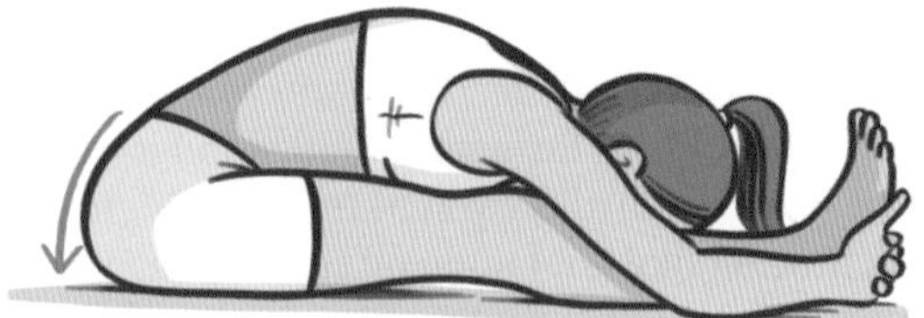

Figure 13.31 For easy forward benders, it is better to think energetically of grounding the sit bones.

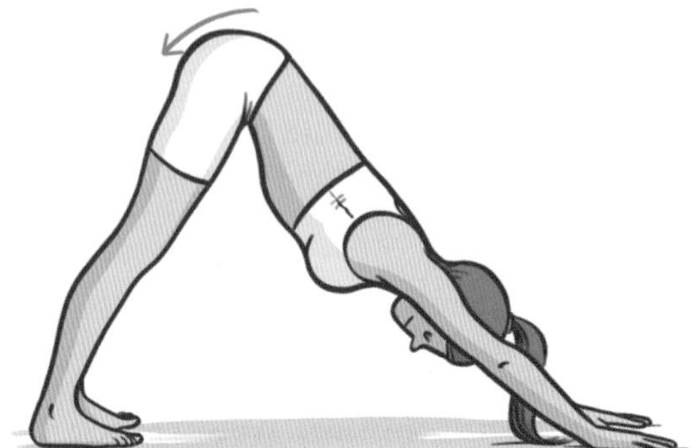

Figure 13.32 Again, the action is bringing the sit bones back toward the floor.

Considering the Comfortable Forward Bender

For some students, forward bending is their "thing" and they fold easily onto their legs in seated postures. If this is the case, we want to change the emphasis of the work. Whereas with challenged students it is all about getting the pelvis to anteriorly tilt, once this movement happens comfortably, there is no need to keep targeting it. The action that ties in with the pelvis tipping forward is the sit bones moving backward, and if this keeps being exaggerated, it may be a contributing factor to the dreaded sit bone pain discussed later.

There is nothing beneficial for the more flexible students to keep trying to take the head closer to the feet. Instead, these students need to create a subtle action of moving the sit bones back toward the ground (Figure 13.31). The pelvis is still anteriorly tilted, but, for example, once the body is on the legs in a seated forward bend, the idea is to ground the sit bones and stop pushing them backward. Energetically there is the essence of a mild increase in lumbar flexion and a pulling back of the legs to where they came from (hip extension).

The same goes when in a posture like Down Dog (Figure 13.32)—once the full expression of the pose is reached, there needs to be an energetic taking of the sit bones back toward the floor. As we have already mentioned, it will be more advantageous for flexible individuals to work on integration and strength rather than seeking out greater ROM.

Hyperextending Knees

It is very easy for students with the ability to hyperextend their knees to fall into that pattern in forward bending postures. Particular attention needs to be taken with asymmetric standing postures, such as *Trikonasana*, where it is especially easy to lock out the front leg.

In seated postures, the heels should be kept on the ground, otherwise it indicates that the back of the knee is being pressed toward the floor. The other main group of poses that I invariably see students lock out in is when the leg is off the floor and held by the hand, such as in *Krounchasana* (Figure 13.33).

One effective method to counter hyperextension is to start in a slightly flexed position, and then using the hamstrings to straighten the leg, engage

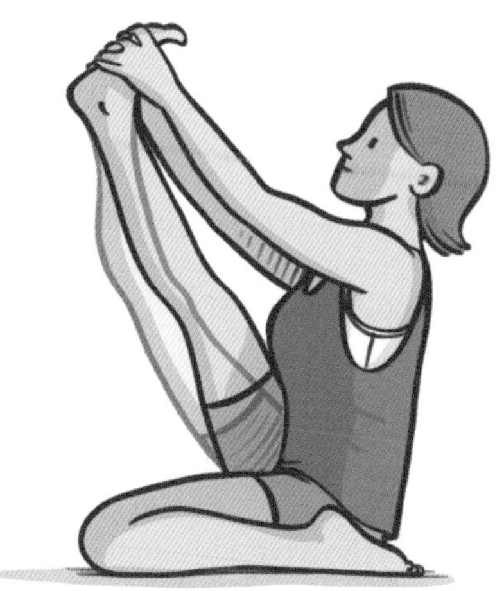

Figure 13.33 Likelihood of hyperextending increases in postures where you can pull on the leg, so extra vigilance is required.

the quadriceps to resist the movement. The student needs to stop straightening the leg when it looks visibly straight, maintaining what is often referred to as a microbend. This may be a subjective feeling rather than a visual positioning, as the leg can be straight just not locked out. The result is plenty of activation on both sides of the knee joint. The student needs to reinforce this positioning with sensory perception so that the same placement can be repeated routinely as well as when the limb is out of sight.

It is only the load-bearing positions that the long-term vulnerability of the knee is an issue, but I think it is sensible to resist hyperextension in all postures. For example, the raised leg in *Virabhadrasana III* should be kept microbent. In this way, there is consistency, and new patterns can be developed that will eventually become the default positioning.

Yoga Butt

It's pretty bad that sit bone pain is so prevalent that it has been given a nickname. Characterized by deep aching right up under the gluteal crease and close to the ischial tuberosity, it may also involve pain radiating into the back of the upper leg. With early intervention, symptoms are likely to subside, but many students just keep hammering away and then the pain will become more intense, often aching when walking, climbing stairs, sitting, and, of course, during and after yoga.

A physiotherapist would probably use the term "proximal hamstring tendinopathy" to describe the condition of chronic pain where the hamstrings join the ischial tuberosity. Unfortunately, I have come across many students where this situation has been going on for several years. One of the problems is that we love what we are doing so don't want to change it, but the other is that once warmed up, it often doesn't feel too bad when doing the postures only to come back with a vengeance afterwards.

In a yoga setting, the cause is most probably an overuse injury associated with the amount of straight-leg hip flexion postures students perform. But as not everyone experiences this immensely frustrating injury, it is obviously not as straightforward as that. The spread of incidence includes beginners and advanced students, both flexible and non-flexible. In other sports, for example, football and running, the trigger is often abrupt movements or dynamically flexing the hip.

As these situations are rare in yoga, I would say that the regularity and intensity of stretching will be one of the main factors involved. There also seems to be some correlation with not strengthening the muscle and tendon. I have read that the forces involved with intense stretching are not enough to cause tendon adaptation by way of getting stronger, but may be sufficient with repetition, to create some tendon degradation. It seems that most successful rehab protocols involve temporarily reducing the depth of the forward bends (stop before pain is experienced) and embarking on a hamstring strengthening program. Also, try pointing the toes.

I think it is a good idea as a preemptive strategy to work on hamstring strength (as well as strength in general) as part of every practice. The proposed activation at end range suggested in one of the previous paragraphs is an excellent place to start, but also refer to Chapter 3, *Strength*, for more ideas.

If you begin to notice a niggly ache near the sit bone, immediately hold back for a week or so and you might be lucky enough to nip the problem in the bud. Be extra careful in wide-legged forward bends, such as *Upavistha Konasana*, because adductor magnus is particularly vulnerable. If it turns out to be this muscle and not the hamstrings, then the discomfort will be felt a little more medially (toward the groin but still on the sit bone).

One other thing worth noting is that sometimes an unrelated incident can trigger the cycle. Things like sitting on a hard floor can start the ball rolling. The situation can then be exasperated by overuse. Be aware that wishful thinking is rarely the answer to sit bone pain, and early intervention is much more effective.

Bent Leg Forward Bends

The posture that springs to mind straight away in this category is *Malasana*, but there are quite a few asymmetric postures such as *Marichyasana A*, *Baddha Parsvakonasana*, and *Akarna Dhanurasana* that all need a deeply flexed hip (Figure 13.34).

There are many postures that also involve additional complications, such as with one foot in a half *Padmasana* or adding a twist. If the leg is maintained close to the sagittal plane (front to back), then the fundamental variation is whether the knee also needs to be fully flexed. We covered the limitations to knee flexion in Chapter 7, *Knee*, and if this is an issue, then sometimes the body will be placed in such a way as to make deeper hip flexion more difficult due to the shift in the COG.

Marichyasana A and *Baddha Parsvakonasana* are probably two postures that students from many styles will come across, so we will use them as examples.

In the first, we have one straight leg, one bent, and a bind (Figure 13.35). Whenever there is a straight leg out in front, then right away there will be the possibility that our forward movement will be restricted because of all the reasons covered above. With the other leg, the ability to bind and eventually travel forward to rest on the straight leg will be dictated by the availability of bent-knee hip flexion. Often, the inability to bind presents itself in students' minds as a shoulder problem, but here, as with most cases, the reason will be the failure to take the torso far enough past the leg to free up the arm to make the bind. And you guessed it, that comes down to bent-knee hip flexion and the same amount of spinal flexion you would expect to see in *Paschimottanasana*.

In *Parsvakonasana*, the front leg starts in a similar position to a wide *Virabhadrasana I*. At this stage, there is not sufficient challenge to knee flexion or hip flexion for that to stop the thigh from lowering to parallel. However, the postures involve the torso and pelvis being taken forward to meet the thigh, and this dramatically increases the amount of

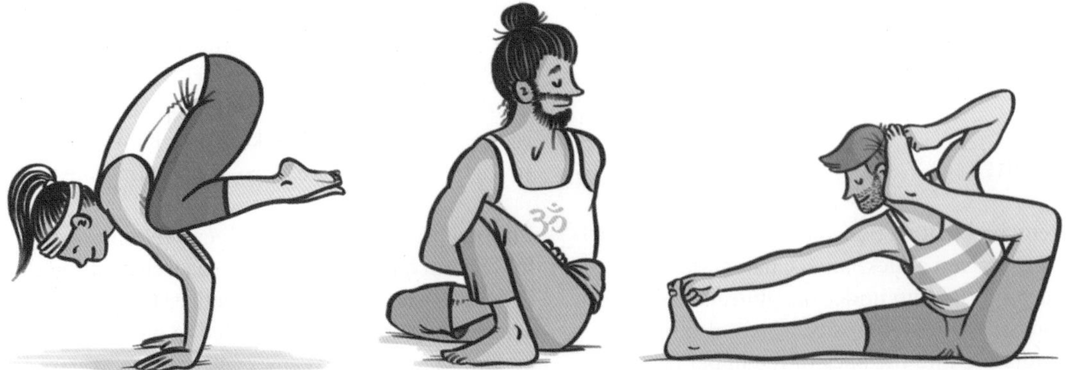

Figure 13.34 Lots of postures call for a deep bent leg hip flexion, luckily the hamstrings are taken out of the equation.

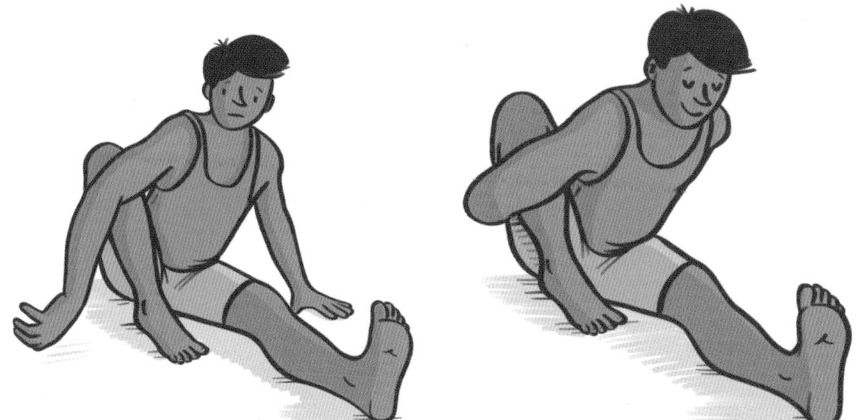

Figure 13.35 If you don't or can't move into deep bent leg hip flexion, the shin will be on the back of the arm rather than in the armpit.

bent-knee hip flexion required. If this is missing, look out for the difference being made up with spinal flexion. In the bound version, if the objective is to get the shoulder below the level of the front thigh, then that will only be possible with an abundance of the same movement.

CHAPTER 14

Hip Rotations

Most yoga postures involve the hips having to do something, but in this chapter, we will focus specifically on those postures where either medial or external hip rotation is an essential factor in the creation of the pose. As I am sure you have gathered from the "Key Concepts," an inability to rotate the hip sufficiently, in the absence of modification, will cause adaptations to be made elsewhere and raise the potential for injury. By understanding where these fundamental movements are necessary, it helps effective sequencing toward peak postures and the avoidance of stressing vulnerable joints. As there are many more postures that involve external rotation, we will look at that movement first.

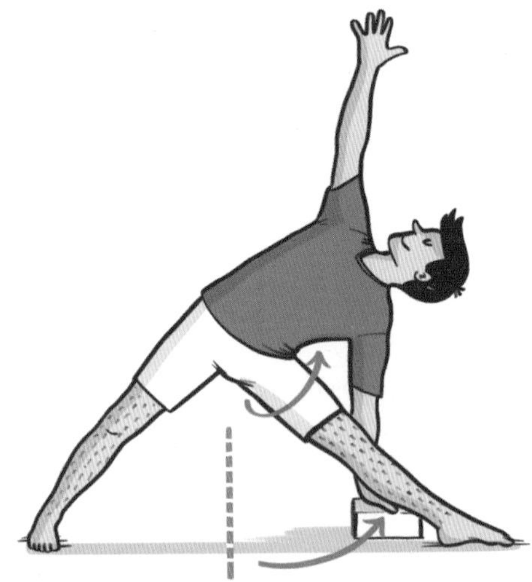

Figure 14.1 Trikonasana, *with the front hip externally rotated.*

Any time the leg is straight and the knee and foot turns away from the body, the action of external rotation has happened at the hip. When the knee is bent, the foot travels in the direction of the opposite side of the body. So, in a standing posture like *Trikonasana*, the front hip is externally rotated (Figure 14.1), and in a seated pose like *Janu Sirsasana*, the bent leg hip has had to do the same. In Chapter 2, *Relational Movement*, we also introduced the idea that when we move the leg relative to the pelvis and afterwards add a pelvis movement relative to the leg, or vice versa, we are often increasing the same original action (Figure 14.2). This combination can add intensity to a rotation if that is what we are looking for, or may, on the other hand, be the limiting factor in completing a pose.

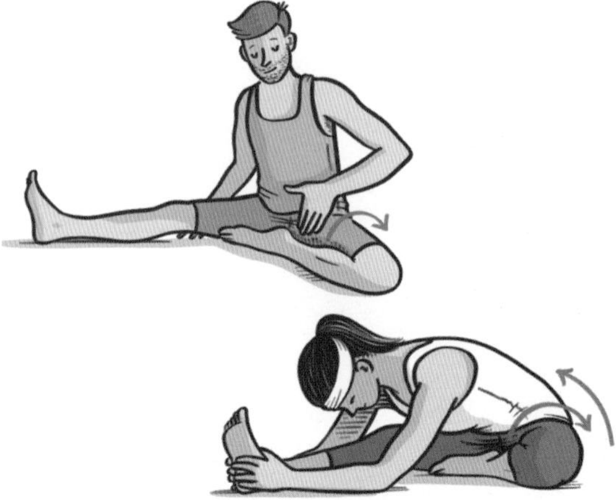

Figure 14.2 When Jasmine moves forward, the pelvis rotates about the femur adding to the external rotation.

Assessing External Hip Rotation

Sukasana

Sukasana is the first stop for determining what level of external rotation is available. In this straightforward cross-legged position, feet should be underneath opposite knees and shins almost parallel to the front of the mat. Looking down, the ground should be seen through a relatively equal triangle of space made between the groin, thighs, and calves (Figure 14.3).

If the knees are not resting on the opposite feet in this position, then we already know some external rotation is lacking because no other movement would be restricting this from happening (Figure 14.4).

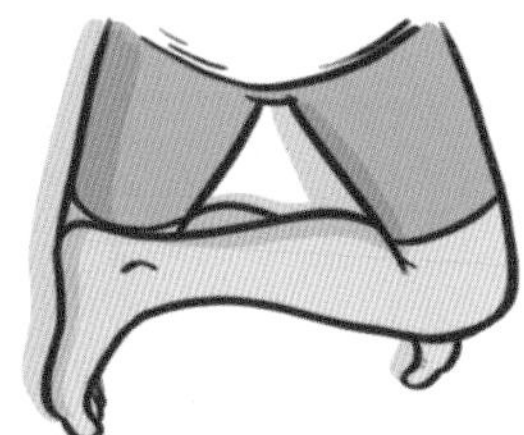

Figure 14.3 Sukasana *from above.*

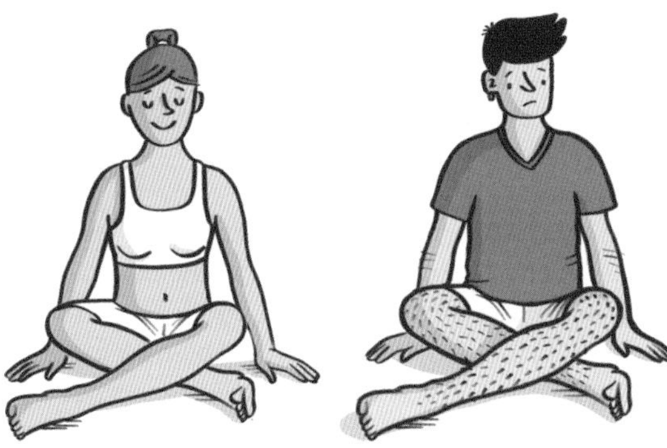

Figure 14.4 Sukasana *is a quick and easy test to show up restriction in external rotation of the hip.*

Always try crossing the opposite leg in front to see if there is a difference between the sides. If this pose still has work available, there is no need to go to the next level, but otherwise, the next posture to try is *Agnistambhasana*. Here the legs are stacked on top of one another, ankle bone to knee, feet dorsiflexed and the shins parallel to the front of the mat (Figure 14.5). If the bottom leg is sitting comfortably on the floor and the top leg on the bottom leg, then there is good external hip rotation available. If it is also possible to fold forward and place the ribcage on the shins and forehead on the floor, then there is probably enough to do all but the deepest postures requiring this movement. When there is space either between the bottom leg and the floor, or bottom leg and top leg, or both, then the amount of space is indicative of the restriction and the degree of opening still required for advanced postures.

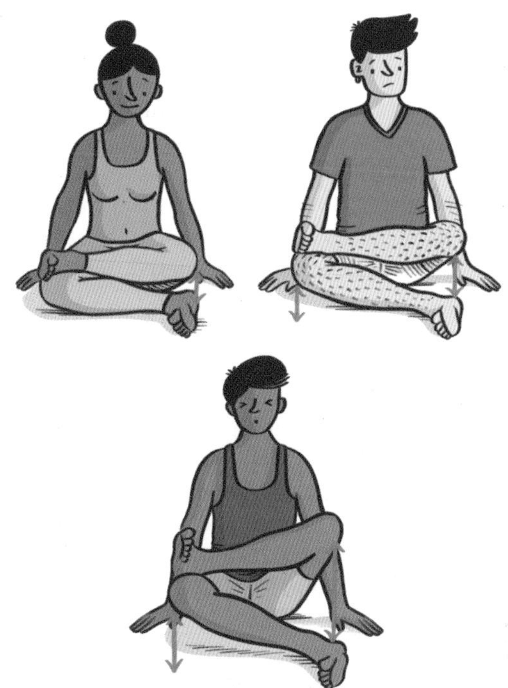

Figure 14.5 In Agnistambhasana, *if the knees are well up in the air like Dave (top right) and Vihan (bottom), it is better to choose a different pose.*

Again, look for imbalances between sides by swapping the leg that is on top. It's pretty easy to cheat in this posture by letting the lower shin scoot back, widening the knees and sickling the ankles, or by not having even weight in both sit bones (Figure 14.6).

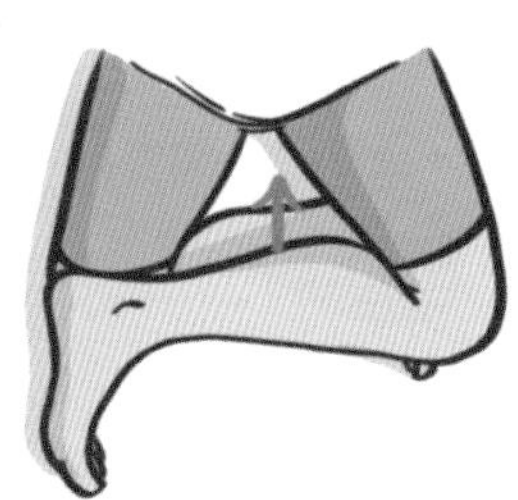

Figure 14.6 Often the bottom shin slides backward.

Janu Sirsasana A

This is one of the simpler shapes, involving external rotation of the hip. There is some abduction and some hip flexion, but only 90 degrees until you move forward. In Chapter 13, *Forward Bends*, we discussed the implications of the straight leg, so here we will think about the bent leg. The basic alignment of the posture will dictate what happens at the bent knee hip.

There are two distinct styles relating to foot placement in this posture. The first has the knee taken back as far as possible, with that side of the pelvis probably moving back also. This creates an obtuse angle between the two legs and allows for the foot to be pointed. The second has the pelvis squared to the front of the mat and the bent leg shin at an angle of 90 degrees or less to the straight leg, and as a result, the foot dorsiflexed.

When it comes to going forward, the position of knee and foot will determine what happens with the bent leg and hence the emphasis of the pose. With the knee taken further back and the foot pointed, the first thing that happens is an asymmetric stretch is placed on the side of the body. As the student moves toward the straight leg, the other leg can roll forward until the thigh is facing the ceiling and the shin is in contact with the floor (Figure 14.7). The bent leg doesn't move into medial rotation of the hip because it started in external rotation, and as the thigh is facing up, it has only returned to neutral.

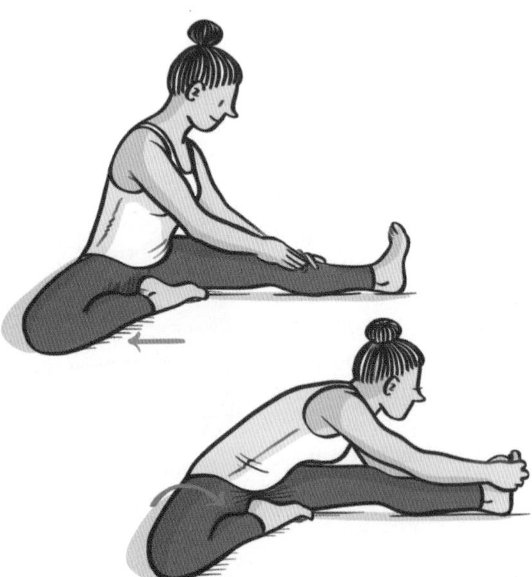

Figure 14.7 With the bent knee taken back and the pelvis deliberately out of line, the thigh can roll medially as the student moves forward.

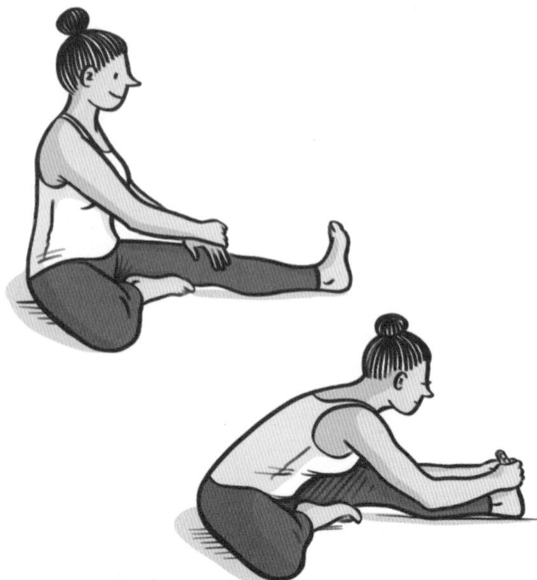

Figure 14.8 In this version, the squared pelvis and dorsiflexed foot creates a need for more external rotation of the hip.

In the other style, the pelvis is square, creating a more even action on both sides of the body. This time when moving forward, the dorsiflexed foot stops the shin and thigh from rolling forward, and so the hip stays in external rotation (Figure 14.8). As more external rotation is required for the pelvis to tilt anteriorly, lack of any more of this movement will stop the student from going deeper into the pose. This version then makes it an excellent way to work on increasing this movement, but as covered in Chapter 7, *Knee*, it also presents the potential for the overzealous student to put pressure on the medial meniscus.

Baddha Konasana

This posture removes any straight leg restriction problems but, as with the second version of *Janu Sirsasana*, highlights the external rotation as both feet are dorsiflexed. The other main movement in this pose is hip abduction. The closer the feet are to the groin, the more hip abduction is required. Therefore, when a student's knees are up in the air, it could be either or both movements that need

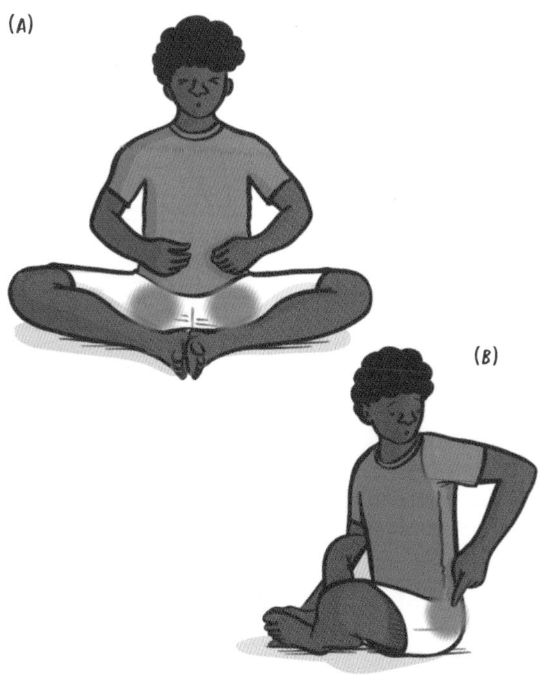

Figure 14.9 Coming forward will accentuate the stretch on the adductors (A), and Gmed and Gmin (B).

addressing. Coming forward will accentuate the stretch on the muscles restricting these movements, namely the adductor group and the medial hip rotators (Gmed and Gmin) (Figure 14.9).

I also feel proportions have a role to play with the height of the knees. In Chapter 8, *Hip*, we talked about the length and angle of the femoral head—as well as the size of the greater trochanter—potentially being responsible for keeping the knees up. But I think there may be even some relationship to the proportions of the femur and tibia length. If the tibia is a little longer than average, as the feet are taken closer to the groin, hip abduction will be increased and the knees pushed higher. Try placing a book between the feet to simulate this and see what happens. Maybe the reverse also happens with a shorter than average tibia.

If a student's knees are up but they can still move the pelvis anteriorly to come forward, that might suggest that it is not muscular tension holding them up. If there is enough tension to keep the knees raised, then it should also resist attempts to go forward as this movement would increase muscular tension. Be aware that this is not the same if the spine is rounded to come forward, as in this situation, the pelvis remains where it is.

We can even learn from the positioning of the knees in *Baddha Konasana* as to where they should be in *Janu Sirsasana A*. If you are in *Janu Sirsasana A* with a dorsiflexed foot and move only the straight leg, bending at the knee to place the sole of that foot next to the other, you will find yourself in *Baddha Konasana* (Figure 14.10). As we have found before, symmetrical postures tend to give a more accurate reflection of ROM because they don't allow

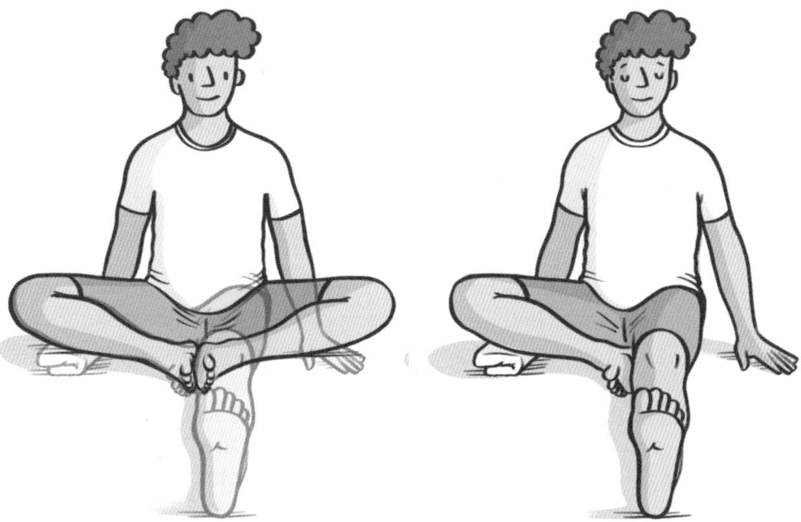

Figure 14.10 Baddha Konasana.

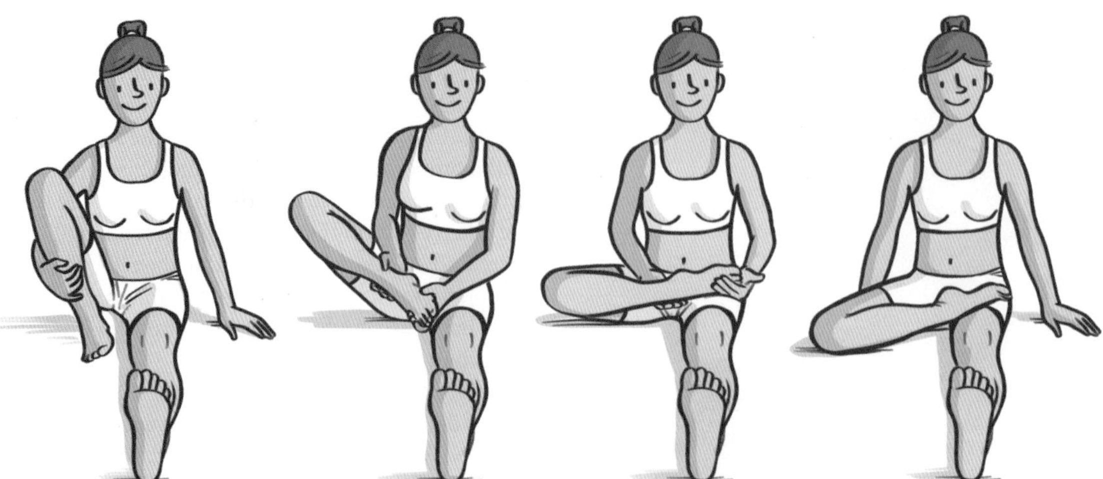

Figure 14.11 Victoria is being very careful in the way she prepares and enters Ardha Padmasana. *We are looking for the knee to be on the floor and a straight line between the big toe and knee, with no sickling at the ankle.*

unobserved adaptations to slip in. Therefore, if the knees are up in *Baddha Konasana*, then in *Janu Sirsasana A*, the knee should be at the same height, as it is really just a half *Baddha Konasana*. A subtle shifting of the pelvis due to the weight of the leg can bring the knee down, but it would be better to prop the knee and keep the weight even on both sides.

Ardha Padmasana

As yoga originated in India, sitting crossed-legged and even in *Padmasana* would have been very natural, but for many people brought up sitting on chairs, they can have immense difficulty accessing this movement. To take the foot into the groin for either *Padmasana* or *Ardha Padmasana*, there needs to be good knee flexion and plenty of external hip rotation. As mentioned in Chapter 2, *Multi-Segmental Movement*, the weak links of the knee and ankle are the places that will be adversely stressed if the required ROMs are not available. *Ardha Padmasana* is a posture in its own right, but also an element of more complicated poses. We will consider the pose first, but the key positioning of foot and leg is relevant to both.

In *Ardha Padmasana*, the ideal positioning of the foot is to have the heel in line with the belly button and the side of the foot in the hip crease. The foot should be plantar flexed, and the toes should only protrude slightly past the hip. There should be no sickling of the ankle. The best way to ensure a healthy placement is to fully flex the knee first, and then cupping the ankle rather than pulling on the foot itself, rotate from the hip and try to take the foot into position (Figure 14.11).

Several things may happen when trying to place the first foot. It may jut out way past the side of the body (Figure 14.12A), or it might only reach to somewhere on the thigh, and the foot might also be sickled (Figure 14.12B).

Once the foot is placed, I think it is a good idea to support the bent leg with the hand under the knee while the other leg is slid underneath. Because the second leg gives support for the top knee and ankle, it reduces the required external rotation and negates some of the importance of exact foot positioning. If the top knee is not resting on the leg below, then additional support should be placed between them (Figure 14.13).

Next, we will consider *Ardha Padmasana* as a pose component. I think I have quite strict views on this as I have encountered so many yoga students with knee issues that can be directly attributed to ragged form. As a starting point, I would say that, for all but a minority of students, if a strict *Agnistambhasana* cannot be performed (external hip rotation test), then they should refrain from

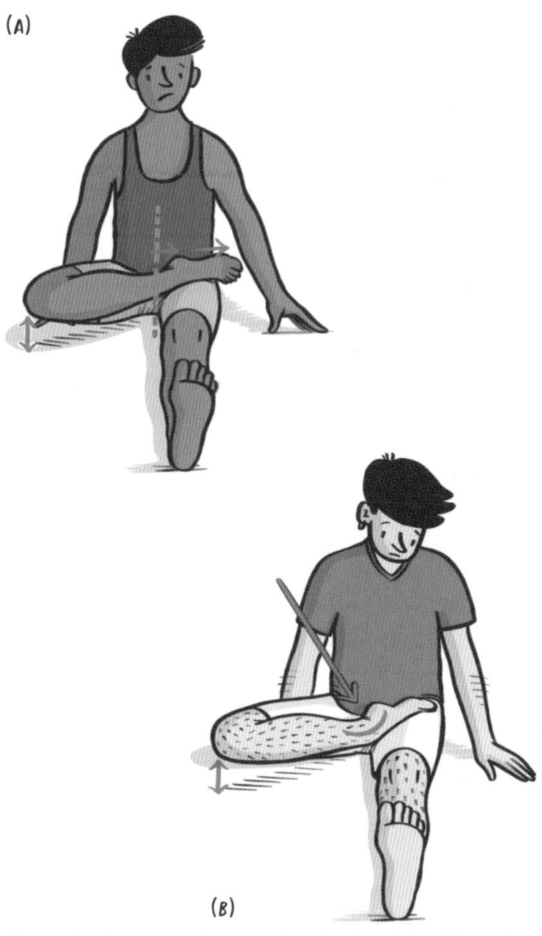

Figure 14.12 Issues when placing the first foot, (A) jutting past side of body; (B) only reaching the thigh, with foot sickled.

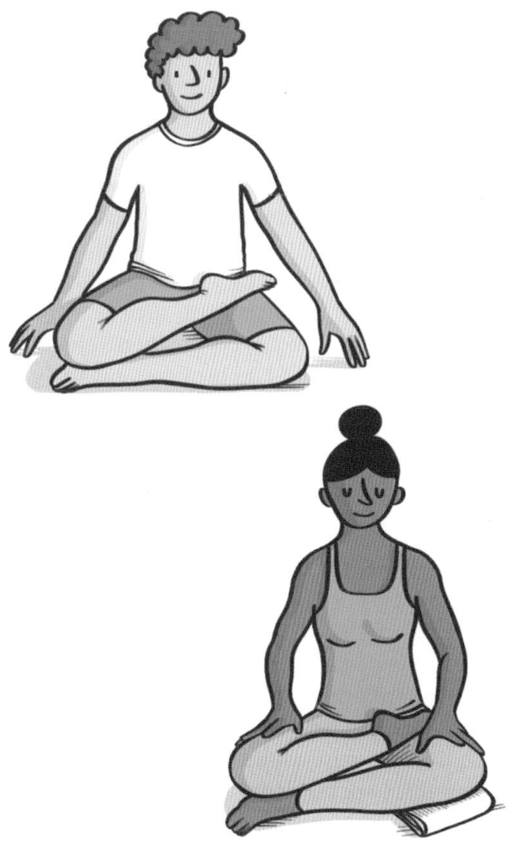

Figure 14.13 In Ardha Padmasana*, it may be necessary to add support under one or both knees.*

placing their leg into the *Padmasana* position. I have added a little confusion because I've implied that it may be ok for some. To clarify that point, I am referring to the odd individual that, due to their particular skeletal geometry or structure, finds more movement in the hip when the shin is not parallel to the front of the mat. I have not come across many such individuals, but the fact that I have encountered some means you can never say never.

The major difference between *Ardha Padmasana* and what we are now talking about is that the bottom leg has been removed. Insufficient external hip rotation will leave the knee floating in the air. If this is happening, then something should be placed under the knee, and no additional complexity should be added to the posture. To proceed further, I suggest the knee needs to be on the floor without weight being shifted off the opposite sit bone. There should be a straight line from the big toe to the knee. I also feel that floor-based poses give a clearer indication of the readiness of the hips, as it is less easy to add in adaptations with the pelvis subconsciously. Therefore, if a good positioning of the *Ardha Padmasana* foot and knee can't be achieved in a seated position, it shouldn't be attempted in a standing position.

For example, if the knee is off the floor in the seated posture *Ardha Baddha Padma Paschimottanasana*, then something should be placed under it, and the student should not proceed to bend forward. This would also determine that in the standing version, *Ardha Baddha Padmottanasana*, the student should either stay standing upright or place the bent leg into a figure four position instead. When further complexity is added by way of flexing the opposite hip or adding a twist, such as with *Marichyasana B* and *D*, a badly positioned foot can add to the stresses placed on the knee and ankle but also introduce some to the spine and SIJ. We will use the two postures just mentioned to explore these ideas.

What I observe in these poses is that many students have a very uneven pelvis, which, in turn, makes the spine flex laterally. The first thing to consider is whether the pelvis can actually remain equally grounded in these poses. This is dependent on the proportions of the upper and lower leg and the degree of bent-knee hip flexion. In most students, it will raise a little, but nowhere near the amount that I see regularly.

It is good to initially test this by keeping one leg straight, bending the other, and placing it next to the hip as if you were in either of these poses (Figure 14.14). Don't lean to the side but try and stay square. If the sit bone raises off the floor, gauge the distance. You are aiming to have the pelvis in as close to this position as possible in the posture. If there is a big difference, the first thing I would look at is the external hip rotation.

What happens a lot is the knee remains off the floor when the leg is placed into the *Ardha Padmasana*. The student then rolls to the side to take the knee down, which is maybe a safer place for the knee but tilts the pelvis. The higher the knee, the greater will be the resulting tilt. On top of that distortion is the likelihood that the ankle will have to sickle considerably because the foot is probably not in the ideal place. Many students put up with the discomfort in the ankle because they want to be in the posture and assume it will help them get better at it. However, this will not help increase the external rotation of the hip, only destabilize the ankle because it has to take up the strain. The knee can also be subjected to strong torquing forces in this scenario.

This is such common practice that teachers regularly allow, and even sometimes suggest, this sort of form. My recommendation would be, as previously stated, if the knee of the leg in *Ardha Padmasana* is not on the floor, the student should go no further with that pose. Instead, the pose should be modified by placing the foot on the

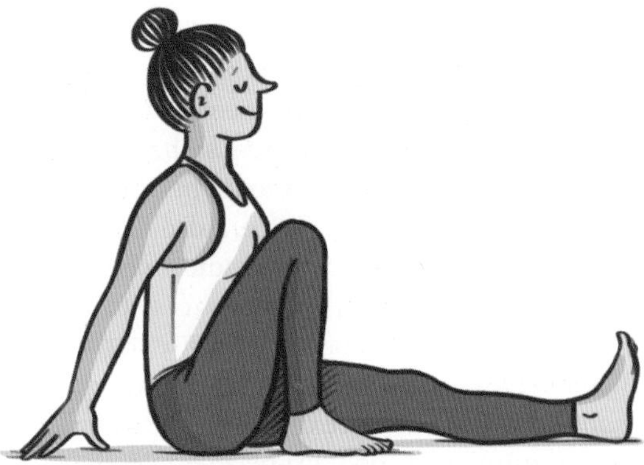

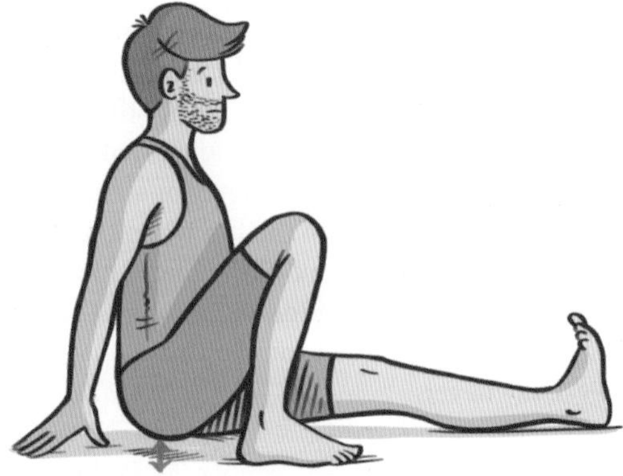

Figure 14.14 Testing to see how high the hip lifts in this way will give a great indication of how much tilt is being added in the posture to make up for missing external rotation in the Ardha Padmasana *hip.*

floor, either next to the opposite hip or adjacent to the other foot. Another telltale sign that this has occurred can be observed when bringing attention to the contact of the *Ardha Padmasana* leg on the floor. In an ideal position, the side of the thigh and calf will be resting down (Figure 14.15).

If the student has had to roll sideways, the top of the thigh will be more in contact. Of course, you can also look at the pelvis itself and the height of the sit bone from the floor of the non-*Padmasana* hip (Figure 14.16).

The same rule applies for all seated postures involving an *Ardha Padmasana*, the knee of the first leg in should be on the floor, while both sit bones remain equally grounded (Figure 14.17). My own feeling about *Ardha Padmasana*, and the full version for that matter, is that it is better to work on the necessary ROM separately and return periodically to check out the positioning. Only when a healthy placement can be achieved is it worth spending any time there as it is so easy to stress those vulnerable knees and ankles. If there is any discomfort, it is more beneficial to put the leg in a figure four position, again with something under the knee, or use another modification (Figure 14.18).

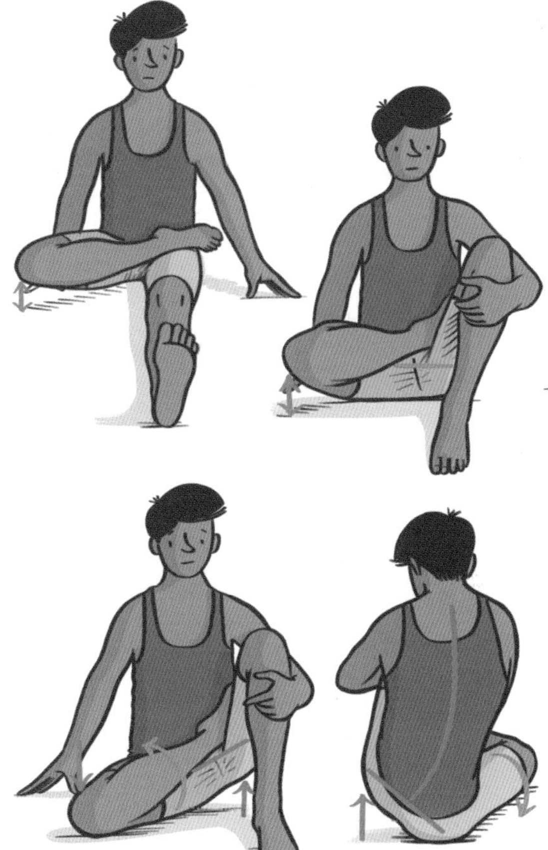

Figure 14.16 Vihan is starting with the knee off the floor and rolls to the side to bring the knee down. This has the consequence of the opposite hip rising and the spine laterally flexing more.

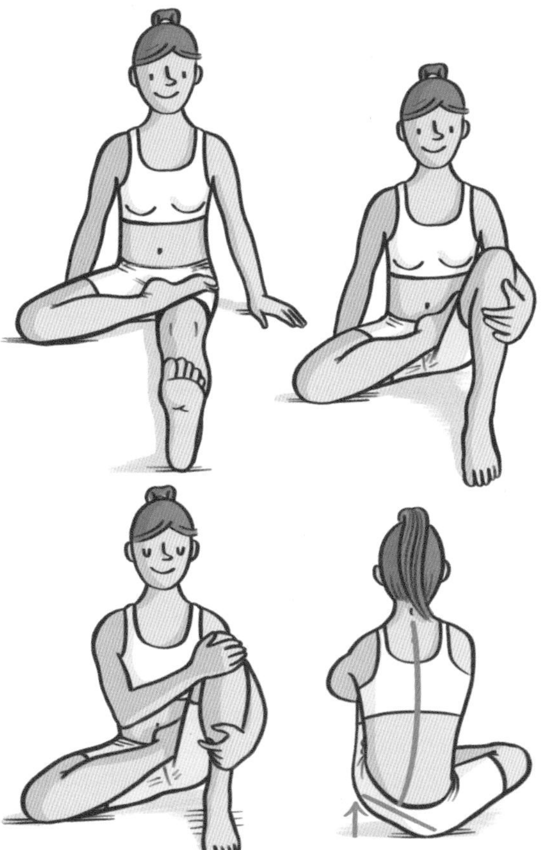

Figure 14.15 Victoria has enough external hip rotation to place the knee on the floor both before and while bringing the second leg in.

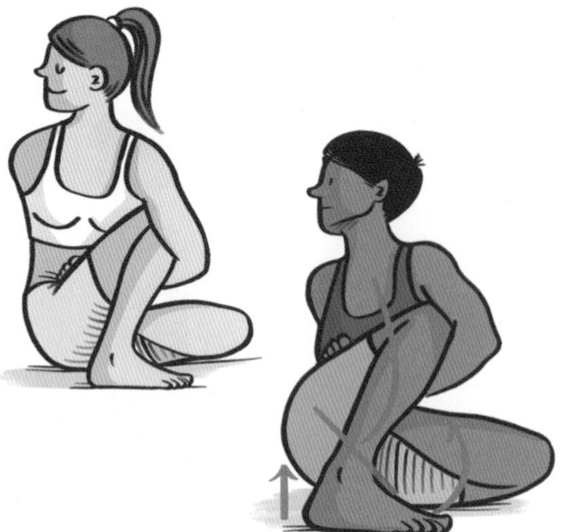

Figure 14.17 Victoria and Vihan are both in Marichyasana D, *but there is a big difference in the quality, and it comes from the original setup. As you can see, Vihan has rolled onto the thigh, the pelvis has a massive tilt, and the lumbar spine will have to take up the slack. The knee and ankle also tend to get more stress taken into them. It is quite rare for a student to be able to keep both hips grounded, but energetically that is a good intention to have.*

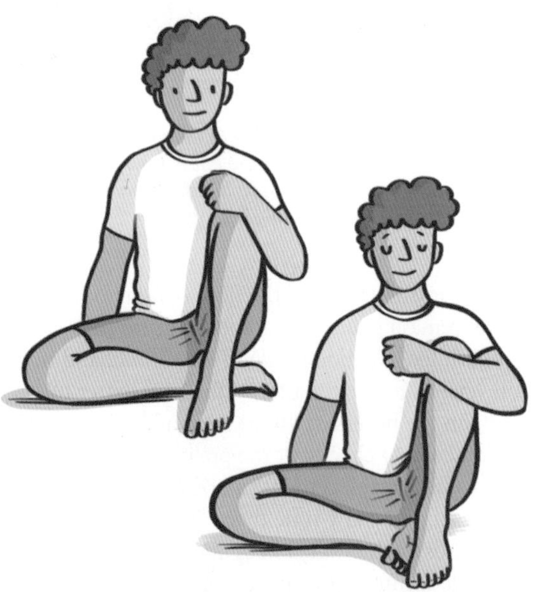

Figure 14.18 Doug is demonstrating two variations of foot placement that can be used if putting the foot into Ardha Padmasana *is not desirable. Placing the sole of the foot against the other foot tends to work on opening the hip more. The same rule goes, however, as with the* Ardha Padmasana: *try not to lean sideways too much, and think of both sit bones working toward being grounded.*

Padmasana

If *Ardha Padmasana* is comfortable, then it may be time to start thinking about a full version. However, the second leg in takes more strain, so it is important that there is plenty of external rotation of the hip available and that in *Ardha Padmasana* the foot is placed correctly, no sickling, and that the knee rests down (Figure 14.19). I am not in favor of lifting the legs to take the position as I feel it encourages bad form and may lead to more strain being placed on the knees. If it can't be performed slowly and methodically, the student is not ready. Similarly, great ease should be experienced in a seated *Padmasana* before one is attempted in an inverted position.

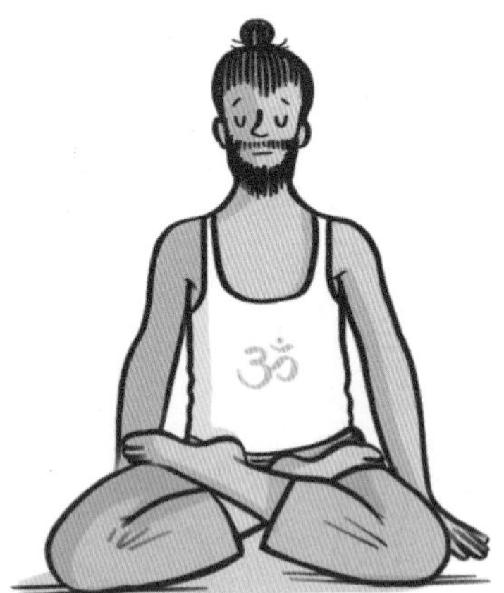

Figure 14.19 Padmasana.

When entering *Padmasana*, the first foot is placed in the opposite hip crease by initializing the movement with a full knee flexion followed by emphasizing the rotation of the hip. The knee flexion of the second leg cannot be maintained because the first leg gets in the way. It is important, though, to keep as much knee flexion as possible and the foot close to the shin while the foot is moved into position. Rather than pulling on the foot, cradling the ankle will reduce the chance of sickling. The knee of the second leg in may not be on the floor, but the whole position should not feel that it is spring-loaded; there should also be absolutely no pain in the knees or ankles. Improvements will not be made by remaining in the posture while suffering—this will only cause damage and reinforce the negative experience of this pose in the brain.

Many sequences only have the one opportunity to do *Padmasana* or have a preference for which leg gets placed first. I would advise that it is best to practice both sides to maintain balance. Because it is not uncommon for there to be a difference in the available ROM between hips, don't feel that this pose should be performed as easily on both sides. Respect the difference, and if necessary, leave doing the tighter way until the body is ready. Of course, do something else instead for that hip.

Foot Behind the Head Postures

Taking the foot behind the head (shoulder), requires a tremendous amount of external hip rotation and hip flexion. In my opinion, for most students, the required ROM to perform this movement goes way beyond anything of functional necessity and most peoples' availability. The second issue I have with this group of postures is the terrible contortions I invariably see in students, consequently placing them right in the firing line of potential injury. Having worked toward these postures myself, I can appreciate the appeal of the challenge, but we also have to consider the journey. Often, what I witness is an uneven pelvis, torqued SIJ, and flexed and loaded cervical and lumbar spine. The forces going into these areas, due to restricted hip ROM and the placement of the foot on the back of the neck, is immense (Figure 14.20).

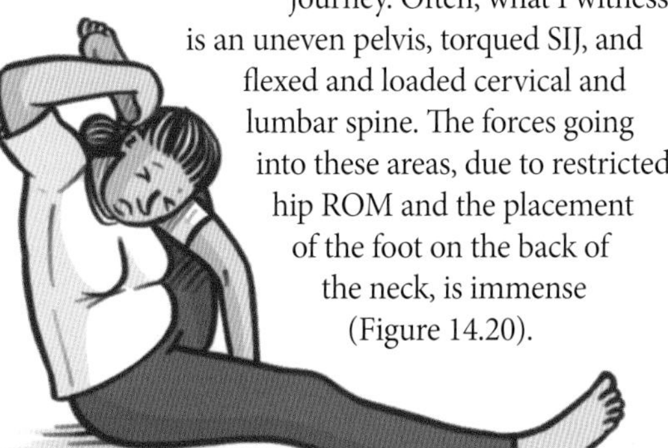

Figure 14.20 If you can do Eka Pada Sirsasana *like Jasmine (top), then you shouldn't be putting any unnecessary strain on the body. But if you are contorting your body like Wendy (bottom), then it is only a matter of time before you hurt something. Stop that nonsense and prepare the body properly or forget the pose altogether!*

In Chapter 8, *Hip*, we talked about the potential for varying the direction of the femoral head, and this could well be one of the determining factors of the likelihood of achieving this movement. Even if you do these types of postures currently, my advice would be to try the following little test to demonstrate your current ROM.

Experiment to Demonstrate ROM

Sit in *Dandasana* with your back against a wall, butt, upper back, and back of the head touching the wall (Figure 14.21). Keeping both sit bones grounded, bring in the right foot, externally rotate the hip, and take the foot toward the face. The distance from the face that the foot reaches is representative of what you would have to make up by distorting the body. It would be even more than this because the foot has to go behind.

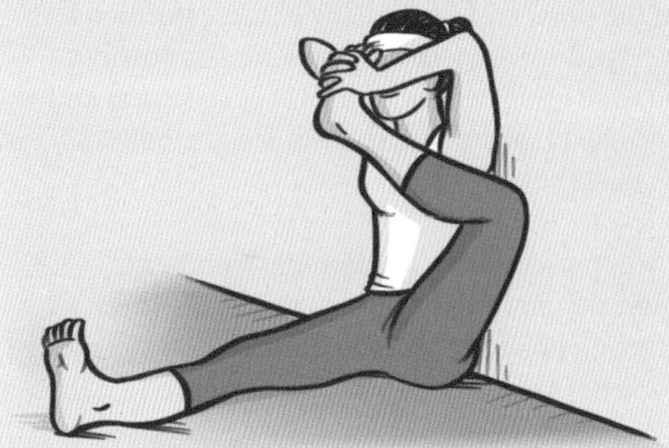

Figure 14.21 Are you ready?

This is a rather strict test because it emphasizes the availability of external rotation of the hip. Those students with an abundance of hip flexion can often get away with less by taking the knee more toward the rear than out to the side. However, the foot won't land up in a very nice position, and the knee will be more vulnerable because of that.

Improving External Rotation

For those who struggle with these rotational movements, it is often not enough to rely just on the postures in your regular sequence. It is good to include both active and passive homework poses that incorporate strict technique. When working passively, the knee is bent because the lower leg is used as a lever to rotate the hip. Actively, it is possible, of course, to rotate the hip whether the leg is straight or bent, but most often a bent leg is used. I think it is actually better to use both as the emphasis on the muscles doing the work changes slightly between the two. I particularly notice in myself that sartorius seems to help more when the leg is bent.

When working with a bent leg, you want to keep the shin parallel to the front of the mat as this makes it harder to escape the rotation work. In each of the following examples, it is necessary to try and isolate the movement in the hip and keep the low back in a nearly neutral position. Otherwise, the rounding spine will make it seem like more is being achieved than it really is. The positioning of the rest of the body will alter the accessibility of the pose. Although many of these positions can be done anywhere in the room, if possible, go to the wall, as it adds a level of strictness and specificity. Make sure you can feel the buttocks against the wall.

I will present these positionings in order of intensity, so find the level that is right. The starting point is *Sukasana*, the position I suggested for external rotation evaluation (Figure 14.22).

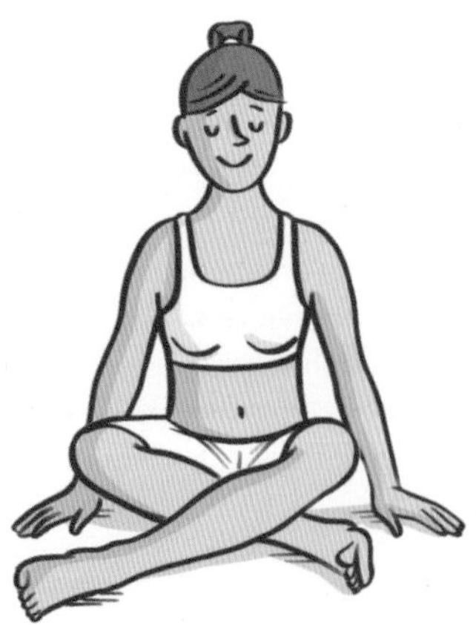

Figure 14.22 Victoria is faking it, but if your knees are up in Sukasana, *it can make an effective opener to spend some time in.*

I gave the details earlier, so just spend some time in this, back on the wall. Don't forget to change the cross halfway through.

Next is *Sucirandhrasana*. Lay on the back, crossing one leg over the other, ankle to knee. Reach through the space between the legs, looping around the flexed knee leg. The hands go either under or over the lower leg (Figure 14.23). The former is suggested for those with sensitive knees. Proceed to pull the leg toward the torso while maintaining the external rotation. Try not to let the knee start pointing toward the shoulder, but instead keep it pointed out. Move only from the hip, maintaining contact with the sacrum on the floor. The head and shoulders should be down and relaxed.

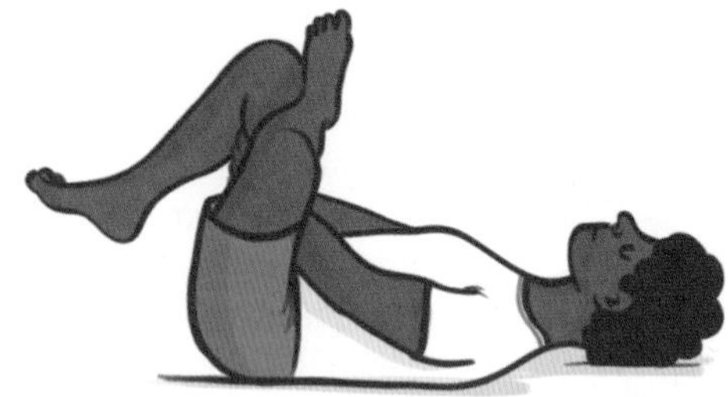

Figure 14.23 Keeping the knee of the crossed leg away from the same side shoulder works best.

If it is strenuous to sustain a comfortable position, instead of holding the leg, one foot can be placed on the wall (Figure 14.24).

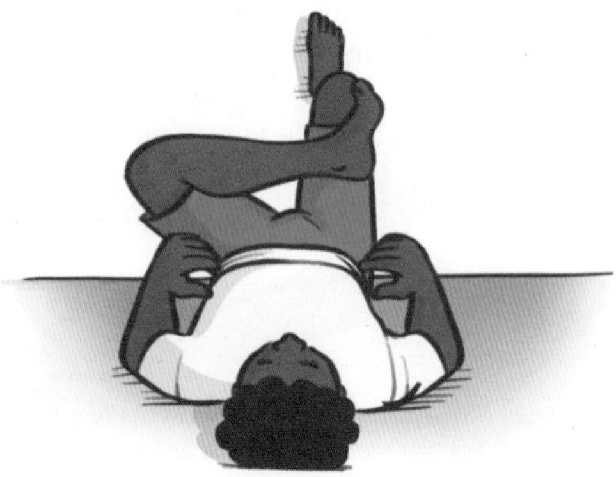

Figure 14.24 The butt is away from the wall, with right thigh perpendicular to the floor.

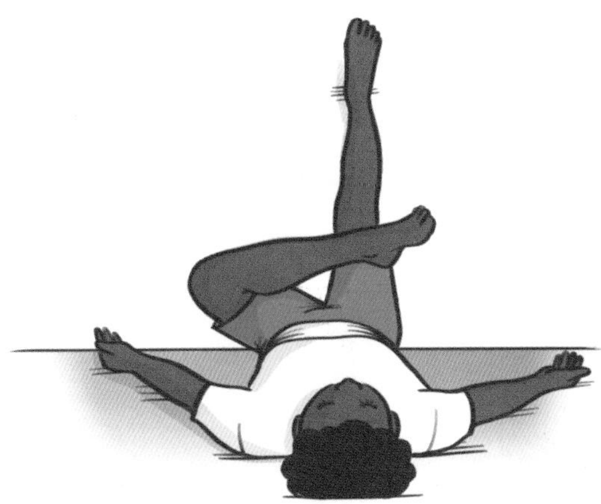

Figure 14.25 The butt is in contact with the wall, and the leg is slid down the wall as far as possible without the butt lifting off the floor.

A little more challenging is to take the leg up the wall with the buttocks also touching (Figure 14.25). The foot is then slid down, stopping when the butt wants to lift off the floor. As before, keep the knee of the rotated leg facing out.

If this seems easy, it is time to sit with the back and butt against the wall (Figure 14.26). One leg is drawn in until the sole is in contact with the floor. Then the other leg is crossed over in a figure four style, ankle bone just above the knee. Again,

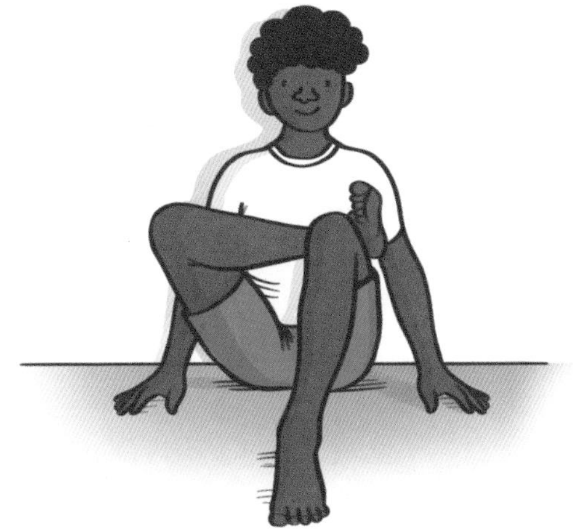

Figure 14.26 In this version, the butt and low back are kept against the wall.

keeping the knee of the rotated hip pointing out, the flexed hip leg can be drawn in to intensify the stretch. If the sole of the foot can't be placed flat on the floor, then hamstring strength will have to be used instead of friction to keep the leg where it is. It will become tiring very quickly, so if this is the case, it would be better to do the previous exercise.

The last passive exercise I will suggest is *Agnistambhasana*. Again, this was also one of my external rotation tests, so the basic technique outline has already been covered. What I will add here is that once you get comfortable with the legs stacked, you can start folding forward. Here, there are also three variations in ascending intensity, straight forward, head to knee, and head to foot.

It is important also to do some active ROM exercises because this helps to reinforce to the nervous system that this movement is useful. This can be done either standing or lying by bringing one hip into about 90 degrees of flexion and then using your muscles to rotate the hip out (Figure 14.27). If the knee is bent, you will be thinking of bringing the foot toward the opposite shoulder. If the leg is straight, the foot turns toward the outside. These sorts of active movements can easily be incorporated into your regular yoga practice. If you are doing these exercises at a separate time, I think it is better to do passive first, then active.

Final Thoughts on External Rotation

Repetition of simple movements can often lead to differences in ROM between sides. One example that crops up in styles such as Ashtanga, where there are a lot of vinyasas to and from seated postures, is that students cross their legs the same way each time they transition. It is important to alternate the cross to maintain balance in the hips. The same goes for sitting in meditation or *pranayama*—change the cross daily.

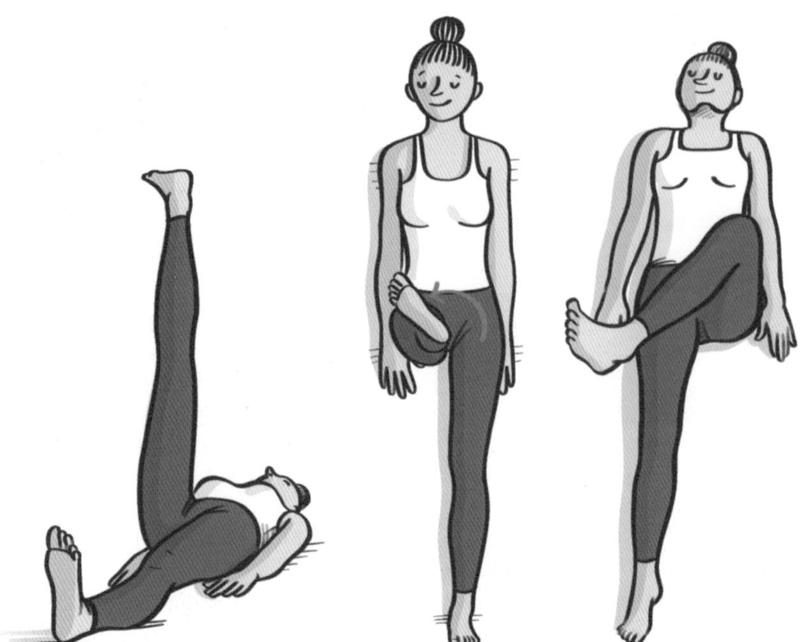

Figure 14.27 These are shown in the lying position, but they could also be performed standing. Hold for 5 to 10 seconds, building up the working intensity and sets over the weeks.

Assessing Medial Rotation

Medial hip rotation isn't used nearly as much as external rotation in yoga postures, but lack of it will definitely affect the comfort in poses where the leg is folded back to the outside of the hip, such as in *Virasana*.

The simple way to see how much is available is to lay on the stomach, place the thighs together, and then, after flexing the knees to 90 degrees, let the lower legs and feet drop out to the side (Figure 14.28). Looking from the back, the thighs are rolling out, but from the front, they would be rolling medially. How far they drop out is a clear

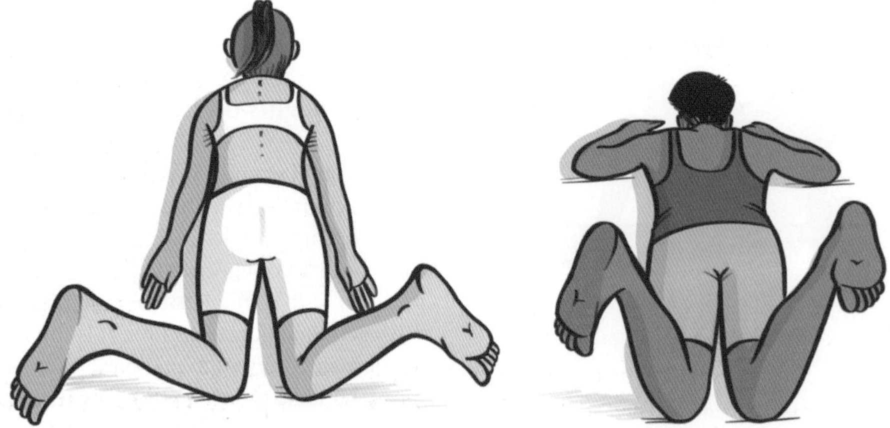

Figure 14.28 On the belly like this is a great way to observe available medial rotation.

indication of the amount of passive rotation. For active rotation, the student can engage their muscles and try and take the feet more in the direction of the floor. Notice I didn't say which muscles. Although we covered the muscles that will do the work earlier, when giving instructions, it is more straightforward to just think of the movement intention.

Improving Medial Rotation

I will share a couple of my favorite passive and active exercises for working on medial rotation of the hip. The active exercises can be done in the same position as detailed previously for external rotation. The difference is that when the leg is bent, the foot will travel away from the body, and when the leg is straight, it will turn toward the opposite side of the body (Figure 14.29). Remember that the foot is just the flag to show you what is happening. Also look at the knee when the leg is straight to make sure it changes the direction it is facing. This will confirm that the rotation is happening at the hip and not being faked by excessive movement at the ankle.

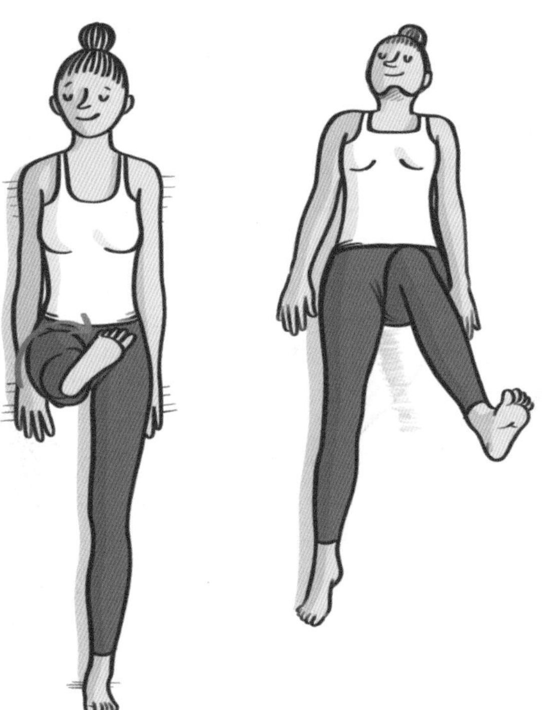

Figure 14.29 When you are not used to the bent leg version, sometimes the TFL, which is a medial rotator of the hip, can start to cramp. If this occurs, ease back on the amount of effort being used. As with the version working on increasing external rotation, build up the time and intensity over several weeks.

For passive work, two exercises spring to mind. The first is to lay on the back with knees and hips flexed and feet just wider than the hips, allowing the knees to drop toward each other (Figure 14.30). If you already have good medial rotation, the knees will rest together, and there will be little value to be had. Within reason, the feet can be moved out to achieve a greater stretch. For the student challenged with medial rotation, this position may even be active work to try and get the knees to meet and keep them there.

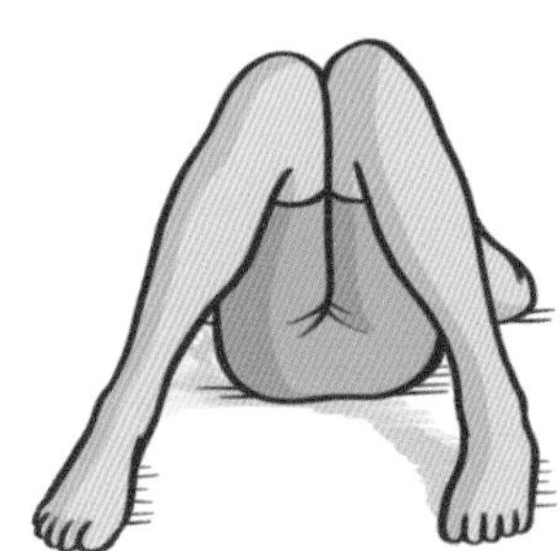

Figure 14.30 Passive work exercise—lay on back, knees and hips flexed, and feet wider than hips.

If this position is too easy, then one leg can be crossed over the other and the weight used to pull the leg toward the floor. The focus will need to be on getting less rotation in the spine and more work in the hip. As mentioned before, if you want a little help from gravity as well, you can use the medial rotation test and actively try and pull the feet closer to the floor.

CHAPTER 15

Backbends

In yoga, the backbending group often divides students into lovers and haters. Generally, this bias is based on how easily they come, existing injuries or vulnerabilities, and fear (frequently associated with vulnerabilities). All, of course, involve the spine moving into extension, but save for the most straightforward, the major joints of hips and shoulders also play a crucial role in the successful completion of the desired shape. Some of the postures emphasize strengthening of the back muscles and others the backbend shape itself. This focus is mostly to do with the orientation of the body within gravity.

Backbending and Orientation in Gravity

To start with, I was going to say that when doing backbends, we can either be supine (face up) or prone (face down). But actually, you can also be on your side, such as *Parsva Dhanurasana*, or at least start perpendicular to the floor as with transitioning from a Handstand, kneeling, or standing position. Therefore, the first principle is to do with whether gravity is assisting you or resisting you (Figure 15.1).

When you are face up or perpendicular, gravity is going to take the weight of your head and shoulders toward the floor. It is doing most of the work in creating the extension in the spine. What the student has to do is control the speed at which the bend occurs using an eccentric contraction of the muscles on the front of the body. All that is needed is an engagement of the back of the body once gravity no longer overcomes the resistance to further backward movement.

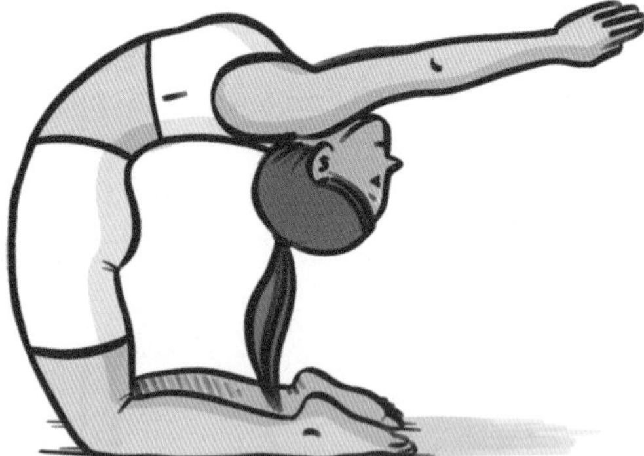

Figure 15.1 Gravity is taking Victoria back.

When you are face down, gravity is taking you toward the floor, so if you want to lift up into extension, you will have to contract the back muscles (Figure 15.2). Resistance to extension from the front of the body will combine with the effects of gravity to determine how hard you will need to work. Therefore, a posture like *Salabhasana* is strengthening for the back, especially as there is no help from the arms or the legs.

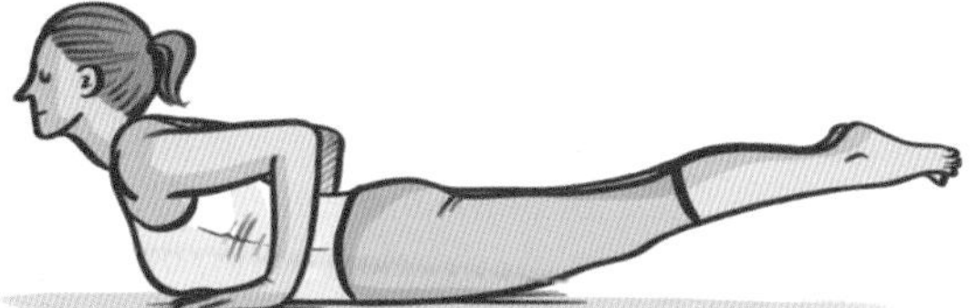

Figure 15.2 The erector spinae muscles are having to work to extend the spine.

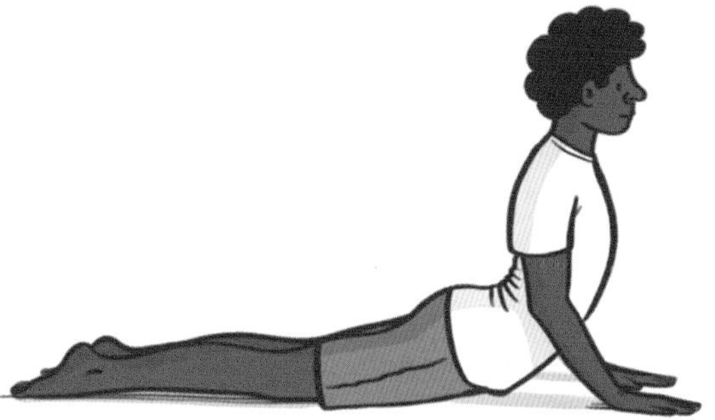

Figure 15.4 In Bhujangasana, *the less Aren uses his hands to support himself, the more active extension work will be needed.*

Side-lying postures are interesting as there is no resistance or assistance from gravity (Figure 15.3A). Therefore, they are an excellent opportunity to work on strength and refinement because you have the backbend without the lift-up. We can add some additional examples to the ones above that change how the body is working.

If you are face down but add in the arms to lift the shoulders from the floor, e.g., *Bhujangasana*, Up Dog, and Cat-Cow, then the effects of gravity change. Now it assists the bend because it is the arms lifting the shoulders, not the muscles that extend the spine (Figures 15.3B & 15.4). The body naturally bends between the foundations of the pose. It is still advisable to press into the tops of the feet and engage the abdominals to smooth the bend.

In a posture like *Dhanurasana*, the arms are in extension and grabbing the ankles, introducing a tensional force between the arms and legs that can be used to increase the backbend. Unless you have a very easy backbend, assisted postures will produce a deeper spinal extension than those against gravity.

It is also possible to aid the backbend when face up by adding in the arms and legs. *Urdhva Dhanurasana* and *Ustrasana* are good examples of how the arms and legs can be used to support each end of the torso (Figure 15.5). The effects of gravity change because the shoulders are being held in place by the arms. The weight of the upper body is no longer a force contributing to the bend, but instead, there is the ability to push the floor away. Here the experience will change dramatically for the student depending on the presence of the

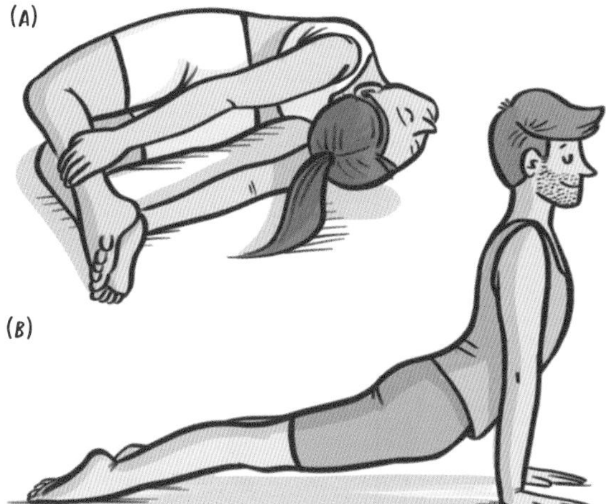

Figure 15.3 (A) Gravity is neutral when side lying, (B) in postures like Up Dog, gravity is assisting the backbend.

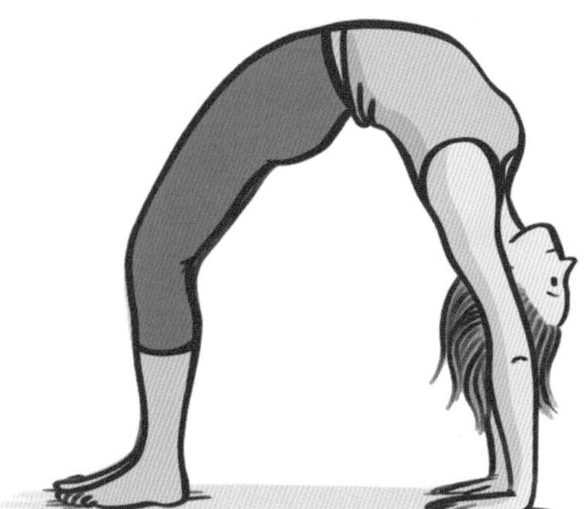

Figure 15.5 The arms and legs can support the arch if the ROM is available to get high enough.

required openness in the shoulders (flexion) and hips (extension).

If there is a restriction, then the depth of the backbend may well be reduced when compared with an open-chain face-up backbend (e.g., standing backbend or from Handstand). *Urdhva Dhanurasana* and *Ustrasana* have the same movement going on at the hips, but opposite movements at the shoulder. So, for *Ustrasana*, restriction in shoulder extension will pull the chest down and reduce the depth of the backbend.

Open-Chain Backbends and Gravity

Open-chain backbends are those where only one end of the arc is in contact with the floor (Figure 15.6). A pose like *Salabhasana* is open-chain, but the middle of the arc is on the floor and it is not gravity-assisted. With open-chain face-up backbends, the weight and length of the moving part of the body can act as a lever on the spine.

For example, in the standing backbend already discussed, gravity and the weight of the head and shoulders can increase the spinal extension. If you fully relax the front of the body, it is possible for the most mobile segment in the spine to accommodate a lot of the movement. If that position is held in an overly relaxed way, the long lever will continue to direct forces to the same area. This same principle goes for a backbend in a Handstand, and it may be even more exaggerated due to the extra weight of the legs and the lever length. Therefore, although it may feel initially advantageous to try and completely relax the front of the body to reduce the resistance to extension, it is essential to protect the spine by maintaining some activation, particularly across the abdomen. This intra-abdominal pressure helps to smooth the curve in the lumbar area and take more emphasis to the hips and shoulders. Ribs flaring is the telltale sign that this integrity is lost.

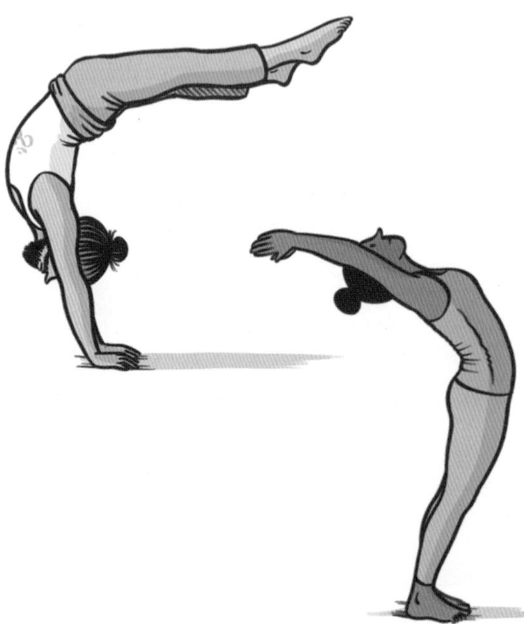

Figure 15.6 Open-chain backbends.

Hip and Shoulder Combinations

Now we can start to think about the hip and shoulder positions in the different backbends (Figures 15.7–15.12). We can have flexed shoulders in combination with either flexed or extended hips, or extended shoulders with either flexed or extended hips. It is also possible to add more complications by considering asymmetric postures, whether the elbows or knees are flexed, or hips rotated.

For example, *Eka Pada Rajakapotasana* is asymmetric, knees and elbows are bent, and the front hip is in varying degrees of external rotation depending on where the shin is.

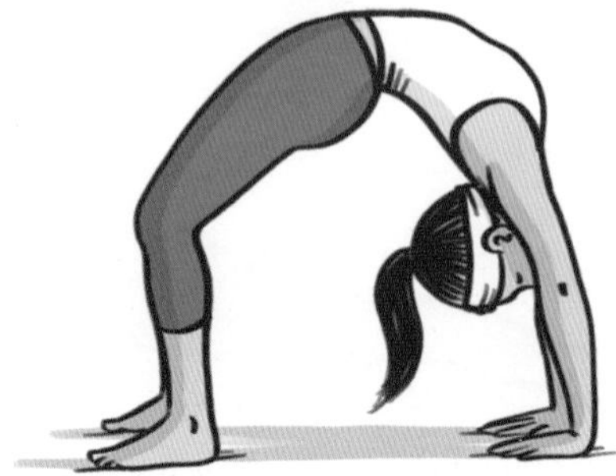

Figure 15.7 Flexed shoulders with extended hips.

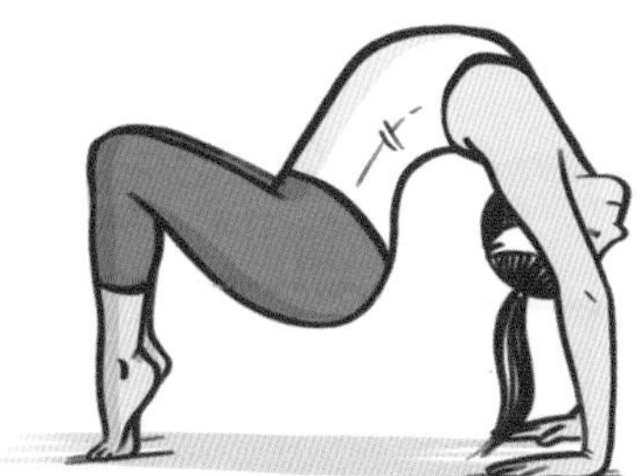

Figure 15.8 Flexed shoulders with flexed hips.

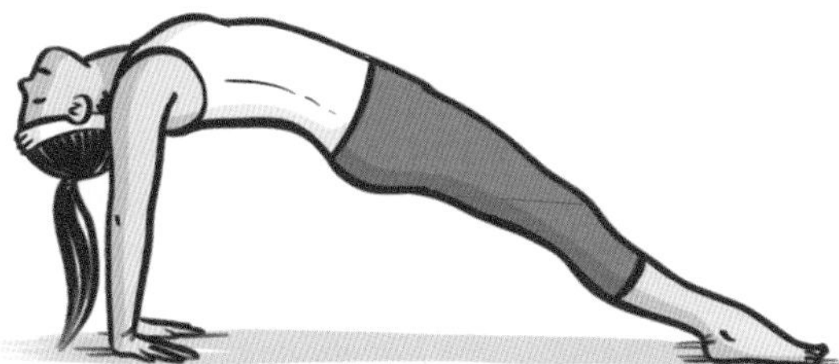

Figure 15.9 Extended shoulders with extended hips.

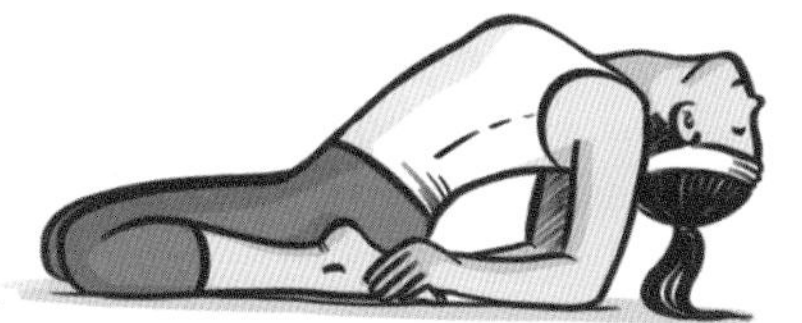

Figure 15.10 Extended shoulders with flexed hips.

Drawing on *Making Shapes* (Chapter 1) and *ROM* (Chapter 2), it follows then that the successful completion of most backbends will depend on how readily the spine extends, and the available ROM in the hips and shoulders (remember direction-specific). We can add in the importance of engaging the muscles in the abdomen to protect the lumbar spine and reduce hinging, leg, and arm strength (for some postures), and incorporating a calm breath as backbends tend to be stimulating. The more of the shape we can create using the hips and shoulders, the less will have to be done with the spine.

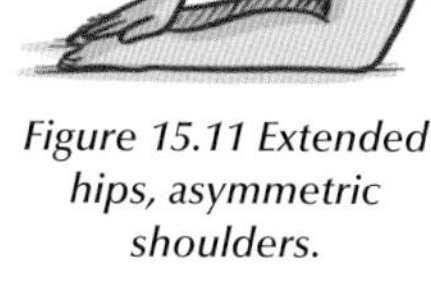

Figure 15.11 Extended hips, asymmetric shoulders.

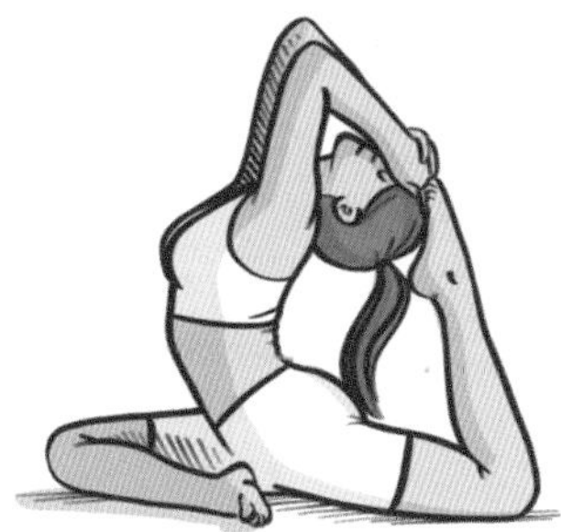

Figure 15.12 Flexed shoulders, asymmetric hips.

The Backbend Arc

When creating backbend shapes, either some or all of the body is used to make an arc (Figure 15.13). The spine is extending, but it is only part of the overall posture. Some poses will require a lot of extension and others very little. What we already know about the spine is that with the majority of students, there will be a minimal amount of extension available in the thoracic region.

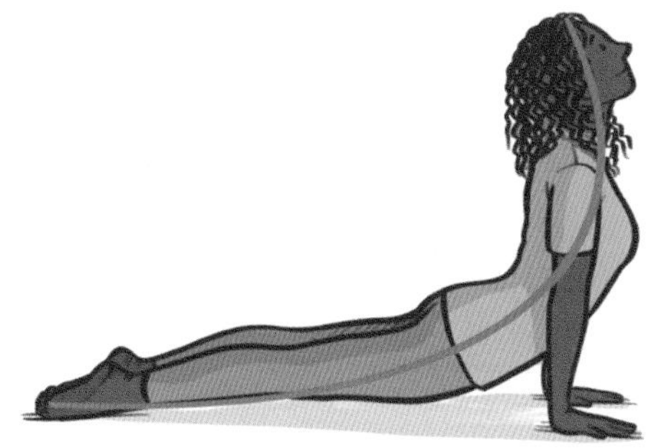

Figure 15.13 It is harder than it seems to create a nice smooth curve like this.

Therefore, when visualizing the part of the backbend pose made with the spine, we know it can't be a smooth curve with a lot more of the curve happening in the lumbar area. If we now include the arms and legs, the shape created more closely resembles part of an oval rather than a circle. The nearer the ends of the arc are to each other, the sharper the curve will be, and the more extension will be called for from the spine (Figure 15.14). The ends of the arc are not always the feet and hands, the knees, butt, head, or elbows, are also possible.

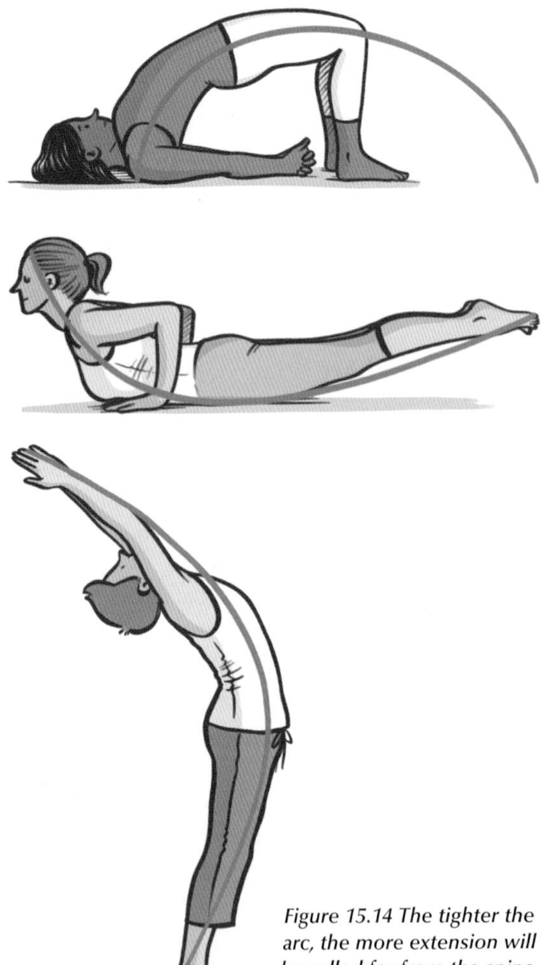

Figure 15.14 The tighter the arc, the more extension will be called for from the spine.

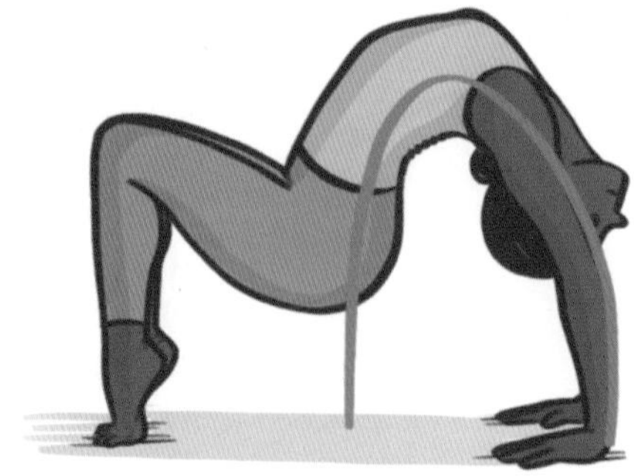

Figure 15.15 Flexed shoulders with flexed hips tend to create the sharpest arcs.

The position of the arms and legs will be one of the major determining factors of the depth of the backbend. If the hips are extended, their orientation contributes to the overall arc of the body and usually leads to less spinal extension needed. When the hips are flexed, the pelvis, in effect, becomes one end of the curve. If this hip position is combined with flexed shoulders, then the resulting shape is likely to call for bucket loads of spinal extension and, frankly, most students won't have it available because of the skeletal structure of their spine. Poses featuring flexed hips and extended shoulders typically exhibit shallower curves.

With a full-body backbend, flexed shoulders allow the arms to make part of the curve and, consequently, often moderate spinal extension will suffice. Of course, that can be overridden if the curve of the arc is exaggerated by bringing the two ends closer (Figure 15.15). Examples would include when the feet are walked toward the hands in *Urdhva Dhanurasana*, *Kapotasana*, or grabbing the backs of the legs in a standing backbend. With this sharp arc, I think most students will have to hinge (Figure 15.16). Considering all the ideas we covered about the role of spinal extension in Chapter 9, *Spine*, I hope you are questioning the benefits of intense backbends.

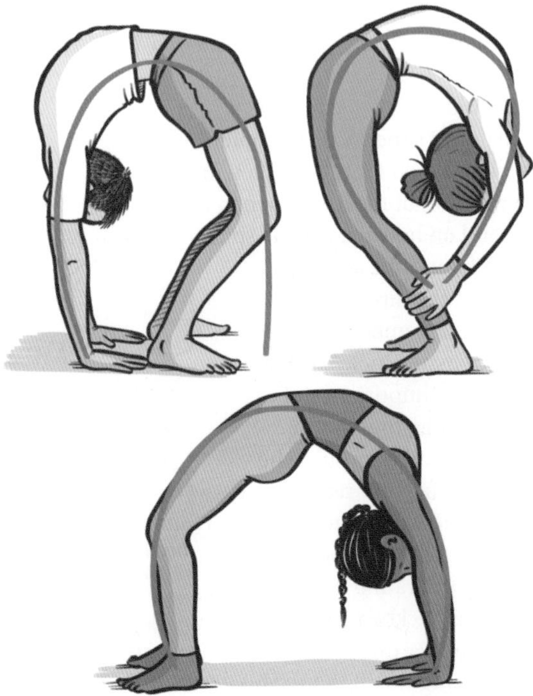

Figure 15.16 The tighter the arc the higher the likelihood of hinging.

Peak Posture or Transitioning Pose

The overall shape of a backbend will determine whether it is a peak posture or something that can be used as a transition or preparation for another more challenging pose. If it is the former, then the sequencing prior to the posture should take into account the movements that will happen at the hips and shoulders, as well as introduce some less dramatic backbends, even strengthening ones.

For example, if the peak posture was *Urdhva Dhanurasana*, then before doing this pose, you would want to have performed some form of lunge variation aimed at finding space across the front of the hip, for example, *Ardha Pincha Mayurasana*, to work on the shoulder flexion while maintaining the external rotation, core activation, such as forearm plank), and preparatory backbends, for example, *Bhujangasana*, *Setu Bandha Sarvangasana*, and *Ustrasana*. Subsequently, when the peak pose is encountered, it will be more likely to spread the curve between the major joints, and there is more chance of controlling any hinging.

The same approach should be followed for all challenging postures, but I think it is especially important when it comes to backbending because of how easy it is for many students to overstress the back. There will be, of course, some students who find backbending super easy and *Urdhva Dhanurasana* might be one of their preparatory postures for a much deeper backbend. I even know practitioners that use *Urdhva Dhanurasana* as a warm-up shoulder opener for their Handstand practice. With all sequencing, it needs to be relevant to the individual.

Upward-Facing Dog

I'm going to explore now a couple more examples, one from each end of the backbend scale, Up Dog and then *Kapotasana*.

Up Dog is a pose in its own right but also often used as a transition in, for example, *Surya Namaskar*. It can be thought of as a gentle/moderate backbend because it is gravity-assisted, and it is easy to control the depth of the bend by firming the front of the body. However, it can also be performed as a pretty deep backbend, and I have seen many students hinge more extremely in this pose than in some more complicated postures. Actually, at the opposite end of the scale (Figure 15.17), when I have managed to tighten up my back, Up Dog can have very little bend at all, we've even nicknamed it "Upward-Facing Plank."

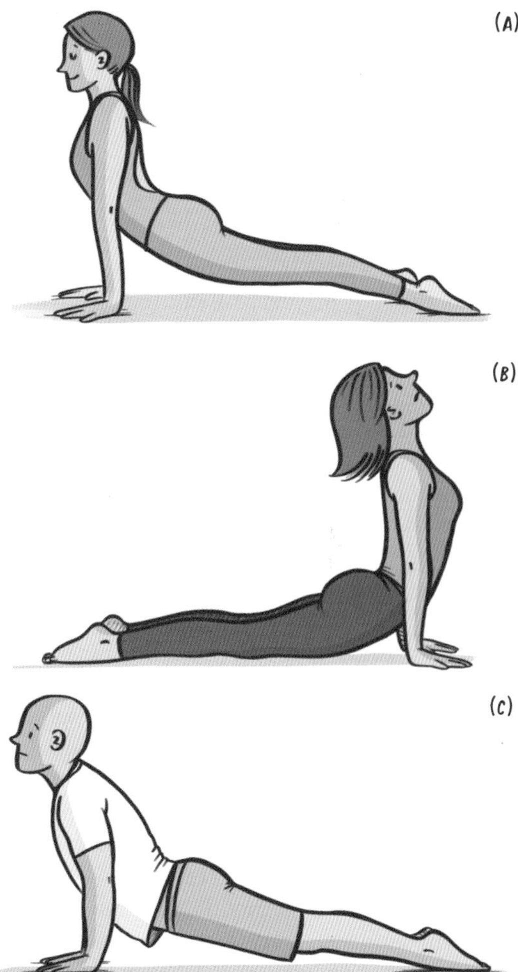

Figure 15.17 (A) The girl in yellow has a very nice line; (B) here, the girl in green is exaggerating the bend by hinging; (C) Upward-Facing Plank due to restricted extension.

What makes a good Up Dog? Here is a list of elements I would look for, but bear in mind they might need to be adjusted for the individual:

- Tops of the feet pressing evenly into the floor.
- Foot, ankle, and shin in line.
- Knees off the floor.
- Engagement of the Gmax.
- Active legs.
- Tension maintained across the front of the belly.
- Shoulders in line or behind the wrists.
- Open across the chest without rolling the arms out or introducing too much retraction of the shoulder girdle.
- Pressing evenly through the hands and depressing the shoulder girdle.
- Face can be looking up, but the head is not hinging backward.

What this adds up to is an active posture, with the front of the body playing a supporting role to avoid just sagging between the two ends of the arc, the feet, and shoulders. Numerous times I see students with their shoulders in front of their wrists, which can place strain on the wrist and shoulders. Many students need to move their feet back before rolling over the toes to come into the posture. This will provide added space and accommodate a gradual curve. The more resistant the student's body to backbending, the further back the feet need to go.

With those students who dramatically hinge, what I tend to see is a short distance between the feet and hands and a nearly vertical line of the spine out from the pelvis. The hinge usually occurs at L5/S1, with gravity just dumping into that area. The student is often just passively hanging from the shoulders. When you get these students to reduce the backbend by moving the feet back, raising the thighs further from the ground, and creating more intra-abdominal pressure through engaging the abdomen, they will remark how much harder work it is (Figure 5.18). And that is a good thing by the way. I mentioned engaging the glutes just now, and I will come back to that after we have considered *Kapotasana*.

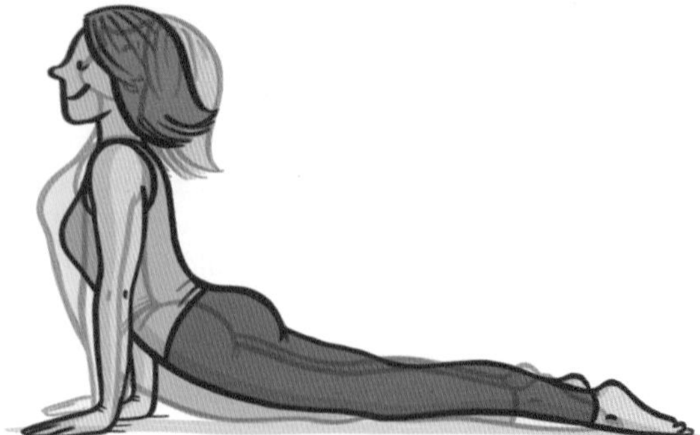

Figure 15.18 That old adage of more is not always better, definitely applies to Up Dog.

Kapotasana

I have seen *Kapotasana* performed with such ease, fluidity, and clean form that it makes you wonder what all the fuss is about (Figure 15.19A). However, I've also seen it attempted and even somewhat accomplished in a way that makes you think that, sooner or later, that student is going to have back problems (Figure 15.19B). I consider this posture an advanced backbend and really beyond the scope of most students to perform healthily.

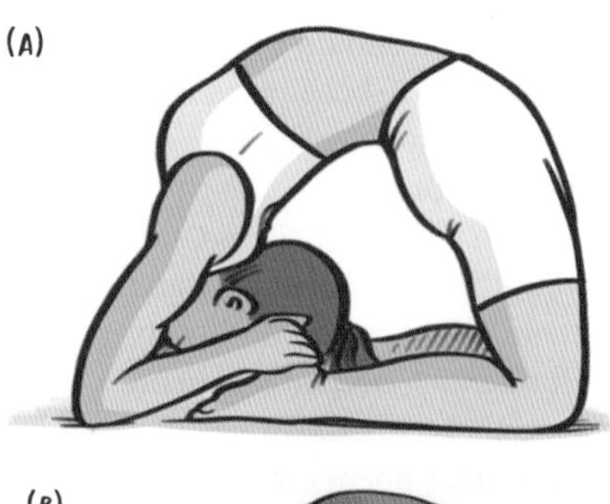

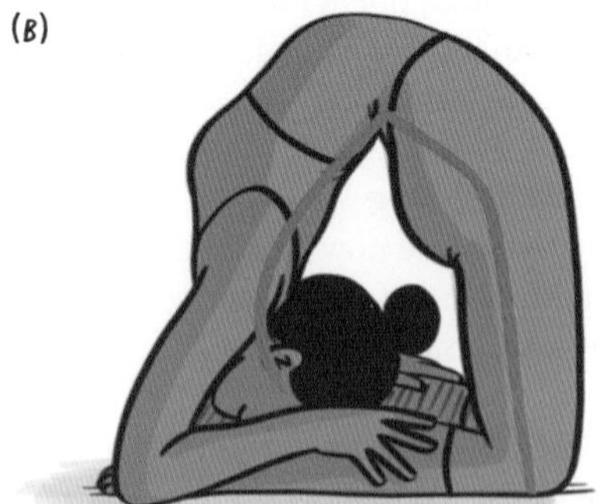

Figure 15.19 Hmmm. I know which body I would rather be in.

That might come as a bit of a surprise considering it is only in the first third of the Ashtanga Intermediate Series. The problems, as I see them, are that the arc of the bend is sharp, a lot of hip extension and shoulder flexion is required, and that the floor or feet can be used to pull deeper into the backbend. It is evident in many students that they don't have the necessary ROM in the hips and shoulders, and in trying to compensate, the knees move further apart, the hips drift back, and the spine hinges. If they can hinge really deeply, they can avoid the work in the shoulders and hips altogether, and just use the hinge.

As a vigilant teacher, you should already have picked up on these avoidance patterns in more straightforward postures. It would be much better for these students to leave this posture, work on the correct ROMs, and then revisit it again several months later. I think it is very hard to clean up an intense backbend posture by simply repeating it and hoping to change the ROM in the hips and shoulders when there is an area of instability in the spine that will give way easily. If an area of instability is not present, then as well as working the individual movements, advancements can be made in the posture itself.

Comparing Some Backbends

If we stick with *Kapotasana A*, we can compare it to *Laghu Vajrasana*, *Ustrasana*, and *Kapotasana B* (Figure 15.20). All four start with the knees hip-width apart, but in *Kapotasana A* and *B*, the shoulders are flexed, whereas in *Laghu Vajrasana* and *Ustrasana*, they are extended. If we look at the arcs of the four poses, they are vastly different. The gentlest backbend is *Laghu Vajrasana*, but

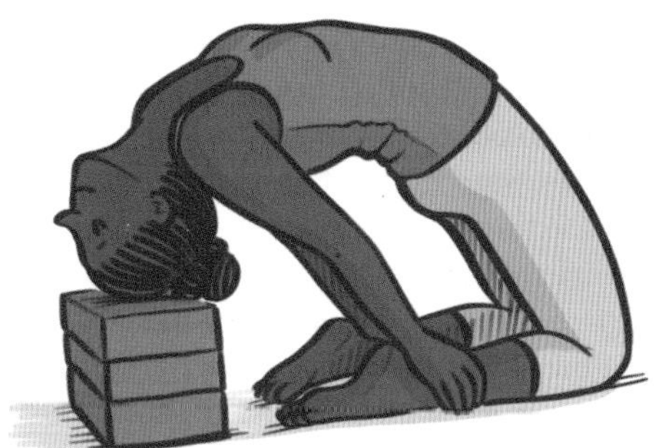

Figure 15.21 Blocks add a level of security and can gradually be reduced over time as strength increases.

that doesn't mean it is the easiest. Because the hips are moving backward and lowering, the posture requires the most strength.

It is better to work on *Laghu Vajrasana* in stages, because the long lever of the body can place a large burden on the quadriceps as they work eccentrically on the lower down and concentrically on the rise back up. I have come across several students who have sprained the patellar tendon (attaches quadriceps to tibia) by overestimating their ability. A good idea is to place a stack of blocks on the mat behind you that you can come down to, reducing the number of blocks over several weeks or months (Figure 15.21). Strong legs are definitely an asset in deeper backbends.

Kapotasana will require the most hip extension to help create the tighter arc, and *Ustrasana* sits in the middle, with *Laghu Vajrasana* typically exhibiting the least. As the COG is lower in *Laghu Vajrasana*, the quadriceps are working more strongly to resist gravity flexing the knees and keep the butt up in the air. Rectus femoris, the quadricep that crosses the hip, will tend to flatten out the amount of hip extension because it is pulling on the front of the pelvis (remember it is also a hip flexor).

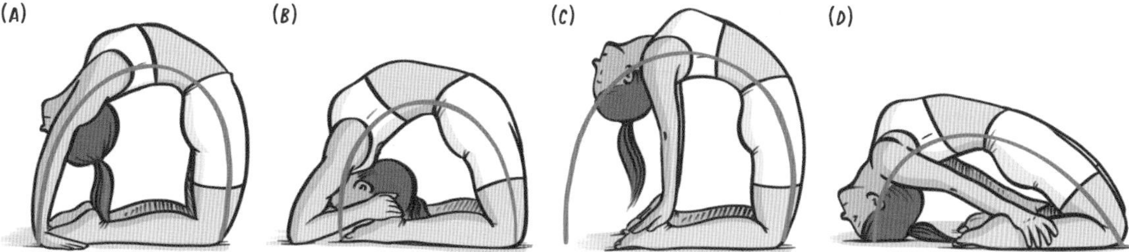

Figure 15.20 (A) Kapotasana B, *(B)* Kapotasana A, *(C)* Ustrasana, *(D)* Laghu Vajrasana.

All postures involve an initial eccentric action of the hip flexors and abdominal muscles to lower the body into position. With *Ustrasana*, you are moving backward the least, but having said that, keeping the thighs perpendicular to the floor is still a challenge for many students, especially if they are restricted in hip extension. In *Kapotasana*, the front of the body will have to work hard to control the descent, but the more open the shoulders and the more easily the spine extends, the tighter the curve will be and the shorter the lever that the body creates.

As already mentioned, the flexed position of the shoulders in *Kapotasana* really adds to the difficulty for most students. Without that ROM to create a straight line through the armpit, the whole posture is pulled flatter, the pelvis will drift back, and the hands will not reach the feet. As we have said, both *Ustrasana* and *Laghu Vajrasana* have extended shoulders, but it is only in *Ustrasana* that the shoulder ROM may be challenging. If this is the case, then it would not be possible to lift the chest as much, which, in turn, will pull the posture lower. Now would be the time to come onto the toes, place the hands on the butt instead, or call in the props and place the hands on blocks (Figure 15.22).

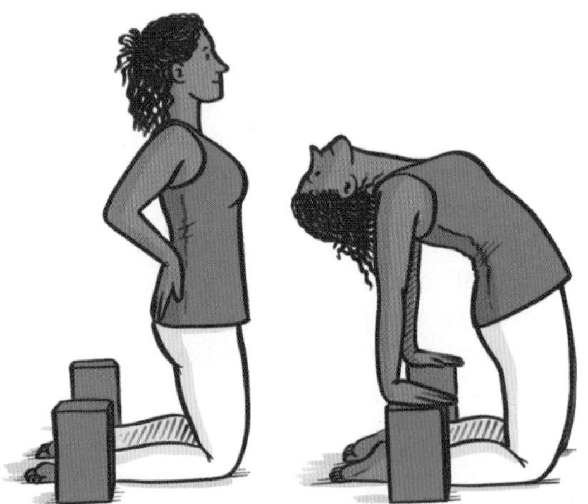

Figure 15.22 When it comes to backbends, I think it is even more important to use props to help position the body beneficially.

Hinging

A lot of students introduce a hinge movement in the spine when doing backbends, either as a way to avoid the work at the other major joints because they are unaware they are doing it, they feel it's perfectly healthy, in an effort to exaggerate the depth of a posture, or because the depth of the posture requires it (Figures 15.23 & 15.24).

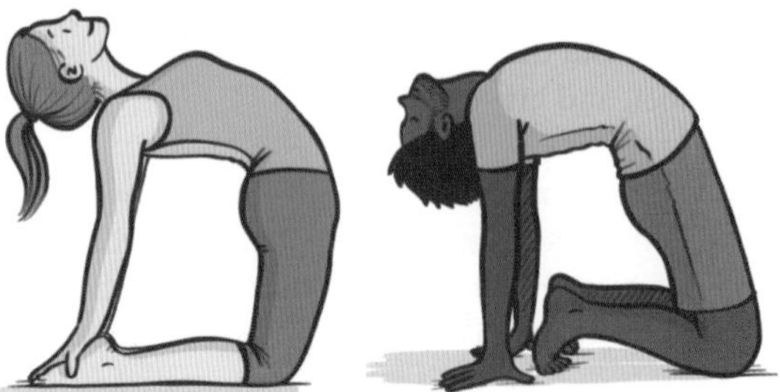

Figure 15.23 Happy hinging in one place, why not add one in the cervical spine as well?

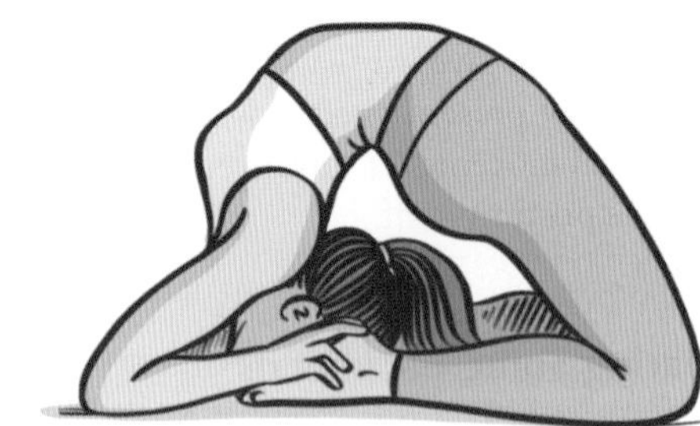

Figure 15.24 The depth of the backbend required to perform Kapotasana *often means students hinge, whether they are aware of it or not.*

You may think this only happens in intense backbends, but when the pattern is there, it will pop up everywhere, even as I mentioned in Up Dog. Just have a look at some Instagram accounts if you don't believe me (Figure 15.25). Actually, if B. K. S. Iyengar was alive and had an Instagram account, I would be sending you there to take a look because, in my opinion, he hinged a lot in his backbends. It looks like one of the reasons for this is that he had a large ribcage and not much room between the bottom of it and the pelvis.

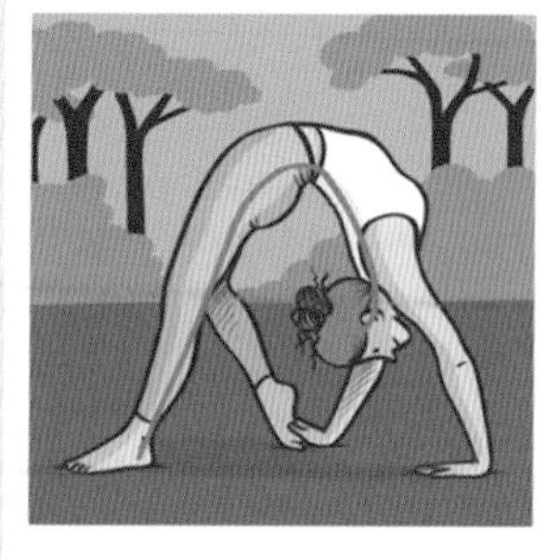

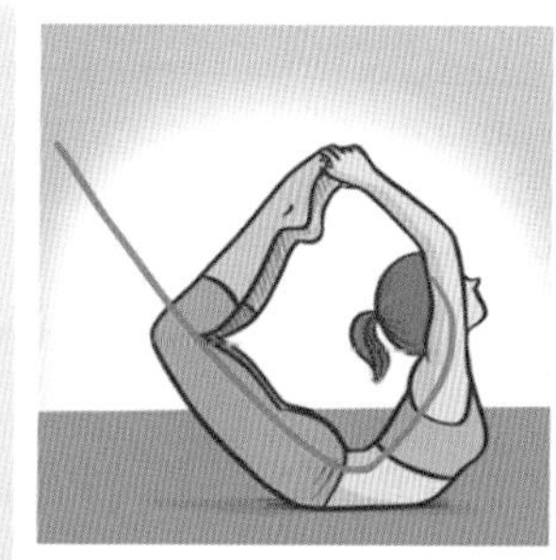

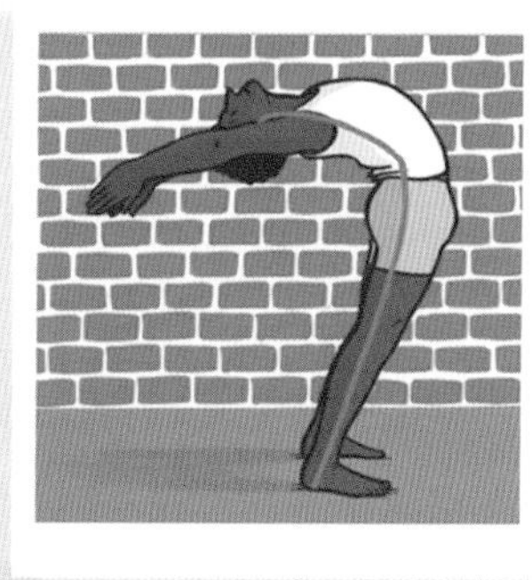

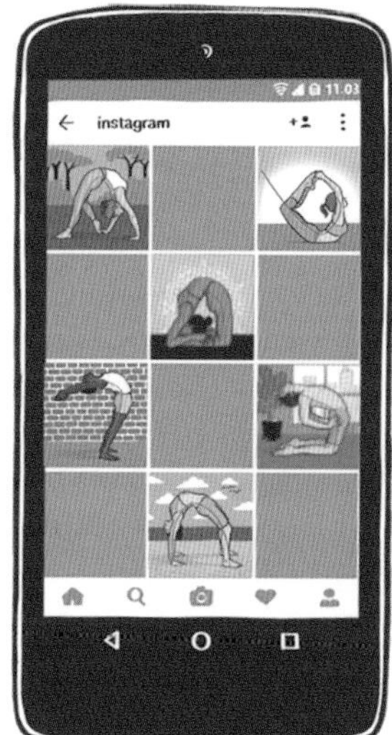

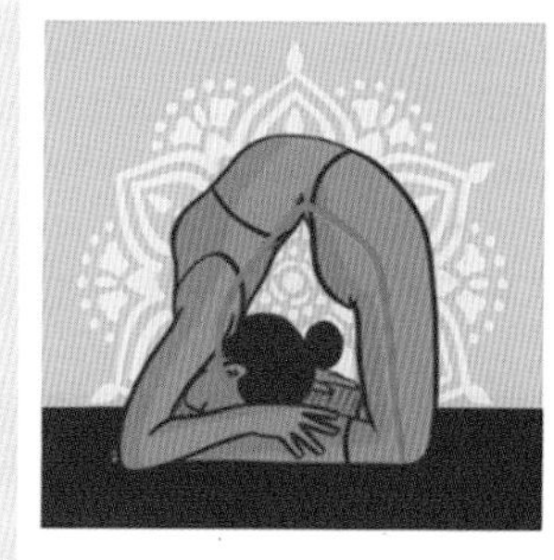

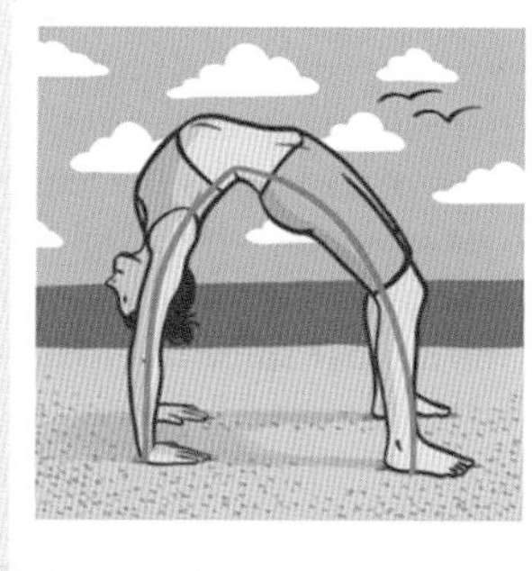

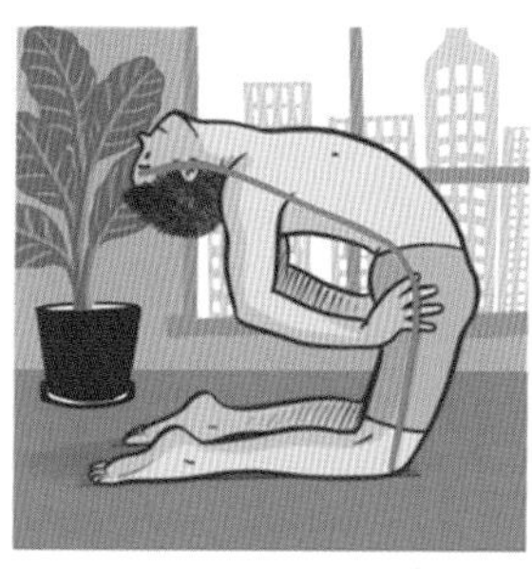

Figure 15.25 With the eagerness to create eye-catching yoga posts on social media, you will have no trouble seeing a plethora of "hinging" yogis.

Just so you know, I'm not bashing any style in particular, there are plenty of renowned teachers from all styles that hinge a lot. If it was good enough for Iyengar, head of possibly the most alignment-based style, why do I keep bleating on about it being a negative thing? Well, it is a view based on the ideas put forward in Chapter 9, *Spine*. Be aware, however, an alternate view goes along the lines that the L5/S1 junction offers the greatest range of extension in the thoracic and lumbar spine, so why not use that area to move into extension? I have no idea why Iyengar chose to hinge, and as with all things, it is up to you to decide if there is value in the ideas I present.

Hyperkyphosis and Backbending Postures

As we discussed in Chapter 9, *Spine*, anyone with a hyperkyphotic thoracic spine is going to have trouble finding a clean backbend line. Although there is very little extension in the average thoracic spine, in a hyperkyphotic spine it will likely stay in flexion. This is particularly true if the shoulders are flexed, as the rounded forward position tends to limit this ROM also. Therefore, all the above postures discussed should be approached wisely and with the necessary propping and modification, with the exception of *Kapotasana*, which should not be attempted at all. What I say sometimes flies in the face of many eager teachers who would like to see students overcoming obstacles, and many students oblivious to the damage they might cause themselves. I would rather err on the safe side than be complicit to injury.

What I have seen many times in students with hyperkyphotic thoracic spines is a hypermobile segment in the lumbar region. The basic premise is if one area is stuck, the adjacent area will sometimes land up taking the strain. The possibility of hinging is exasperated when combined with an area that won't extend at all, and as mentioned, probably stays in flexion. When we have been using the term "hyperkyphotic," it is not in a clinical way (that might be much more extreme), but a milder version due to primarily poor posture patterns. However, to give you a real-life example, I will recount a tale for you.

Case Study: A Troubling Tale

Several years ago, I came across a lovely student who was easily recognizable as hyperkyphotic and experiencing lower back pain. The student happened to practice near me in the subsequent days, and I saw them perform *Urdhva Dhanurasana* with the inevitable deep hinge. The next time I saw the student, I advised them that I felt the root of their pain was due to doing backbends in this way and that, because of their condition, they should refrain from deep backbends and work on strengthening the core instead.

Not wishing to take my advice, the student went on to tell me that they loved doing backbends and even earlier that year their primary teacher had managed to get them to catch their ankles in a standing backbend. As you can imagine, I almost fell over with horror. To take someone into an extreme posture in which there is no alternative but to hinge aggressively is ludicrous, and negligent both by the teacher and the student themselves.

Let's change that! Postural yoga can cause harm.

The Role of Gluteus Maximus (Gmax)

Time to think about the role that the butt—or specifically Gmax (hence referred to as the butt or glute max, even though it is only part of it)—plays in a backbend. Firstly, if the backbend is one with flexed hips, it really doesn't play any role at all, apart from the fact you might be sitting on it. The reason we want to consider Gmax is because of its primary action of hip extension. When we are creating an arc that includes the legs as part of it, we want to have as much hip extension as possible so that, as we have mentioned, the amount of extension the lumbar spine has to do is reduced. As Gmax is the strongest hip extensor, it would make sense to use it to perform the task. But some possible consequences are worth considering.

The major concern with actively using the Gmax is that, by so doing, stress may be directed inadvertently toward the SIJ or low back. So initially, we will discuss why this might happen and then how it can be avoided.

The first thing that can be addressed is the force of contraction. When the cue is to engage the butt, it does not mean to squeeze the hell out of it like you are trying to juice a potato. For a lot of inexperienced students, trying to separate engaging the butt from the low back is difficult; an overly strong contraction can lead to a jamming up of the whole area. This is common in postures like *Urdhva Dhanurasana*, where the student can barely lift the head off the floor, and it seems like the intense contraction is the only way to keep the hips up. When you can lift higher, you can properly use the power in the legs, keeping the butt sensitively engaged and low back more relaxed. For this reason, I suggest it is not worth students creating tension just hovering off the floor (Figure 15.26). It is better that they release their restrictions first and return to this posture some months later when they are better prepared. In the meantime, they can work on more accessible poses, such as *Ustrasana*.

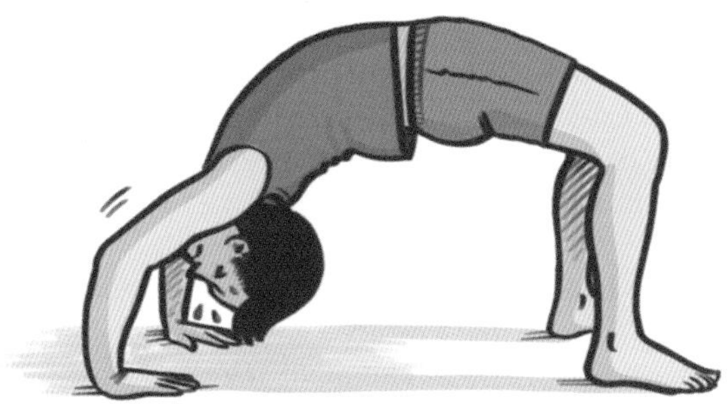

Figure 15.26 If the student is struggling to get off the floor, they are much more likely to create tension. Greater ROM will help.

There is more to this story than just over engaging. If you can remember from Chapter 8, *Hip*, other actions of Gmax are external rotation and abduction. The fear is that an unchecked engagement could send the knees out and with them the feet, resulting in energy being directed into the SIJ and low back. I have a feeling this compensation is also linked to trying to escape the restriction of the iliacus and psoas to hip extension. The answer to this scenario is twofold. If the body is open enough to do the posture, then Gmax won't need to work too hard and, with awareness, it should be easy enough to keep the legs tracking parallel. If more work is required, then more active control is needed. It is not so easy for the legs to widen unless the feet turn out as well. The feet won't turn out unless the grounding is lost and there is a pivoting action on the heel.

Therefore, working backward, the actions I would recommend are to firm the foundation of the feet before pushing up. Keep weight across the whole foot and especially into the base of the big toe. Go up slowly and with control, peeling the hips off the floor first, ensuring that the feet don't move (Figure 15.27). This is performed while, at the same time, creating a sense of adduction at the hip, not to go into adduction but to neutralize any forces of abduction. The thighs stay parallel. This can always be practiced in *Setu Bandha Sarvangasana* first to establish the pattern and then progressed into *Urdhva Dhanurasana*. If sufficient shoulder

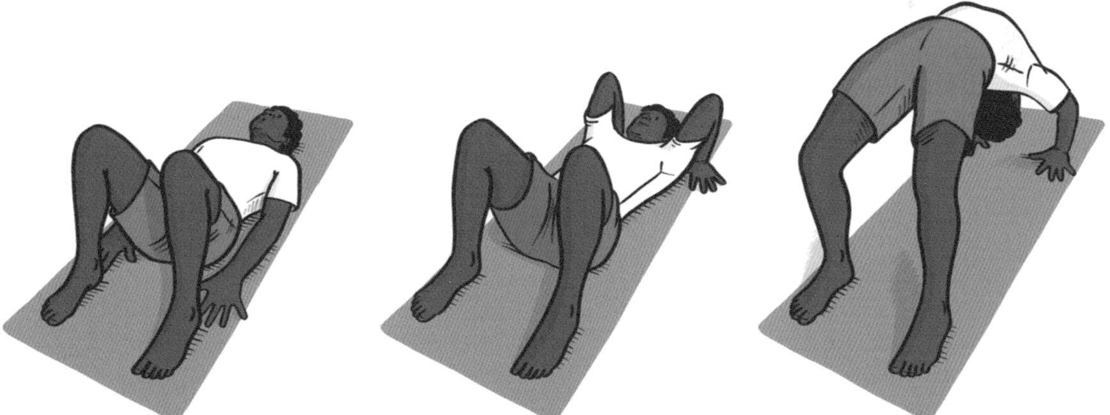

Figure 15.27 Keep the feet fully and evenly grounded, and the knees similarly spaced the whole way through the process from setup to being in the posture.

flexion is missing, there will be more temptation to compromise at the hip end. Keep it real and only go as high as it is possible to do so without losing the form.

In postures such as Up Dog, *Bhujangasana*, and *Salabhasana*, the butt can again be engaged. This time, the corrective cueing to prevent the hips rolling out will be to keep the soles of the feet facing the ceiling. There will be a tendency for the little toe side of the foot to be higher. If the hips are medially rotated slightly before starting, it can help to get the right action. In Up Dog, don't let the ankles drop out and keep the weight evenly distributed across the top of the foot.

The upside of engaging the glutes in postures is that they will become stronger. Gmax is a big muscle, and big muscles are meant to do lots of work. Weak glutes are also often contributing factors to postural issues and pain patterns, and another plus is that along with strength comes tone.

Core

The good news is that you don't need to be able to do a thousand sit-ups. Nowadays, the concept of what constitutes the core is broader than developing a six-pack or continually activating transversus abdominis. Predominantly, the first thing that still comes to mind is the area between the ribcage and pelvis, but really we can expand that area up to the shoulders and throughout the pelvis at a minimum. It is probably better still to include the whole body (Figure 15.28), as we know how much instability in one area will trigger overcompensation in another. So, what the hell do we focus on now that we have the whole body to think of?

What we need is to feel integrated and secure in many different orientations and planes when performing multi-segmental or whole-body movements. Therefore, it is those types of combined actions we want to test ourselves in.

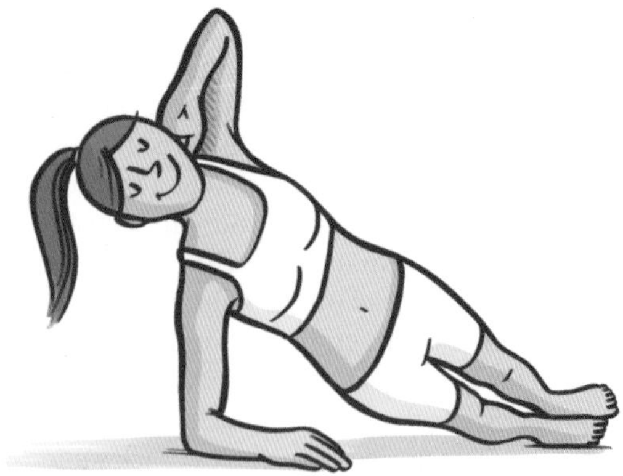

Figure 15.28 Use the whole body to strengthen the core.

Forearm planks and high planks are great but so too are all sorts of balancing postures. The more precarious, the harder the whole body works. But you still don't want to fall awkwardly, so build it up progressively. Take standing postures you can do comfortably and add an element of challenge. Explore playfully to find your stability strengths and weaknesses. For myself, I found it was the spinal extension and the side body that were weak. Some of this was due to avoidance and some to sequence programming.

With a history of back issues from a previous work injury, I found that I avoided a lot of active spinal extension work because it made my back ache at the time. In recent years, I revisited holding postures like *Salabhasana* for longer periods because I wanted strength in that movement for some particular arm balances I was working on. What I found was that contrary to making my back ache more, after an initial getting-used-to-the-work period, my back ache in general reduced and holding extension positions no longer caused aching. I now do a wide-legged variation of *Salabhasana* on blocks (two side by side) to reduce the amount of support from the floor, also engaging the glutes and hamstrings strongly as it happens (Figure 15.29). Not just for summer posing, you understand. The right exercises, of course, depends on each individual's etiology. Case in point that more stretching is not always the answer.

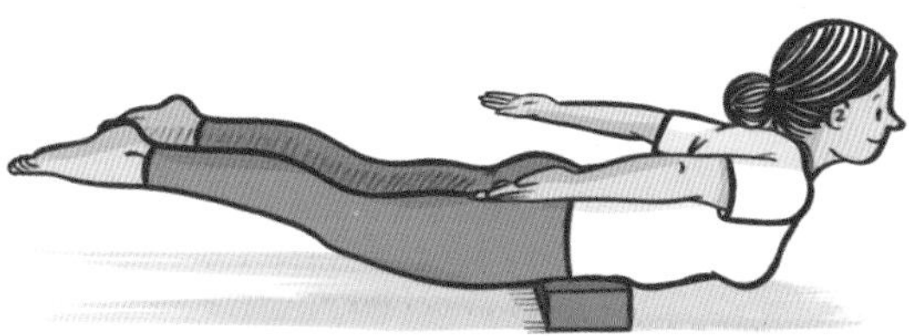

Figure 15.29 With less of the body as a BOS, more stabilization work will be needed. I usually do one set of 15 breaths like this and then turn the block on its side for another two sets of 15 breaths. You can have the hands under the shoulder also, but not out in front.

As a cautionary note, working on active extension is not going to be suitable for everyone. A lot of valuable work can be done in positions like Bird Dog, because it is an excellent way to develop that stability cylinder from which you can move the legs and arms independently (Figure 15.30).

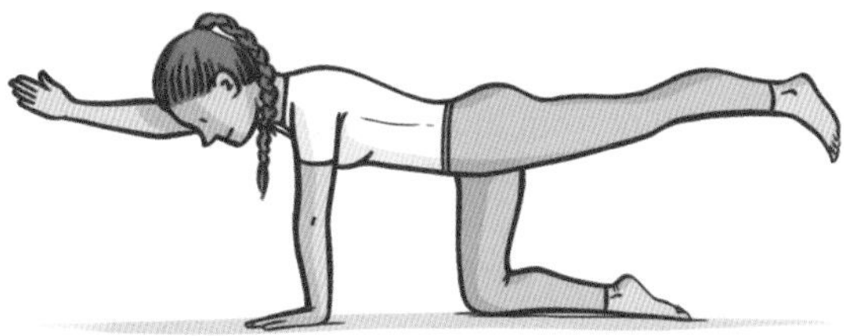

Figure 15.30 Bird Dog is an excellent exercise that can easily be slipped into a yoga practice. Only lift the leg as high as you can without the low back going into deeper extension.

As the hands move in front of the shoulders, the lever length increases, and the back muscles will need to work harder. When the arms are outstretched past the head, sometimes called Superman, the forces can be quite significant on the lumbar spine (Figure 15.31). This positioning would undoubtedly be too much for anyone with back issues, and unnecessary unless you are looking to recreate this position within another posture. It is preferable to keep them in line with the shoulders.

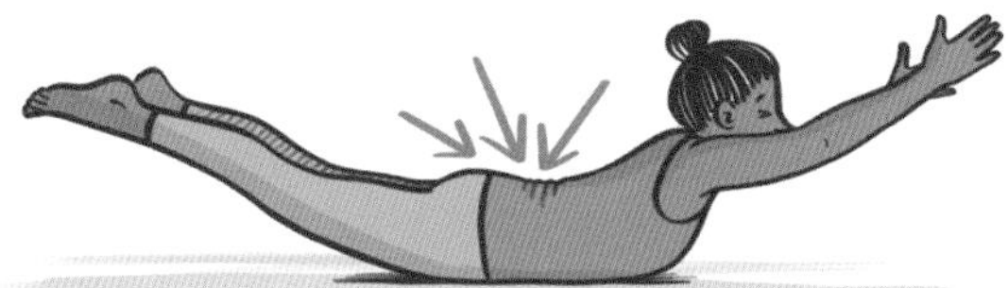

Figure 15.31 To have the arms reaching forward is not sensible for most students.

After many years of doing Ashtanga primary and intermediate series (modified), I decided to try some of the postures in Advanced A series, with the first being *Vasishtasana*, a side plank variation (Figure 15.32). When I tried it, I was really surprised how weak I was lifting away from the floor in this position. It makes plenty of sense though, because there is nothing like that action in the first two sequences. Working on this position and other more simplified versions has really helped my overall sense of integration. This worked for me, but each person has to discover what they need and the right way to get it.

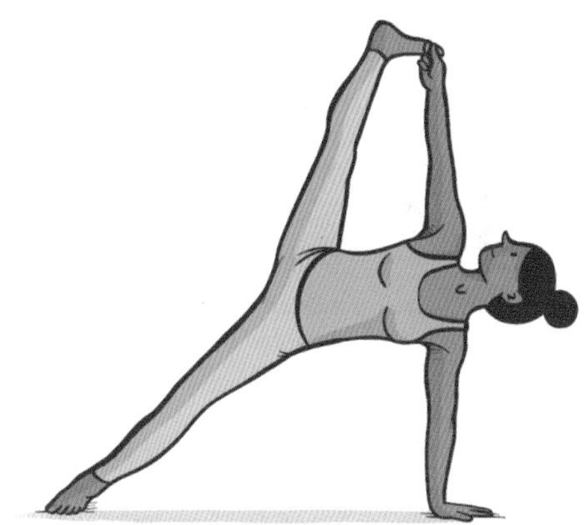

Figure 15.32 Vasishtasana *and its variations are a good way to incorporate side body strength.*

Proportions

As we have talked about before, our general proportions make a big difference to how we create our postural yoga shapes. The same goes for whole body backbending when there is a marked variation between upper and lower body length. The shorter part of the body can tend to shift the curve and stop the opposite end moving through the full ROM available. For example, if the torso and arm length are proportionally shorter than the pelvis and leg length, then it's possible that the hips won't be able to extend as much. By placing blocks under the hands, you can, in effect, create more balance and allow the hips to realize the full ROM available (Figure 15.33). If the proportions were reversed, then blocks could be placed under the feet instead.

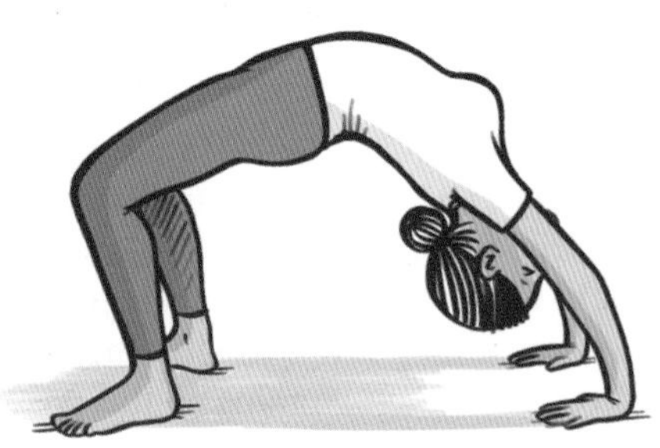

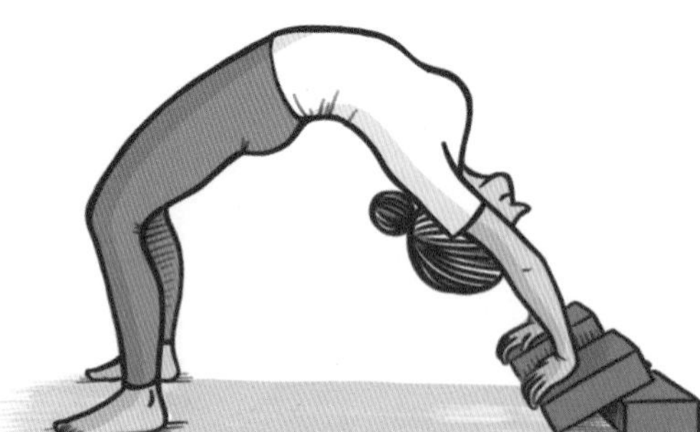

Figure 15.33 Using blocks and other props can help address proportional differences.

Side Bends

As well as the side body strength mentioned above, an important posture group that is not included in many sequences is side bends. Either standing or seated are ideal for creating space between the ribcage and pelvis. Many students find more freedom in both twisting and backbending poses after having done a side bend. It makes sense because a lot of the muscles around the waist, for example, obliques and QL, can restrict freedom of movement of the lumbar spine or resist the ribcage moving relative to the pelvis.

A side bend with the arm above the head will also put latissimus dorsi under a stretch because it originates in the thoracolumbar fascia and travels up the back to attach to the front of the humerus near the shoulder. It is one of the muscles that can easily resist the student finding sufficient shoulder flexion in postures such as *Urdhva Dhanurasana* and *Kapotasana*. It is also very often the muscle responsible for the elbows going out in those same postures because of its secondary action of medial rotation of the shoulder. See Chapter 3 for more information.

Cat-Cow

I really like Cat-Cow transitioning as a spinal warm-up as well as to work on refinement and assess movement restrictions or hinging. Of course, you can't see your own back when you are doing this, but you can always get feedback or set up video (side and top view are useful). As there are no complications, balance, or fear associated with this pose, it's worth trying to be specific with the movements. Working from one end of the spine to the other is quite a helpful exercise, swapping the start point from thoracic to lumbar alternately. It is relatively easy to see if there is an area that doesn't want to move much, and if one side of the body shortens during the transition from flexed to extended or vice versa. Take this time to observe the common hinge segments of T12/L1 and L5/S1.

Breath

Backbending can be stimulating to the nervous system. I do sometimes wonder whether this is because the brain is worried about what the hell you think you are doing. Nevertheless, regardless of my skepticism of intense backbends, we do know how closely tied the breath is to the nervous system. If you struggle to find ease in a backbend, it is well worth focusing on calming the breath and tuning into the natural undulation of the spine with the inhale and exhale. A more relaxed breath also feeds into a calmer mind and a less tense body. You can even team this up with positive visualization that you are light and floating rather than heavy like a sack of spuds.

CHAPTER 16

Twists

The twisting action itself should be generated by muscular contraction, primarily the obliques, rather than levering or pulling oneself around. In this way, it is unlikely the twist will go too far, and active ROM will be increased. It is fine to do a passive twist as we would for many other areas but forcing is inadvisable. We have discussed already the potentially detrimental outcomes of using the likes of the elbow on the knee to force twists deeper.

When we twist, it is the gross, more superficial, muscles that do most of the work, primarily the obliques, with those close to the spine doing more refined and stabilizing work. I did read somewhere that the aptly named rotatores muscles that go from the transverse processes of each thoracic vertebrae to the spinous process of the one above, don't actually rotate the spine. However, as most anatomy books still list them along with the multifidus as assisting rotation, feel free to lump them in.

Many students have pretty good proprioceptive awareness when it comes to contracting the hamstring or quadriceps, but when it involves the obliques, it's trickier, especially as there are two layers on each side. The way I remember it is as follows: the external oblique draws the same side shoulder forward, and the internal oblique draws the same side shoulder backward. As an example, if we wanted to twist to the right, then the right shoulder goes forward and the left shoulder goes backward. This means right external oblique and left internal oblique are contracting and right internal oblique and left external oblique are lengthening (Figure 16.1).

Maybe you will be glad to hear me say, "But who cares, what are we going to do with this information." As long as we twist in both directions, we will balance things out. I think the intention of twisting is sufficient.

Drawing from Chapter 9, *Spine*, we know that most of the twist needs to happen in the thoracic region as that is the area of the spine designed to twist (Figure 16.2). As a reminder, the directionality of the articulating processes (the bits that stick up and

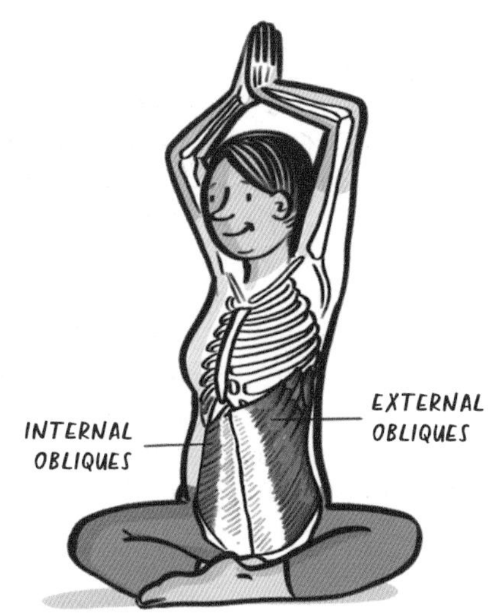

Figure 16.1 The obliques.

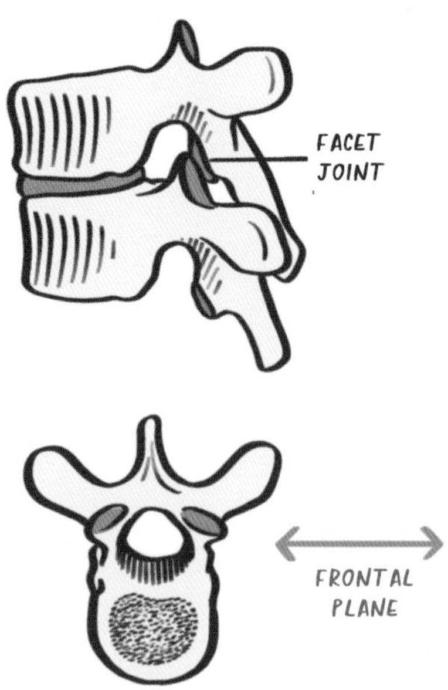

Figure 16.2 The thoracic spine is designed for twisting.

down) is such that they are aligned in the frontal plane, facilitating vertebral rotation. Those in the lumbar region are aligned in the sagittal plane and resist rotation. So, when twisting, the lumbar area should be moved first, but only a little, then firmed and stabilized. Next from the thoracic area comes the majority of the rotation. And lastly, the head is turned as far as is comfortable toward the direction of travel. It is important not to lead with the eyes or head as this can place strain on the more fragile cervical area.

We do want to be able to rotate the head, and many students who suffer from neck tension—often due to workspace ergonomics—will find that their ROM is restricted. There is also a tendency to want to drop the head back to find the extra rotation. I would say we can work consciously within the postures to encourage rotation, but it is probably better to just sit on the heels and work on actively turning the head and holding for a number of breaths (Figure 16.3). I am always in favor of deconstructing gross movements, working on simple actions, and then recombining everything again.

The average cervical rotation changes between the age groups and reduces with age but is somewhere

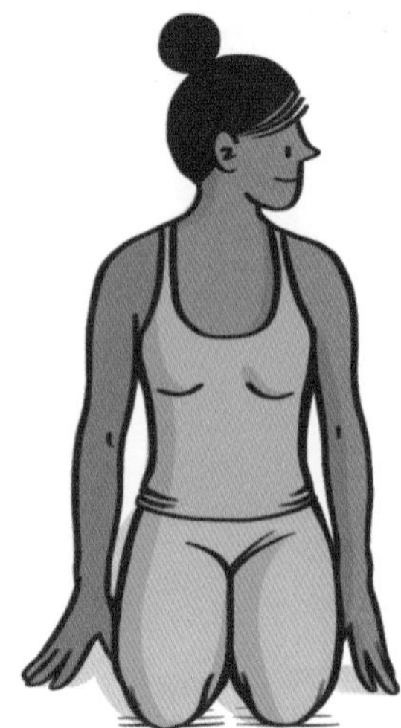

Figure 16.3 Gentle active cervical twist.

in the region of 70 to 90 degrees. It will also be altered by regular activity. For example, sport swimmers who perform front crawl often have better neck rotation because the breathing pattern dictates that they turn their head a lot. I would say that many office-based workers have a rotation ability nearer 70 to 80 degrees. This means that when the head is turned in a twist, the chin won't reach the line of the shoulder. The rest can be made up with the eyes but doesn't look so good in Instagram pics. By the by, I once met a lady who could turn her head about 110 degrees and extend it easily 90 degrees (average is 70 degrees), most bizarre, reminded me of a snake. I also met another lady who could lick her own elbow, but that is a story for another day. Try it now.

I think we should, as much as possible, aim toward twisting around the vertical axis of the spine and not unintentionally introduce flexion. It may seem that when the spine is rounded, a greater degree of rotation can be achieved, but I feel that this is probably due to the lumbar facet joints (between the articulating processes) allowing more rotation because the flexion has pulled them more open. Taking the twist down into the lumbar area could then make the intervertebral discs and lumbar ligaments more vulnerable. There are several instances when spinal flexion might be unnecessarily introduced into the shape of a pose, including a student's proportions, when binding around a leg, if the pelvis is tilted sideways, and in

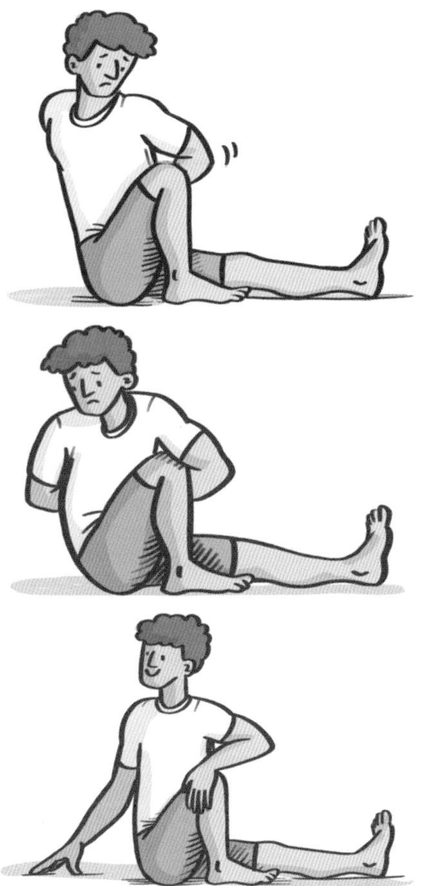

Figure 16.4 Do you remember Doug from the early chapters? His long torso means it is healthier for him not to try and bind.

multi-plane movements (Figure 16.4). We will think of these next.

When we considered individuality, we introduced the idea that a proportionally longer torso would mean that the student would likely not be able to bind in twisting postures such as *Marichyasana C* without hunching down and detrimentally rounding the back. It would be better instead to hug the knee and sit up straight. A posture such as the simple supine twist that is not influenced by proportions would make an ideal alternative. The same will go for standing postures if the lower body is longer. Without props, such as a block to place the hand on, more hip flexion may be called for, and if not available, the student would have to flex the spine to reach the floor (imagine *Parivrtta Trikonasana*).

If there is something to twist around, like a leg (e.g., *Marichyasana C & D*), we want to consider where it is in relation to our center line. If the leg is in line with the hip, then it would be necessary to flex the spine to reach past the leg. I think it is advisable to take the leg to be bound around across to the center line of the body. Ideally, the twisting action would then take the shoulder clear of the leg, allowing for a comfortable bind. In this way, the spine can rotate about its vertical axis. Sometimes the leg may resist being moved to the desired location either due to hip muscles resisting adduction or a less than ideal *Ardha Padmasana* foot placement. If this is the case, then hugging the leg is again the preferred option. In my opinion, there are no marks for getting into a posture by any means, it is all about the quality of the chosen positioning.

The pelvis is the seat for the spine, so as it moves, the orientation of the spine will change also. The pelvis might be thought to be unlevel if laterally tilted (one side lifted) or rotated (one side forward) (Figure 16.5). We are not referring here to postural dissymmetry of the pelvis but rather when the pelvis has been moved. In Chapter 14, *Hip Rotations*, we discussed how insufficient external hip rotation in *Ardha Padmasana* causes lateral flexion of the spine due to an uneven pelvis. It is also possible for the sit bone to lift as one leg is brought in and the foot placed near the hip, for example, *Marichyasana C*. So now we might consider that flexion could be added into the mix if reaching forward or across from that laterally tilted position.

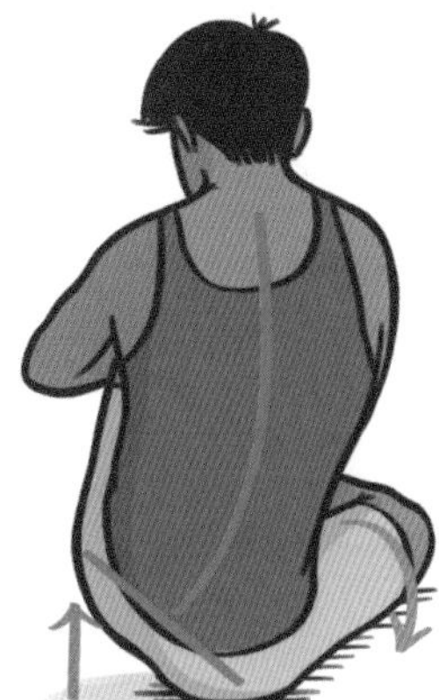

Figure 16.5 Vihan's spine is laterally flexing because his pelvis is so uneven.

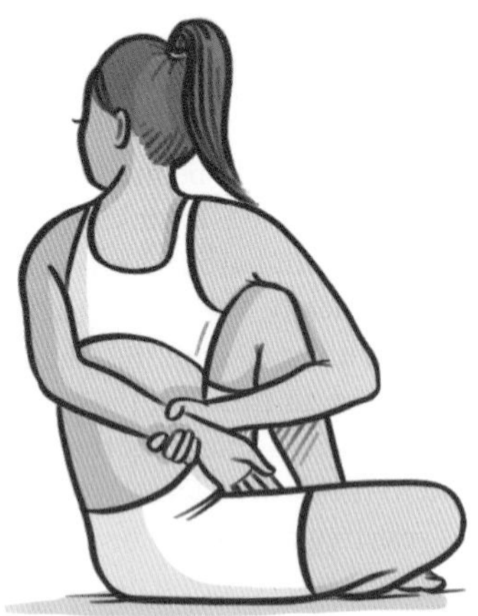

Figure 16.6 Victoria is being lazy here and letting her pelvis drop back.

Another positioning I have observed quite a lot, is to allow the pelvis to drop back when twisting (Figure 16.6). This may again seem to make the twist easier, but I think for the same reasons mentioned above. If there is a posterior tilt to the pelvis, the lumbar spine will round, and the facet joints will be more open. I feel then it is more advisable to keep the pelvis neutral and sit tall.

It is easy to oversimplify things and think the pelvis should always be aligned to the front or side of the yoga mat. Although this makes for easy cueing and in many symmetrical postures may well be the case, in some circumstances, it is acceptable or even desirable to have a rotated pelvis. Again, what is important is that we have chosen to do so rather than it happens through disconnectedness. In a forward bending posture, a rotated pelvis will usually result in a side bend and a more intense stretch on one side of the torso. Whereas in a twisting pose, a rotated pelvis can reduce the intensity of the twist. Let's consider some examples.

Paschimottanasana is a symmetrical forward bend, so if the pelvis is uneven, it might indicate a tensional pattern or postural issue. *Janu Sirsasana A* is an asymmetrical forward bend and the choice of keeping it level or not will alter the experience of the pose. If the pelvis is aligned parallel to the front of the mat when the bent leg is taken in, as the student takes their chest forward, there will be a minimum of lateral flexion introduced. The emphasis will be mostly on the back of the straight leg and the hip of the bent leg.

If, on the other hand, the hip of the bent leg is taken further back, then that side of the torso will have to lengthen more as the student moves toward the leg. Likewise, the destination of the chest will alter the amount of lateral flexion. If the center of the chest is taken to the outstretched leg, then lateral flexion will be introduced because the upper body also has to move to the side (Figure 16.7). There is no negative inference from introducing the lateral flexion in this circumstance because we are not twisting at the same time. However, did the student choose to take the hip back or did it happen to go back as they brought the bent leg into the inner thigh?

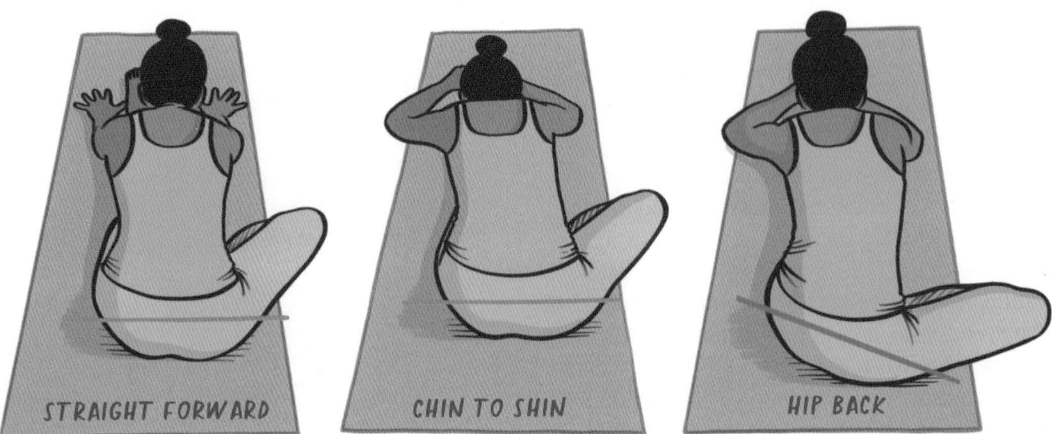

Figure 16.7 Taking the chest to the leg will introduce a bit of a side bend, but more so if the opposite hip is taken back.

If we use *Marichyasana C* again as an example, I think it is perfectly acceptable to choose not to keep the pelvis parallel to the front of the mat. We are not talking about lifting one side but taking one side back. So if the rotation is to the left, then the left sit bone could move back. The pelvis is starting the body turning, and the relationship between the lumbar spine and the pelvis can still be maintained. Less twisting of the spine happens overall because the body is turned in the direction of the twist (Figure 16.8). The same principle still applies that most of the twist will happen in the thoracic area. As the student's ability to twist increases, the pelvis can be brought back toward a squared position.

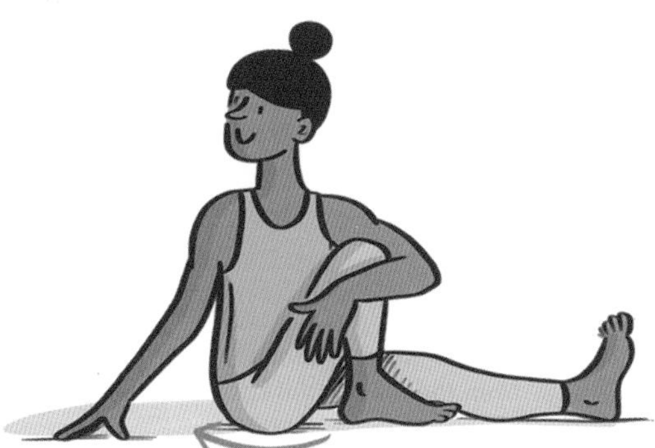

Figure 16.8 Myra has taken her right hip back and so needs less spinal twist.

The same sort of movement can happen in *Parivrtta Trikonasana* (Figure 16.9) and *Parivrtta Parsvakonasana* (Figure 16.10). In these examples, instead of the same side moving back, the opposite side of the pelvis moves toward the floor a little. The movement is the same, a turn of the pelvis toward the direction of the twist, but the orientation in space has changed. Again, while in the posture, the action can be to try and move back toward a level pelvis (up), at the same time, making sure any additional twist comes from the thoracic spine.

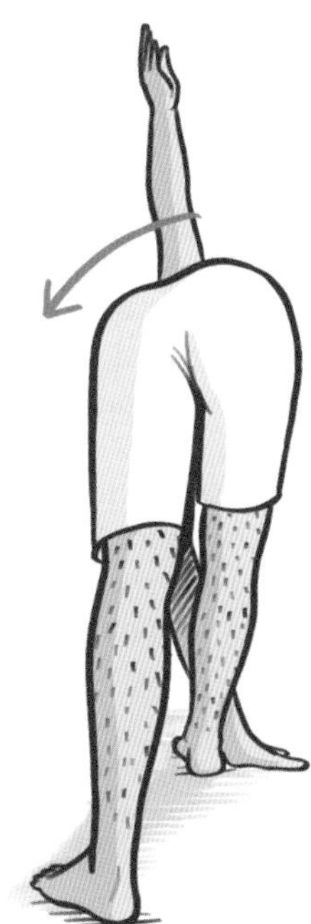

Figure 16.9 An uneven pelvis isn't always a bad thing.

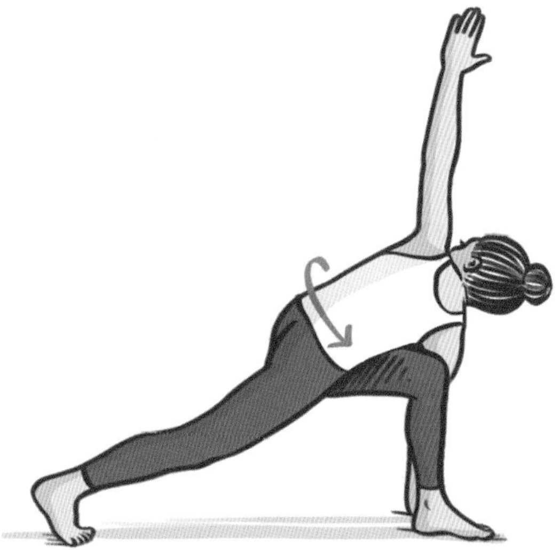

Figure 16.10 Here, the right hip is dropping, and so again, less spinal twist.

As before, there is a difference between tilting the pelvis without realizing and choosing to do so. In the first scenario, the student thinks they are twisting further than they really are and may also be less aware of the lumbar-sacrum-pelvis relationship. In the second scenario, awareness of the difficulty of twisting is established, and modification is being made to find a more comfortable position, knowing at the same time that the long-term goal is to move back toward the blueprint of the pose.

Parivrtta Parsvakonasana also has the potential for using the elbow outside the thigh as a lever. When a student can comfortably twist sufficiently in the thoracic spine to place the arm outside the front leg, then there isn't a problem. However, observing many classes, this is not very common. If the hand is away from the side of the foot, or it is a struggle to place it there, then that is a good sign that levering is taking place (Figure 16.11). A safeguard would be to allow the arm to cross in front of

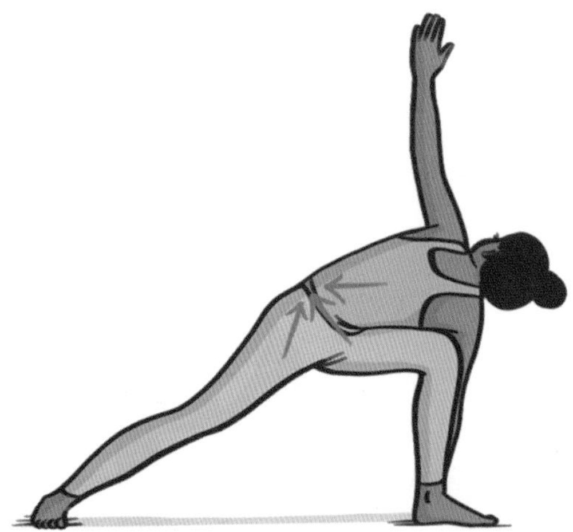

Figure 16.11 With the foot turned out and the arm on the other side of the knee, a levered twist has the potential to take stress into the SIJ.

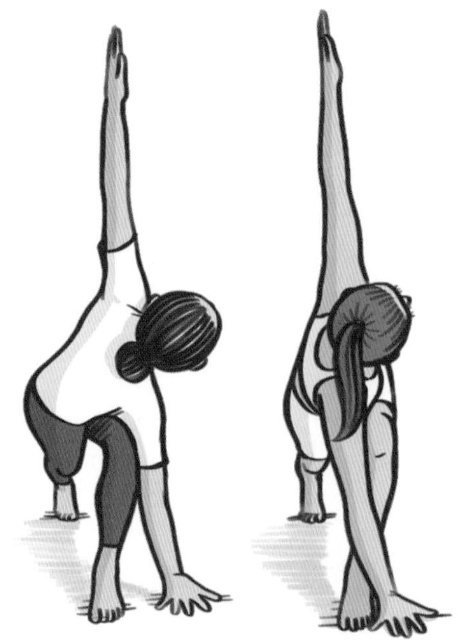

Figure 16.12 Trouble twisting shows up as the hand being placed away from the foot. In this case, it would be better to cross in front.

the shin rather than placing the shoulder on the outside of the knee (Figure 16.12).

We will now use the simple supine twist to reiterate the same concept. If the knees are stacked one on top of the other with kneecaps level, then the pelvis will be perpendicular to the floor. When that position is maintained and the far shoulder can also be grounded, a good twisting ability has been demonstrated. If the shoulder doesn't reach the floor and is left dangling in the air, then the weight of the body is used to increase the twist. It is also not very nice for the shoulder as the weight of the arm will be levering the shoulder joint (Figure 16.13). In this situation, it is better to let the top knee slide back and the pelvis rotate (top side goes back) to bring the shoulder down. If the legs come apart, then something can be put between them or under both.

When combining movements in different planes, it is harder to be precise and land up in the right place. This time we will use the example of *Parivrtta Trikonasana*. It makes a smooth movement to spiral down into this pose by taking an outreached arm forward and across the front leg, while at the same time, the pelvis tilts anteriorly and the spine rotates (Figure 16.14). However, what I usually observe is that students are less aware when the pelvis stops moving and introduce spinal flexion as they reach across. The giveaway is that the head and shoulders are no longer in line with the feet, but past the center line (Figure 16.15). I think a better line can be achieved by isolating the forward bend from the twist, even if one move blends into the next. The pelvis can be tilted forward, and the twist can be initiated while keeping the head over the front foot.

It is essential to appreciate the relationship of the lumbar spine, sacrum, and pelvis. If the three are moving in the same direction, then there won't be any torquing. Consequently, a squared pelvis combined with allowing too much rotational force to travel down from the desired thoracic area and into the lumbar and sacral area is potentially more detrimental than having a rotated pelvis. It is useful to get to grips with this concept so that different alignments can be assessed as to why the student

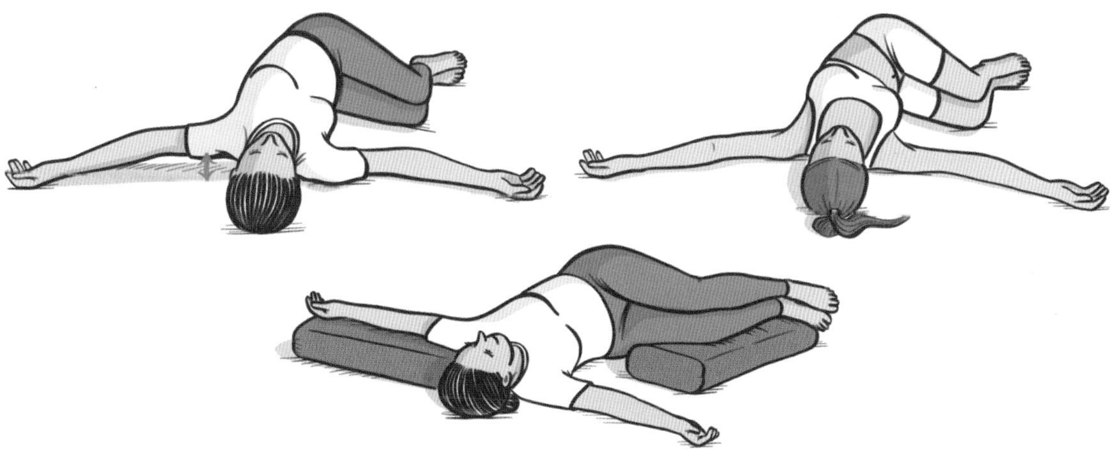

Figure 16.13 Victoria (right) has everything grounded, but if not, it is better to use propping than to have the shoulder or knees floating in the air.

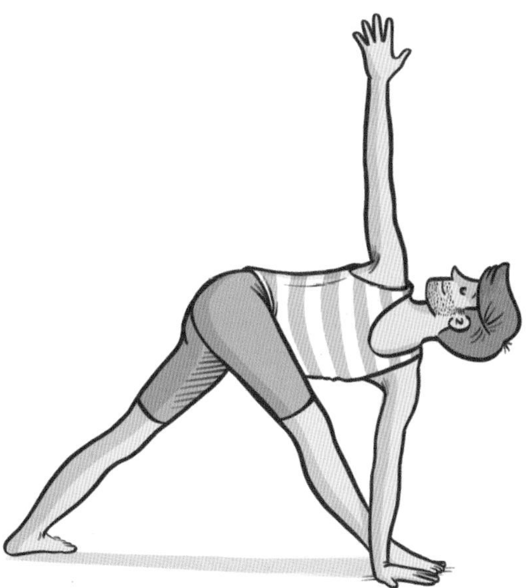

Figure 16.14 Parivrtta Trikonasana.

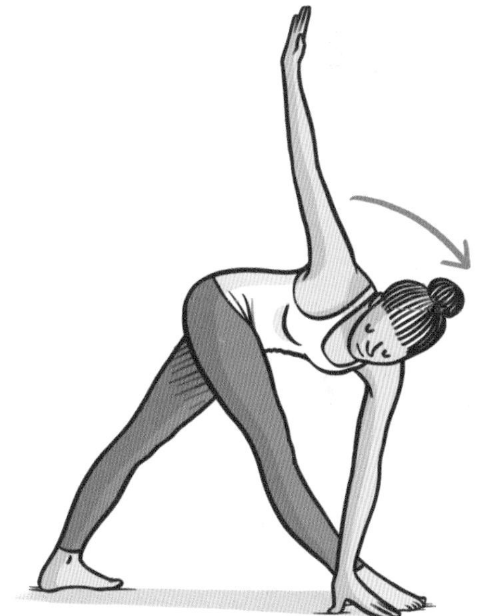

Figure 16.15 Next time you are in Trikonasana, *turn your head and look down at your foot to see if you have flexed the spine and traveled across the center line.*

has placed themselves in a particular way, as well as to appreciate any potentially harmful forces. At the same time, we don't want to encourage extreme rotations of the pelvis as this may introduce stress further down the chain (e.g., knee).

Although most of the twisting action happens in the thoracic area, tightness in the lower back can somewhat anchor the ribcage to the ilia and severely limit twisting prowess. Spasming or tight QLs and/or erector spinae will be the culprits, so aim to sort this area out before thinking of deep twists. If this is the case, it may be that some side bends before twisting poses might create more freedom.

In postures like *Pashasana* and *Parivrtta Ardha Chandrasana*, if a solid foundation can't be achieved, then it's dubious whether an uninhibited twist will happen. Instability and fear of falling will result in the body stiffening, especially if the twist results in the head looking at the ceiling. Turning the head often adds a fun challenge, but it is really fluff, so it would be better to get a decent twist with a less adventurous gaze before going for glory. One thing that works well when combining balance and gaze shifting is to trace a line with the eyes as you move the head.

If you are binding or reaching as well as twisting, then generally the shoulder girdle on the leading side protracts and on the trailing side retracts. However, this doesn't influence the twist in the spine as the scapulae just slide on the ribcage, serratus anterior doing the protraction work, and the rhomboids the retraction. I think if you over-exaggerate the protraction in a bind, it can make the shoulder jut forward, so think toward drawing that side back again to neutral once you are where you want to be. For example, when I am in *Marichyasana D*, I think of retracting both scapulae and opening across the front of the chest.

CHAPTER 17

Postures Involving the Shoulders

The shoulder has all the same movements available as the hip because it is a ball-and-socket joint, but also consider the shoulder girdle. I would say the most useful ROMs in relation to yoga are flexion and external rotation, followed by extension and medial rotation. The movements of abduction, adduction, and the horizontal variations, although used, are unlikely to be critical elements as far as creating postures go. However, for the shoulder girdle, I would say issues probably revolve more around weakness rather than flexibility.

Shoulder movements are generally components of a posture rather than the focus, as is the case in many backbends, when binding, or for inversions. However, there are postures that could be considered as specifically targeting the shoulders, such as *Garudasana* and *Gomukhasana*. Poses such as *Pincha Mayurasana* and Handstand, although not thought of as addressing the shoulders, will be compromised most by restrictions there.

What I find with many students is that they identify more easily with the hips and can often sense the restrictions around that area that stop them from going deeper. However, when it comes to the shoulders, there is generally some confusion as to what they need to work on, resulting in unspecific openers. But the shoulders follow the same fundamental "Key Concepts" as everywhere else. If you require more shoulder flexion, you need to do preparatory poses that target that movement, rather than random shoulder postures.

Assessing Flexion and Extension

There is a straightforward way of testing active shoulder flexion and extension using the wall. First, to evaluate flexion, stand with the back on the wall but with the feet about 8 in (20 cm) away with knees bent (Figure 17.1). Pull the ribcage down using the abdominals and flatten the low back against the wall. Place the back of the head on the wall as well. Make two fists, straighten the arms, and have the palms of the hands facing each other. Now, keeping the low back on the wall and the ribcage pulled down, take the arms overhead in an arc, only moving from the shoulders. Keep the arms parallel and let the shoulder girdle move up naturally. If the hands touch the wall without bending the elbow or tilting the wrist, it shows good ROM in that direction. On the other hand, the distance they stop from the wall is an indication of how challenging that movement is.

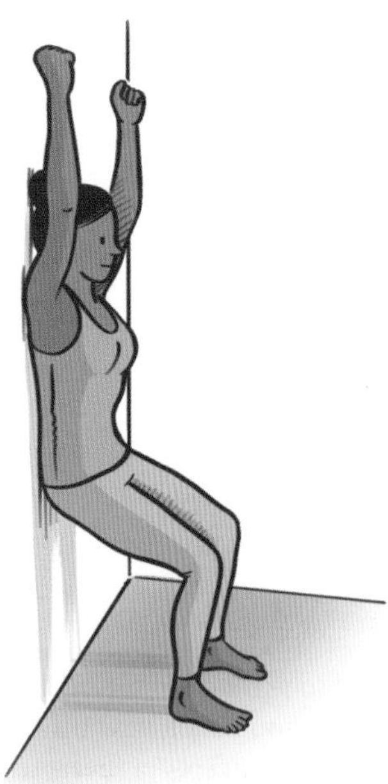

Figure 17.1 Where do the arms stop when ribcage is fixed?

To test active extension, turn to face the wall and place the forehead, ribcage, and thighs on the wall (Figure 17.2). With the same orientation of the arms used previously, take them in an arc toward the rear. The expectation for ROM in this direction might be somewhere between 40 and 90 degrees.

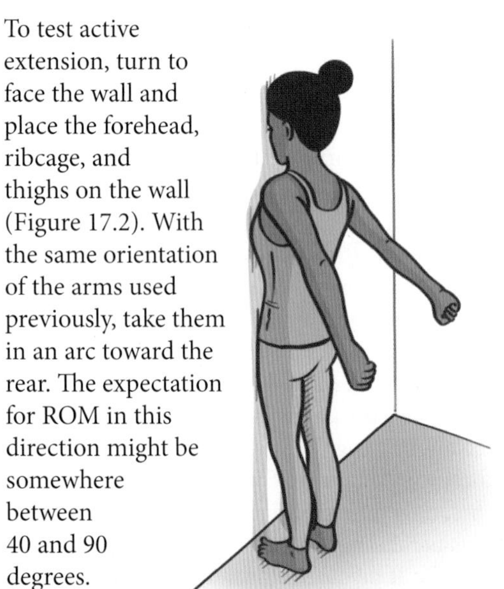

Figure 17.2 Shoulder extension test. Keep the pelvis, forehead, and chest on the wall.

To evaluate flexion passively, we can do something like *Uttana Shishosana* (Figures 17.3 & 17.4). The key here is to try and keep the spine in slight flexion as this will isolate the movement in the shoulder. The angle across the armpit can then be observed.

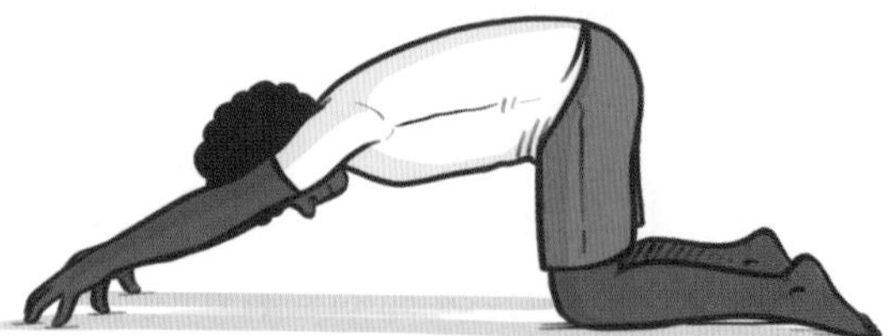

Figure 17.3 In this shoulder flexion exercise, Aren can't get a straight line through the armpit. This means he has restriction in this movement.

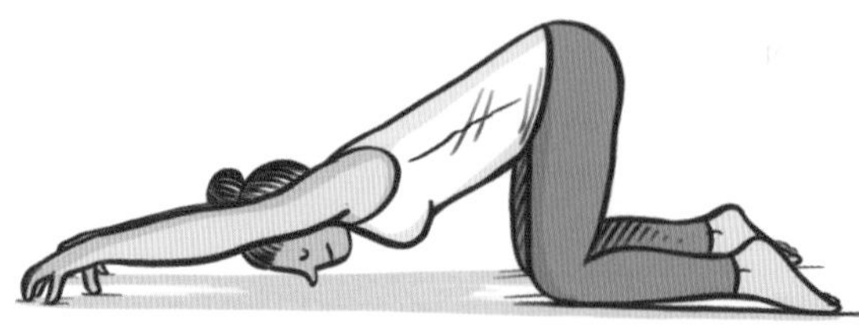

Figure 17.4 This movement is a lot easier for Sasha, and it will show up in postures that require shoulder flexion.

A handy test for extension is *Prasarita Padottanasana C*, although it only has the benefit of gravity rather than something to press against (Figure 17.5).

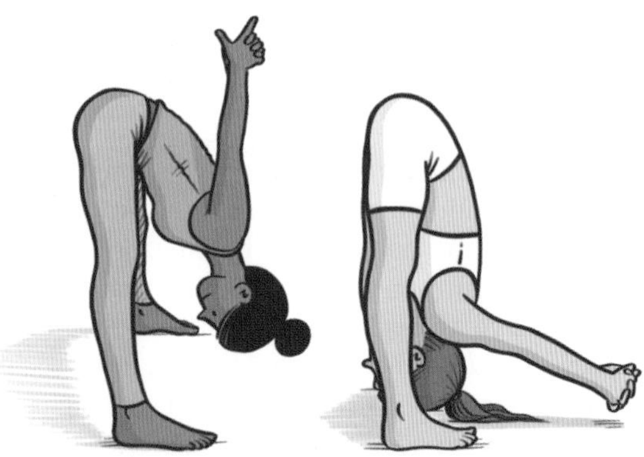

Figure 17.5 To observe the amount of shoulder extension available, we want to look at the arm torso angle, rather than how far forward they have gone (hip flexion).

Assessing External and Medial Rotation

When testing or working on rotation at the shoulder, we never want to move into a painful position. This goes for anywhere on the body, but the shoulder is particularly complicated and prone to impingement issues. Moving into pain will only increase soft tissue irritability. If these movements are found to be uncomfortable rather than just restricted, it is better to undertake a more in-depth functional assessment of the shoulder. Actually, the same goes for shoulder flexion.

Active external rotation can be evaluated starting in the same way as above with the back on the wall. This time the arms are kept close to the sides with the elbows bent 90 degrees (Figure 17.6). The backs of the hands are taken toward the wall, moving only from the shoulder. It is important to keep it strict by maintaining a pulled down ribcage and a straight line across the wrists. Someone who has plenty of external rotation available will touch the wall comfortably with their lower arms (Figure 17.7). More restricted individuals will find they stop someway short. Extending your wrists (tilting your fists back) doesn't count, by the way.

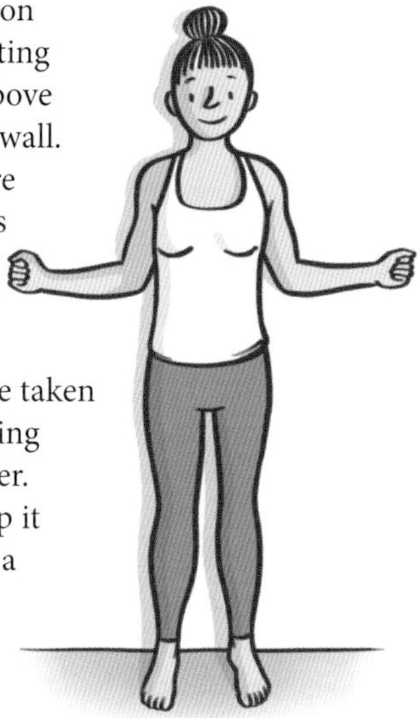

Figure 17.6 Keep the elbows close to the sides and externally rotate at the shoulder.

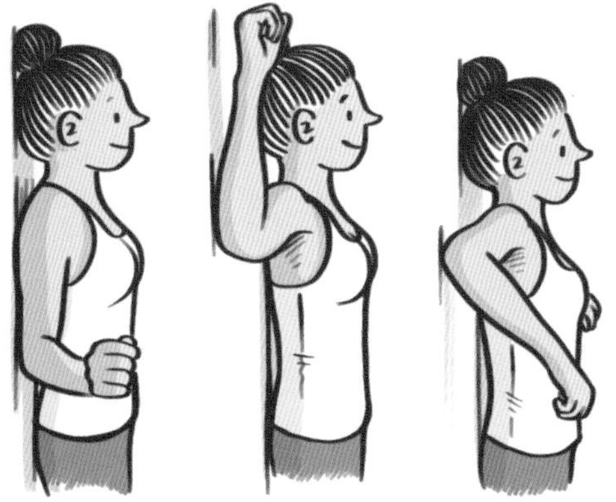

Figure 17.7 External rotation can be assessed or actively worked either with elbows by the sides or in line with the shoulders.

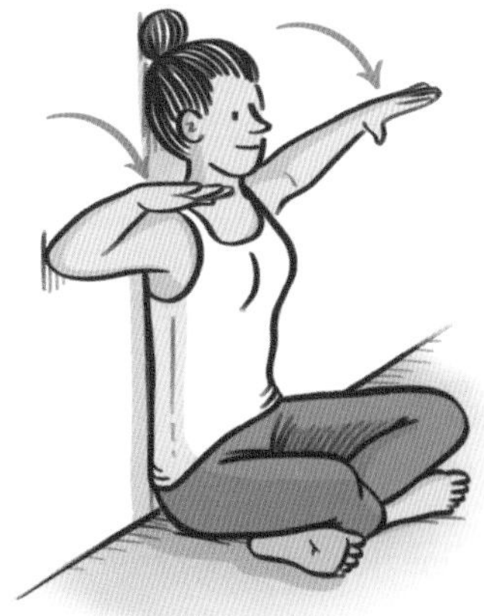

Figure 17.8 Moving toward the floor is medial rotation. All exercises can be done standing or sitting but keep the spine neutral.

For medial rotation, we can use the same wall position but shift the arms to shoulder height (Figure 17.8). The start position is with the elbows bent to 90 degrees, shoulders externally rotated, and back of the forearms on the wall. This position may again highlight if external rotation is a challenge, but they don't have to be on the wall to start as we are testing in the opposite direction. The lower arm then moves in an arc toward the floor while keeping the elbows at shoulder height and on the wall. If they stop before parallel with the floor, then it demonstrates a significant restriction. It is important not to let the scapula to rotate off the back (Figure 17.9).

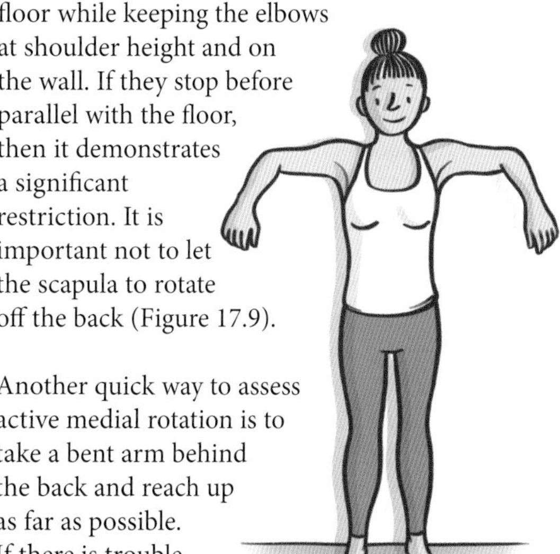

Figure 17.9 Keep the scapulae on the wall and wrists straight.

Another quick way to assess active medial rotation is to take a bent arm behind the back and reach up as far as possible. If there is trouble touching the bottom of the opposite scapula, then this reveals difficulty with this movement. On the other hand, some students will be able to place their lower arm up their spine with the fingertips reaching to C7 or further. It is a good idea also to observe the scapula here because if the medial border markedly comes away from the ribcage, then the movement is achieved not just at the shoulder joint (GHJ).

Although this test also involves the shoulder moving into some extension, I think it is relevant to the way the movement is mostly used in yoga, such as when binding, Reverse Prayer, or *Gomukhasana* arms.

Assessing Flexion and External Rotation

In the same way that medial rotation seems to be used mostly in combination with extension, flexion is often combined with external rotation, although not in quite the same way. Here I often use the phrase "moving into flexion while maintaining external rotation," but this is not really correct. For the most part, what is needed to keep desirable alignment in yoga postures is to resist the shoulder from moving into medial rotation, and hence the elbows going out, so the arm is trying to be kept neutral.

As we covered in Chapter 11, *Shoulder*, there are big muscles, such as latissimus dorsi and pectoralis major, whose secondary action of medial rotation may be exhibited when taken into a stretch. Also, there are the smaller muscles that perform medial rotation, subscapularis and teres major, which will also be placed under a stretch as the shoulder is taken into flexion. Evaluating the combined movement will give a good indication of what is likely to happen in postures such as *Urdhva Dhanurasana* and *Pincha Mayurasana*. If a student already demonstrated difficulty getting the lower arms to the wall in the external rotation test, then they will also have trouble with this one.

For this assessment, we need something to keep the arms at shoulder width. Using two large blocks normally works well. Remember, of course, that individuals will have different width shoulders, so it may be necessary to make some adjustments. The priority is to isolate the shoulder movement and not take the spine into extension, which, as before, means keeping the ribcage pulled down. I have found that using a helper ensures strictness.

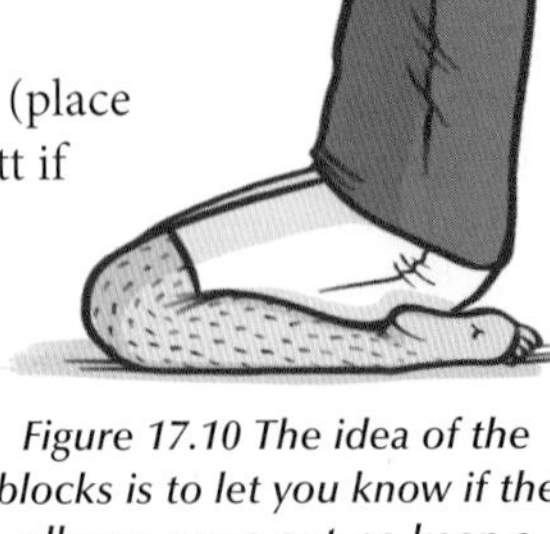

Figure 17.10 The idea of the blocks is to let you know if the elbows move out, so keep a strong grip with the forearms on the blocks.

Start sitting on the heels (place something under the butt if necessary), place the two blocks between the forearms and hands, with elbows bent to 90 degrees (Figure 17.10). The blocks can be oriented to suit the width of the shoulders, but for most students, the longest sides will be going across.

The helper places one hand on the lower ribs (below the chest) and the other between the shoulder blades. The hand on the back should be higher than the one on the ribs. Now moving from the shoulder only and keeping the elbows bent, the arms are taken over the head. More restricted students will find the elbows being pulled away from the blocks as the arms move upward. This needs to be resisted, and a firm grip of the blocks maintained. An individual with above-average ROM will be able to take their elbows to face the ceiling. At the other end of the scale, I have seen students that only manage to get the arms halfway up, demonstrating a very restricted ROM in this combined movement. These students will face problems with any posture that heavily draws upon this particular ROM.

Increasing Shoulder Flexion

In Chapter 11, *Shoulder*, we introduced the idea of working on active shoulder flexion during the Sun Salutation. This same principle can be used in a whole variety of positions where the arms are over the head. As mentioned, the key to isolating the shoulders is to keep the ribcage still. Many body placements can be used for both active and passive work. One of my favorites, as it doesn't require any equipment, is simply placing both hands on the wall and taking the chest toward the floor (Figure 17.11). I think it is worth trying different heights and widths with the hands to see what feels intense. It is possible to be very passive in this position or to work on pulling yourself deeper actively. I have also found it helpful to strongly push the wall away as you move the chest toward the floor. Maintaining a slight rounding of the spine will ensure the focus stays in the shoulders.

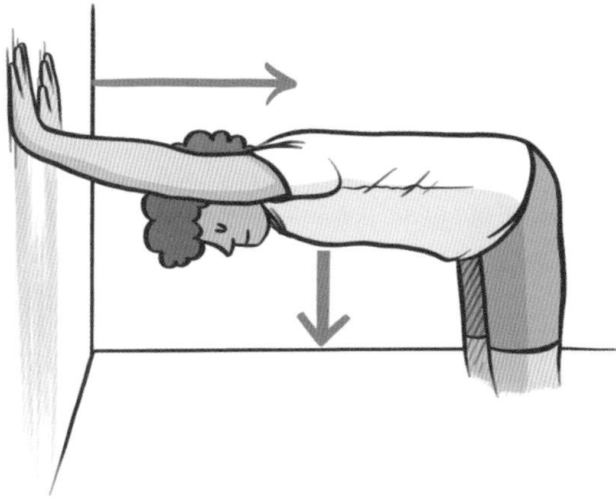

Figure 17.11 Keeping the arms straight, push away from the wall at the same time as trying to take the chest in the direction of the floor.

Another popular placement is lying supine over a block placed between the shoulder blades. I have discovered more comfort can be experienced by switching the block for a roller or bolster. Here again, the arms can be actively pulled toward the floor or for a more passive experience, a wooden block or another weighted object can be held (Figure 17.12). It is also possible to combine the assistance of the weight with muscle engagement. The tendency is for the back to arch over the block, so it makes it very strict if the knees are pulled to the chest.

Often the upper back and shoulders are combined in one exercise, so for example in the exercise just

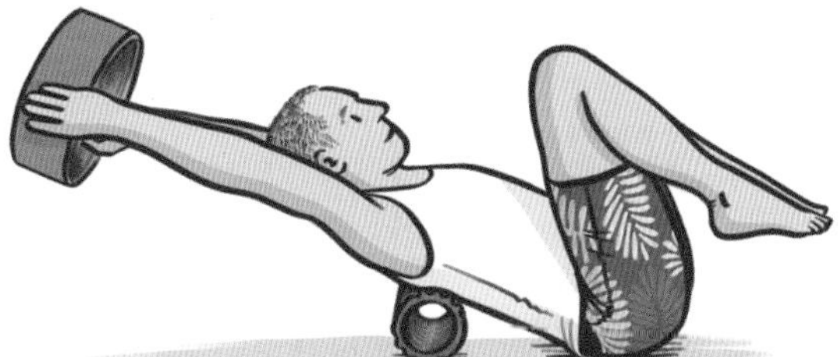

Figure 17.12 Bringing the knees up isolates the shoulders better.

detailed it is possible to alternate between letting the ribs flare and pulling them down.

When doing openers with straight arms, I think it is harder to control the external rotation. If the object is to work on the combined movement of "moving into flexion while maintaining external rotation" then, as with our evaluation test, bent arms and a spacer will prove useful. Another go-to exercise is the "butcher's block," where a strap just above the elbows and a block between the hands keeps the arms parallel to each other. With the elbows on a raised platform, such as a chair or table, the chest can be taken toward the floor (Figure 17.13). Of course, the same principle applies, to isolate the work in the shoulders, the back would be kept slightly rounded.

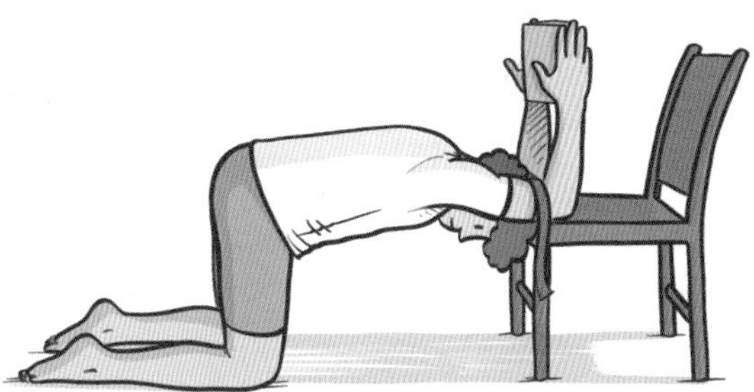

Figure 17.13 Butcher's block or block and strap work if you don't like that imagery.

We have mentioned that pectoralis major and latissimus dorsi can cause the shoulder to medially rotate as the arms are taken above the head, and they can also resist flexion. The ideal way to place pectoralis major under a stretch is with the arms in a cactus shape. I much prefer using a bent arm because I think it removes potential stress from the elbow.

There are two variations that I use most often, one on the wall and the other on the floor. The principle is to introduce horizontal abduction by turning the body away from a fixed arm. For both versions, the starting position is to have the upper arm at 90 degrees (or slightly more) to the torso. With the arm on the wall, the body can be lunged forward, or on the floor, it is turned away using the assistance of the leg and opposite hand (Figure 17.14).

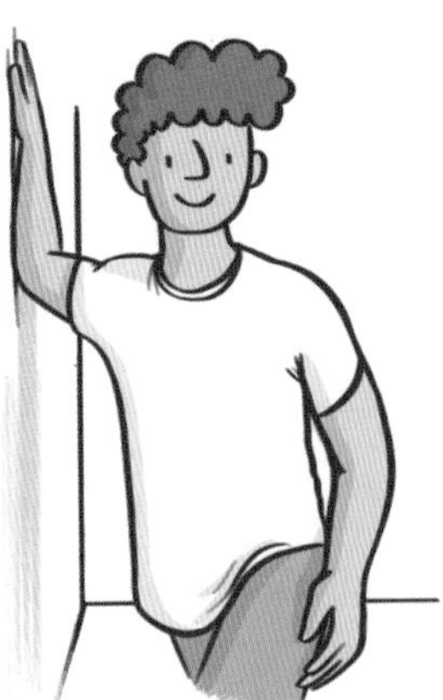

Figure 17.14 This can be done with a straight arm, but I feel it can take some stress into the elbow, so I prefer a bent arm, with the elbow the same height as the shoulder.

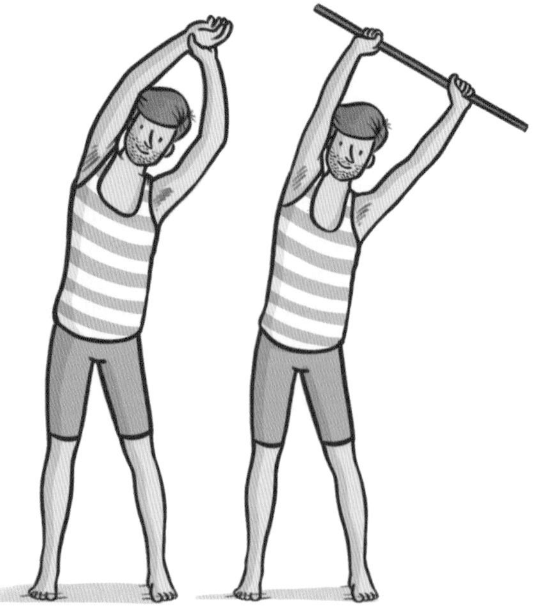

Figure 17.15 When trying to isolate the latissimus dorsi as against the whole side of the body, keep the hips square and reach out of the pelvis. Bring the arm of the outer curve closer to the head.

To access latissimus dorsi, the body needs to be taken into a side bend, focusing on hips to fingertips (or elbow), and to avoid accessing the QL, it is necessary to make sure that the shoulder plays a large part in the movement by taking the arm toward the center line and keeping it externally rotated (Figure 17.15). An easily accessible version is to take one arm over the head, bring the biceps next to the ear, grasp the wrist with the opposite hand and then move into a side bend. Although not always available, I find a deeper stretch can be achieved when holding on to something like a pole or pillar and hanging away from it.

Increasing Medial Rotation

For active work, the same position can be adopted as for our wall test, trying to draw the lower arms deeper through the arc while maintaining strict form. The same exercise can be performed in a lying position, with the hips flexed and feet on the floor to flatten the spine (Figure 17.16).

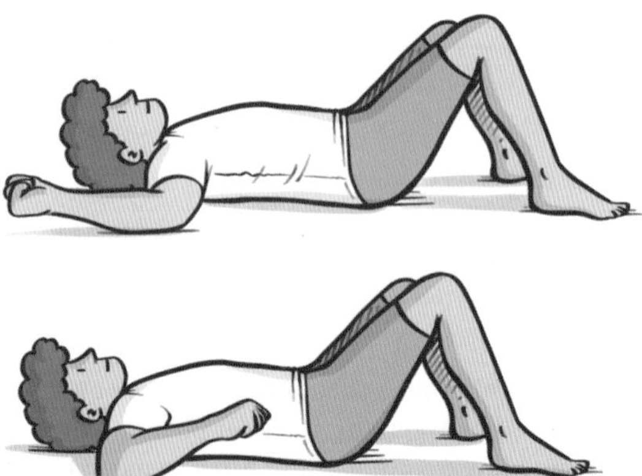

Figure 17.16 If you are restricted in medial rotation, this can be a way to actively work that movement. Keep the shoulder down.

Another useful exercise is to come into *Gomukhasana* with a strap between the hands. Now a contract-relax technique can be used. First, walk the lower hand up the strap as far as is comfortable. Now using no more than 30 percent

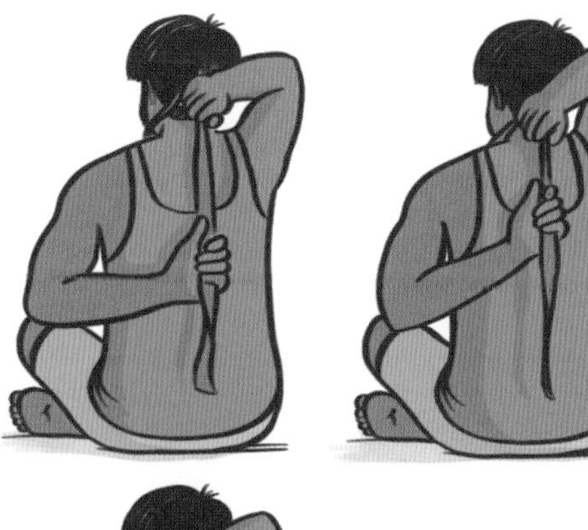

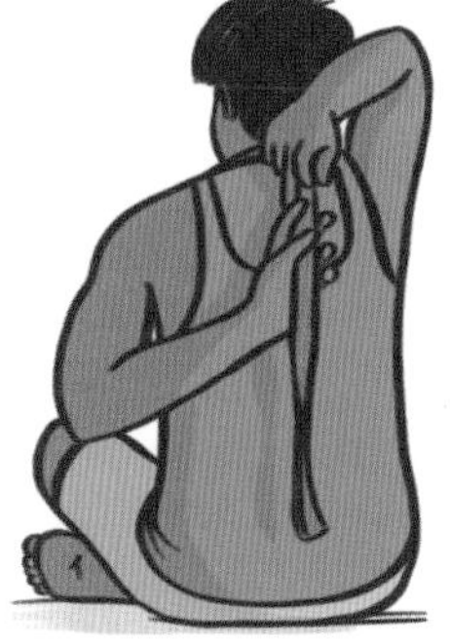

Figure 17.17 Gradually work the hand up the strap after each repetition. It is important not to experience any pain.

effort, pull the lower arm down while providing enough resistance with the upper arm that no movement occurs. Maintain this work for 8 to 10 seconds and then walk the lower hand further up the strap (Figure 17.17). This can be repeated for three cycles. As mentioned above, if this creates pain, it should not be done.

Increasing Extension

This is a movement where I feel large ROM has limited real-world application. I also mentioned in Chapter 11, *Shoulder*, that it is easy to take stress into the ACJ. For this reason, I would mostly advise working actively to take the arm behind the body. The shoulders often have a tendency to ride up around the ears, so keep the shoulder girdle depressed.

Hanging

An exercise that has found popularity in recent years is hanging. Not only will it help to stretch some of the muscles restricting shoulder flexion but also, over time, may help create some space under the acromion process. It will improve grip strength, provide mild traction to the spine, and may help with wrist discomfort.

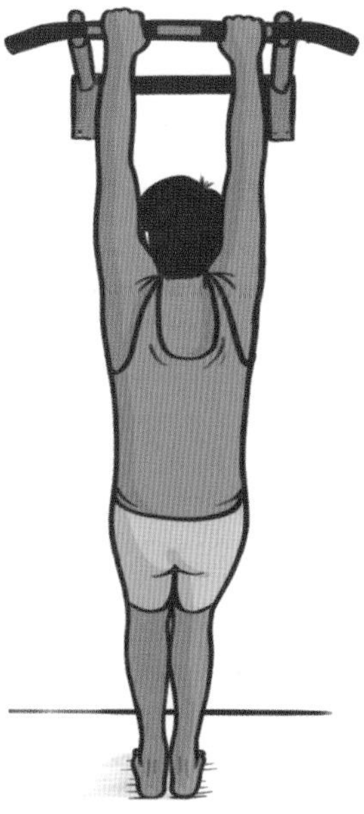

Figure 17.18 The feet can take some weight.

It is normally sufficient to start by keeping the feet on the floor, otherwise it won't be very long before you can't hold on anymore. Some people work toward several minutes but be happy initially to hold for closer to 30 seconds. From what I understand, it seems to be more beneficial to have short hanging periods dotted throughout the day rather than one longer session. Keep a tight overhand grip on the bar, and as the hand starts to open, come down (Figure 17.18). Hanging can be performed both actively and passively. If you are suffering from an upper body injury, such as in the shoulder or wrist, seek professional advice first.

With the passive hang (Figure 17.19A), the grip is tight, but the rest of the body is relaxed. The arms

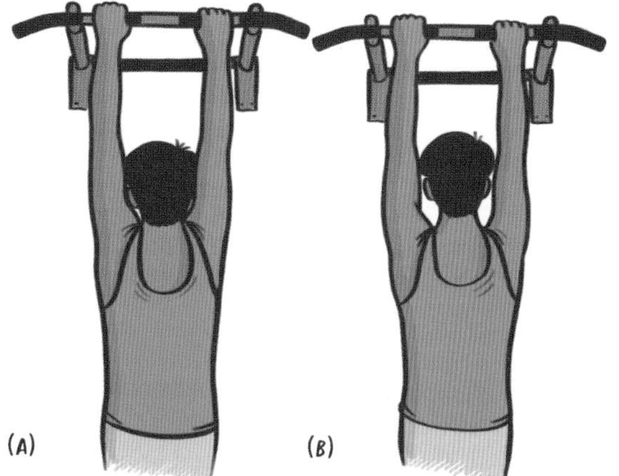

Figure 17.19 Passive (A) and active (B) hanging. Pull the shoulder girdle down for active hanging. Keep a tight grip for both.

are straight, hands shoulder-width apart, and the shoulder girdle is allowed to elevate. If you are already very flexible around the shoulders or have a tendency toward hypermobility, it would be sensible to do the active hang instead.

In the active hang (Figure 17.19B), the same body position is kept as in the previous example except for the shoulder girdle being pulled down. Again, the elbows don't bend, and the back doesn't arch. There are a lot more varieties of hanging techniques, so if this is something that interests you, it would be worth researching the subject further.

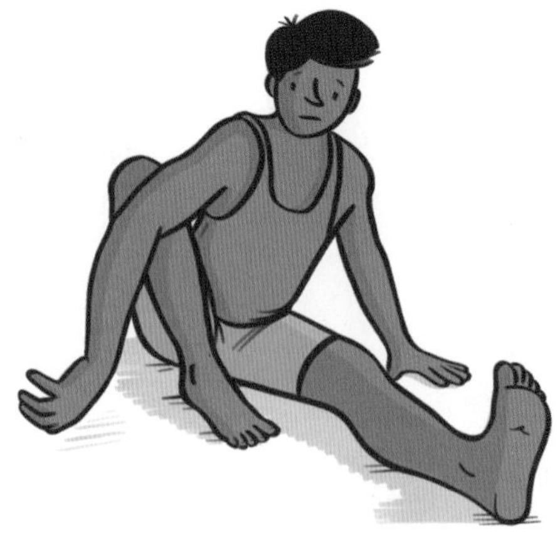

Figure 17.20 Normally an inability to bind is due to proportion or hip flexibility rather than a shoulder restriction.

Binding

It is very common for students to have difficulty binding, and often they blame restrictions in the shoulder. Unlike the Reverse Prayer positions, I feel most students have enough ROM at the shoulder to bind. What they are lacking is the ROM in other areas, such as the hips, to get them in the right position to bind, or their proportions are the issue.

We can use *Marichyasana A* as an example. The shin of the bent leg needs to be in the armpit of the binding arm so that the shoulder is free to rotate. If the torso cannot be taken far enough forward, then the shin lands up somewhere on the upper arm between the elbow and shoulder. In this position, the upper arm is pushed outward rather than being allowed to travel backward, so it comes down to lack of mobility in the hips rather than the shoulder.

On the other hand, the student may be able to position their shoulder in the right place but if they have a stockier body type, with thicker legs and torso, and shorter arms, then they will have trouble just because there is more to get around (Figure 17.20). Time for a strap.

Students reporting discomfort at the front of the shoulder when in bound positions is also widespread. This is often experienced in postures like Reverse Prayer and *Gomukhasana*. I feel the discomfort comes about due to an over-emphasis of medial rotation of the shoulder, causing some impingement. Quite regularly, it can also be observed that the top of the humerus is jutting forward and there is a deep crease between that and the chest. Next, I will detail an alternative approach to binding that I think most students will find more beneficial.

Taking *Ardha Baddha Padmottanasana* as an example, the arm wraps around the body to take hold of the foot. This is definitely one of those postures that I refer to as "congestion around the front of the shoulder." Generally, students just roll the shoulder medially and take the arm behind the back. Here is what I would suggest instead.

After the foot has been placed in the hip crease, the shoulder is rolled *externally* (Figure 17.21A). It helps initially to turn the forearm outward (supinate) at the same time so the hand faces away from the body, as it assists in getting enough rotation at the shoulder. While maintaining the external rotation, the shoulder is then extended as much as possible (Figure 17.21B). This positioning is held while the forearm is now rotated medially (pronated) so that the hand faces to the rear (Figure 17.21C). The fourth step is to flex the elbow (Figure 17.21D), which will bring the arm behind the waist. Lastly, the hand can be slid the rest of the way to take hold of the foot by adducting the shoulder (think of elbow moving toward the center of the back), Figure 17.21E. At the same time, make sure the openness across the front of the chest and shoulder is not lost.

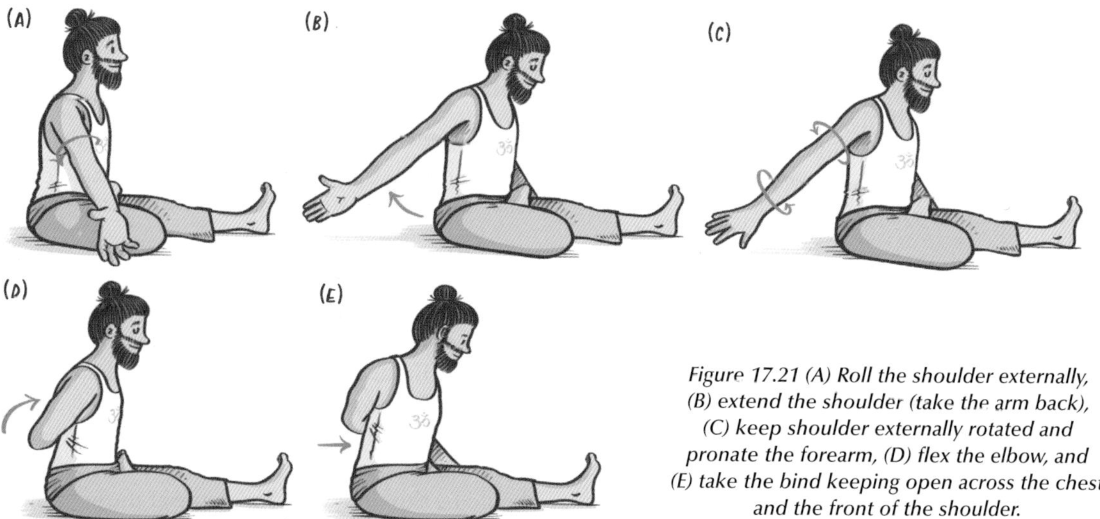

Figure 17.21 (A) Roll the shoulder externally, (B) extend the shoulder (take the arm back), (C) keep shoulder externally rotated and pronate the forearm, (D) flex the elbow, and (E) take the bind keeping open across the chest and the front of the shoulder.

Of course, this example uses a posture involving *Ardha Padmasana*, so safe placement of the foot is still essential. In addition, if the foot is not placed correctly, it may well put it out of reach.

Exactly the same technique can be used for *Gomukhasana* and Reverse Prayer. It might not be possible to stick to this sequence precisely when binding around a leg, such as with *Marichyasana C*, but the move can certainly be initiated with an external rotation rather than medial.

Upper Body Strength

Some postures, such as arm balances, definitely need upper body strength, but this section is about trying to create some balance in the body. Due to the easy access to food for the majority of our species, without the need to hunt, forage, or till the land, most people are weaker than they should be unless they actively seek out strength work. As I travel around yoga studios, what I come across, very often, are students who are particularly weak in the upper body. Barring injury, I feel as a bare minimum we should be able to support our body weight, whether on straight or bent arms. This is not only necessary with respect to making transitions and supported positions safer but also for overall body integrity.

If a student cannot hold a plank or lower themselves down from High Plank to *Chaturanga* under control without putting the knees down, then they are not strong enough. This doesn't mean that everyone should have their knees off the floor for this transition, but it is a wake-up call that there is some work to be done. Of course, there will be times that extra care needs to be taken to assess the appropriate intensity when, for example, working with the elderly or injured.

Chaturanga seems to be the go-to exercise when yoga students think of strengthening the upper body, but it is not sufficient on its own. Remember that strength is direction-specific as well as muscle-specific, so the *Chaturanga* position and transition needs to be only one element of a broader approach to strengthening the upper body. Side planks, Bird Dog, Supported Handstand, and shoulder girdle stabilization drills (introduced further on) are just some examples of adding variety. There are also many opportunities to challenge the shoulder muscles when not using the arms to support oneself. An example might be to hold *Virabhadrasana B* for longer, because this will build stamina due to the outstretched arms. In *Virabhadrasana A*, the arms can be squeezed toward the ears. This might be quite simple for students who have less restriction around the shoulder, but otherwise, it can be a considerable amount of active work.

Chaturanga Dandasana

Although *Chaturanga* gets a bad rap for causing shoulder injuries, I think that these are most likely to be due to either bad technique, muscular strength, and ROM imbalances, or perhaps too much repetition.

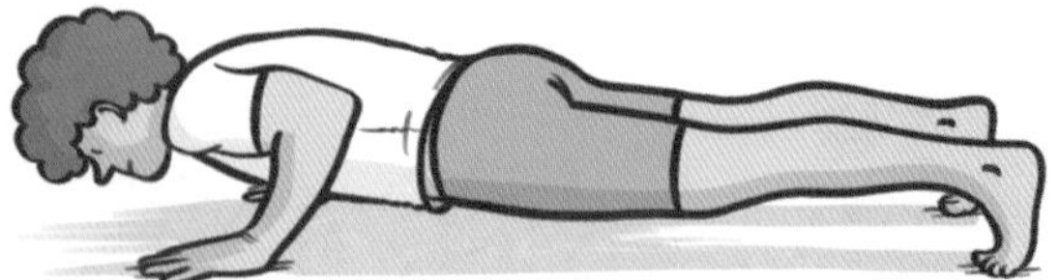

Figure 17.22 You might notice the elbow is behind the wrist, and we will cover that in a minute.

There are many different thoughts on the lower down to *Chaturanga*, generally focused around achieving a specific position at the bottom, so let's first consider what the *Chaturanga* position itself might look like.

I mentioned above that I feel *Chaturanga* needs to be done off the knees if possible. The explanation for this is that the core integration and leg activation experienced are nowhere near the same when the knees are down. The challenge is much reduced, and from what I have witnessed, students seem to get stuck forever on their knees once it has been introduced. The reasons behind not progressing are probably to do with the on-knee option not being difficult enough to cause muscular strength adaptation and the jump in workload needed to be off the knees.

Of course, it is unfair to expect weak students to be able to hold the bottom position straight away, so there must be some form of progressions. I would suggest, rather than starting a student on their knees, swap it for not going so low instead. In this way, the depth can be increased as strength, control, and stability gains are made. Even before an attempt to lower is encouraged, a solid High Plank is crucial. We will come back to the High Plank in a moment.

It is important to be strong and stable in the chosen lowest position. Especially until strength has improved, it is imperative to stop in a position that can be held for several breaths without gravity forcing a continuation of the downward journey. For those particularly precarious students, it is worth using a bolster to lower toward. Whatever the depth of travel, the elbow should maintain a position close to the body, but without clamping it (Figure 17.22). I often use the description of feeling the inner arms brushing the sides of the ribcage.

Regularly, *Chaturanga* is used as a transition rather than a position that is held, but in this scenario, it is easy to avoid the work by stopping short and being in the work zone for no more than a moment. To effectively initiate strength changes, we must draw on our understanding that time under tension is crucial. As a transition, the lower down should be slow and include a pause at the bottom position. Quicker improvements will be made if the *Chaturanga* position is held for 5 to 10 breaths at a depth that presents a significant challenge.

The major disagreements voiced concerning how *Chaturanga* should be performed are to do with the relationship of shoulders to elbows and elbows to wrists, as well as how low one should go. There is a tendency to prefer positions of stacked joints and specific angles because it makes teaching cues easier, and the body often has less muscular work to do when the joints are stacked. However, we are not always looking to make exercises easier and to elicit change; we need to find the positions that make the body work. What we do want to consider is whether a particular positioning places the body in a vulnerable state. But as we have mentioned before, even that is not straightforward because, with the right strength and stability, we can find integrity and safety in challenging positions and may even choose to seek them out. What I will do next is to present what I feel are the important aspects of *Chaturanga* and consequently, how that might determine the alignment.

If we isolate the *Chaturanga* position from any transition for the moment, I feel the following points will provide substantial body integration and adequate challenge (Figure 17.23). Heels over balls of the feet, thighs and abdomen engaged, straight body with no sagging or buckling, shoulders protracted but with a broad chest, elbows over

STRONG STRAIGHT BODY
HEELS OVER BALL OF FOOT
REACHING OUT THROUGH
THE TOP OF THE HEAD
REACHING OUT
THROUGH THE
HEELS
LOOKING STRAIGHT DOWN
THIGHS AND BELLY ENGAGED
ELBOWS BEHIND WRISTS

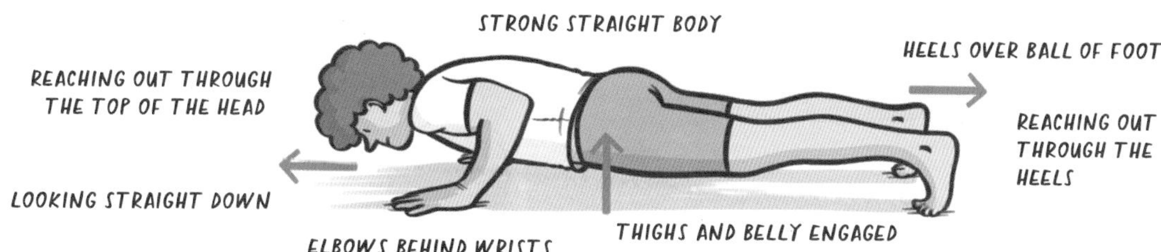

Figure 17.23 Substantial body integration and adequate challenge can be achieved by following these points.

wrists if at 90 degrees or behind if lower, arms close to the body, and head neutral. If the elbows are kept over the wrists, and the bend increased more than 90 degrees, the shoulders would go below the elbows and would also have to move into extension. This positioning might be too much strain on the front of the shoulders for some individuals. Therefore, I would suggest that if you want to take a low *Chaturanga* position, just hovering over the ground, it would be preferable to take the elbows back as far as is necessary to keep them at the same height as the shoulders.

In a High Plank, the initial positioning of shoulders over wrists and heels over balls of the feet is important. The shoulder girdle should be protracted (wrapping the shoulder blades around the body) but without taking the head toward the floor or exaggerating the thoracic curve. This maintains broadness across the chest. The head can be kept neutral, which is more pleasant for the cervical spine, as well as allowing for the opposing forces of reaching away in two directions, from the top of the head and the heels. The thighs should be engaged, and if there is a tendency toward an increased lordotic curve, a mild tucking of the tailbone can be introduced (Figure 17.24).

Figure 17.24 High Plank ideal positioning points.

I like to envisage a straight stick from the head all the way to the heels. The butt up in the air means some core work is being escaped from because it is a much easier position to hold than a straight body. The belly sagging toward the floor indicates more engagement between the ribs and pubic bone is required. I think it is better to make sure a clean and stable High Plank can be held for 5 to 10 breaths before incorporating the lower down. This will ensure that when lowering is attempted, there will be enough strength to hold the shoulder girdle position and allow the arms to move independently.

When lowering from the High Plank to *Chaturanga*, only the arms need to move. The rest of the body should remain stiff and stable. The position of the heels over the balls of the feet should be maintained, and this will decide the final placement of the elbows and shoulders. The length of the body from heel to shoulder is a constant (if shoulder girdle elevation or depression is stabilized), so the arc traveled by the upper arm will determine whether the elbow needs to move behind the wrist.

If the elbows remained over the wrists and the heels were allowed to move as the body was lowered, the longer the upper arm of the individual, the further forward the shoulders would go and the heels with them. It is my perspective that once the heels are in front of the balls of the feet, it is harder to press back through them and to maintain a strong engagement of the thighs and abdomen (Figure 17.25). Consequently, it is better to maintain the position of the heels and adjust the position of the elbows as necessary.

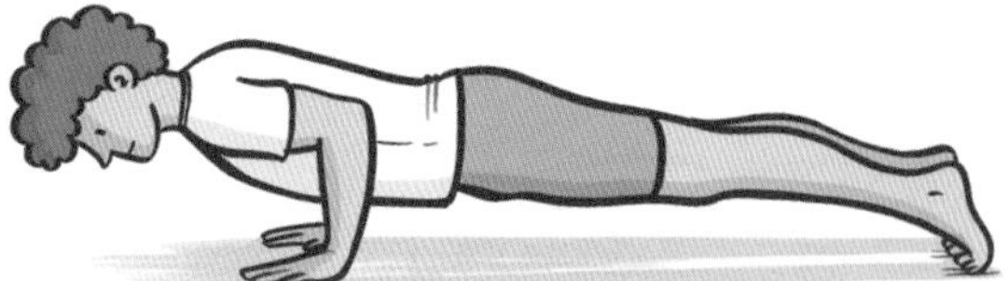

Figure 17.25 Here, Doug has kept the elbows over the wrists but that means the heels travel forward.

The student should only lower to a depth where they can keep the integrity of the rest of the body, going further down as their strength improves. This approach to *Chaturanga* adjusts the positioning relative to the individual's strength and proportions. If the shoulder blades come together or wing away from the ribcage during the lower down, it indicates that the student is not stabilizing the shoulder girdle and would be better off spending more time working in High Plank to build up their strength.

Chaturanga is used in the Sun Salutation sequence, and one of the questions often asked about this is whether it is better to jump to the bottom position or jump back to High Plank and then lower. From my point of view, jumping to *Chaturanga* avoids most of the work unless you can make a very controlled descent. The dynamic nature of catching the body at the bottom also adds a greater likelihood of overstressing the stabilizing muscles around the shoulder. My recommendation for all but accomplished practitioners would be to jump back to High Plank and lower to *Chaturanga* from there. There should be an effort made to make the landing with straight arms soft and controlled.

The Transition from Chaturanga to Up Dog

One of the positions that most often follows on from *Chaturanga* is Up Dog. In Chapter 15, *Backbends*, we covered the key points for a healthy Up Dog, so here we will focus on the other issue raised there, which was the need for most students to move the feet back. The intention is to move smoothly into an Up Dog, where the shoulders are not in front of the wrists (Figure 17.26). Those students with a very flexible spine will probably be able to roll over the toes without adjusting their

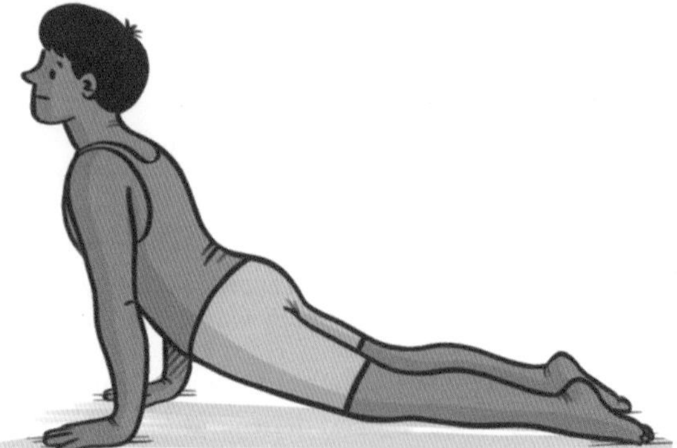

Figure 17.26 In Vihan's Up Dog, his shoulders are in front of the wrists. This will place stress on the wrists, shoulders, and low back.

position in *Chaturanga* but, as already discussed, this invariably lands up with a very steep Up Dog and the consequential hinging.

There are three straightforward ways to move the feet back. The first is to forget rolling over the feet altogether and instead come on to the tops of the feet, one at a time. The other two options offer a smoother transition but involve more strength in the bottom position.

The easier of these is to hold the position of the body static and just push the toes back by plantar flexing the feet. Before the toes flip out, start the movement forward by rolling over them (Figure 17.27).

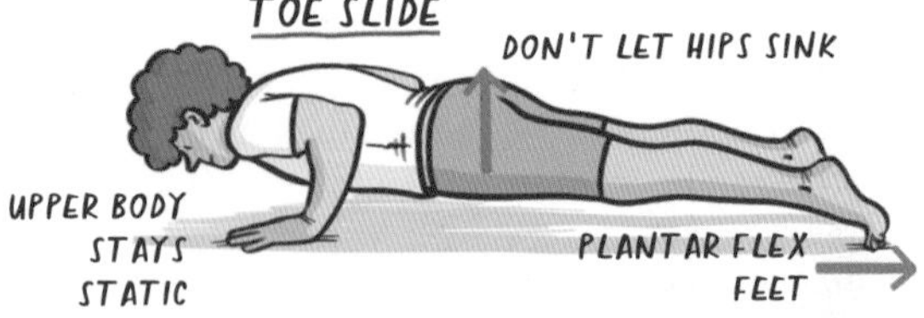

Figure 17.27 Plantar flexing the feet.

The last option involves pressing into the hands and sliding the whole body back while keeping the feet dorsiflexed, then rolling over the toes as normal (Figure 17.28). Both these options involve adjustments in how far to take the toes back according to the individual's proportions and resistance to spinal extension. The less easily you backbend, the further back you will need to slide.

Initially, there will need to be a little bit of trial and error to arrive in the desired Up Dog position, but once established and repeated a few times, it will become the ingrained pattern.

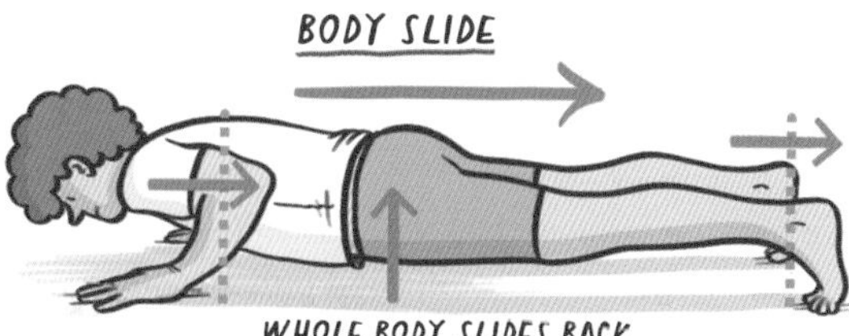

Figure 17.28 Sliding the body back.

Bent-arm Strength

Chaturanga is an essential position to master if you hope to be able to hold arm balances, perform low-level postures such as *Nakrasana* and *Bakasana*, and clean up those jump backs. My suggestion is to build up the time under tension by first slowing the lower down to around a count of four. Work up to achieving this for every transition from High Plank to *Chaturanga* while also gradually increasing the depth until the upper arms can be comfortably taken parallel to the floor or lower. Now some static 5 to 10 second holds can be introduced into the practice, not for every transition, but as a pose in its own right. Once there is a feeling of stability, the challenge can be added of pushing slowly back to High Plank rather than Up Dog. A good goal to aim for is to lower for a count of four, hold for four, and push back up for four.

For all the above progressions, it is important to keep a watchful eye on technique, particularly as the body begins to tire. The most common sloppiness that creeps in is on the push back to High Plank. If the body is not held ridged, then the shoulders will come up first with some amount of spine extension introduced. It often lands up resembling a half Up Dog, half push up. If working alone, it is always worth using a camera to capture the technique because the body is very crafty at improvising to get out of the work, and many cheats can go unnoticed. Working on strict form in this more stable orientation will also pay dividends in postures where there are less foundational elements and a need to control the relationship between the upper and lower halves of the body, for example, *Sirsasana*.

Shoulder Girdle Stability

As we introduced in Chapter 11, *Shoulder*, the scapula moves on the ribcage to allow the arm to be taken through a greater ROM, particularly in flexion, abduction, and horizontal adduction. However, there are times when we want to be able to keep it stable so that the arm can move independently, as I suggested is the case with the lower down. The main muscles that produce retraction (rhomboids and mid trapezius) and protraction (serratus anterior and pectoralis minor) can be isometrically contracted to hold it in place, making it easier for the muscles that cross the shoulder to control the arm.

High Plank is an ideal position to address scapula stabilization. Initially, as suggested, maintaining the position for 5 to10 breaths with protracted scapulae will begin to build strength. Transitioning from protraction to retraction and back is another beneficial exercise (Figure 17.29). Keep the arms straight all the time, and alternate between wrapping the scapulae around the body and drawing them medially toward the spine. Actively exaggerate both movements, strongly pressing the arms away when protracting the scapulae and squeezing the scapulae together when retracting.

Hand hovers are also a useful stabilization drill (Figure 17.30). Starting in a protracted High Plank, one hand can be lifted just enough so that it is no longer in contact with the floor (½ in/1 cm only). Alternate between the hands every 5 to 10 breaths. Be aware that if you lean the body away from the lifted hand, you must bring it back to neutral because the rest of the body should stay in precisely the same position.

Another variation is to take the lifted hand to tap the opposite shoulder, place it down, and swap

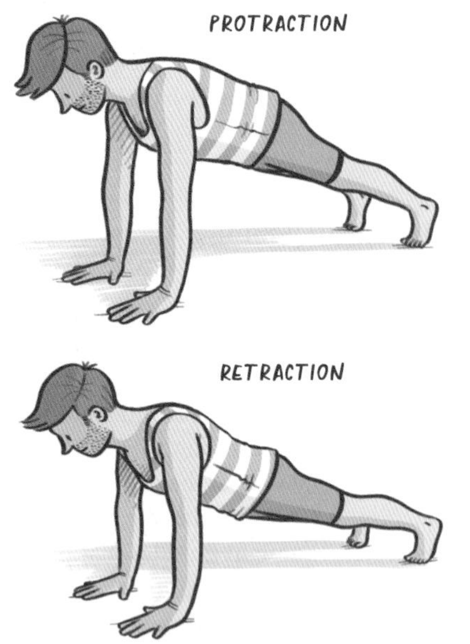

Figure 17.29 The whole body stays exactly the same apart from drawing the scapulae around the body (protraction) and back toward the spine (retraction).

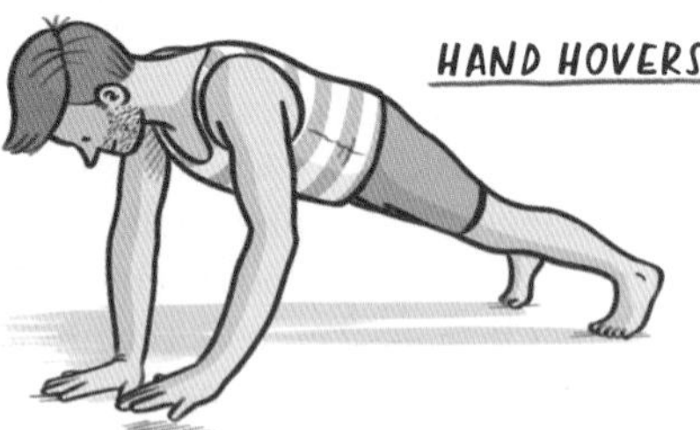

Figure 17.30 Keep the rest of the body in exactly the same place as the hand is lifted only a couple of centimeters from the floor.

(Figure 17.31). Most students I have observed doing this drill tend to rush, but it is preferable to move slowly. Remember that crucial concept of "time under tension."

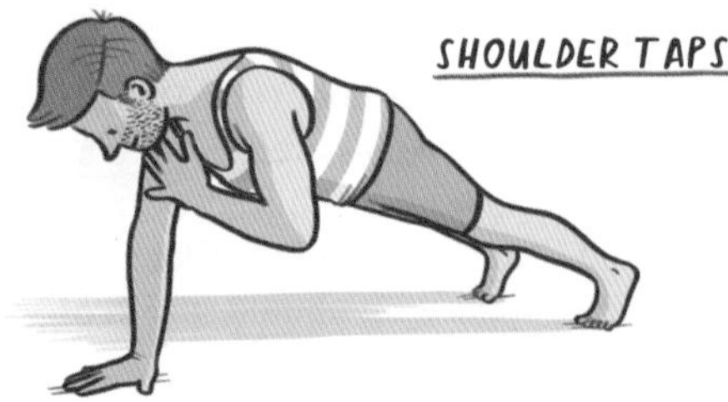

Figure 17.31 Same here, keep the body still as alternate hands tap the opposite shoulder. Move slowly and with control.

If confident in a Handstand, a face-to-wall position is perfect for working between elevation and depression of the shoulder girdle. For those who already feel strong and confident on their hands, alternate shoulder taps can also be performed here.

Pulling

We have mentioned that yoga has an inherent imbalance between pushing and pulling actions, so I will also introduce some worthwhile pulling exercises for yogis to complement the hanging introduced earlier in this chapter.

Resistance bands are a great addition to the yogi's toolkit because there are straightforward strengthening exercises for every part of the body. Of course, we could fill another book with conditioning exercises, but I want to introduce them because, unlike other actions that can be worked in some fashion within the yoga practice, for pulling, there is a need for equipment.

Choose a thickness of band relative to your strength. It is always best to start with a lighter band than you think. In the start positions, hold the band so there is already some tension in the band but not so much that you can't stretch it.

The first exercise is performed in *Dandasana*. The starting position is with the resistance band looped around the feet, scapulae protracted, and with the arms straight and parallel to the floor (Figure 17.32A). The arms do not bend as the scapulae are drawn toward the spine (retraction), Figure 17.32B. This position is held for a count of five while continuing to squeeze the scapulae together. When returning to the start position of protraction, additional work can be done by resisting the pull of the band and moving as slowly as possible (eccentric contraction). Aim for 10 repetitions.

This exercise uses the same movements of the shoulder girdle as in the High Plank protraction/retraction exercise previously but targets the rhomboids and mid trapezius (the retraction muscles) rather than serratus anterior and

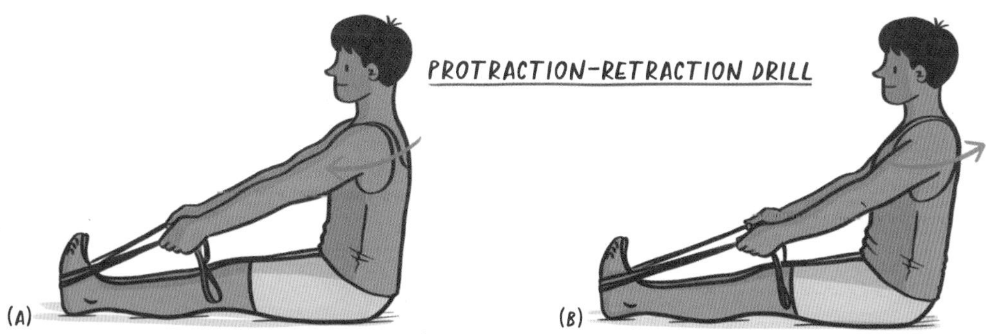

Figure 17.32 (A) Start sitting upright with a tensioned band. Let the band pull you into protraction but slow the movement down by resisting, (B) keep the arms absolutely straight, maintain the same position with the pelvis, and draw the scapulae toward the spine.

pectoralis minor (the protraction muscles). The difference is that the orientation has changed, and the resistance band provides the force to work against instead of gravity. In the High Plank position, gravity takes the body toward the floor, which means protraction will work against this force, and retraction will happen through relaxation of serratus anterior and pectoralis minor. The squeezing of the scapulae toward the spine at the end of the movement will be the only significant work for the rhomboids and mid trapezius. However, in this exercise, the work is exactly the opposite, with the rhomboids and mid trapezius providing the pulling action and serratus anterior and pectoralis minor not doing much.

The second exercise starts in the same position but without the protracted scapulae (Figure 17.33A). This time, the arms bend and the hands are pulled toward the waist. Hold here against the resistance for a count of five and then, under control, return to the start position (Figure 17.33B). Again, use the eccentric contraction by going as slowly as possible when returning to the start position. With this exercise, the upper arm moves relative to the scapula (shoulder extension) and the lower arm relative to the upper arm (elbow flexion), so we are getting a rare chance to work latissimus dorsi and the biceps, as well as the rear head of the deltoid.

The last exercise might be termed more of a remedial exercise and seems to be particularly useful for individuals suffering from shoulder pain due to excessive overhead pushing, for example, someone who does a lot of overhead presses in the gym or perhaps a lot of Handstands. The focus is on bringing some balance to the shoulder area, but this time the target is the smaller muscles, primarily the posterior head of the deltoid.

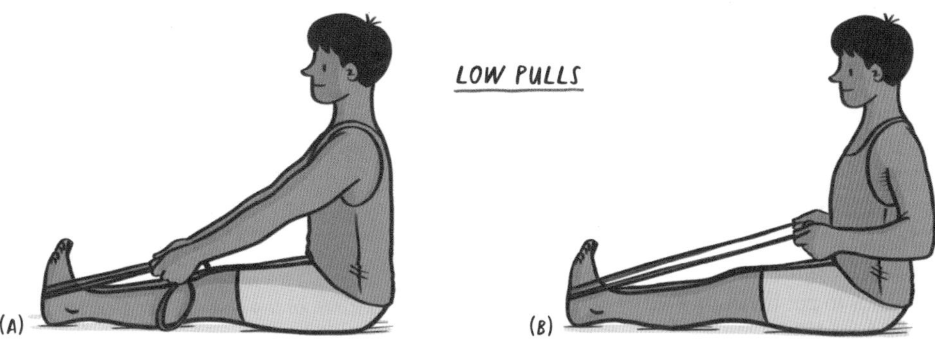

Figure 17.33 (A) Start sitting upright with a tensioned band, (B) pull the hands to the waist, nothing else changes. Then resist the band as it pulls you back to the start position.

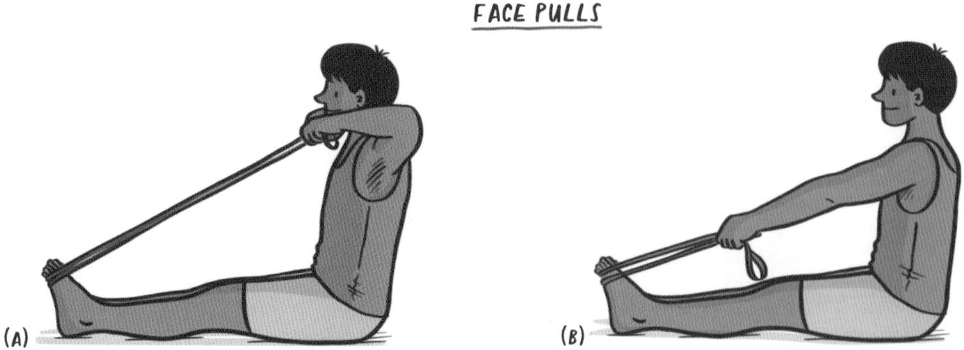

Figure 17.34 (A) Slowly pull the band to the face and then resist it back to the start, (B) get a better grip with the feet as you will be pulling upward and away. Use a lighter band as the targeted muscles are smaller.

The technique is to keep the body sitting straight up with arms straight, then pull the band to the chin or face without moving the rest of the body (Figure 17.34A). It is important to use less resistance in this exercise and keep the form strict as the muscles are weaker compared with the big ones reached before (Figure 17.34B). They may also be out of condition. You may also need to take care that the band doesn't slip off the feet as you are pulling on an incline.

Finally, if there is a suitable place to hang from, two other pulling exercises become available, the chin-up and the pull-up. The chin-up uses a shoulder-width underhand grip and the pull-up a wider overhand grip. In these exercises, unless modified, the weight of the body must be pulled toward the hands. I would predict that most yoga students who don't do any other forms of strengthening exercise would not be able to pull themselves up, because, of course, that movement is lacking in yoga. Luckily there is plenty that can be done.

The first option is to use one or two resistance bands, depending on their thickness, to give the extra lift. Don't go for so much help that it becomes a joy ride—try and find the right amount of assistance that allows 6 to 10 repetitions to be achieved. Whether going for the chin-up or pull-up, the starting position is with a firm grip and hanging at arm's length with one or both feet in the band. The aim is to get the chin slightly above the height of the hands (Figure 17.35A & B). Make the movement slow and smooth, with no swinging. On the lower down, remember as before to slow

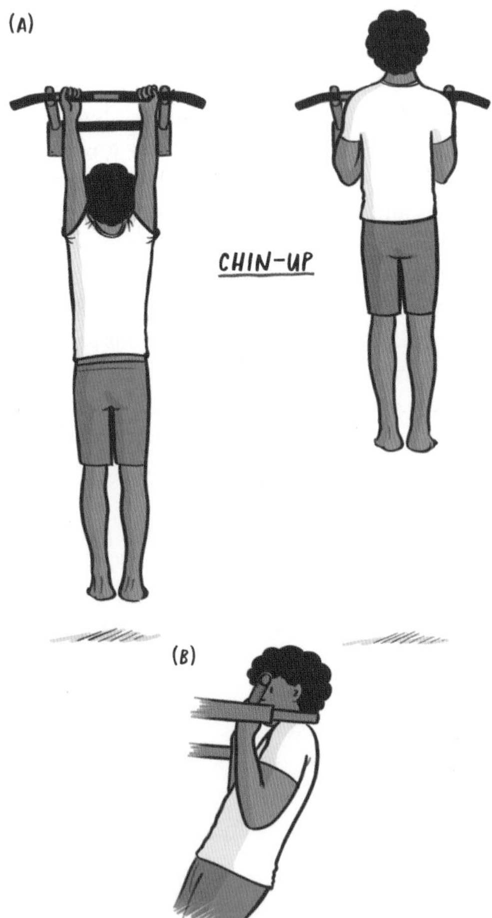

Figure 17.35 (A) It's tempting to keep a bend in the arms at the bottom of the chin-up, but that is cheating as you don't travel through the full ROM. Pull the chin above the bar, (B) this will work those neglected biceps and latissimus dorsi.

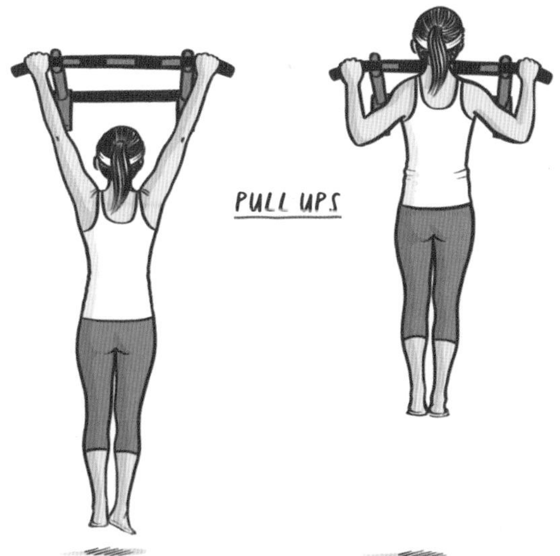

Figure 17.36 With the wider arms, there is less help from the biceps, so it may well feel harder. If you can't pull up, do the negative instead, going down as slowly as possible.

the descent and return to a position where the arms are completely straight. Reduce the amount of help as strength gains are made. Just because you are strong in *Chaturanga*, don't expect miracles—there is no correlation between the two exercises.

In the event that there are no resistance bands, the second option is to work the negative instead (Figure 17.36). In this variation, the starting position is at the top, so stand on something stable that allows the chin to be taken above the hands. The work is to lower as slowly as possible.

Once at arm's length, climb up and start again, looking to achieve the same number of repetitions. Even this option may be a big ask for a weak student, so it can be sensible to start with keeping the feet on the support and when lowering down, take some of the weight of the body by pressing up lightly with the legs. The amount of help from the legs can again be reduced over time.

CHAPTER

18

Inversions

In this chapter, I will focus on *Pincha Mayurasana*, *Sirsasana*, *Sarvangasana*, and *Mukta Hasta Sirsasana A*, all of which have also been partly discussed in other chapters.

Inversions come bundled with all sorts of envisaged physiological benefits, such as improving the immune system and venous return, reversing the aging process, preventing illness, toning the internal organs, and removing toxins. I must admit that the physiology of yoga postures has never interested me as much as the functional anatomy, mostly I think because the effects can't be seen and purported claims are hard to substantiate. I did read somewhere that they are also a natural facelift. Well, that can be seen, and they for sure have not done that for me. Joking apart, I do believe they improve venous return, at least for the time you are upside down anyway, in the same way that you would raise your arm if you cut your hand. Because of gravity and the inverted position, they will also increase the blood pressure in the head while in the posture. This might be a consideration or contraindication for someone who suffers from high blood pressure.

I am not going to say that most of the reported physiological effects are untrue, but I am skeptical, and not the person to advise on such stuff. If this is your area of interest, I would recommend that you look for rigorously performed case studies.

As with all postures, the intention for doing them is important. If it is the physiological benefits of being upside down that you are after, maybe keep it simple and do *Viparita Karani*. In Chapter 9, *Spine*, we looked at its construction, and I covered some of the potential negative consequences of resting on the head or flexing the neck too vigorously, so in this chapter, I will concentrate more on shape making.

Pincha Mayurasana

This pose looks like a pretty straightforward shape, but it can present a tremendous challenge to create and maintain. I would say the blueprint for this pose is to have the forearms parallel and a straight line from elbow to heel (Figure 18.1A). It is also like a Handstand in that it is possible to do it with less shoulder flexion and a banana back (Figure 18.1B). In fact, the second variation would be necessary if the purpose was to continue over into a *Vrschikasana* variation. Whenever there are style differences, my stand is always: are you choosing which shape to make or do your limitations dictate what you are doing? As the curvy one is easier, I would suggest aiming for the straight one as this will inform about the body better.

I reckon everyone can place their forearms parallel on the mat when resting on the shins (Figure 18.1C). However, the problem is when the butt is lifted and the angle between the torso

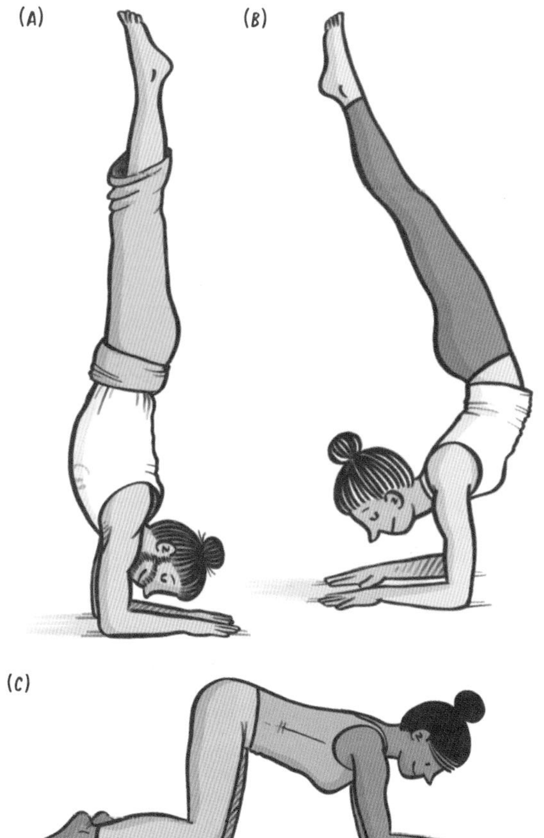

Figure 18.1 Pincha Mayurasana. *(A) Forearms parallel with straight line from elbow to heel, (B) banana back, (C) forearms parallel on the mat when resting on the shins.*

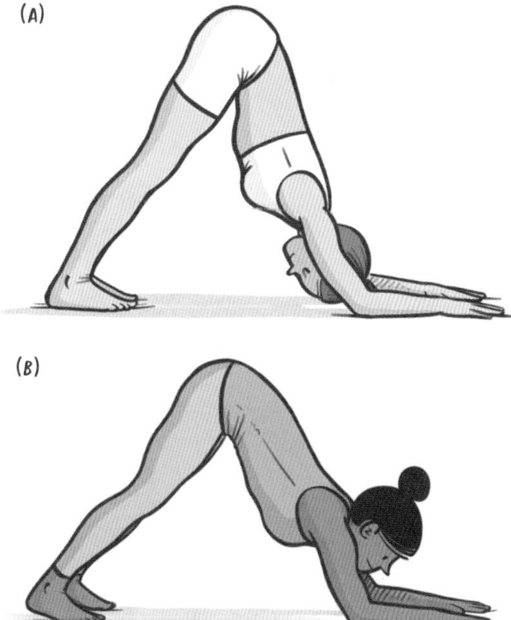

Figure 18.2 Ardha Pincha Mayurasana. *(A) Victoria can walk in a long way, but (B) Myra gets stopped by muscle tension in the shoulders.*

and upper arm is increased. We have referred to this before as shoulder flexion while maintaining external rotation.

What will happen if there is restriction is either the shoulders will medially rotate, bringing the hands toward each other, or if the arms are kept in place, shoulder flexion will be stopped before a straight line through the armpit is achieved.

The first step to assessing the availability of this movement is to do *Ardha Pincha Mayurasana*. Here, the shoulder movement can be recreated without the worry of balancing. The arms must be kept parallel, otherwise the exact movement that is trying to be resisted is being allowed to happen (medial rotation of the shoulder). The restriction will be easily demonstrated by the break in the line between elbow and hip (Figure 18.2).

Of course, it is perfectly acceptable at other times to do *Ardha Pincha Mayurasana* with the hands together if that is what makes it comfortable, but it is of no use for this purpose (Figure 18.3A). As well as the visual feedback, the subjective experience will also alter vastly. For those that are more open in this ROM, it can be quite relaxing, and a way toward working further on that same ROM. Conversely, if this ROM is a challenge, then it can seem like something out of a "hang tuff" competition, and unless you get some help, finding a position of relaxation is impossible (Figure 18.3B).

This little test tells us a lot about the expected performance in *Pincha Mayurasana*. No straight line on the ground means no straight line in the air, and a curved spine is the only option. The hands could be moved, but that will compromise the foundation. If it is possible to have a good alignment in *Ardha Pincha Mayurasana*, then there is no ROM excuse for not being able to find the straight line in the posture. There is either a lack

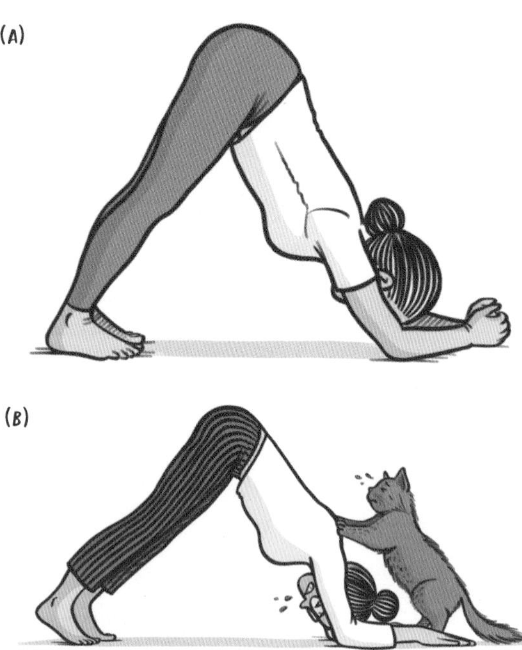

Figure 18.3 (A) Hands together will make shoulder flexion easier, but also avoids the work necessary for Pincha Mayurasana, *(B) Gerald is happy to help, but it can be hard to overcome the resistance.*

of shoulder girdle and arm strength or instability in the midsection. If this is the case, then it's time to go back to the forearm plank drills. Of course, there may still be psychological reservations as the possibility of falling is real. If this is the case, start by the wall. For the setup, have the fingertips touching the wall to prevent introducing too much curving of the spine.

The most glamourous entry into *Pincha Mayurasana* is a press from a sharp *Ardha Pincha Mayurasana*. For this to be on the table, there needs to be the shoulder ROM spoken of before as well as good hip flexion. If these elements are present, then the hips can be walked into a position where they are over the shoulders, the feet will feel light, and there is no more issue with raising the straight legs up than there would be in *Sirsasana*.

Resistant shoulders or hip extensors will prevent the hips from reaching the right place and mean a kick up is the only option left (Figure 18.4). It is still important to walk in as far as possible and reach the leg in the air as high toward the ceiling as it will go. The further in it is possible to walk, the less momentum needs to be generated with the kick up, and the quicker balance will be found.

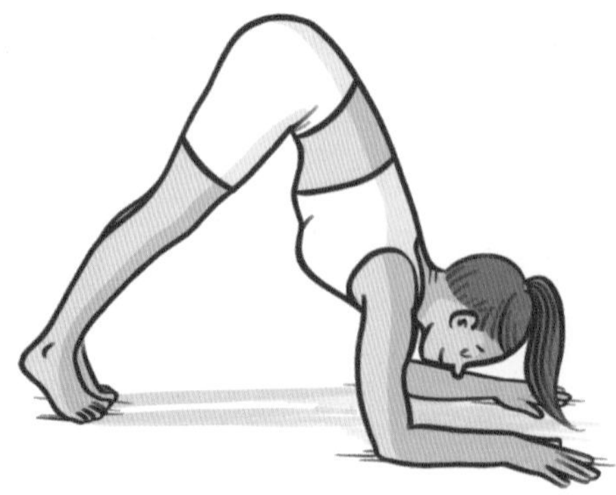

Figure 18.4 Where Victoria has stopped walking in, the hips are not far enough forward to lift into Pincha Mayurasana, *and she would have to kick up.*

If the legs can be walked in so far that the leg in the air is pointing to the ceiling, and the other leg can be lifted with muscular engagement rather than hopping, the full two-leg press is very close to happening (Figure 18.5).

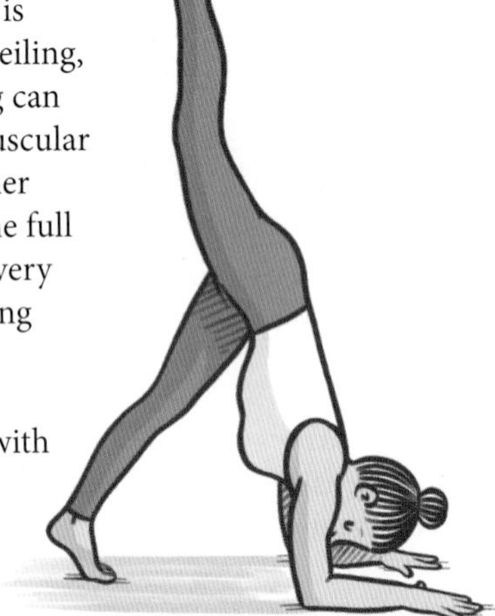

Figure 18.5 From this position, Sasha could probably shift her weight to draw the second leg off the floor. Also, a two-leg press would be very close.

Those students with a bendy spine often like to go into a straddle with the legs and then find balance from there. In some ways, it is a little easier to get the initial balance because of the lowered COG, but the backbend that has been introduced is hard to get rid of fully, and we are back in banana land. My recommendation is to keep a firm belly with the ribcage pulled toward the pubic bone, only take the leg over the head as little as possible, and find the straight line quickly by allowing the second leg to follow on and up.

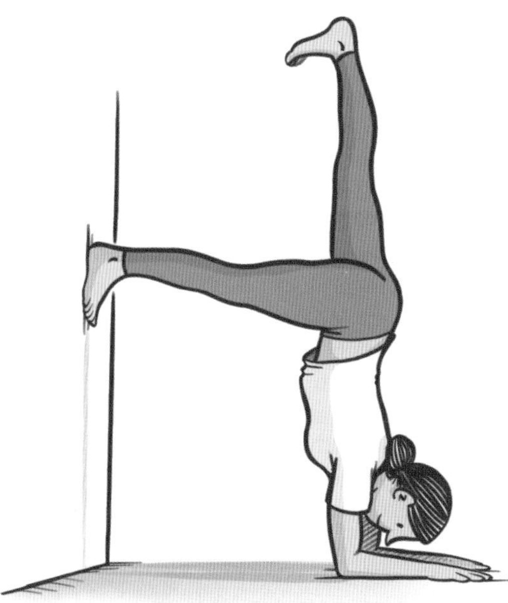

Figure 18.6 The security of the wall is the perfect place to find a straight line and work on the strength in the shoulders.

If there is instability or sinking in the posture due to strength, then the single-leg version using the wall is worthwhile doing (Figure 18.6). This allows much more strength-building time under tension because the balance element is minimized. It is also very useful for working on good alignment, so when spacing the setup, have the leg on the wall perpendicular to the wall and the rest of the body straight. The stability that the wall provides also means that it will be easier to maintain the forearm position while pressing the shoulders away from the floor. This sort of active work into the ROM will be easier the less resistant the muscles are, so it may be necessary to supplement it with a gravity-assisted exercise such as the butcher's block detailed in Chapter 17, *Postures Involving the Shoulders.*

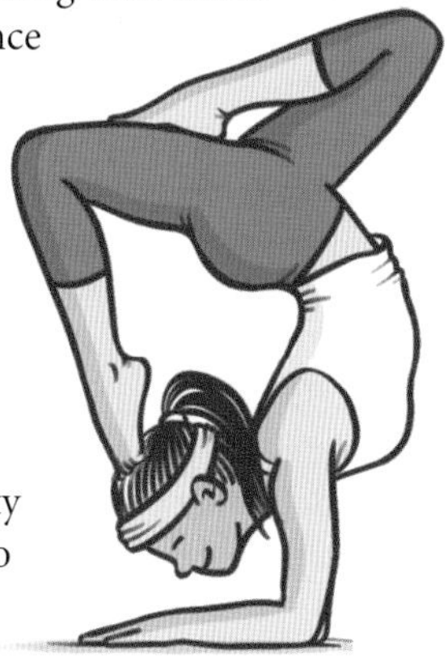

Figure 18.7 Once a strong foundation can be relied on, all sorts of shapes can be explored.

The last thing I will talk about regarding *Pincha Mayurasana* is a tip for keeping the arms aligned. When the foundation moves, the ROM work is avoided, and the posture is less stable. Extra grip can be created by setting up the arms to face the ceiling and then rolling them to face the floor. It is essential to then fight hard to not allow the foundation to slip as the walk in begins—pressing the hands and forearms into the ground will help (Figure 18.8).

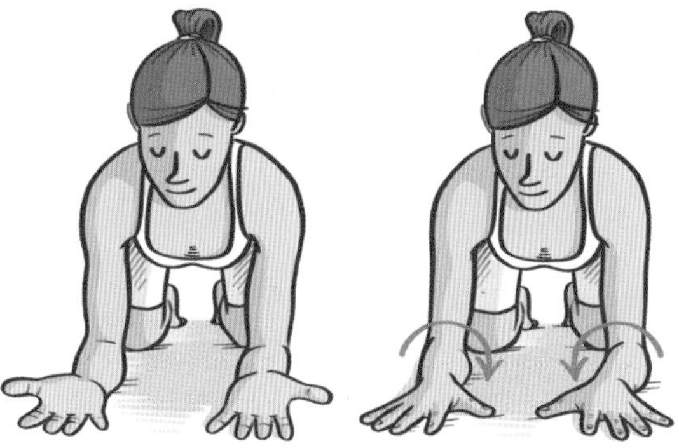

Figure 18.8 Create extra grip.

Sirsasana

I have to repeat here that good alignment of the spine in normal posture and freedom from other neck issues is paramount before considering *Sirsasana*. The other major requirement is strength in the arms and shoulder girdle. It is my recommendation that students should be able to perform a minimum of 25 breaths in a head off the floor "L" hold against the wall before being allowed to try *Sirsasana*. This will ensure that strength and stability are available (Figure 18.9).

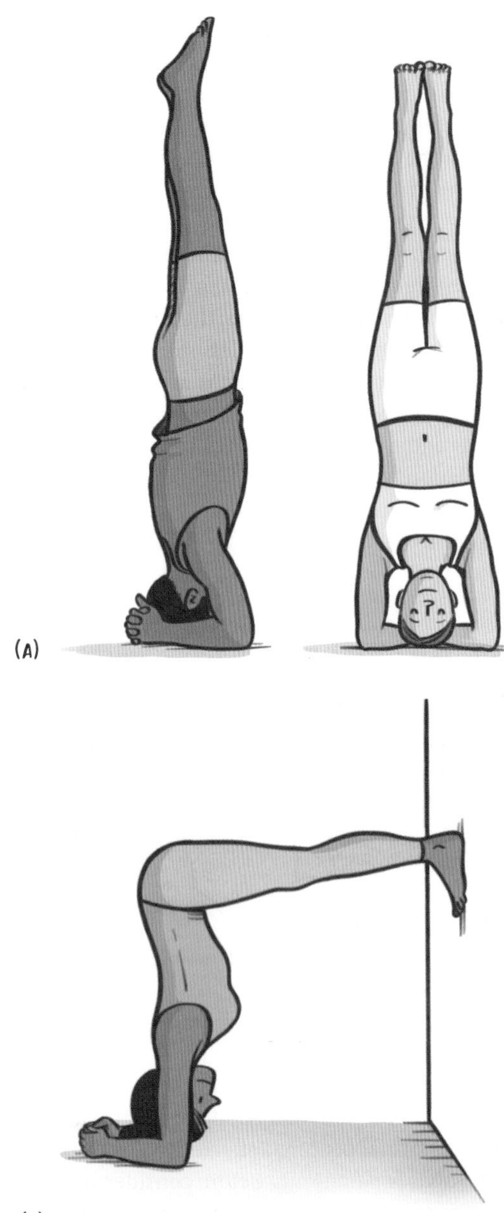

Figure 18.9 (A) Sirsasana, *(B) the "L" wall hold is perfect for building strength.*

The fact that the hands are together in this posture means that it will be much easier than *Pincha Mayurasana* to get the necessary shoulder flexion. In addition, less is required because the alignment is not with a straight line through the armpit. When it comes to the hands, I think it is preferable to have a clasped grip as against an open grip, because it provides greater stabilization of the foundation, and is more suitable for lifting the head off the floor. As I prioritize cervical spine health, I advise pressing the head clear of the floor and, if this is not possible, only spending a minimum amount of time in the posture. I do appreciate the allure of *Sirsasana*, but it is probably better to do something else instead if the head cannot be raised.

Another contraindication is to do with proportions. If a student's upper arms are not long enough for the elbow to protrude beyond the head when the bent arm is taken next to the ear, then even with elevating the shoulder girdle, it would be hard to remove weight from the head (Figure 18.10). If this is the situation, I would leave *Sirsasana* altogether or use a specialist prop where the weight can just be taken on the shoulders.

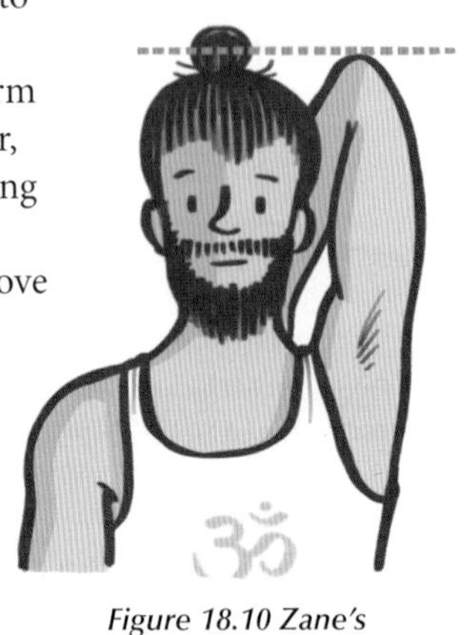

Figure 18.10 Zane's elbow clears his head.

One of the most vulnerable times for the neck is during the entry and exit phases. It is advisable not to jump, and when loaded, the cervical spine should not be rounded. This, again, is impossible to achieve without the necessary hip flexion to walk the legs in and get the hips over the shoulders. When the hips are in the right position, the feet will feel very light on the floor. It is the stabilization of the body that then allows the hip extensors (hamstrings and gluteus maximus) to raise the legs. To reduce the work initially, one leg can be raised toward the ceiling, followed by the other. However, the second leg should not be kicked up, but instead raised with muscular engagement. It can help to draw the foot just off the floor by shifting the hips a little beyond the head. This is achieved with the muscles of the shoulder and back extensors.

Sarvangasana

I did cover in Chapter 9, *Spine*, that the sensible setup for *Sarvangasana* to reduce stress on the cervical spine is with a block of blankets (Figure 18.11). As the hips can be taken closer to the floor also to lessen the amount of neck flexion needed, the remaining concern is the support from the arms. The hands should be on the ribcage rather than the butt to provide a supportive framework behind the body. The elbows also need to be in line with the hands. This will be hard to achieve if there is restriction across the front of the chest that resists horizontal abduction. If this is the case, what will tend to happen in the pose is that the elbows will gradually slide apart, causing the foundation to weaken and sink.

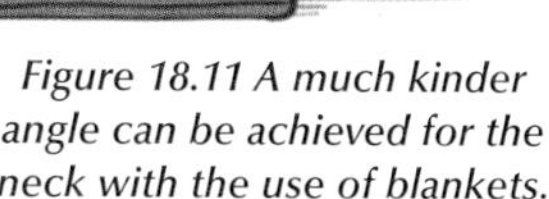

Figure 18.11 A much kinder angle can be achieved for the neck with the use of blankets.

When in the more upright position, the weight on the arms can be reduced by reaching the legs toward the ceiling and engaging the abdominal and back extensors to bring firmness to the body. It is possible to work actively on improving the elbow position when standing (Figure 18.12). In exactly the same way the arms are taken behind the back, and then the elbows are drawn toward each other, and an isometric (static) contraction held for a number of breaths.

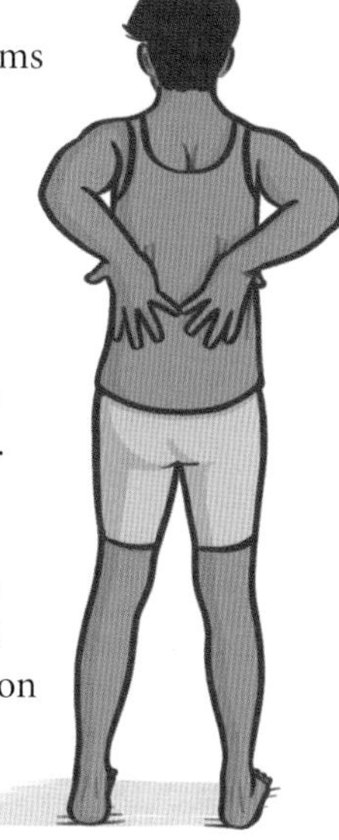

Figure 18.12 This is quite a nice way to open across the front of the chest.

Please refer again to Chapter 9, *Spine*, for anatomical insights relating to *Halasana*, often sequenced to follow *Sarvangasana*.

Mukta Hasta Sirsasana A

There are several *Sirsasana* variations where the arms move away from the head and, subsequently, there is no choice but to take weight onto it. *Mukta Hasta Sirsasana A* is the variation most used because it provides an excellent position for many transitions to other poses such as arm balances (Figure 18.13). It can also be entered into from poses like *Prasarita Padottanasana*.

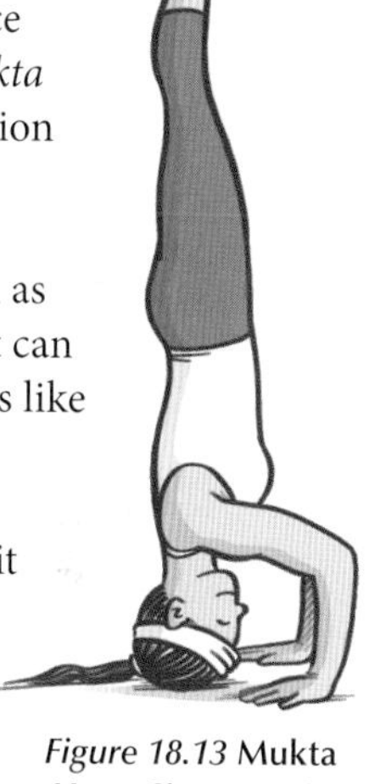

Figure 18.13 Mukta Hasta Sirsasana A.

However, as fun and as useful it may be, it comes again with the warning over alignment, strength, stability, and weight-bearing on the head. All the same entry advice goes as with *Sirsasana* regarding not hopping and ruling out erroneous neck movements. I will share my thoughts and experiences, but ultimately, it is up to you to make a decision over the potential risks to your body, or, more importantly, that of your students.

At least 10 years ago, I had an X-ray of my spine and found that I had several disc bulges in my cervical spine. I had been suffering from neck pain and stiffness, which I had attributed to too much time on the computer. The scan was not actually to investigate this, but to look for signs of a hereditary condition, which turned out to be absent. I was, at this time, practicing the Ashtanga Intermediate Series, which has seven *Sirsasana* variations, six of which remove the possibility of lifting off the head. Although disc bulges are not that uncommon and may, on occasion, have no associated pain, I decided that armed with this knowledge, the most sensible course of action was to stop doing *Sirsasana*.

Over the coming months, my neck discomfort subsided and has not come back since. Now, this is only my experience and is far from scientific proof, but I feel happier prioritizing the longevity of my yoga practice and health in general. If you follow me on social media, you will know that I love arm balances, and it is super fun to try and transition into them from *Mukta Hasta Sirsasana* A. My compromise is that now and again I will work on this but keep my time down to only one breath in *Sirsasana*.

If you are going to perform *Mukta Hasta Sirsasana A*, make a triangular foundation with the head and hands, keep the neck neutral, resist wobbling around, don't stay up very long, and come down in a controlled way.

Books, videos, and online classes can never replace the presence of an experienced teacher, and this is particularly pertinent when it comes to inversions that include weight-bearing on the head. Especially if any of these poses are new to you, or you have any doubts about the quality of your alignment, wait until you can be in the company of the right teacher before you experiment.

CHAPTER 19

Arm Balances

Arm balances are so much fun, but they can place quite a workload on the body (Figure 19.1). It is sensible to gradually build up the number of variations or the time spent doing them. Having started yoga after many years in the gym, I naturally gravitated toward arm balances as it seemed more attainable for me compared with the pretzel postures. But although there is definitely a strength element to arm balances, many of the shapes will be unavailable if the required ROM, usually hip-related, is missing.

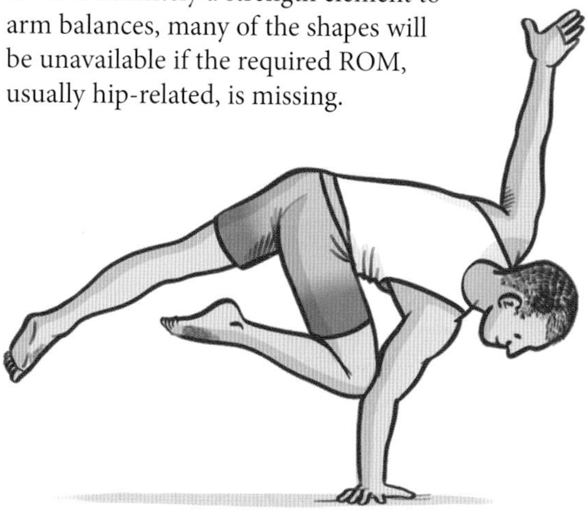

Figure 19.1 Arm balances are fun!

I must admit that when I started, I would just keep doing the ones I could manage and see improvement over time. As I become more flexible, a greater variety of positions became available. Although I often say, you won't get better at something unless you do it—this approach favors neurological adaptation and tends to take longer than a methodical breakdown followed by training specific elements. Understanding arm balances can be approached in the same way as we have considered any other yoga shape. What is required to allow the body to be positioned in space in this particular way? The four main components I focus on for this group of postures are upper body strength, wrist health, hip flexibility, and balance. Also, you don't really want a lot of extra weight to be heaving around the place. Accordingly, if you can be at what I refer to as "fighting weight," these poses will already be more accessible.

We will consider some specific posture examples to work through later, but there is also plenty of common ground. We can say that the foundation is reduced to either one or two hands, the arms are bent or straight, and the legs will make it look pretty but also create challenges through their placement, both relative to ROM requirements and COG shift. I will start off by narrowing the focus and shifting hand balancing (Handstands) to the end of the chapter. This leaves us with a group of postures that are all pretty close to the ground.

Wrist Health

The interface between our hand foundation and the rest of the body is the wrists, and arm balances will definitely highlight any issues already going on there. The wrists should always be warmed up thoroughly through mobilization and simple load-bearing before testing them with precarious body positions. Also, build up the time spent on the hands gradually to allow the structures of the wrist to adapt and get stronger. The average active wrist extension is around 70 degrees, which increases to around 90 degrees when applying force. It is essential to have a comfortable 90 degrees of passive wrist extension, with more required for some straight-arm variations. If this is not available, it would be sensible to use a wedge to remove the strain and avoid those variations that are particularly challenging for the wrist. The wrist extension exercise detailed in Chapter 12, *Elbow and Wrist*, makes an excellent element to add to the warm-up as well as for working on ROM increases. For straight-arm variations, turning the hands out slightly (10 to 15 degrees) may reduce the required wrist extension.

Balance

The body is pretty low to the ground in this group of postures, so I feel that balance is influenced mostly by having the strength to maintain your position. When on two hands, the side-to-side movements are not really an issue, but the forward and backward will be the challenge. When it comes to one arm, then you have all directions to deal with and especially the chance of rotating. As we talked about in Chapter 1, *Gravity* and *Balance*, a stable position is all to do with getting your COG over your BOS. It is possible to be in a position where this is not the case for a while, but it will require a lot more strength.

Shifting the COG doesn't always have to be forward or backward, it can also be upward. For example, in *Bakasana* with straight arms, a lot of wrist extension will be needed if the goal is to keep the torso parallel with the floor. The butt and legs are heavy, so to get the COG level with the hands (BOS), the shoulders need to move forward. If this position is a little frightening or the required amount of wrist extension is missing, then the butt can go up instead. This action also shifts the COG forward. Bending the arms will reduce the amount of wrist extension required, so in many cases, the posture lands up in a middle ground with the arms not fully bent or straight (Figure 19.2).

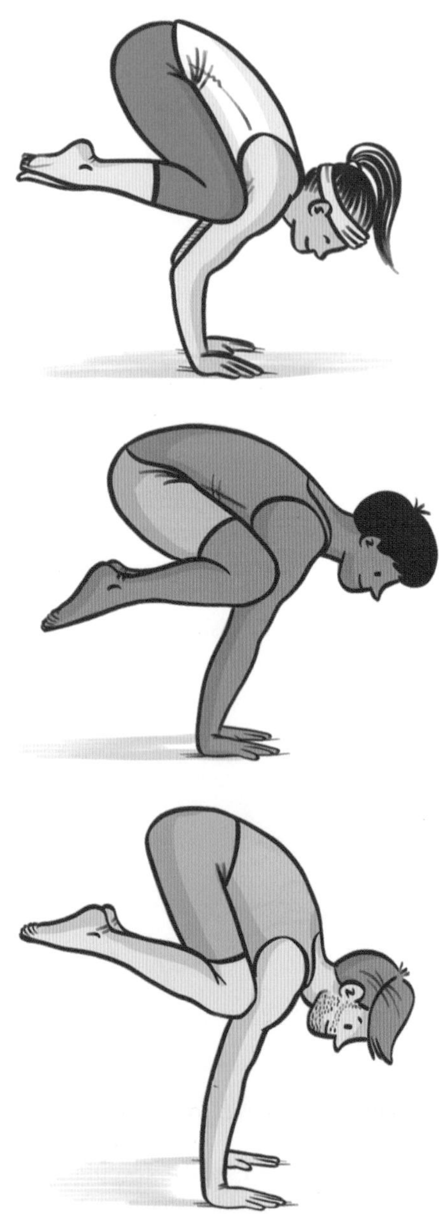

Figure 19.2 Bending the arms and lifting the butt in the air shifts the COG forward, reducing the amount of wrist extension required.

Tittibhasana, on the other hand, doesn't need as much wrist extension in either of the two butt positions, because the outstretched legs act as a cantilever and distribute more of the body weight in front of the foundation (Figure 19.3).

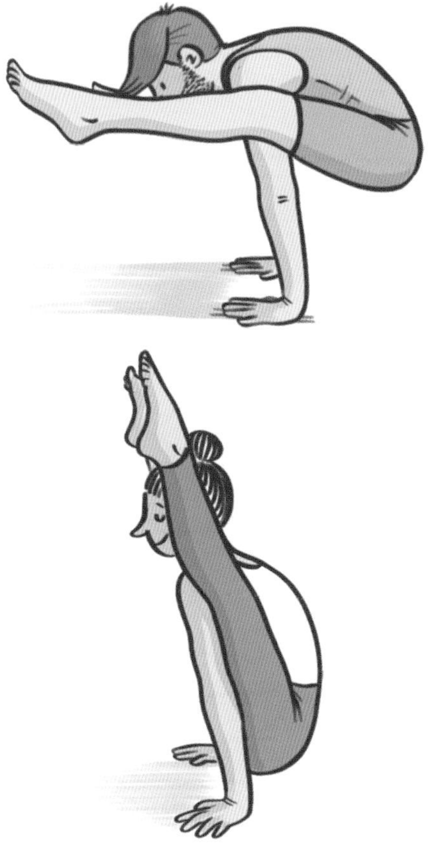

Figure 19.3 In Tittibhasana, *the legs act as a cantilever, shifting the COG forward.*

Bent-Arm and Straight-Arm Strength

Most arm balances fall into the bent-arm strength category, and the easiest way to work on this within a yoga setting is in *Chaturanga*. If you can be super strong in the bottom position, then if you have the hip ROM for the posture shape, it doesn't really matter what you are doing with your legs. In the final arm balance position, I often observe uneven shoulders. Sometimes this is an aesthetic choice, but more usually it's because it's the easier option. When the legs are out to one side using the seesaw action of dropping one shoulder to raise the legs certainly does the trick, but the work is being avoided (Figure 19.4). Having that strong bottom position opens up the possibility of keeping square and isolating some work in the hips. I also think it looks better.

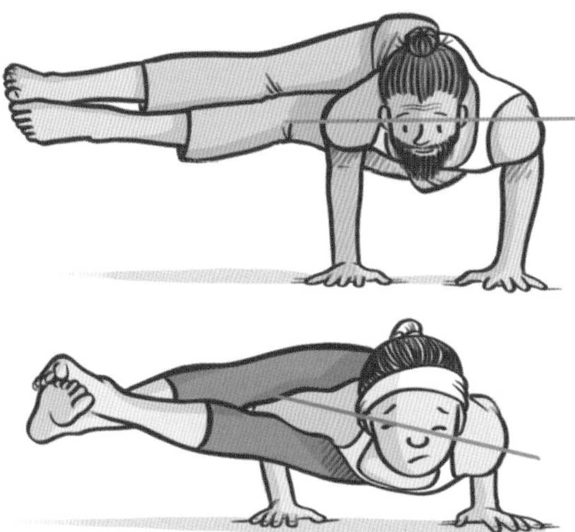

Figure 19.4 I think dropping one shoulder should be avoided unless aiming to form a specific geometry or aesthetic appearance.

A good start for building that bent-arm strength is to increase the time in *Chaturanga*, but you need to recreate the position you want to maintain in the poses. That means being down with the upper arms parallel to the ground. If you have skipped through the book, take a look back at Chapter 17, *Postures Involving the Shoulders*, for my tips on *Chaturanga*. What tends to happen as the body tires is to either sink toward the floor or raise up to a less challenging position. A worthwhile strategy to ensure strict form is to place a block under the shoulders and hover above it (Figure 19.5). This will give immediate feedback, even if the body is working in stealth mode.

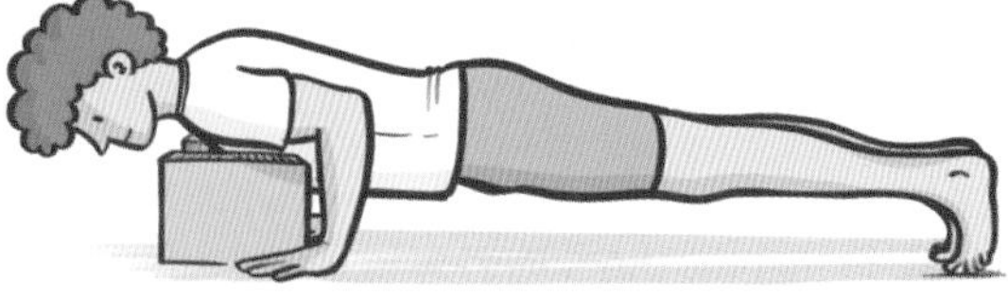

Figure 19.5 Hovering over a block gives great feedback.

Just holding *Chaturanga* is the initial test, but then once this can be done comfortably for 10 breaths, it is time to step up the difficulty. Controlled raises and lowers from High Plank to *Chaturanga* are next, aiming for multiple repetitions, and then comes the fun. When you become competent at moving up and down, it is possible to play around with halfway stops and random direction changes. For example, from High Plank to *Chaturanga*, halfway up and hold, back to *Chaturanga* and hold, all the way up and hold, halfway down, back to High Plank, down to *Chaturanga*, etc. This level of strength frees you up to focus on the technique and body placement of the arm balance rather than worrying about face planting or collapsing.

Although we have been specifically talking about working on strength gains, the same understanding can be applied to sequencing and student preparedness. Placing some static hold *Chaturanga* before arm balance poses will help ensure the arms and shoulders are ready, as well as highlight any students who may need a modification of the intended pose. As already mentioned, the shoulders are inherently unstable and relatively easy to overwork, so I would recommend that anyone not able to hold the bottom position in *Chaturanga* for five breaths should not challenge the body further with arm balances.

Straight-arm strength makes transitioning more secure and is needed for postures such as *Bakasana*, *Tittibhasana*, and *Eka Pada Bakasana*. Like increasing bent-arm strength, the first step is purely to increase the hold time in High Plank, keeping the shoulder girdle somewhat protracted, and not sinking between the shoulder blades. Building up scapula protraction strength can be included by using the High Plank retraction-protraction drill, again detailed in Chapter 17, *Postures Involving the Shoulders*.

As most of the straight-arm balances are with the shoulders in front of the wrists, it can be worthwhile training this position in isolation. In calisthenics, they call this position "planching," and it involves taking the weight forward while in High Plank so that the shoulders are in front of the wrists (Figure 19.6). This can be extremely challenging, so

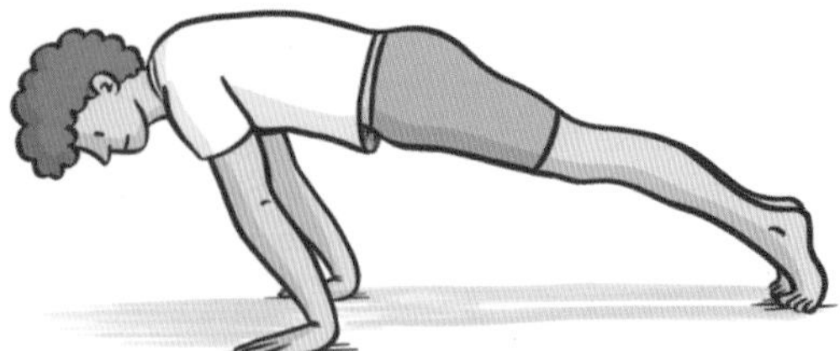

Figure 19.6 Here the hands can be turned out a little to reduce stress on the wrists.

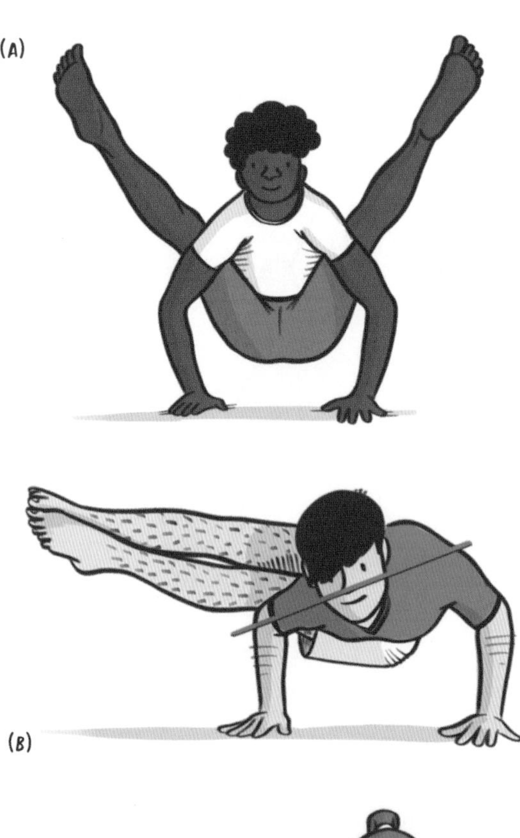

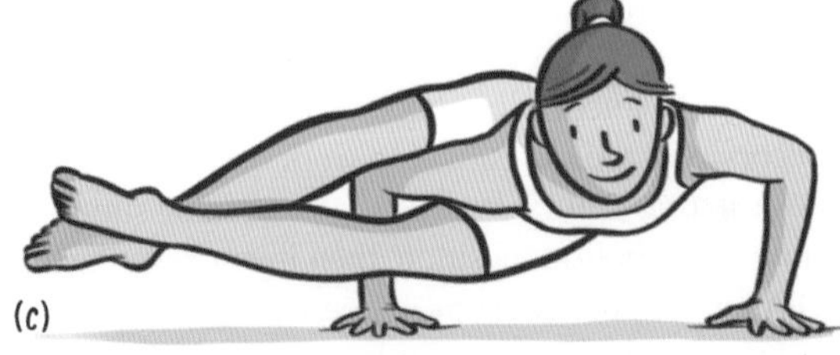

Figure 19.7 Faulty technique. (A) Aren has let his chest collapse in, (B) Dave has let one shoulder rise up with less bend in that elbow, (C) Victoria has taken her hands way too wide, which will make transitioning more difficult.

build up the time gradually and initially don't go too far forward.

Common sloppiness I observe in technique that may place additional stress on the body in arm balances, involves changes to arm and shoulder position due to accommodation of lacking ROM or insufficient strength (Figure 19.7). We have mentioned the uneven shoulders already, but they may also jut forward too much, the elbows can drift away from the body, and the width across the chest diminishes. As with many yoga postures, the answer often lies in opposing actions, energy distribution, and awareness. If you are fighting to survive in a pose, this is when the erroneous movements are easily overlooked, so work on that strength!

Hip Flexibility

I am singling out hip flexibility as the major ROM challenge for arm balance shapes, but there are also a few that call for an ample twisting ability. Until you come on to Handstands, there is nothing that tests shoulder ROM, except if we are including *Pincha Mayurasana*, but maybe we can call that an inversion. Where we need to place our legs for an arm balance will present the same issues as any other yoga pose. The various arm balance shapes will call for specific movements at the hip. Sometimes, as with *Bakasana*, it won't really be a limiting factor. But other times, if there is a problem with hip flexion, external rotation, abduction, or any of the other hip movements, it may severely disrupt the completion of the shape or even make it unavailable. Depending on the entry into the arm balance, hip restrictions may even lead to a less than ideal setup.

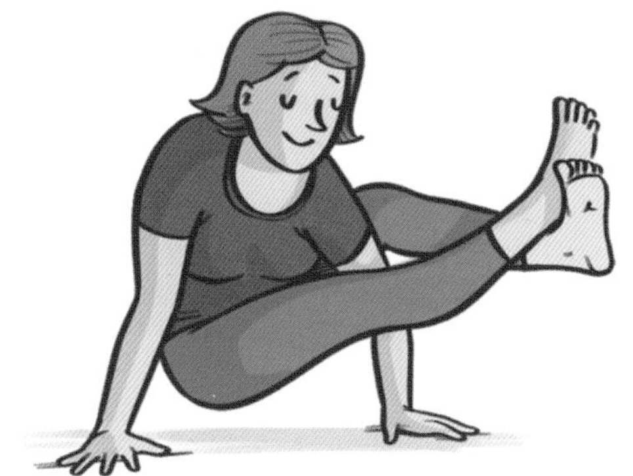

Figure 19.8 Bad setup can land up as one big nasty mess.

For example, if we consider *Astavakrasana*, the hip position in the final pose is no big deal, with some degree of hip flexion only. However, the standard non-flashy (i.e., not from *Mukta Hasta Sirsasana A*) entry is by hooking one leg high up over the arm and clamping it into position between the upper and lower leg. If bent-knee hip flexion is a challenge, the knee will land up too far down the arm, and the whole posture will go down the drain (Figure 19.8). Of course, for the following discussion, we are presuming that shoulder and arm strength are sorted.

Let me give you a few more examples and the ROM that would be a limitation. *Bhujapidasana* suffers the same as *Astavakrasana* in the setup if there is not enough bent-knee hip flexion (Figure 19.9). The knees will land up too far down the arms. If external rotation of the hip is poor, then it will be hard to cross the legs, and even if they do, the feet will catch on the floor because of the resulting

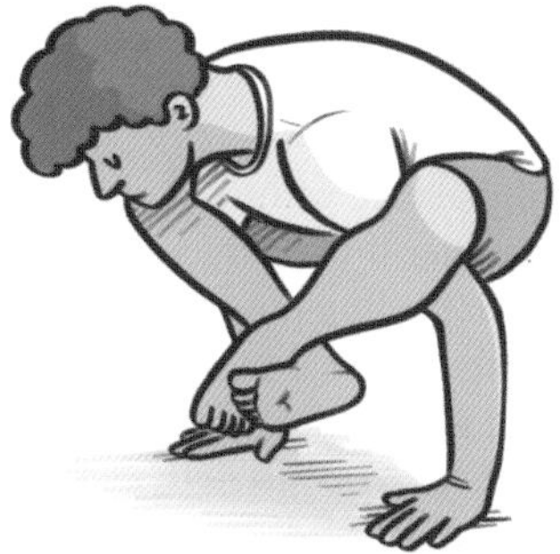

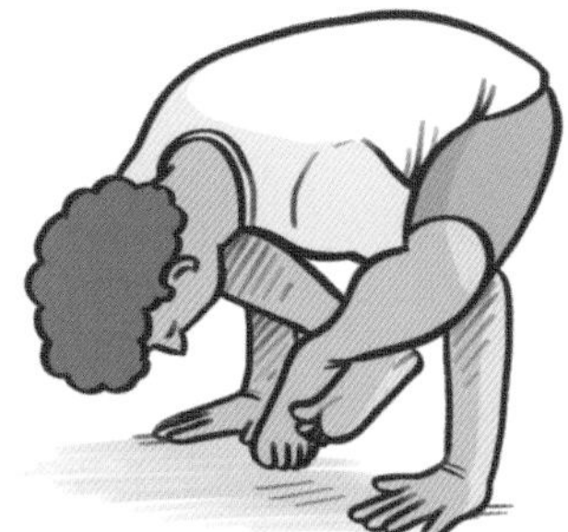

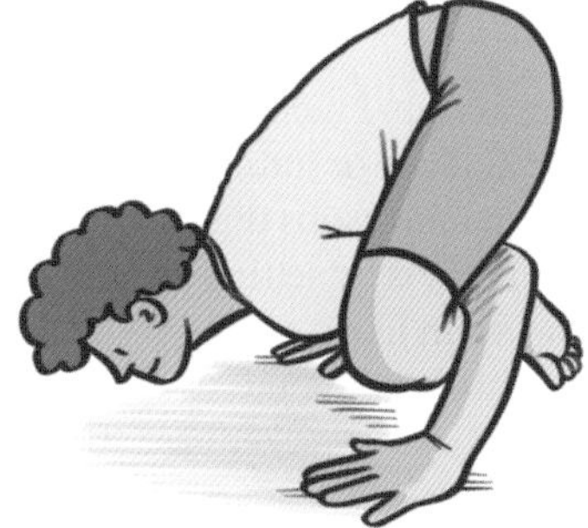

Figure 19.9 Bhujapidasana *requires plenty of external hip rotation to get a good enough cross to get the feet through.*

lower leg angle (Figure 19.10).

If you are having trouble visualizing that, the way it works is as the hips externally rotate, the lower leg will rotate away from the floor; maintaining that position will allow the feet to go through between the hands as the head tips forward, and the butt rises.

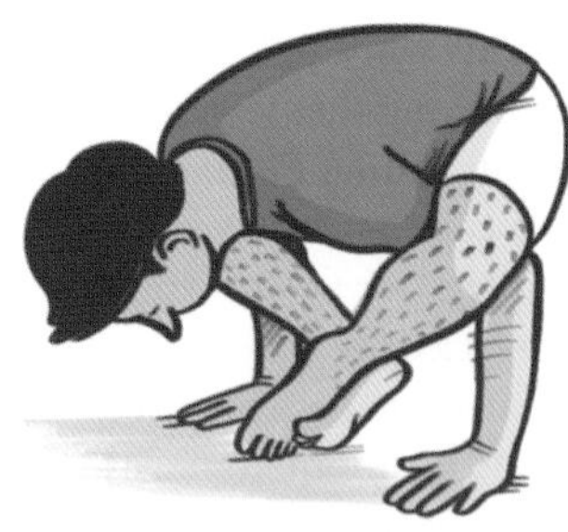

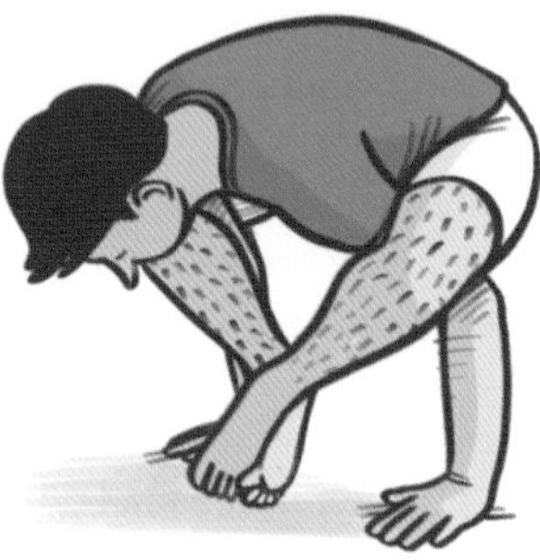

Figure 19.10 Dave can't get his feet off the floor because of the restrictions in his hips.

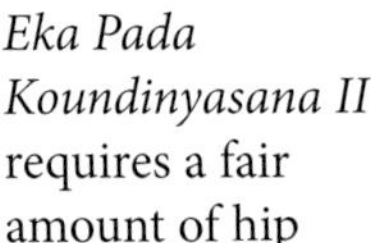

Eka Pada Koundinyasana II requires a fair amount of hip flexion and horizontal abduction, otherwise it will be difficult to keep the leg on the arms (Figure 19.11). As before, breaking down postures in this way and recognizing what movements make them up will allow for the right poses to be sequenced before them.

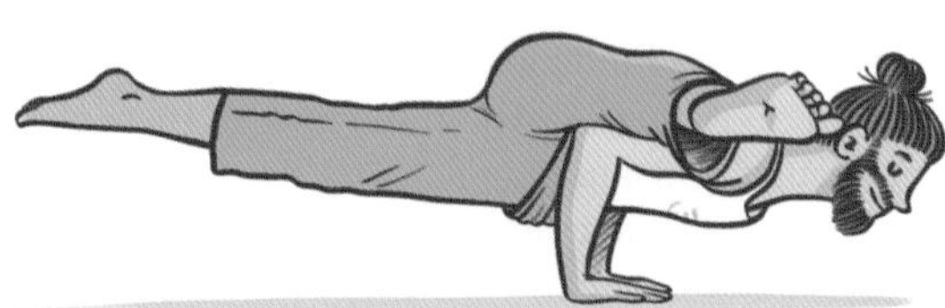

Figure 19.11 Zane has good bent-arm strength and hip flexibility. Fancy poses are a breeze.

Hand Position and Arm Angle

Further up, I mentioned about elbows going out and uneven or jutting shoulders. I think one of the main reasons this can happen, besides lack of strength, is by setting up with hands too wide. It can seem like it will be easier with the hands wider, especially when the setup is a struggle, but actually, it provides a weaker base. The hands want to be shoulder-width apart.

I'm a bit of a purist when it comes to arm balance shape, but I feel if it is a bent-arm version, the upper arm should be parallel with the floor and if a straight-arm version, the arms should be straight, not somewhere in the middle ground. That is not to say that this is always going to be possible, but to know where you are trying to get is important. There are also more than just aesthetic reasons.

If the arms are meant to be straight in the pose, there is minimal support from the arms for the legs, which will require more engagement of the core (abdominal muscles plus other stuff) and legs to maintain their position. Bending the arms escapes some of this work.

On the other hand, in a bent-arm pose, the upper arm provides an excellent platform for the leg, knee, or foot to rest on. Moving up from that parallel to the floor position is less secure and leaves the pose more likely to slip apart (Figure 19.12). If you find yourself in no man's land, try and establish why that is and then work on those elements. To start with, it is fine to be happy with just being in something that resembles the pose, but then as with every other posture, the refinement needs to commence.

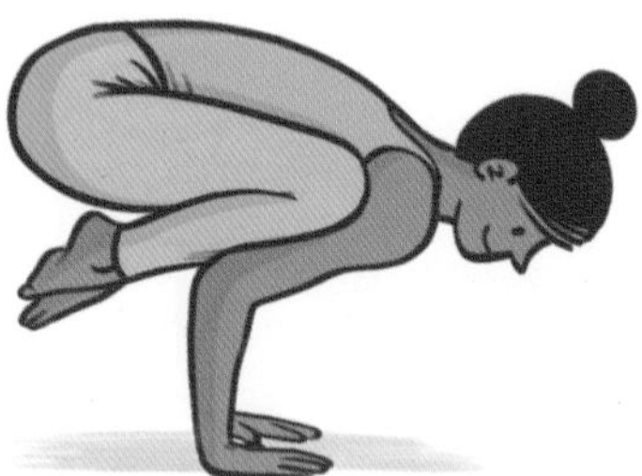

Figure 19.12 This position will require more of a tuck action but provides a nice platform for the shins.

Examples

If you are placing an arm balance within a sequence, it will make it easier if you target the key movements with the preceding poses. By now, you might recognize the actions that make up different shapes, but I will go over a few to help with the process. Lack of bent-arm strength will be a limitation to all of them.

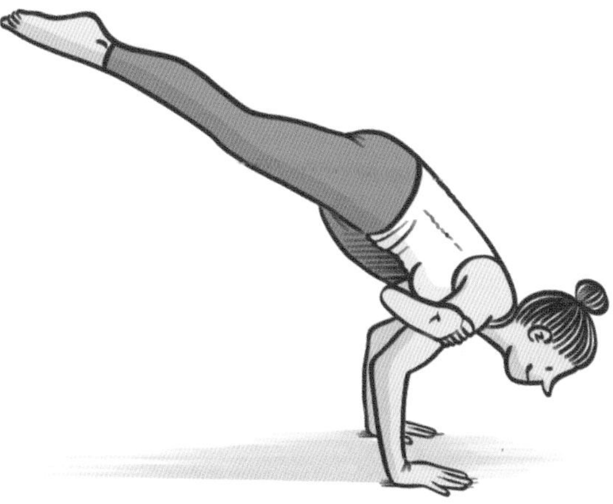

Figure 19.13 Galavasana *will stress the knee if there is not enough external hip rotation.*

Galavasana is dominated by the need for oodles of external hip rotation because without it, the correct leg placement is not possible, the knee can be stressed, and the pose will slip apart (Figure 19.13). Look at the orientation of the crossed leg in Figure 19.14—it needs to be parallel with the floor.

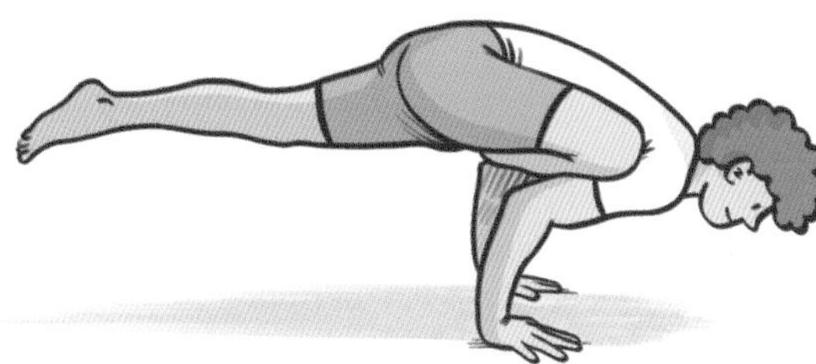

Figure 19.14 Doug will need more strength to hold this low Galavasana *than the more spectacular high leg diving duck version.*

As this is the same positioning as in *Agnistambhasana*, it would make an excellent preparatory pose but could also be an indicator of whether the arm balance should be attempted. I am always extra careful when it comes to the potential for injuring the knee, so if there is more than a small gap (1 to 2 cm) between the legs, I would advise not to do it until that ROM has been realized.

On the setup, another warning sign will be if the torso cannot lay flat on the leg with the shin in both armpits. If the foot end is down the arm or the torso doesn't rest on the leg, it is time to abort as there is insufficient external hip rotation. I have seen all sorts of directionality for this posture, and they are of no anatomical consequence apart from the fact that the workload will change, and the chest should be kept on the shin to protect the knee, even in the higher angles. One of the things you will see happen in this posture is the foot sliding down the arm toward the elbow (Figure 19.15). In this position, it won't be long before the pose falls apart. The key to preventing this is to make sure you have sufficient external hip rotation in the first place, and then grip the arm with the foot by maintaining strong dorsiflexion.

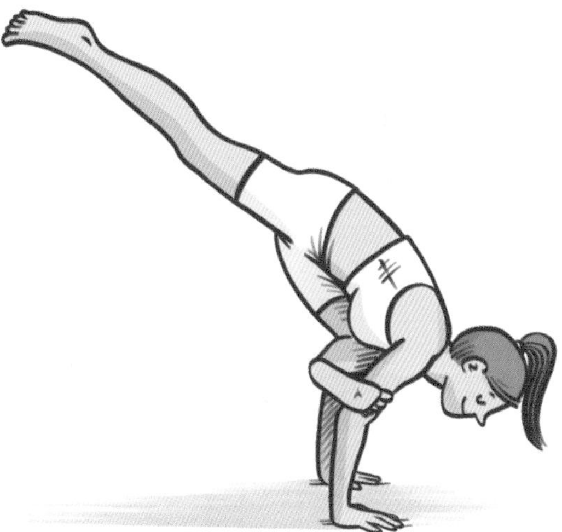

Figure 19.15 You might remember that Victoria has good external hip rotation, so the foot is sliding down the arm because her active dorsiflexion is failing. Finally, it will slide off.

Parsva Bakasana is one of the most accessible arm balances as there are no real ROM limitations apart from a half-decent twist. It comes down to arm strength and confidence that the head won't be cracked on the floor. Those students with good twisting ability and the right proportions will find that they can place the thigh on both legs, but others (like myself) will feel more comfortable with just the knee end on the arm and the hip end free (Figure 19.16). Because it is quite a compact pose, it is usually relatively easy to control the forward and backward movements. If you get used to this

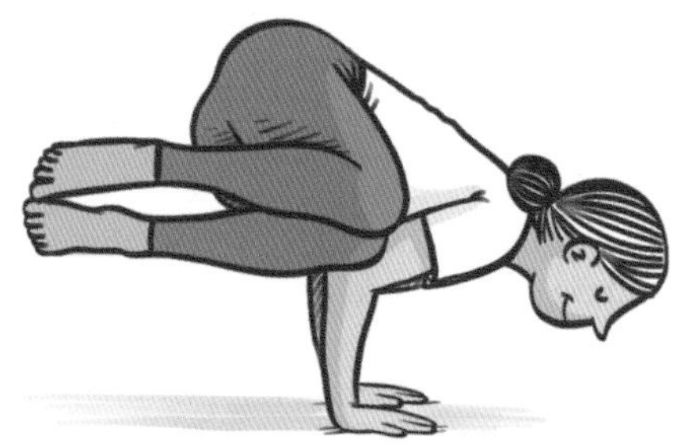

Figure 19.16 Students can be pleasantly surprised by the accessibility of this arm balance.

pose, try the clam version where the top knee is taken toward the ceiling while keeping the feet touching.

Dwi Pada Koundinyasana is often entered from *Parsva Bakasana*, but what differs here is the change from bent-legged hip flexion to straight-legged hip flexion (Figure 19.17). There needs to be greater than 90 degrees of hip flexion available otherwise, either it won't be possible to straighten the legs, or they will get pulled off the arms as the hip flexion decreases with the straightening of the legs.

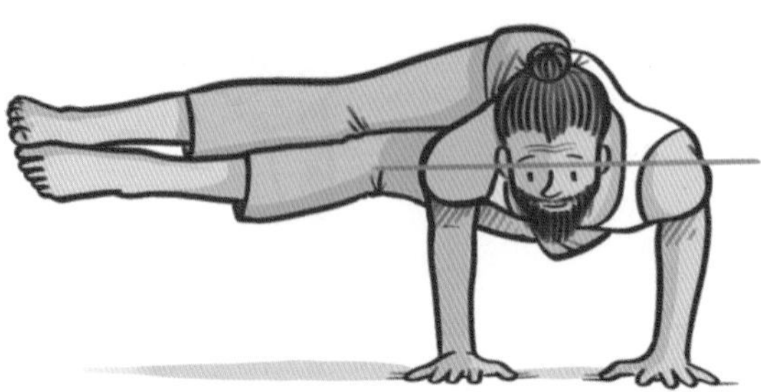

Figure 19.17 Dwi Pada Koundinyasana *is a super pose because it opens up the possibilities of lots more leg positions.*

As a side note, my normal standpoint is to always avoid pain in poses, but I do remember that when you are not used to this pose, the pressure of the arm on the ITB down the outside of the leg can smart a little. It does go with practice and shouldn't cause any damage. This is just a sensitive area on the leg, but do use common sense.

Eka Pada Koundinyasana I is often transitioned into from *Dwi Pada Koundinyasana*, where generally a degree of spinal flexion reduces the amount of hip flexion required (Figure 19.18). However, now the top leg is taken back, it will straighten the pelvis and torso, requiring more straight-legged hip flexion to keep the bottom leg on the arm. It also involves some horizontal adduction of the hip and a small spinal twist, but they are not limiting factors. The back leg position means there is more weight behind the wrists than in front. The COG will have moved back, and it will take more strength to maintain a straight position than to tip the head and shoulders toward the floor.

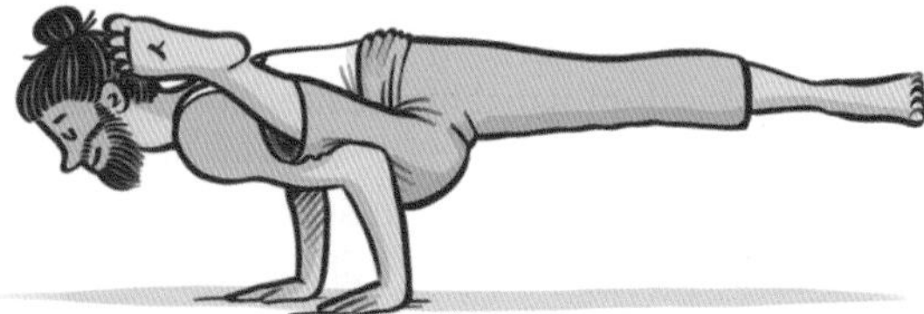

Figure 19.18 It can be a fun challenge to sequence the Koundinyasana *variations together.*

Super fun but tricky pose, *Parsva Bhuja Dandasana* requires good bent-knee hip flexion and external rotation to place the foot on the arm (Figure 19.19). There is a twist in the spine and a minimum of 90 degrees of hip flexion for the straight leg, although more is better. Furthermore, if the supporting arm cannot be bent enough due to lack of strength or stability, the foot will just slide off the arm and take the straight leg with it.

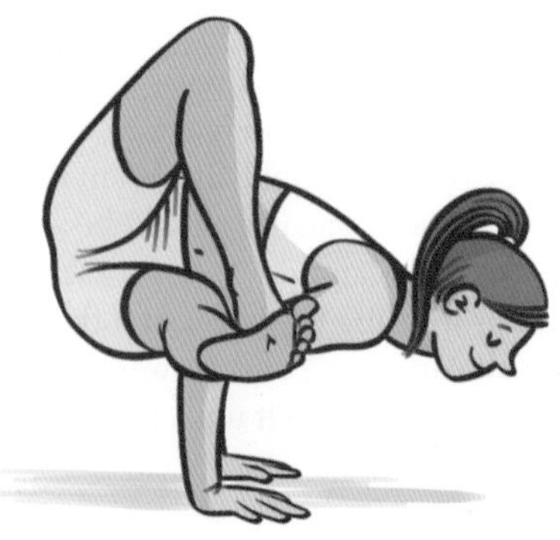

Figure 19.19 From this angle, you can see the external rotation of the top hip.

I would say that *Bakasana* is the arm balance that finds its way into most yoga classes. It can definitely be called an "entry-level arm balance" because the setup is relatively straightforward, and there are so many progressions available, like just rocking in and out, lifting one leg, squeezing around the outside of the arms with the inner thighs, or touching the toes down. It also has the potential of simple scaling for multi-level classes.

There really aren't any ROM limitations, although proportions have a role to play, as a heavy lower half of the body will require more effort to shift the COG. Failure to bend the arms enough and fear of welting the noggin on the floor again comes from lack of bent-arm strength. Friction of the legs or knees on the arms is greatly overused in this posture because it is the easy option, but this avoids the valuable work that occurs (Figure 19.20). That feeling of precariousness, with the chance of the legs slipping off the arms, can be countered by developing more of a lifting action. Rounding the spine and imagining moving up and away from the arms rather than resting on them changes the experience of the pose. I have found that working on this action on the floor can help carry the intention into the pose.

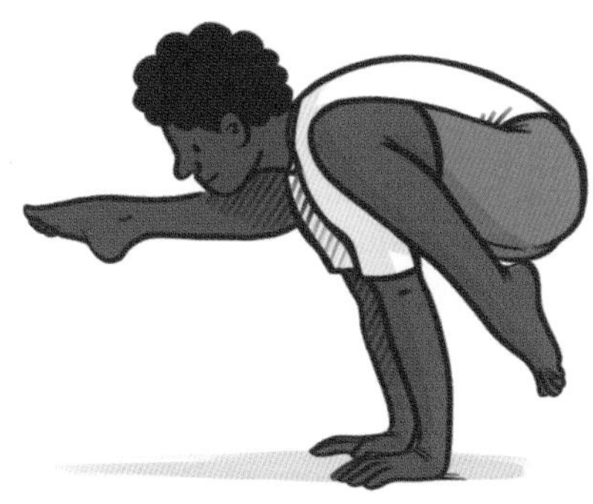

Figure 19.20 To pull this one off, you can't just rely on the knees resting on the arms.

Bakasana can be recreated on the back without the struggle of supporting the weight so that the focus can be on the core engagement. Lay on the back with bent knees, pressing the hands toward the ceiling while protracting the shoulder girdle (Figure 19.21). Now allow the spine to round as the knees are strongly pulled toward the armpits or backs of the arms. This action should pull the sacrum off the floor. Hold this position for 5 to 10 breaths and then repeat. It is surprisingly hard work. Then redo *Bakasana* and try and find the same actions.

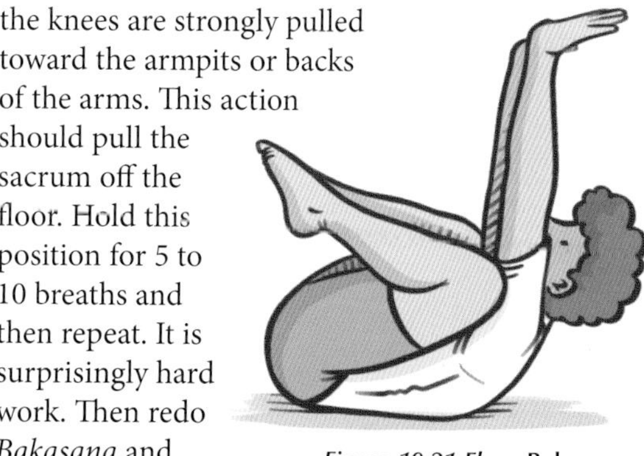

Figure 19.21 Floor Bakasana *is excellent for refining the actions.*

Handstands

Handstands are a passion of mine, but I still wouldn't consider myself a Handstand teacher; it is a specialty of its own. That said, I will lay out the anatomical insights as I see them.

To start with, we can say that the COG is much higher than in the other arm balances discussed so far. Because of this, balance becomes much more of a primary element. With a small BOS, the long lever of the body and high COG, it doesn't take much to disrupt stability. There also needs to be the strength in the arms and shoulder girdle to hold the body weight. Another critical factor is that the minimum requirement of 90 degrees of wrist extension can't be avoided unless wedges are used. My advice is that anyone who has trouble supporting themselves in High Plank for less than 10 breaths should work on this before considering a Handstand.

There has been a massive surge in the interest in hand balancing in recent years, and with it, much greater refinement of desirable positioning. Initially, a posture doesn't have to be perfect, but it should be safe. It is beneficial as well if the technique provides a foundation upon which to build progressions and variations. What I will call the "old style" or "banana" Handstand is more easily achievable for many students, but there is not much you can do with it (Figure 19.22).

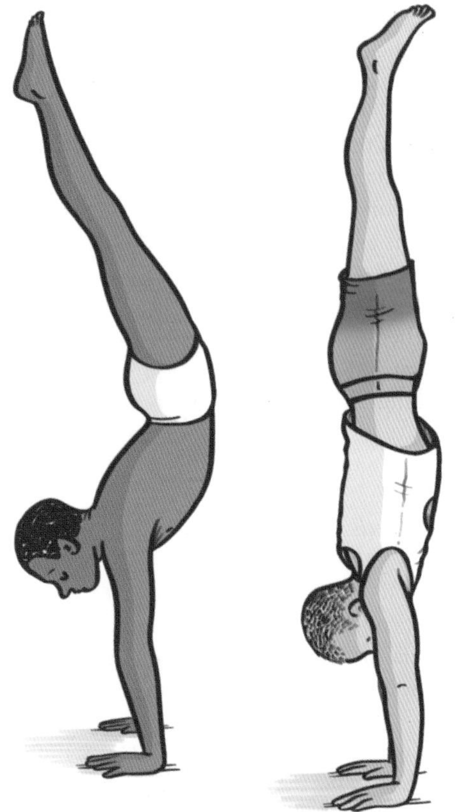

Figure 19.22 Handstands, showing "banana" (left image).

The backbend is not much deeper than in Up Dog, so as long as any hinging is controlled, it shouldn't be detrimental. However, adopting this curved positioning is avoiding much of the work and discovery that can be found when trying to create a straighter line. That said, there can be a long road to clean form, and mild bananas are absolutely acceptable as part of the journey. Being on the hands and balancing, even for a short time in any way possible, gives the body a welcome jolt of energy.

Modern technique has drawn substantially from gymnastics and performance hand balancers, and this has provided insights on gaze point, grip, shoulder, and pelvis position.

When using both hands, the side-to-side balance is not really an issue, it is the forward (overbalance) or backward (under-balance) movement that needs to be controlled. The standard yoga spread-hand isn't the best tool for this particular task, and most serious Handstand practitioners adopt a tiger paw-type grip (Figure 19.23). This has the finger bases and tips on the floor, but the middle knuckles raised, providing much more control.

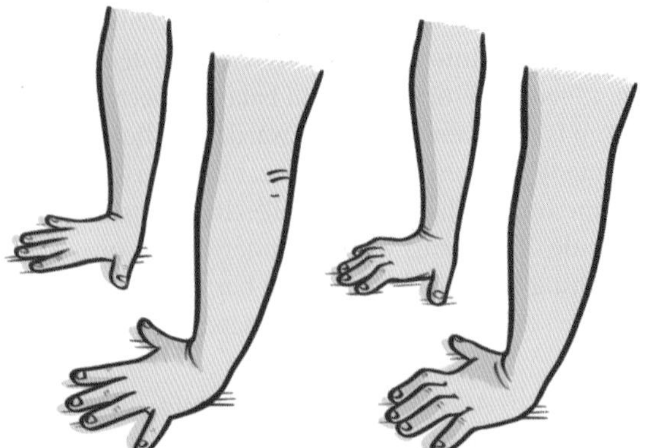

Figure 19.23 Using a tiger paw-type grip gives much better control.

Working up the body, one of the most noticeable differences at the shoulder is the amount of shoulder flexion. In the straight Handstand, the shoulder girdle is elevated maximally, bringing the inner arms close to the ears, and there is a straight line through the armpit. The elbows can then be locked straight, reducing fatigue in the arms (Figure 19.24A). The ROM of shoulder flexion is an essential ingredient to the modern Handstand. If a straight line between torso and arms cannot be achieved, balance can only be maintained by introducing an extension in the spine to bring the legs over the head (banana) and the line of gravity over the hands (Figure 19.24B). To create shapes where the legs are on the under-balance side of the body, such as with a tuck, even more shoulder flexion will be required (Figure 19.24C).

The homework for most Handstand addicts involves plenty of shoulder flexion ROM work (Figure 19.25).

There is plenty of discussion about how strong the abdominals need to be for maintaining a straight line, and I fall into the camp of "not so much."

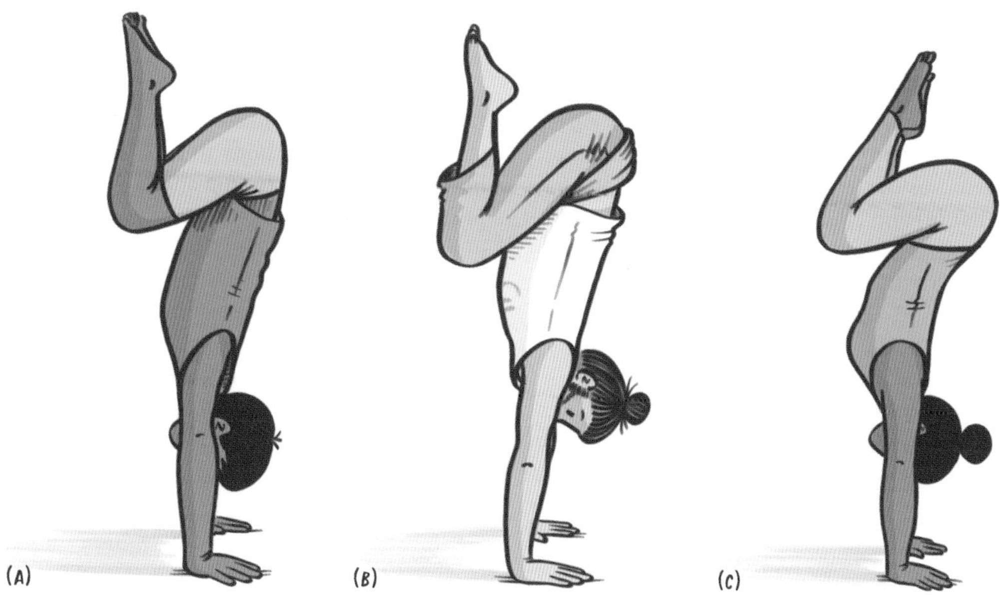

Figure 19.24 As more of the body weight is shifted toward the under-balance side, something must be done to keep the COG over the BOS. (A) Vihan has flexed the shoulder more, (B) Zane has extended the wrists more, and (C) Myra has extended the lumbar spine.

If you think of the work that goes on in the abdominal area when you are standing up, Handstands are similar, just upside down.

Having said that, if you are naturally a "bendy Wendy," then working on core stabilization drills like forearm plank and hollow body hold should certainly help. There is generally a slight tuck of the pelvis in the straight Handstand, which helps keep the ribs from flaring, the legs are seamed together, and the toes reach toward the ceiling. These actions can be explored in the hollow body.

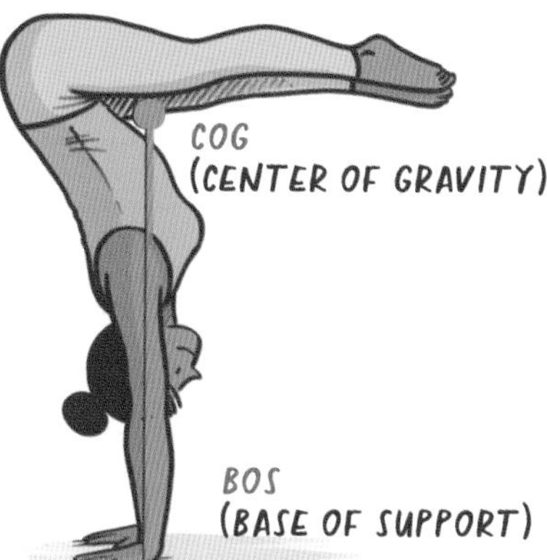

Figure 19.25 In a pike position "7," more adaptation will need to be made to maintain balance.

The key to this exercise is to keep the low back pressed into the floor because this dictates the height of the legs. I find it works best to start with the legs at 90 degrees (pointing to the ceiling), raise the shoulder blades off the floor, and then lower the legs slowly, stopping at a point before you lose the low back contact (Figure 19.26). Now the hold begins. Gradually build up the time until you can do something like three sets of 20 to 30 seconds, or several minutes, depending on your aspirations.

Kicking up does not need to be like heaving a sack of spuds onto your back. In the same way as moving the hips over the shoulders in *Sirsasana*

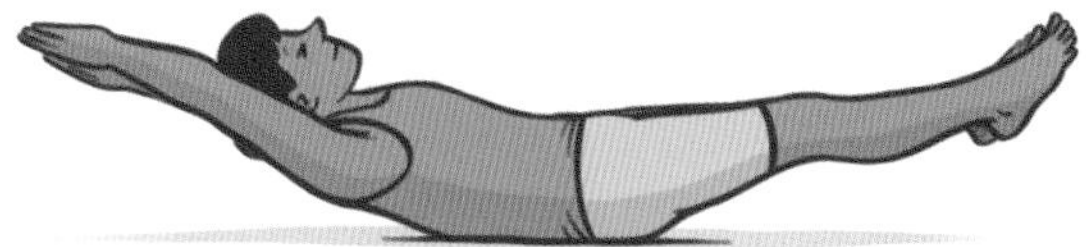

Figure 19.26 In a hollow body, raising the arms or legs will reduce the intensity.

makes the feet feel light, going up in Handstand is about the transition of weight. As the leg goes up, the shoulders should be over the hands. A minimal amount of effort will make it much easier to control the stopping point. Using the wall as a guide removes the fear factor of going over the top (overbalance) and crashing onto your back like a felled tree, but it should not become a crutch that you can't do without.

The solution to this is to learn to save yourself, which involves doing a cartwheel. This is not something you should learn from a book, so seek out a teacher if you want to go free standing. Once you know you can always land on your feet, the fear is gone. I don't advise to save a crash by dropping over into *Urdhva Dhanurasana* as it is easy to hurt yourself if it goes wrong.

If you want Handstands to be part of your practice, you need to give the body time to figure out how to gauge where to stop and how to hold the position. Repetition of structured work is the key. There is little point in keeping throwing yourself up against the wall in the hope that one day you will suddenly balance. As with other postures, seek calmness, insight, and patience. By fighting hard to maintain balance, your nervous system will reinforce the successful interventions. Within the limitations of wrist healthcare, the more time you spend trying to balance, the quicker you will improve.

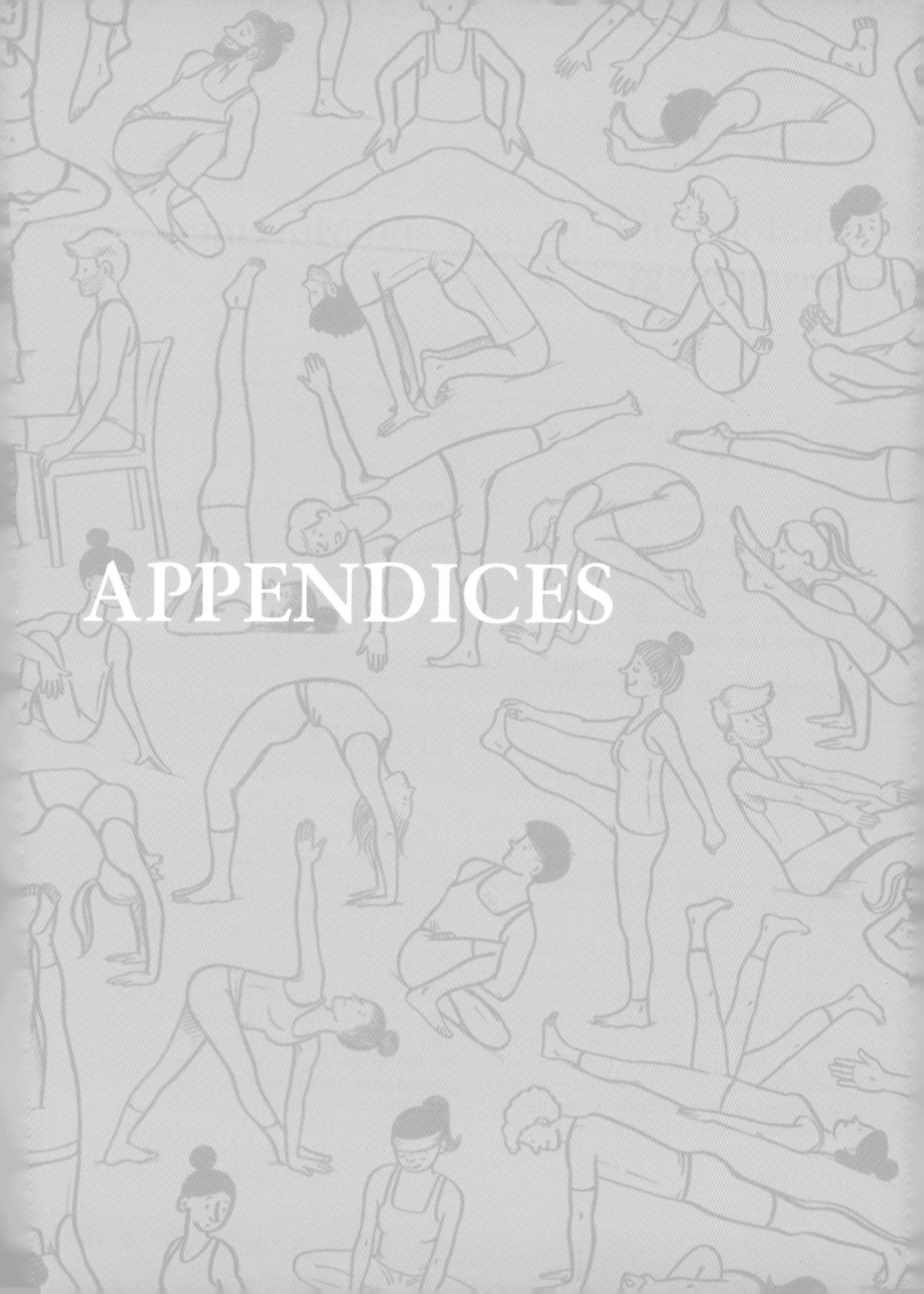

APPENDICES

Anatomical Language and Movement Terminology

The idea of this book is to provide knowledge based specifically on its implementation into the physical practice of yoga, so as you will be aware, we just started straight in with the "Key Concepts." However, some students will want or need more formal anatomical background information. Appendix 1 provides quick reference material for those struggling with terminology, bone, or muscle names. There will also be the answers to questions posed during earlier chapters.

The *anatomical language* introduced below is used to describe or talk about how one structure relates in space to another, directional movement, and the position of a specific area or surface on something. Once you learn the terms, you can start combining them in different situations to be precise and concise.

Anatomical position looks similar to *Tadasana*. This is the traditional starting point from which we can describe movement or structural relationships. The head, hands, and feet are all facing forward, with the arms a little out to the sides, and the legs parted to about shoulder width. Initially, we will just concern ourselves with terms that relate mostly to position or structural relationship, but then we will start combining some of these words with others to describe joint movements, for example, medial rotation.

Directional Terminology and Planes

When we are investigating the structures of the body, it is sometimes useful to take a slice (plane) through the body in a particular way that allows us to view these structures as they relate to those around them (Figure A1.1).

A *sagittal plane* divides the body down the middle into left and right sides. At right angles to this is a *frontal plane*, separating the body into a front and back section. A *transverse plane* divides the body into an upper and lower section.

More useful for us when thinking of yoga postures is that we may also relate movement to planes. To step out for *Virabhadrasana* A, we would be moving in a sagittal plane. Taking our legs apart for *Prasarita Padottanasana* would involve movement in a frontal plane, and twisting relates to the transverse plane.

Planes are not that important for our uses, but they do crop up now and again, for example, when defining some specific joint movements. Flexion is often described as a forward movement in the sagittal plane. Try and think about what that looks like and why knee flexion doesn't work with this definition. There are only three planes, so it is worth trying to remember them. Most of the words used to describe the relative position of a

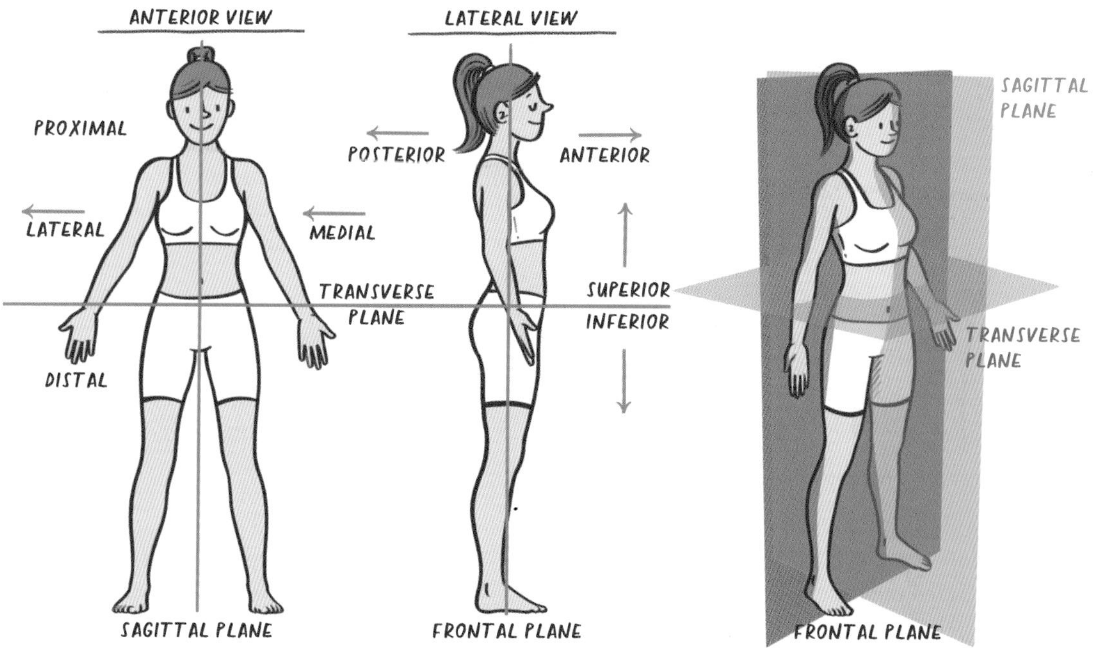

Figure A1.1 Directional terminology and planes.

structure will be familiar from normal vocabulary, apart from proximal and distal, but consider the similarity to proximity and distance (Table A1.1).

Table A1.1 Directional terminology.

Term	Definition
Superior	Toward the head, or the upper end of a structure
Inferior	Away from the head, or the lower end of a structure
Anterior (ventral)	Toward the front of the body
Posterior (dorsal)	Toward the back of the body
Medial	Nearer the midline of the body or structure
Lateral	Away from the midline of the body or structure
Proximal	Closer to the attachment point of a body part to the trunk, or the part of a structure nearer its origin
Distal	Further from the attachment point of a body part to the trunk, or the part of a structure further from its origin

Location Can Make a Difference

In this book, I have not been particularly specific about the exact area on a bone that muscles attach. I feel it is sufficient for our purposes to know a rough location. But it does matter which side or surface that attachment area is because it will influence the actions a muscle can perform.

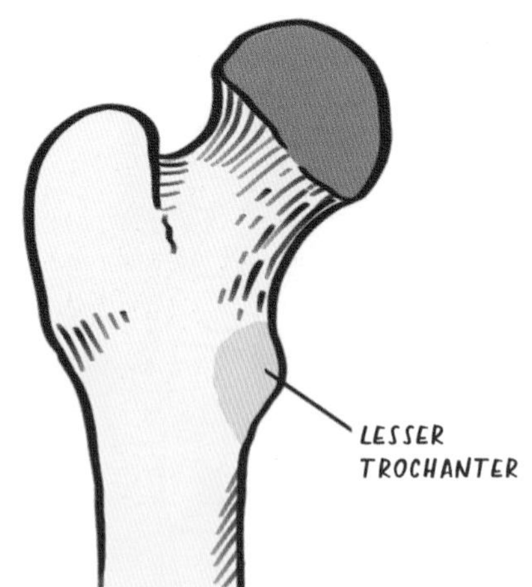

Figure A1.2 Lesser trochanter (left leg, posterior view).

For example, in Figure A1.2 of the top of the femur (upper leg bone), you will see a bony landmark highlighted called the lesser trochanter (don't worry about what that means at the moment), The image is of the left leg looking from the back, and that rounded area at the top is what fits into the hip socket. You can see that this particular bony prominence is a bit around the back and on the inside of the leg, so we could say it is at the proximal end of the femur on the posteromedial aspect. The psoas muscle attaches here, so when it contracts, the directionality of pull will make a difference to the actions it has on the femur and hence the movement at the hip joint.

If you are reading a more formal book, you might need to translate this type of positional information so that you can understand the area that is being referred to.

Bone Names

For our purposes, knowing around 20 bone names will make your anatomy journey easier. It is useful to divide the bones into two groups:

The *axial skeleton* (reddish color in Figure A1.3): skull, vertebral column (spine), and ribcage (ribs and sternum).

The *appendicular skeleton*: bones of the upper and lower extremities (arms, legs, hands, and feet), shoulder and pelvic girdles.

It is hard to fathom when we look at a body standing right in front of us, but the only place the upper appendicular skeleton attaches to the axial skeleton is where the clavicle meets the sternum (SCJ).

The axial skeleton has two main roles:

- **Protection**—forming cavities to protect vital organs, such as the brain, heart, lungs, and spinal cord.
- **Support**—allowing us to stand upright by means of the vertebral column, aiding some organs in maintaining their positions by providing solid structures to attach to, and providing areas from which the appendicular skeleton can hang.

Appreciating these roles helps us to understand the resistance to deformation that the axial skeleton will elicit when we try and proceed deeply into some postures. The spine will only want to bend so far to make sure the spinal cord is not compromised. The ribcage will resist being flattened or squashed too much because it is protecting some vital organs. If you have a large ribcage, you may also find it can impede hip flexion when it comes into contact with the legs or even acts as an obstacle in certain bound twists. The ribcage is also one of the factors that limit backbending.

The appendicular skeleton, on the other hand, is more involved with locomotion and manipulating our environment (Figure A1.3). From this standpoint, we can conceive that the elements of the appendicular skeleton will try to find a balance between stability and ROM. The appreciation of the need for mobility also informs us that if we use those same structures for support, such as when doing a Handstand (I'm thinking wrists here), then

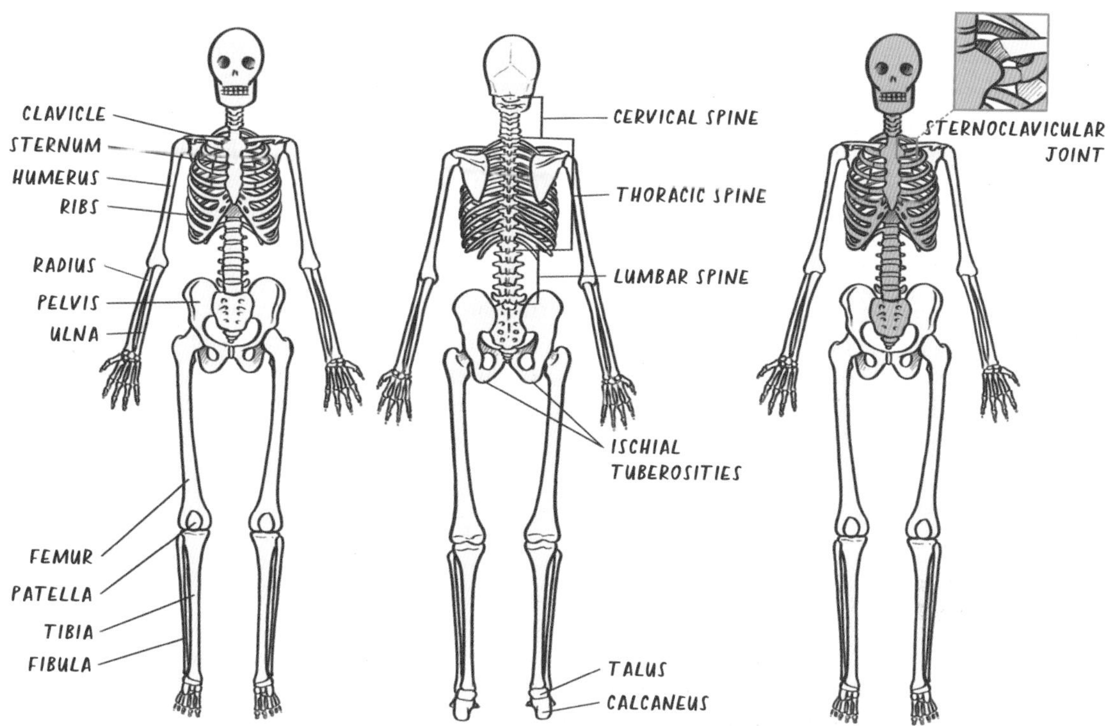

Figure A1.3 The axial and appendicular skeleton.

there will be an inherent vulnerability that we need to take care not to overlook.

As part of the appendicular skeleton, the legs play the dual role of support and locomotion. We would expect, therefore, to see less ROM in its associated joints when compared with the arms, which are for interacting with the environment. These ideas help inform us when we start contemplating how much ROM is desirable in specific areas of the body, considering what we might ask of them and what they are designed for.

One of the nice things about yoga is that we place demands on the structures in many different ways, allowing us to get in touch with our bodies and sometimes challenge the limits. However, it is also easy to destabilize areas by focusing on too much ROM and not enough strength.

Bony Landmarks

No bone is smooth or even straight. Most of them twist and bend along their length and have many lumps and bumps (Table A1.2). Luckily enough, unless you were made on a Friday afternoon, this has been taken into account and generally, the two articulating surfaces where bones meet each other butt up quite nicely. That's not to say you could pop out my clavicle and slot it into your body. Even if they were the same length, the chances are my twists and turns would mean that the two ends that form joints with the scapula and sternum would be a bad fit. Paul Grilley has some great images on his website that demonstrate the potential differences.

Therefore, if the structural geometry of a joint can vary even slightly between individuals, then we can surmise that there will be configurations that predispose a person to greater stability or ROM at that particular joint and vice versa. For example, when we looked at the shoulder, we discussed that there could be certain shapes of the converging bones that may severely limit movement in one or more planes. Physically we are not all equal. Therefore, our expectations of what our body can do and the way we need to work also requires us to take this into account. This is not the same as saying we should not shoot for the stars, just that on the way there we should respect the bodies we have. You will find this theme of individuality intertwined throughout the book.

What about the lumps and bumps? Well, for the most part, these areas of thickening and/or protrusion are there either to create the required structure for the joint or to form areas where muscles attach. For example, the distal end of the femur has the characteristic "dog bone" shape. This not only provides a larger articulating surface than if it had stayed the same size as the shaft, but also the shape itself accommodates the function required at the knee joint. Areas for muscle attachment will be more pronounced where the muscles are larger and stronger and again, between individuals, particularly influenced by gender.

Table A1.2 Bony landmarks.

Term	Description	Example	Function
Tuberosity	Large, rounded projection	Radial tuberosity	Attachment sites for ligaments and tendons
Crest	Narrow, prominent ridge	Iliac crest	
Trochanter	Large, blunt, irregular process	Greater trochanter of femur	
Tubercle	Small, rounded projection	Greater tubercle of humerus	
Epicondyle	Raised area on or above a condyle	Medial epicondyle of humerus	
Spine	Sharp and slender projection	Spine of scapula	
Head	Expansion from neck or shaft	Head of fibula	Projections that help form joints
Facet	Smooth nearly flat surface	On articular processes of vertebrae	
Condyle	Rounded projection	Lateral condyle of tibia	
Ramus	Arm like projection	Inferior ramus of pubis	
Sinus	Cavity within a bone	Nasal sinus	Depressions and openings that allow room for nerves and blood vessels to pass
Fossa	Shallow depression	Glenoid fossa scapula	
Foramen	Round or oval opening in bone	Nutrient foramen of femur	

Depending on their size and shape, these bony forms are given names such as tuberosity, condyle, epicondyle, ramus, etc., and then generally used in conjunction with the name of the bone they are on to give a location. For example, you have pubic ramus, femoral condyle, and ischial tuberosity.

We can take the ischial tuberosity as an example, as it is a good one to know because those beloved hamstrings attach there. A tuberosity is a large, rounded projection—this one is on the ischium, which is one of the bones of the pelvis—so we have a *tuberosity* that is large relative to a *tubercle*, a small, rounded projection. I think you will be glad to hear that, apart from some significant landmarks, we can consider the terms as just different sized bumps and projections. The main point for bringing them up now is so that if you do further reading about a particular muscle, you won't be deterred by the terminology. I have put a list of markings in Table A1.2, just read through it once or twice, so you have come across the terms.

Movement Terminology

In the human body, movement occurs where two bones meet—what we refer to as a joint (Table A1.3). We will talk more about the characteristics of joints themselves a bit later, but for the moment, we want to think of what types of movement might be available. We have introduced terms that help describe the relative position of structures (e.g., anterior, inferior, distal, etc.), and likewise, we need terms that clearly indicate the direction of joint movement. Movement is described relative to anatomical position.

When reading about movement and talking in an anatomy-based environment, the joint will be referenced, not the limbs involved. For example, we would say "internal rotation of the shoulder" not "internal rotation of the humerus," or "flex the hip" not "flex the leg, thigh, or femur." You will find that the previously learned terms of medial and lateral will be used in conjunction with the new terminology of rotation.

When deconstructing postures or transitions, we might want to consider the movement that is needed to take us from point A to point B and from there, what muscles would I need to use to achieve that, or even what movements are required at a particular joint to perform a given posture. Once we know the movements needed, we can investigate what might be stopping us achieving it. Is it insufficient strength to perform a certain action or is it something restricting that movement?

Of course, the movements required to enter a posture will invariably not be the same as when we are staying in the posture. We may, for example, need to flex our hip to proceed into a posture, but once in it, we may decide to engage those muscles that extend the hip. Not with the intention of coming out of the posture, just stabilizing and being active rather than passive.

Table A1.3 Movement terminology.

Movement	Description	Example
Flexion	Angular decrease	Elbow flexion brings the forearm closer to the upper arm
Extension	Angular increase	In standing position, hip extension takes the thigh to the rear of the body
Adduction	Movement toward the midline	Thighs move toward meeting in the middle
Abduction	Movement away from the midline	Arm moves sideways away from the body
Rotation	Movement around an axis in one plane	Turning head to left or right
Lateral rotation	Rotation away from the midline	You laterally rotate the hip when doing *Baddha Konasana*
Medial rotation	Rotation toward the midline	You medially rotate the shoulder when binding in *Marichyasana C*
Circumduction	Circular movement	Making circles with the arms
Inversion	Plane rotation medially (refers only to feet)	Sole of the foot rotates so that it is facing inward
Eversion	Plane rotation laterally (refers only to feet)	Sole of the foot rotates so that it is facing outward
Dorsiflexion	Superior plane shift (refers only to feet)	Pointing the foot up. The top of the foot comes closer to the shin
Plantar flexion	Inferior plane shift (refers only to feet)	Pointing the foot down. The top of the foot moves away from the shin
Protraction	Forward movement	Drawing the mandible forward
Retraction	Backward movement	Drawing the scapula back
Elevation	Upward movement	Drawing the shoulder girdle up
Depression	Downward movement	Drawing the shoulder girdle down
Supination	Anterior plane shift	Turn palm to face up or to the front
Pronation	Posterior plane shift	Turn palm to face down or to the back

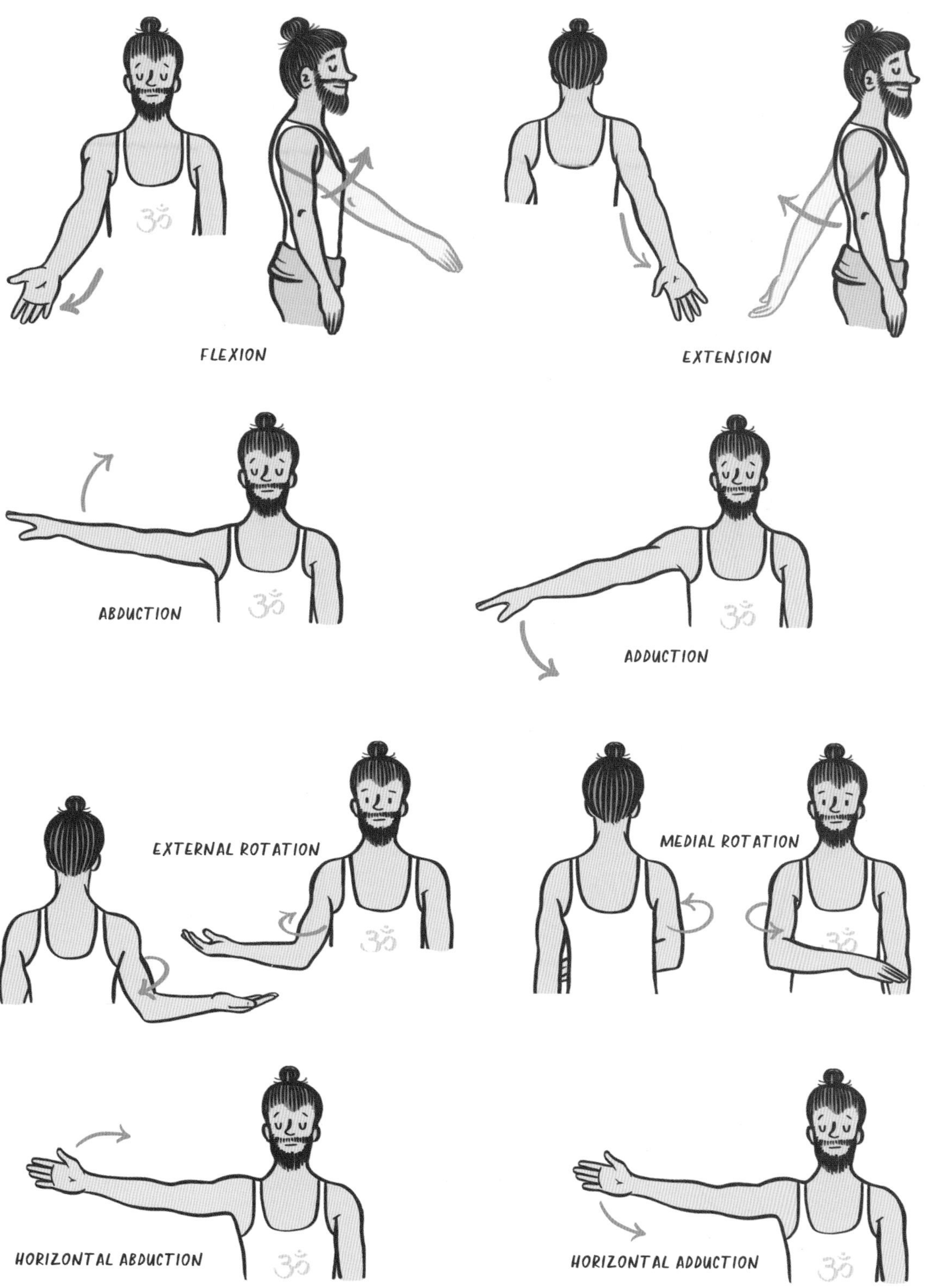
FLEXION
EXTENSION
ABDUCTION
ADDUCTION
EXTERNAL ROTATION
MEDIAL ROTATION
HORIZONTAL ABDUCTION
HORIZONTAL ADDUCTION

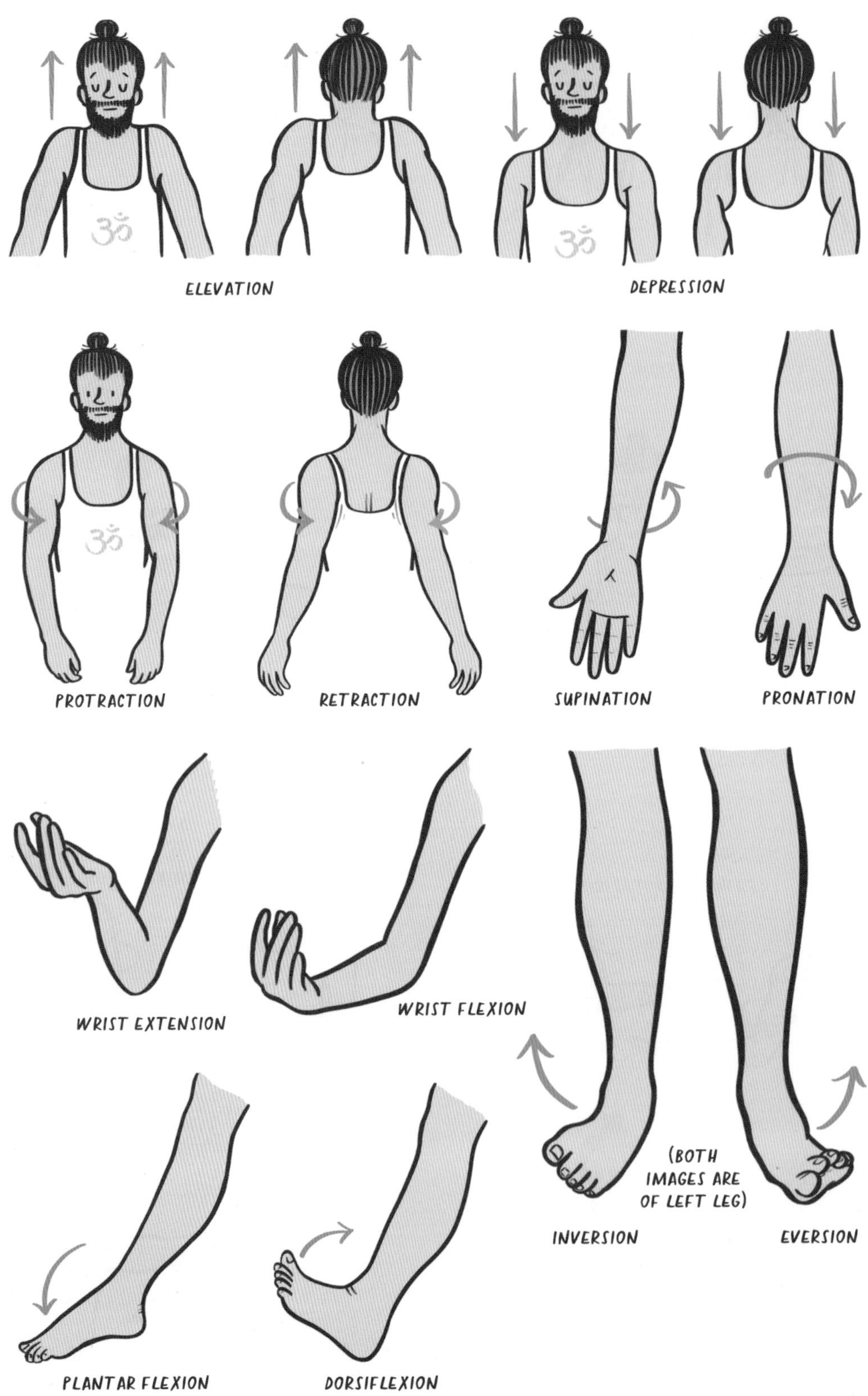
ELEVATION
DEPRESSION
PROTRACTION
RETRACTION
SUPINATION
PRONATION
WRIST EXTENSION
WRIST FLEXION
(BOTH IMAGES ARE OF LEFT LEG)
INVERSION
EVERSION
PLANTAR FLEXION
DORSIFLEXION

Breaking Down a Posture by Joint Movement

In anatomical texts, movement is relative to anatomical position, but when looking at yoga poses, we will often be in a much more convoluted positioning. We need to be able to take those thought processes off the paper and apply them to the physical body and movement relative to different starting positions. In addition, we may be fixing in place various parts of the body and need to think a little laterally to visualize what is happening (Figure A1.4).

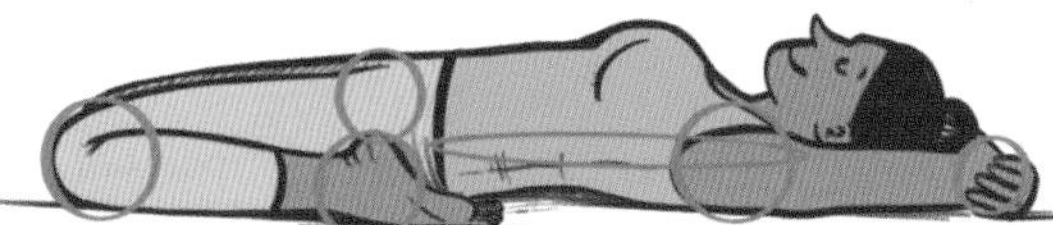

Figure A1.4 You want to be able to look at a posture and know what joint movements are happening to create the shape.

Let me give you an example of this last point. If we are moving from a starting point of *Dandasana* into *Janu Sirsasana A* on the right side, we first need to flex the right knee and then externally rotate and abduct the right hip. This will bring the foot to the inside of the left thigh and the outside of the bent leg laying on or close to the floor. Those movements have occurred by the leg moving relative to a static pelvis (we are still in *Dandasana* as far as the pelvis goes).

If now we decide to fold forward, the movement is still going to happen at the hip, but because the leg is now on the floor, we are moving our pelvis relative to the leg, thus increasing the external rotation at the hip (Figure A1.5). This is covered in Chapter 2, *Relational Movement*.

If you are guiding students into postures in a yoga class, much of this type of terminology may not be appropriate. You will need to use your own judgment to determine what is helpful. In anatomically minded situations, we reference the joint, but for students, this may not work. To avoid confusion, it is likely you will be referencing the limb being moved.

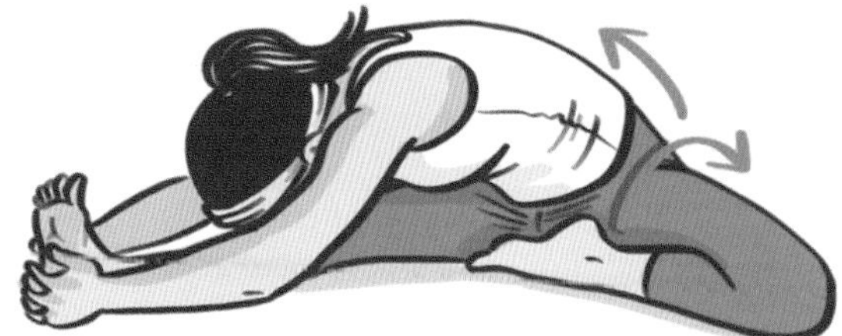

Figure A1.5 In Janu Sirsasana A, *the leg rotates relative to the pelvis and then the pelvis relative to the leg.*

There is also a standard vocabulary that can be used outside anatomical texts: thigh (upper leg), leg (lower leg), arm (upper arm), and forearm (lower arm). Often, you will hear people say "extend the spine" when they are trying to give instruction to create space. As we can now see, this may be taken to mean initiate a backbend. It is better to use a word like "lengthen" in these situations. With the popularity of medical and science television programs, you may be surprised by how much anatomical terminology has entered the public domain. How you teach is really a side issue, because the purpose of this book is to prepare you to make informed decisions based on a certain level of analysis.

Joints

The junction where two bones meet is called a joint. Not all joints allow movement, and functionally, they are divided into immovable, slightly movable, and freely movable. They may also be classified structurally based on whether or not there is a synovial cavity. Fibrous and cartilaginous joints have no synovial cavity and provide little or no movement. Synovial joints, on the other hand, freely allow movement, although not in all planes as differing joint design determines what can be done. It is this last group (synovial joints) that is of most relevance to yoga (with the exception of the cartilaginous joints between the vertebrae).

There are six types of freely movable joints, and each design will have different ranges and directions of movement available, the least with gliding joints, and the greatest with ball-and-socket joints. Movement around a joint is dictated by the way the articulating bones are shaped, the tension in the surrounding ligaments, and the arrangement and tension of associated muscles.

Look at Table A1.4 to see the differences. In some places, like the elbow and ankle, there are two joints very close to one another to create the functionality required in that area. While in other places like the knee, joint design sometimes allows for some extra movements. If you have a play with your knee, you will find that although we consider it a hinge joint, when flexed, there is some rotation available.

It is important to know what we should expect from the different joints so that we can protect them from specific movements they are not designed to perform. An example of this would be the unfortunate habit of students trying to use their lower leg as a lever to pull themselves into *Padmasana* when they are not sufficiently open in the hips. This places tremendous stress on the structures of the knee and, with repetition, will invariably result in injury.

To make the shapes with our body that we may consider constituting the physical representation of a yoga posture, we need the gross movements at the major joints, ankle, knee, hip, spine, shoulder, elbow, and wrist. Of course, there is some adaptation throughout the other joints in the body, but generally speaking, it won't stop us doing a posture if, for example, your finger extension is somewhat limited.

In yoga, it is the major joints that we actively seek to increase ROM and strength. How much is too much is also an important question? If we look at Table A1.4 and think about the major joints mentioned, we can see that the types of joints we are most interested in are ball-and-socket, hinge, and pivot. In this section, I am only giving you an overview of joint types. In Part II, *Body Bits*, we look at each of the major joints separately.

The naming of joints is often by placing an "o" between the names of the two bones (or parts of), that are meeting. They are then, for ease of use, often referred to by the starting letter of those two bones. Common examples are: sternoclavicular joint (where the sternum and clavicle meet), acromioclavicular joint (where acromion process of the scapula and the clavicle meet), and sacroiliac joint (where the sacrum and ilium meet). They would be referred to as SCJ, ACJ, and SIJ respectively.

We tend to refer to the major joints of the body by body location, shoulder joint, knee joint, etc., but

Table A1.4 Joints and their movements.

Joint Type	Movement	Example
Gliding	Sliding back and forth, side to side. No rotational or angular movement	Between carpal bones (wrist)
Hinge	Flexion and extension	Knee
Pivot	Rotation	Between atlas and axis
Ellipsoid	Flexion, extension, adduction, abduction, and circumduction	Between radius and carpals (wrist)
Saddle	Same as ellipsoid but with freer movement	Between trapezium and metacarpal of thumb
Ball and socket	Flexion, extension, adduction, abduction, rotation, and circumduction	Hip and shoulder

you should realize that if you needed to read more in-depth, the same type of naming convention would appear once again. This is necessary because joints are rarely straightforward and may comprise multiple articulations, creating the need to be able to specify the area you are talking about. For example, the knee is not a straightforward hinge as we have the patella in front, and that dog bone end to the femur creates two semi-separate articulations with the tibia. If you started to delve deeper, you would find a reference to the femoropatellar articulation and medial and lateral femorotibial articulations.

Don't freak out, you shouldn't need that sort of detail, this is just so you know there is a consistency to naming things, and if you come across this terminology, you can work out where they are talking about.

Ligaments

A ligament is a band of connective tissue that connects one bone to another, and its role is specifically to create joint stability and protect the structures from movement in undesired range or direction. They are somewhat elastic but not as much as tendons and only be able to withstand about 6 percent stretch deformation before damage occurs. That sort of makes sense because if you are trying to use something to create stability, it's no use if it is too stretchy, but you also need some give for adaptability. In weight-bearing areas such as the hip, the ligaments are much thicker and stronger than areas where more mobility is required. When someone is termed hypermobile, in simplistic terms, it means that their ligaments are more elastic than average, allowing for greater joint ROM but, of course, liable for less stability.

There will be a varying number of ligaments around the individual joints depending on the amount of stability required, design characteristics, muscular support, and degree of load-bearing. When we damage a ligament, it is referred to as a sprain rather than a strain, which is used to refer to muscle or tendon damage. There are some ligaments that are regularly damaged in sports, such as the anterior cruciate ligament in the knee and the anterior talofibular ligament on the outside of the ankle. I think, as a teacher, it's helpful to know the names of those commonly injured, so you don't have a blank face when someone tells you they damaged it, but actually, it's more important to have an appreciation of the possible ramifications.

If a ligament has been damaged recently, the pain will normally stop people from doing anything too excessive. As we heal and return to regular activity, the area will be more fragile and sensitive to reinjury. If we understand that the ligaments are there to stabilize a joint, then we can avoid postures that may place a lot of strain on that area and make them work too hard in their weakened state. It is not beneficial to rule out all postures involving the affected area because they need to be working on rehabilitating.

Unless you have a background in medicine, I don't imagine you will know how to do that, but what you can do is modify a sequence so that the healing ligament is not placed under too much stress. To accomplish that, you need to know where the damage is, so just ask a student to point to the spot where they hurt. If you are not sure, back it up by asking what movements are uncomfortable to perform. With a repeated injury to the same area (as often happens with ankles) an individual will develop greater instability in that area.

Let me give you an example—someone sprained their ankle tripping over a few weeks ago and is coming back to class for the first time since it happened. Most ankle sprains occur with the foot pointed (plantar flexed) and the sole facing toward the center line (inverted), Figure A1.6.

As weight comes down on the foot in this position, it places strain on the ligaments on the outside of the ankle. Nearly 80 percent of all ankle sprains occur with the foot in this position, and it is likely that the main ligament involved is the one mentioned above, the anterior talofibular ligament. If this was the case, you would want to avoid, for the time being, postures where the foot would be placed in a similar position to when it was injured.

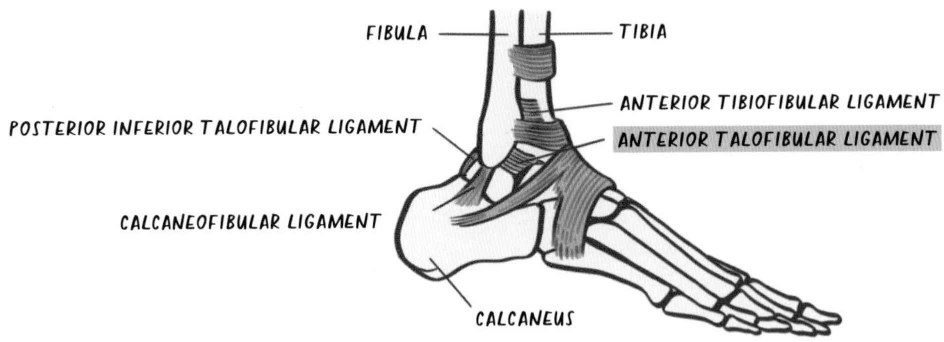

Figure A1.6 Ankle ligaments.

This is the position of the foot in *Padmasana*, for example, and somewhat similar in *Baddha Konasana* if the knees are up in the air. Also, thinking in terms of stability, the demands on the ankle would be much greater in a single-legged balancing posture than with both feet grounded.

There will, however, be many postures where the ankle feels just fine. You don't want to be jumping to conclusions when someone says they have sprained their ankle because the mechanism of injury may have been in the opposite direction and, as such, would have damaged something on the inside of the ankle and thus contraindicate different postures.

See the slight difference in the name of the two ligaments shown on the right: tibiofibular and talofibular. The former goes between the tibia and fibula the latter between the talus and fibula. You may have noticed something familiar about the way the ankle ligament in the example above was named (anterior talofibular ligament). In the same way that we name joints, in most cases, reference is made to the two bones the ligament connects, in this example, the talus and fibula.

As there are many ligaments around a joint attaching to the same bones, some reference to the position is also needed to distinguish the exact one, such as the use of anterior here. The image is not there for you to learn all the ligaments around the ankle, just to demonstrate naming convention. The point is if someone told you the ligament they had hurt, knowing the names of the bones should allow you to pretty much determine where it is and hence what movements to limit. Not all ligaments are named in this way, for example, cruciate in ACL reflects that there are two forming a cross shape (the other is the PCL).

It is important in yoga that we do not overly stress ligaments when trying to get into a pose, mistakenly thinking we are increasing our flexibility. If we unnecessarily stretch ligaments, a joint will become unstable. Particularly vulnerable are the ankle, shoulder, and knee.

Muscles

As with the bones, there is no need to know every muscle in the body, somewhere between 20 and 30 will suffice. There are numerous chapters in Part I, *Key Concepts*, that relate to muscles, and more detailed anatomical images in Part II, *Body Bits*, so there is no need for me to go into extra detail here. Figure A1.7 is an ideal quick reference or learning tool to familiarize yourself with the rough location of muscles.

If you want to learn about sliding filament theory which explains muscle contraction at a molecular level, you can go ahead and "Google" it. The main thing I would like you to seek to understand from this book is that as well as movement, muscles also stabilize and help protect joints. Learning how to work on strength within the yoga practice is key to maintaining a healthy body for anyone that does not perform strength training exercises.

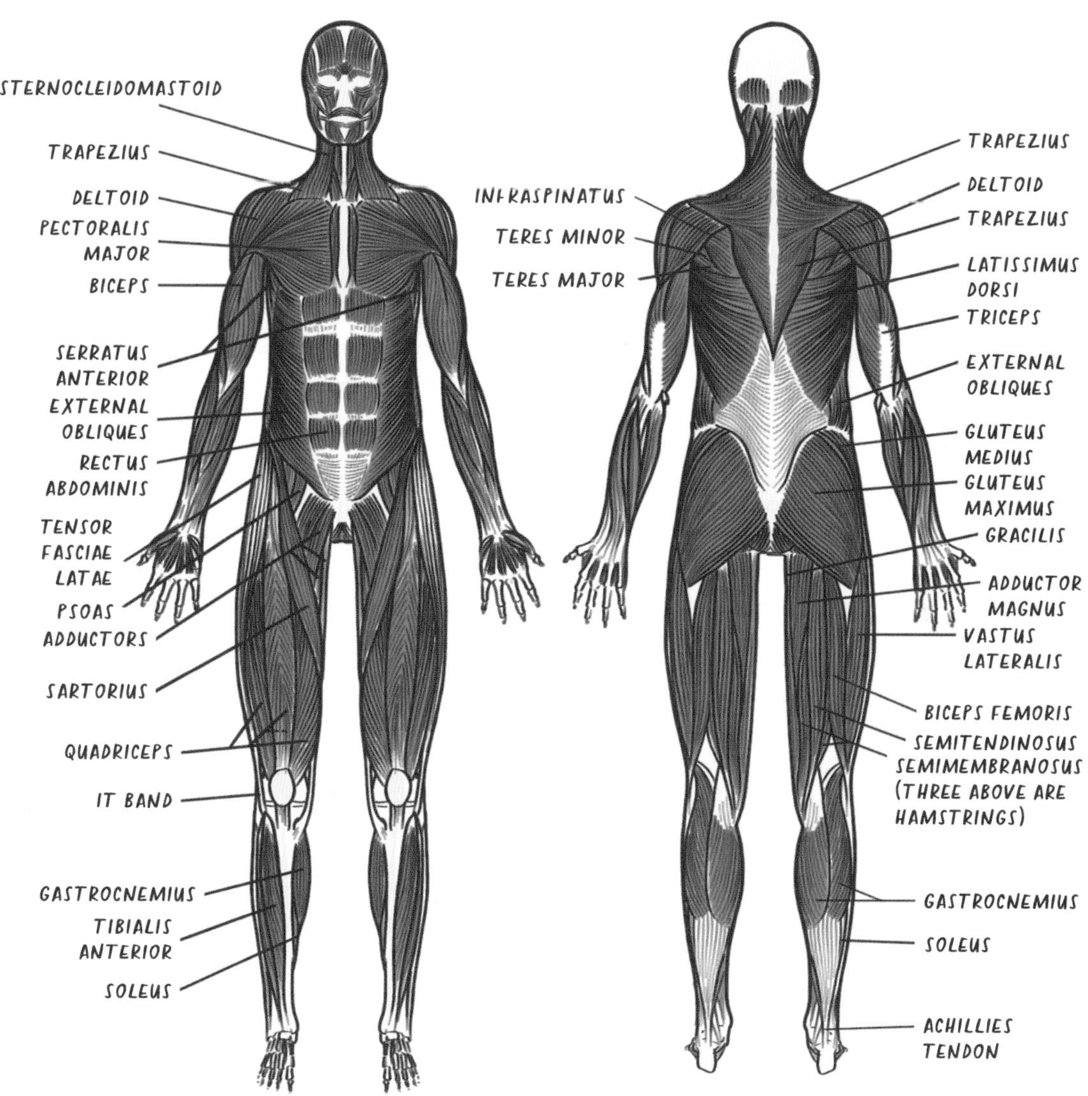

Figure A1.7 Main skeletal muscles of the body.

Answers to Questions

ROM Question 1: What is happening to allow a student to do *Hanumanasana*?

Answer: The back leg is extended, but because hip extension is limited to about 30 degrees or less, the pelvis is in an anterior tilt. This increases the amount of hip flexion required for the front leg. To sit up, the low back will need to extend again due to the pelvis being anteriorly tilted.

ROM Question 2: How is dorsiflexion at the ankle influenced differently depending on whether the knee is extended or flexed? Think Down Dog versus squat.

Answer: The question is aimed at considering muscular restriction to dorsiflexion. This would be due to the muscles that perform the opposite action of plantar flexion: gastrocnemius, and soleus. Both attach distally to the Achilles tendon, but proximally the gastrocnemius crosses the knee joint, but the soleus doesn't. This means that when the leg is straight (e.g., Down Dog), either muscle could resist dorsiflexion, but when the knee is bent (e.g., squat) gastrocnemius would not provide resistance because as the knee bends, its attachments get closer to each other. This means that if you are looking to improve dorsiflexion when squatting, it is good to do other bent-knee dorsiflexed postures, such as *Utkatasana*.

Multi-Segmental Movement Question 1: The elbow is another area where many students can move excessively in a particular direction. Can you think of a few postures where you are moving the arms intending to access the wrist or shoulder, but that can be accommodated in the elbow instead if the student is not attentive?

Answer: If you are trying to increase wrist extension, it is common to see students exaggerating the extension at the elbow (Chapter 12, *Elbow and Wrist*). In a posture like *Kurmasana*, often students don't have enough hip flexion to get the shoulders on the floor and can land up overextending the elbow as the legs press down on the arms.

Strength Question 1: What muscles would be concentrically contracting to take us from a squat to standing?

Answer: The quadriceps will extend the knee, and the gluteus maximus and hamstrings will extend the hip.

Strength Question 2: What muscles control us down from High Plank to *Chaturanga*?

Answer: Working eccentrically, it will be the triceps controlling elbow flexion and the anterior deltoid controlling shoulder extension.

Strength Question 3: What muscles are you using to lower your legs from *Sirsasana* to the floor?

Answer: Working eccentrically it will be the gluteus maximus and hamstrings.

Secondary Action of Muscles Question 1: Right at the start, we also mentioned the potential for elbows moving out in postures with the arms overhead, and that two common postures where you might see this are *Urdhva Dhanurasana* and *Pincha Mayurasana*. This is due to medial rotation of the shoulder joint. There are two large muscles potentially responsible for this happening, latissimus dorsi and pectoralis major, and two smaller muscles, subscapularis and teres major. Look up now where they attach and see if you can apply the same concept used above to explain this.

Answer: Pectoralis major and latissimus dorsi attach around the front of the humerus and have a secondary action of medial rotation of the shoulder. Subscapularis and teres major also attach around the front of the humerus, and their primary action is medial rotation of the shoulder. For the postures mentioned, the shoulders have to move into flexion, and in doing so, will place these muscles under a stretch. This can pull the shoulder into medial rotation which in turn causes the elbows to point outward.

Stu's Simple Model of Infinite Complexity

This model encompasses the possibilities of moving from a basic understanding of a pose to in-depth consideration by adding multiple layers of detail (Figure A2.1). There is no hierarchy, because most of the elements are interactive and interrelated. The idea of the model is to provide a framework for breaking down and exploring postures. We may have multiple intentions for doing this, such as appreciating our challenges in performing a particular pose, assessing potential risk, the building of balanced sequences, or how we can improve the quality or

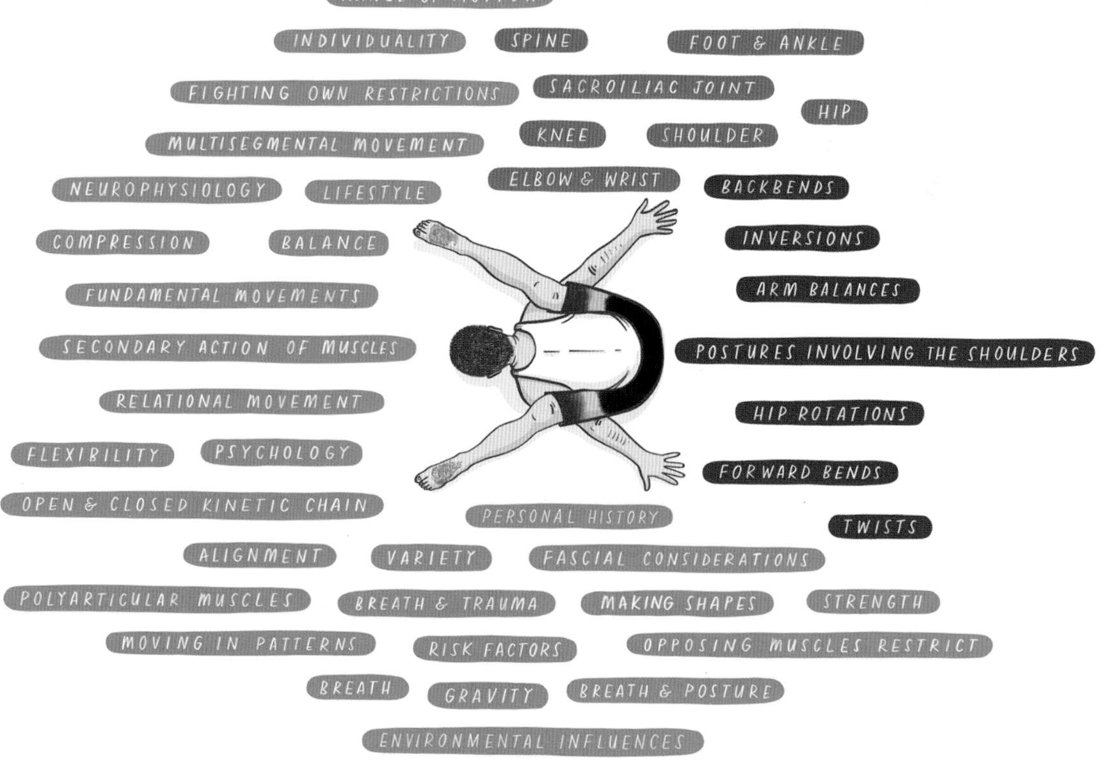

Figure A2.1 Stu's simple model of infinite complexity.

alignment appropriate to the individual. We might wish to understand why a pose is difficult for some people and not for others, what is being worked on, how to go deeper or create progressions, and make it more comfortable or less daunting.

The human body is infinitely complex and interwoven at every level. To explore a particular topic, it is useful to have a working model that helps define the way you approach it. Whatever model you choose will have its strengths and limitations, but at least it will send you off down the path of gaining insight. I like it to be simple initially because you can always work toward more complexity as your understanding grows. If you start with something too complex, you can land up lost in the jungle before you get going. The downfall of a simple plan is that you are going to be leaving things out, how important they are, only time will tell.

Intention

An individual's reasons for doing a physical yoga practice can vary from purely a vehicle for spiritual transformation to a replacement for aerobics or going to the gym, and of course, all things in between. For whatever reason, generally, students start from the positive mindset that yoga is therapeutic and, therefore, whatever they do in yoga is going to be good for them, which I'm afraid it isn't. I feel it is essential to understand the physical implications of postural yoga for the body, even if that is not the intention of someone's practice.

We could use the posture *Eka Pada Sirsasana* to clarify what I am getting at (Figure A2.2). To get the foot, or even both feet for that matter (*Dwi Pada Sirsasana*), behind the head, a much greater than average ROM is required at the hips. If we are intent on achieving this pose, we may embark on a program that targets the hips with a view to getting the necessary freedom.

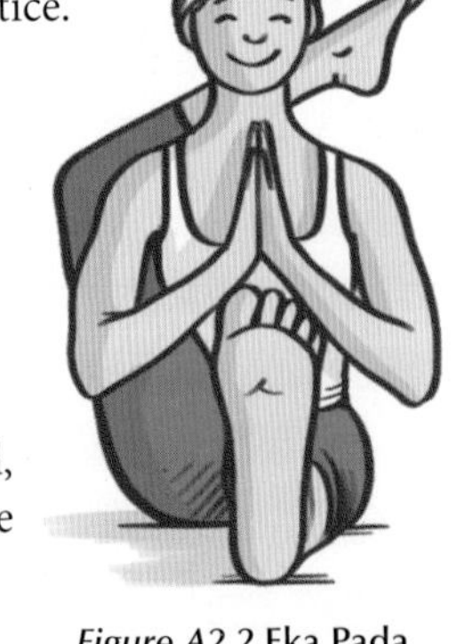

Figure A2.2 Eka Pada Sirsasana.

Looking at how the body is made we will find that there are strong structures (ligaments) in place to limit motion in this ball-and-socket joint, which is mobile by design. As it is a weight-bearing joint and needs to be able to transmit locomotive forces from the legs to the pelvis, the body has decided that this is an area that, although mobile, needs also to be constrained and stable. The ROM required for this posture is so far beyond what is required to function fully in everyday life it is hard to see the potential benefits to the body. Even the journey toward achieving this posture can land up placing strain on other vulnerable areas, such as the SIJ (where the spine meets the pelvis). We may have chosen this posture as a challenge or be working on it because it is the next one in our set sequence (it is about halfway through the Ashtanga Intermediate Series), or even just because we can.

What I am suggesting is that even though yoga lives within the realm of a therapeutic exercise, it doesn't mean that everything will be the right choice for all individuals. For the vast majority of students who reside within the middle ground of human potential, the space, strength, and freedom that yoga can promote will generally increase their wellbeing. It is as we push the boundaries that things become less clear. Of course, how do we know where our boundaries are until we push up against them.

Diving Deep

During the progression through this book, we have discussed good technique and how to perform postures safely. Hopefully, you will have gained an understanding of the way particular postures influence parts of the body, being able from that to determine if a sequence is balanced. That should bode well for the long-term effects of the practice, but we will remain unsure how all the elements will play out as each individual starts from a different place, responds in their own way, and has a multitude of environmental factors, movement patterns, and predispositions stirred into the mix.

If we look at any pose, we can try and determine what we need to do to achieve it to a given depth. "Key Concepts" can help to unravel this as well as any potential risks. They aren't in any specific order, as each posture will be influenced by more or less of the different elements and, of course, many will interact with each other or even be co-dependent. For example, you might decide that a particular posture needs greater psychological fortitude, feeling you have gained some strength and slowing down the breath might bolster that. There will also be a tendency to try and accommodate an element that you lack in (not missing, just need more of) by intentionally or otherwise using more of another element. I remember when I first started yoga, I came from 20 years in the gym, so I subconsciously tried to compensate for everything else with strength.

To start with, we may just consider a few factors at a time, but as they become more familiar, we will appreciate how interlinked they are and be more comfortable with the patterns of interaction. If we take flexibility as an example, this is linked to the ROM of a joint, and many of the other "Key Concepts," such as compression, environmental influences, neurophysiology, and strength.

When we look at a posture in this way, we are, in effect, using the model to reverse engineer it. Which elements it is made up of and how much of each do we need (roughly, of course)? The model is not meant as a scientific style investigation or analysis, but more of a vehicle to ask valid questions about poses and perhaps give some ideas for direction or emphasis of practice. Through looking at postures in this way, you can start to see what different postures have in common and sometimes how one posture might help another, even though on face value they seem very different. We can then use the same model to go from point A (what our pose looks like now) to point B (our blueprint of the pose) or think why a particular option might be more suitable for an individual.

Putting it all Together

We need to bear in mind that we can use the model in a general way but it is also specific to an individual or outcome. The idea is not to try and consider every concept, only those that are appropriate to the pose. Sometimes, a bit of lateral thinking may uncover associations you had not even thought of. Factors may be interconnected for one person and not for another, or potentially a primary influence, or barely important. Different concepts may become more prominent as the yoga journey unfolds. The model is what we might consider plastic, meaning it adapts and changes over time. At the center of everything is the individual. Try and remember what you can about the different "Key Concepts," and if there are some that I don't mention that you think are appropriate. We will use four examples to illustrate some of the thought processes, *Svarga Dvijasana*, *Parivrtta Ardha Chandrasana*, *Malasana*, and *Adho Mukha Vrksasana*.

Svarga Dvijasana

This pose is a bound single-leg balance with a simple and elegant shape but with the raised leg's positioning adding the difficulty element (Figure A2.3). What makes this pose an extra challenge is that straightening the upper leg involves active knee extension. There are numerous variations in style, such as levelness of pelvis and angle of the leg, which will influence both accessibility and ROM requirements. Luckily, there is a bent-knee version that makes it suitable for multiple levels of flexibility.

We could start by describing a proposed blueprint where the pelvis is relatively square, minimum lateral flexion of the spine (side bend), leg close to the body (30 degrees-ish from the center line), shoulders level, and open across the chest. In reality, many of these components will be adapted, so when we break down the pose, we can explain why this might happen.

Whether the pose is transitioned into from another bound posture like *Baddha Parsvakonasana* or set up individually, essentially it is entered from the

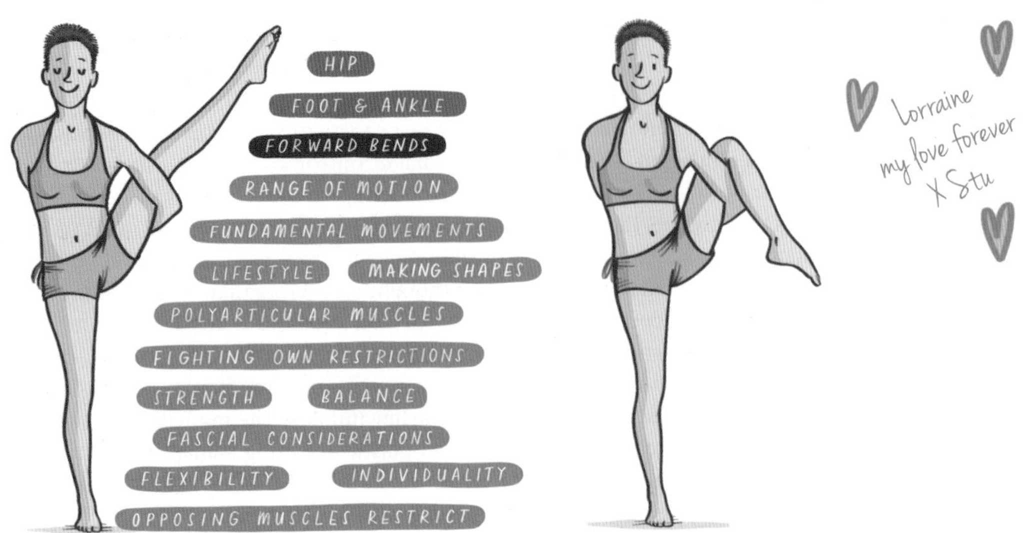

Figure A2.3 Svarga Dvijasana.

Forward Fold

same starting place of a bent-legged forward fold. The weight is mostly on what will be the standing leg, and the leg that is bound is on tiptoes. The bind wraps from the inside of the leg, and a student's proportions may dictate the need of a strap. Even the starting position may present challenges for some students, so a kinder option can be to have the foot of the leg to be bound raised on a couple of blocks (Figure A2.4).

Individuality

The first test will be to maintain balance while standing up. Anyone who tends to overpronate may well collapse on the medial arch, and an extra

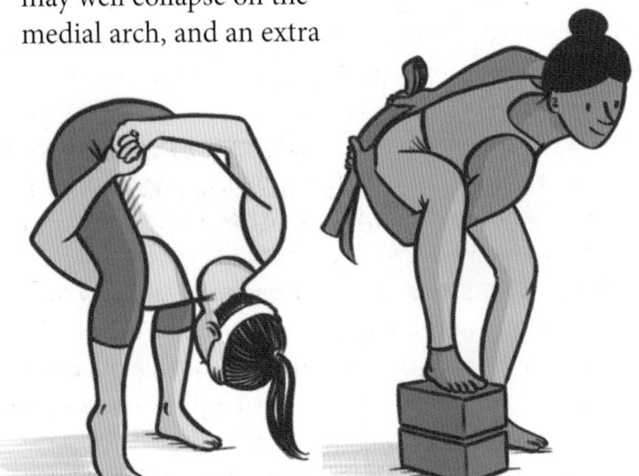

Figure A2.4 The standard entry and assisted with blocks. The tighter the bind, the more closely it will hug the leg to the body, adding difficulty.

effort will be needed to sustain a solid foundation. A fixed gaze point will help reduce any wobbling around. The leg's weight will pull the upper body forward, so the erector spinae muscles are engaged in an isometric contraction to keep the spine in neutral. The raised leg side of the pelvis is likely to lift a little, even if that is not the intention, and it will probably be rotated toward the rear as well. Only those students with extremely flexible hips (we will cover in which directions in a moment) would be able to position the leg in such a way that it was behind the line of the torso. Consequently, the shoulder of the bound arm will also tend to get pushed forward by the leg, so an extra effort is directed at counteracting that, even though it will probably stay forward.

Foot and Ankle

Hips

In the initial standing position, the hip is flexed and slightly horizontally abducted. Because the knee is also flexed at this stage, the hamstrings won't provide any resistance as they are polyarticular. Although the hip is in deep flexion, the bent knee will reduce the tension as it would in any forward bend.

Polyarticular Muscles

Do you remember an experiment in Chapter 1, *Fighting Own Restrictions*, where the thigh was held in place in *Ardha Ananda Balasana* while an

Fighting Own Restrictions

attempt was made to straighten the leg? The posture we were talking about at the time was *Tittibhasana*, and although you may think they look nothing like each other, the similarities are there. Imagine if the butt was lowered down to the floor in *Tittibhasana* and the freed-up arms were then bound behind the back, you would have something like a Double Bird of Paradise. So, the same issues with trying to straighten the leg will present here. The hip has been flexed so deeply that only those students with plenty of straight-legged hip flexion available will be able to straighten the leg fully. The chances are that if a restricted student makes a valiant effort, as the leg is straightened, it will pull the thigh away from the body. It is a matter of finding a happy place to work in, more hip flexion and less knee extension or less hip flexion and more knee extension.

Strength

The quadriceps will have to concentrically contract to extend the knee (straighten the leg), and the presence of strong tensile resistance from the hamstrings will stop that from happening. The leg is not meant to point straight up, so there is also some horizontal abduction in this pose, but unless the angle of the pelvis is changed dramatically (Figure A2.9), the adductors (opposing muscles) won't be the greatest source of defiance. We also talked about the property of stiffness as it relates to MTUs in Chapter 2, *Flexibility*. If this is the type of tissue a student has, it is likely they won't be able to reproduce the same depth of ROM that they would be able to perform passively. Translated, that means they won't be able to straighten the leg completely.

Flexibility

ROM

Another similarity could be found with *Supta Padangushtasana B* if the leg was taken slightly to the side of the torso and toward the floor. Rather than taking the leg straight out to the side, it would be useful to attempt to recreate the same angle of the raised leg in *Svarga Dvijasana*. This makes it a great prep or homework pose because the ROM and body positioning can be worked on independently to the balance element. As the raised leg tries to mimic the position in the standing pose, the floor will also give excellent feedback on changes in pelvis and torso position (Figure A2.5). Work the leg on the floor also, because that would be the standing leg, by keeping it straight and pressing firmly away. This is the beauty of thinking in shapes. It will give you ideas of accessibility, preparatory, or homework postures.

Making Shapes

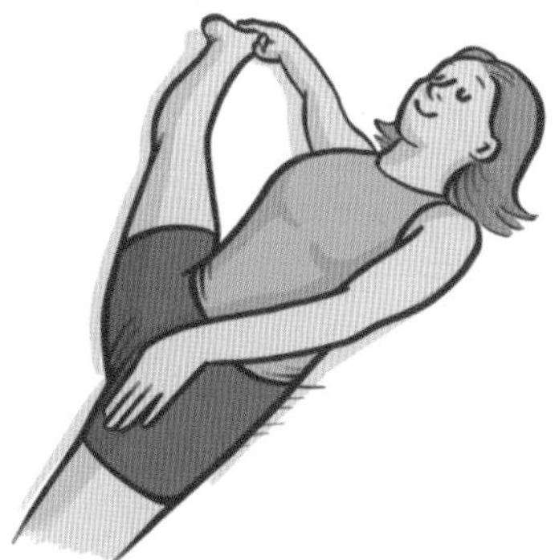

Figure A2.5 Imagine spinning this up to standing and adding a bind. It's very similar.

I have mentioned *Ardha Ananda Balasana*, and I think this also makes for an excellent preparatory posture to work on the hip flexion. Again, also be active in the free leg. Flip this posture from supine (face up) to prone (face down), and you have *Utthan Pristhasana* (Figure A2.6). I like to be on the ball of the back foot as this helps build leg strength, but swap between that and knee down pressing into the top of the foot as necessary. Have the front foot only turned out enough to mirror the directionality of the thigh.

If we kept adding to the *Utthan Pristhasana* shape by coming up a little, taking an inside bind, externally rotating the hip, and grounding the back foot, we would be in *Baddha Parsvakonasana*. Now we get to recreate a similar position to *Svarga Dvijasana* but side facing. Of course, the front knee is flexed, but we are getting into the hip and working that bind (Figure A2.7).

I would consider the full version of *Svarga Dvijasana* as a peak pose and, as such, the body will want to have been sufficiently prepared before

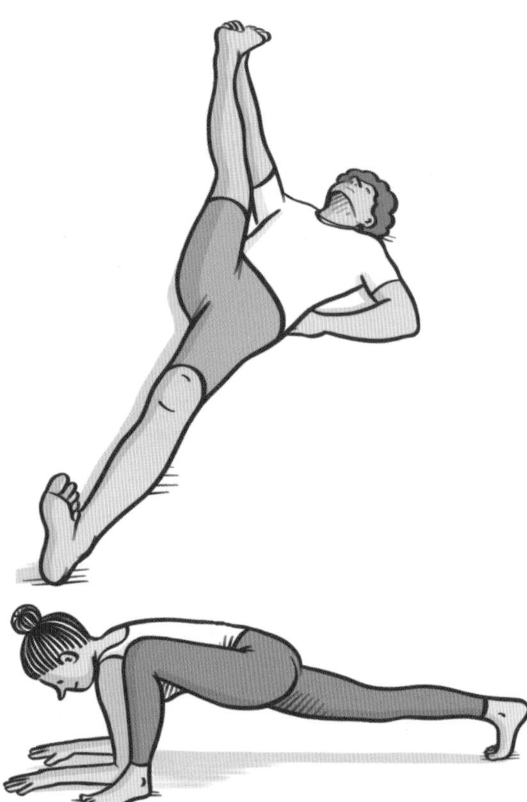

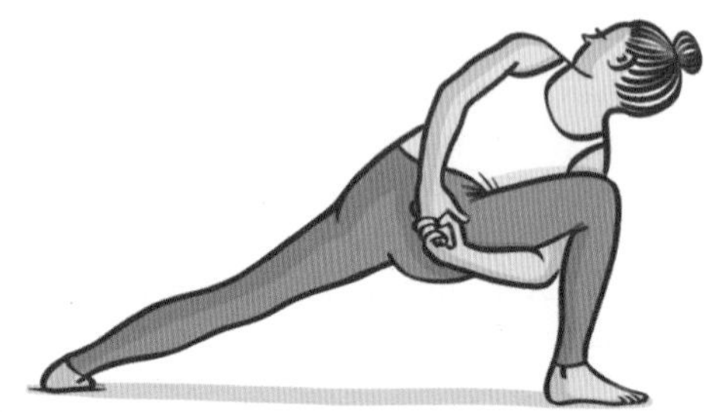

Figure A2.6 Both Ardha Ananda Balasana *(top) and* Utthan Pristhasana *(bottom) are ideal for working on the hip flexion.*

Figure A2.7 Such a similar bind without the worry of balance.

Opposing Muscles Restrict

attempting it. Because we are trying to land up with a deep straight-legged hip flexion of the raised leg, the hamstrings will be the muscles that resist the most. As we are placing this pose within the forward bends posture group, we might like to think back to all those aspects that influence forward bending in general. It would be worth preceding this pose with more gentle forward bends, hip rotations, and adductor stretches. If we also consider that idea of a backline of the body, we may also want to experiment if it makes any difference whether the foot is plantar flexed or dorsiflexed.

Fascial Considerations

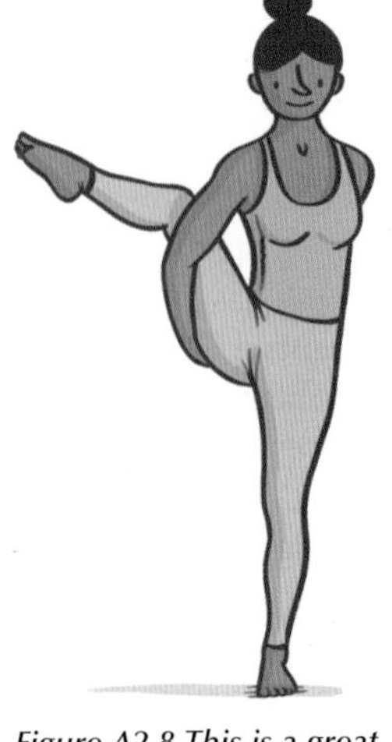

Figure A2.8 This is a great place to be, consciously working on straightening the leg while maintaining good form.

Also, being a balance, all the same guidelines apply, repetition, a fixed gaze, firm but giving body, focus, foundation, and ease. You will have no free hands, so the magic fist is a no go. The quality of comfort is a central aspect. There is little point in going for glory if you are just going to fall out of the posture. Instead, frequently expose your body to the posture and let it figure out what the hell it has to do. Find stability, strength, breath, and balance, and over time, work on straightening the leg more (Figure A2.8).

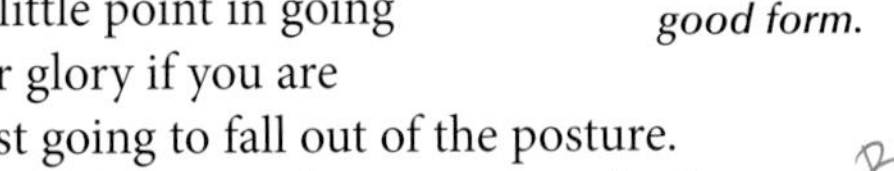

Balance

Our guest student in Figure A2.9 is extremely flexible and is demonstrating the version where one hip is raised. This makes it more like a standing slide split, and with that, the willingness of the adductors to lengthen becomes a key element. The spine will also have to do more of

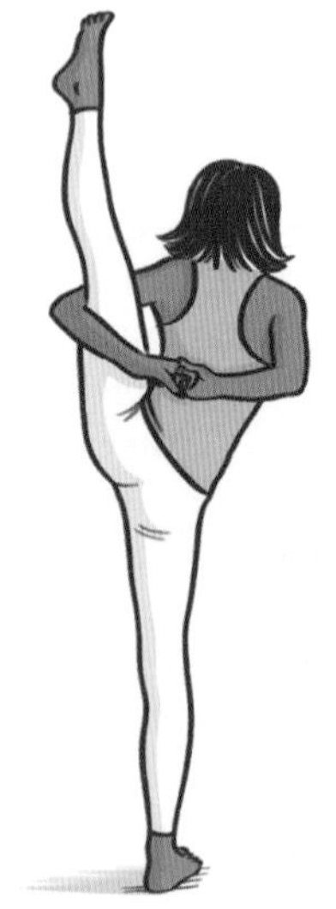

Figure A2.9 As the shape is changed, the joint movements are also, and the influences of particular muscles.

a side bend to bring the body upright from a slanted pelvis.

Lifestyle :)

Although it is a challenging posture, plenty can be done to make it accessible and worthwhile. Use blocks to raise the body, a strap to help the bind, keep the raised leg bent, even swap to hugging the knee instead. Think of incorporating the pose into everyday life, such as when waiting for the bus or chatting with friends.

Parivrtta Ardha Chandrasana

Oh dear, this one can be well tricky (Figure A2.10). We have a single-legged balance again, this time with a 90-degree forward bend on the standing leg, an active twist, and a free back leg that can wave around like a weathervane. As long as someone has the flexibility to sit upright in *Dandasana*, they have enough hip flexion for this pose, but do they have the strength?

Gravity

As the head, torso, and arms usually weigh more than a leg, gravity will be taking the top end of the body toward the floor, pivoting around the fixed point of the standing leg hip. The muscles that do hip extension (hamstrings and Gmax) will be in an isometric contraction trying to maintain the L-shape relationship between the upper body and standing leg. The erector spinae, running up the back, will be likewise in an isometric contraction, this time working on maintaining the natural spinal curve and preventing upper body sagging. The job of the quadriceps is to keep the knee of standing leg extended. As with the previous balance, a good foundation and active arch of the foot are essential to keep unnecessary swaying to a minimum.

Strength

Balance

Gravity

Gravity will also be influencing what needs to happen for the back leg, which, essentially, is an upside down *UHP* C lifted leg. In other words, parallel to the floor, knee face down instead of knee face up. The actions are then going to be the opposite. Instead of working to keep the hip flexed, it will have to be kept extended (hamstrings and Gmax). The knee is straight in both postures but whereas in *UHP*, gravity means the quadriceps have to maintain the knee extension, but in this posture, gravity is doing that work. This would be one of those occasions—for students who tend to hyperextend the knee—to be vigilant of the standing leg but also the leg in the air. Even though it is not weight-bearing, keeping a microbend will help enforce healthy patterns.

Moving in Patterns

Before we think of the twist, we will stay with gravity and consider the body's relationship to the BOS. We have already decided that we will be more likely to need to resist tilting forward, but now we can think about side to side.

Hip

HIP
SPINE
TWISTS
ALIGNMENT
MAKING SHAPES
SECONDARY ACTION OF MUSCLES
STRENGTH
BALANCE
BREATH
GRAVITY
MOVING IN PATTERNS
RELATIONAL MOVEMENT
ENVIRONMENTAL INFLUENCES
REACHING THROUGH BOTH HANDS
REACHING OUT THROUGH HEAD & FOOT
HAMSTRINGS & GLUTEUS MAXIMUS ENGAGED IN BOTH LEGS
THORACIC TWIST
BROAD CHEST
CALM BREATH
QUADRICEPS & HIP ABDUCTORS ALSO ENGAGED IN STANDING LEG
MINIMAL WEIGHT IN HAND
ACTIVE FOUNDATION

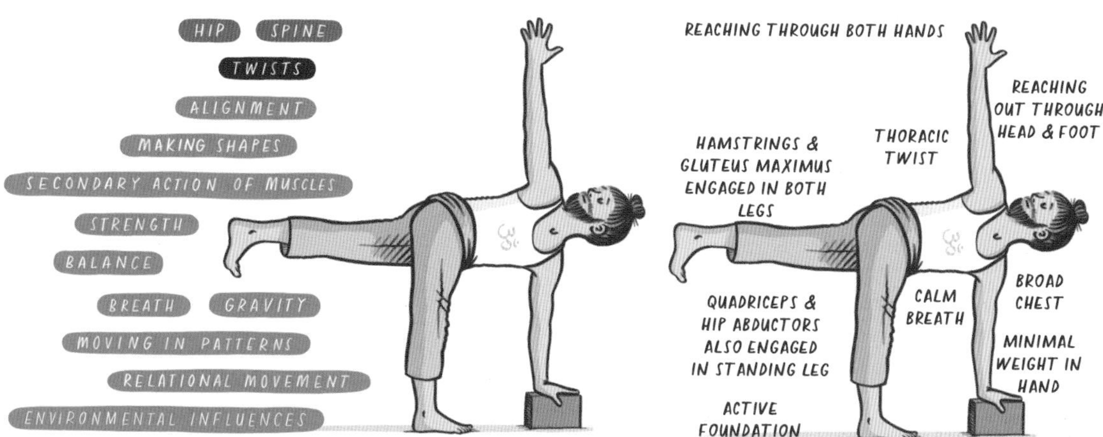

Figure A2.10 Parivrtta Ardha Chandrasana.

The foot of the standing leg is our BOS, but unless we do something, that isn't going to be central to our width. Because we are on one leg, the opposite side of the pelvis is not supported and will be pulled toward the floor. This would equate to the hip of the standing leg incorporating some horizontal adduction (the pelvis would move relative to the standing leg). To keep the pelvis level, the hip abductors will have to resist this force (isometric contraction). However, unless we shift the pelvis across toward the standing leg side, our COG will still not be over our BOS, and they will have to work that much harder.

Again, the lessons learned in *UHP* of shifting the COG sideways can be applied here. If we move the pelvis toward the standing leg side enough so that the belly button would be roughly in line with the big toe, we should near enough have the same amount of weight either side of our BOS.

Something else you might observe is the lifted leg hip adducting, bringing it across the center line. This is your body trying to help out. The action again brings more weight across to the standing leg side but distorts the shape of the posture. As such, it is something to look out for and counter with a contraction on the abductors of that same extended hip.

Secondary Action of Muscles

The muscles that abduct, adduct, flex, and extend the hip, often have secondary actions of rotation, or maybe even have a primary role of rotation and a secondary role of abduction or adduction. For example, some of the deep external rotators can also help abduct the hip when it is in certain positions, and Gmax that extends the hip can also help externally rotate the hip. This means that in a posture like this, we will invariably notice that some rotation has been introduced. Usually, the standing leg is corrected because we reference our surroundings, but the raised leg is out of sight and often lands up externally rotated. Bring attention here and counter with some medial rotation to keep the knee facing the floor.

I imagine that these last few paragraphs have presented quite a challenge to comprehend fully, and that is to be expected as we are trying to apply our concepts to a shape that is not in the same orientation as when we may have learned the movements. If you are struggling, you are normal. It should help to think of what the mentioned movements would look like in standard orientation and then visualize keeping that same relationship as you rotate the body. Remember, we can move the pelvis on a static leg, or a leg on a static pelvis, the joint action is the same, even if gravitational pull and orientation determine which muscles are working. If need be, digest a little at a time.

Making Shapes

Relational Movement

We haven't added the twist yet, and so the posture more closely resembles *Virabhadrasana C* than it does *Ardha Chandrasana*, as the pelvis is parallel to the floor rather than perpendicular (Figure A2.11). This makes it ideal for working on all the same stabilizing actions and alignment without having to worry about the twist. I think if you can get good and strong in *Virabhadrasana C*, then the finished shape of *Parivrtta Ardha Chandrasana* stands some chance of resembling the blueprint.

In Chapter 16, *Twists*, I suggested that often it can be healthier for the lumbar and sacral regions to let the pelvis travel in the same direction as the twist. However, in this posture, although it would present no contraindications, letting the pelvis rotate as the torso turns toward the standing leg side would distort the posture by pulling the unsupported side toward the floor. I suggest that the pelvis remains level and the rotation is restricted to

Twists

Spine

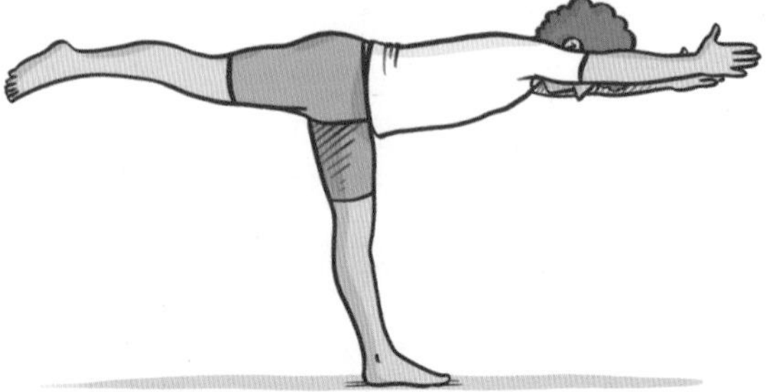

Figure A2.11 Virabhadrasana C *is the perfect pose for working the same leg actions. Bringing the arms to the sides makes this pose easier to balance and gives the chance to incorporate the shoulder movements without that troublesome twist.*

the thoracic spine. With the lack of levers, this pose can be an ideal reflection of genuine spinal rotation. It is better to focus on clean form than set a goal of pointing the top hand to the ceiling.

Alignment

As we don't wish to add any shortening on one side or spinal flexion, it helps to reach out through the top of the head and the foot of the raised leg, keeping the body long. A block can be used under the hand to make up for the difference between leg and arm length. Grounding but lengthening out of the hand on the block, while reaching away with the other hand and depressing the shoulder girdle, will create space across the chest and upper back. Resist the urge to use the friction of the bottom hand on the floor or block to help pull you around, using active engagement of the obliques instead.

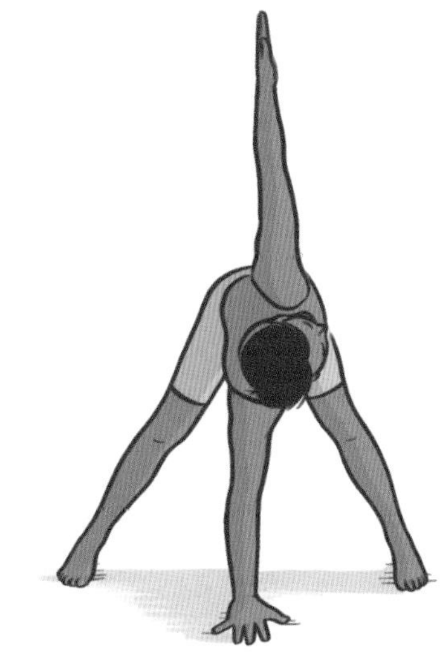

Figure A2.12 The stricter the alignment in this pose, the closer it will tie in with our target posture.

Spine

Having scoliosis that restricts me when turning to the right, I find this sort of pose highlights the difference between the sides much more than a seated position. Not only is it an active twist, but the reference of how close the hand is to pointing toward the ceiling seems easier to judge than how far you have turned behind you. Having worked separately on the balance and stability element, we can also experiment with a similar twist without the balance. A posture such as *Parivrtta Prasarita Padottanasana* fits the bill as the shape and orientation from the pelvis to the head is the same (Figure A2.12). As the wide stance drops the height of the pelvis, a block under the hand probably won't be needed. The major difference when it comes to the twist is that it will be harder to notice if the pelvis starts to rotate as well. Pay close attention to the telltale sign of a change in tension between the two sides of the inner groin (adductors) or have someone give you feedback.

Twists

Environmental Influences

Finally, this is the perfect posture to make use of your environment if you have a wall handy (Figure A2.13). The foot of the lifted leg can be placed hip height to reduce the balance element dramatically and allow the twist to be securely explored. It is also great training for the alignment of the leg. Changing position so that you are side

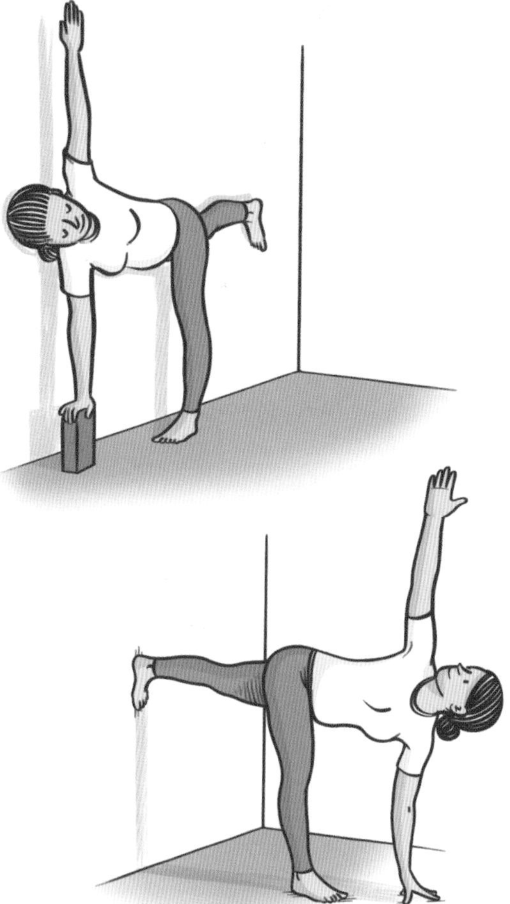

Figure A2.13 Making use of the environment to perfect your technique.

on will alter the feedback, helping with proprioception of hip placement and any introduction of flexion, as the back can be placed on the wall. Diminishing the need to balance both variations allows more time to be spent in the posture, helping to strengthen the legs and hips. Although the bottom hand is on the block, I think it is preferable to envisage that you could remove the hand and still maintain the same position. This will again make the legs have to work harder.

Breath

Although the breath is central to the whole yoga practice, I particularly sense my connection to it in twists and balances. Having both elements combined in the same posture gives plenty of opportunities to seek out a refined quality of ease and evenness, and observe its influence on body position.

Malasana

Fundamental Movements

Squatting seems to come so naturally for some students and looks like the most awkward of things to do for others. I introduced it earlier in the book as one of the fundamental movements, as well as the idea of incorporating this sort of posture into your lifestyle. It is a good warm-up pose if you can do it comfortably but equally a pose in its own right (Figure A2.14).

Balance

A quick anatomical breakdown reveals that it involves deep knee and hip flexion, ankle dorsiflexion, and some spinal flexion. We can place it in the bent-knee forward folds group of postures. What happens with the arms won't restrict the squatting movement but will influence the COG and consequently balance. If the arms are out in front of the knees, they act as a counterweight, shifting the COG forward. Conversely, placing them behind the body and the backward shift of the COG can add a significant challenge.

Gravity

Forward Folds

Have a play next time you are squatting. Bringing the feet and knees together as you would need to do for a squatting twist like *Pashasana* stops the ribcage from moving between the legs, which will emphasize the need for good dorsiflexion. If a student's proportions include thick legs or a large ribcage or butt, it will then additionally add to the struggle to shift COG over the BOS.

Hip

Individuality

Alignment

We can appreciate from our look at the hip joint that for some individuals, their specific combination of femoral head length and angles, pelvis width and orientation, and depth of acetabulum (hip socket), may make specific foundation width and thigh angles more sensible. However, alignment wise, I think the positioning to aim for is with the feet a little wider than the hips, turned out as least as possible (about 10 degrees) unless intentionally targeting the inner thigh. The further the thighs are abducted (taken wider), the more the stretch will be taken into the groin (adductors), Figure A2.15.

The advantage of trying to keep the feet and knees facing forward is that it is a more functional

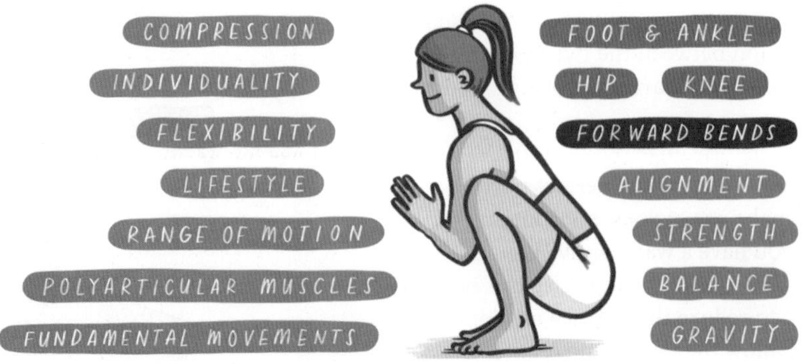

Figure A2.14 Malasana.

positioning from which to transition to standing or to prepare for postures like *Ardha Padma Prapadasana*. But it is perfectly fine to play with different angles to explore how the intensity shifts.

Often, when I see students with their feet pointing out because restrictions dictate that is all they can do, they generally drop in on their medial arch or their knee is not traveling in the same direction as the foot. This will place unwanted stress in these areas as well as make for a shaky foundation. Whatever angle is chosen for the feet, the priority must be for the knees to also point in the same direction.

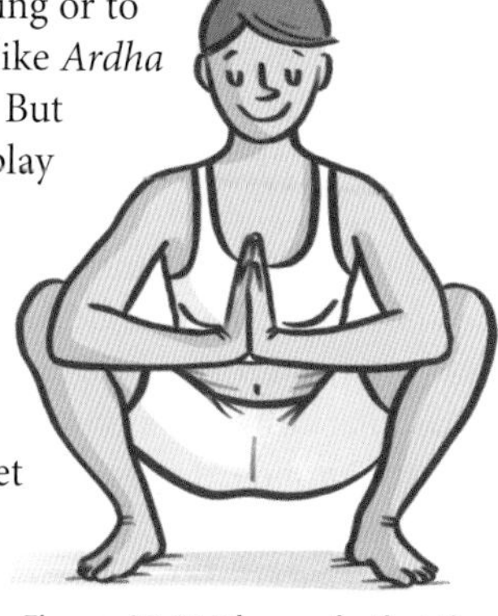

Figure A2.15 The angle that the knees and feet are turned out will change the stretch on the adductors.

The low back will be in a degree of flexion, but this area shouldn't be used to escape from restrictions elsewhere by exaggerating this movement. Instead, it is desirable to lengthen out of the pelvis and sit tall. Once the freedom is found to do this, the arms will no longer be needed to maintain balance, and many different arm positions will then be available to add variety to the pose.

Compression

Whenever a pose requires joints to be near their end ROM, it is worth considering if compression has a role to play. I won't go over all the detail again because we have covered it in Chapter 2, *Compression*, and the relevant *Body Bits* chapters. If we work from the foundation up, there could be hard compression at the front of the ankle, tibia on talus bone, soft compression at the knee (flesh on flesh), or soft (torso to thigh) or medium compression (between ASIS and femur) at the hip. If this can be ruled out, we can continue to proceed deeper into the pose, if not the current depth would be maintained or reduced.

Ankle

Flexibility

When addressing the positioning in this pose, several aspects are usually easily identifiable: the heels can't be rested on the floor, the squat is not very deep, or balance is a struggle to maintain as the student feels they will fall backward at any moment.

Lifestyle

I have observed gardeners in Thailand squatting for many hours and even shuffling around without bothering to stand up, so it is the type of posture that in some ways is self-supporting if everything can be adequately aligned. Unlike many other postures where fatigue would set in. I remember watching some Iyengar students holding *Virabhadrasana B* for many minutes and thinking, "Rather you than me!"

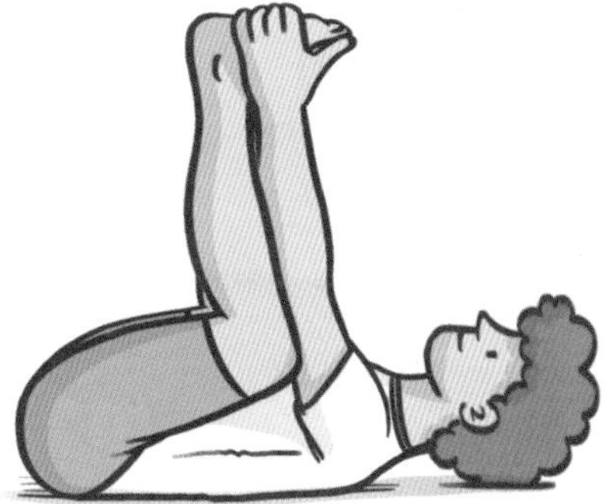

Figure A2.16 Accessing that deep hip flexion.

When setting out to gain a greater depth in this pose, we want to consider if any of these elements are present in similar poses and where restrictions are likely to be. For example, *Ananda Balasana* has a comparable positioning of the hips, but the pose has less knee flexion, no dorsiflexion, and is without the need to worry about balance (Figure A2.16).

We know that if the knees are not level with the ribcage or lower in *Ananda Balasana*, that same restriction in the hips will translate into *Malasana*, regardless of what needs to additionally happen at the knees and ankles. If there is trouble with bent-knee hip flexion as described above, this will shift the COG further backward and make staying in the pose difficult. The other joint movements essential to this posture are knee flexion and ankle dorsiflexion, and lack of either will also shift COG further back. The availability of sufficient knee flexion can be assessed by taking the heel to the butt when lying face down, and dorsiflexion by taking the knee in front of the ankle in a low

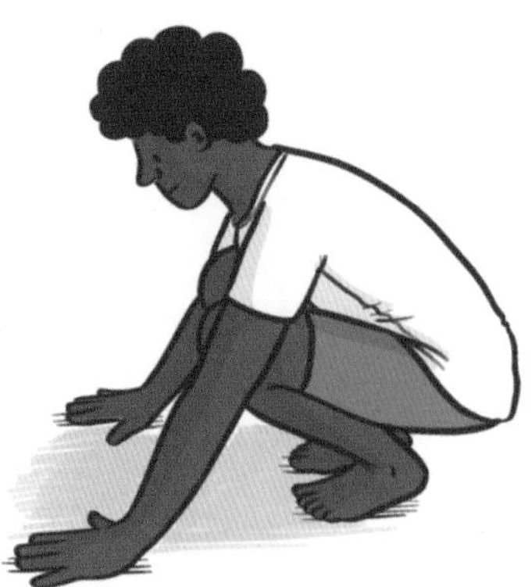

Figure A2.17 I call this a tilted squat. The idea is to lean forward and let your weight take the heels in the direction of the floor. Good as a test of ankle dorsiflexion as well as something to stay in for a number of breaths.

lunge (back knee on the floor) or tilted squat (Figure A2.17).

Similar postures to observe could include sitting on the heels with the shins on the floor, or *Virasana*, for knee flexion, and *Utkatasana*, for dorsiflexion (Figure A2.18).

This pose involves extensive ROM at the adjacent joints of hip, knee, and ankle, so it is always worth considering if there are any polyarticular muscles that may be under a significant enough stretch to restrict ROM. As it happens, there aren't, but I will explain why. To challenge a polyarticular muscle with a stretch, both or more joints that it crosses must be positioned in a way that lengthens the muscle.

In *Malasana*, the combination of joint movements is such that this is not the case. As detailed, the movements we are interested in are hip flexion, knee flexion, and ankle dorsiflexion. Rectus femoris (a quadricep) and the hamstrings cross the knee and hip, and gastrocnemius crosses the knee and ankle.

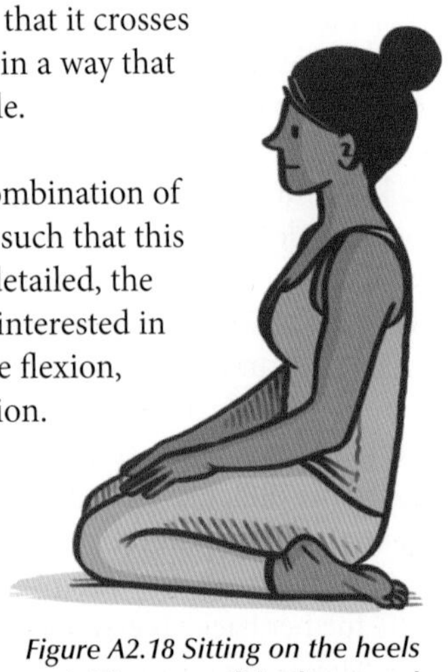

Figure A2.18 Sitting on the heels or in Virasana *will both test and work the deep knee flexion used in squatting.*

However, the combination of knee flexion with hip flexion means that the stretch is reduced in all of them because one end of the muscle is taken closer to the other. For rectus femoris to be under a significant stretch, the hip would need to be in extension, and for the hamstrings, the knee would have to be extended. For gastrocnemius, the knee would have to be in extension, not flexed. Drawing from that we can ascertain that if there is a muscular restriction to ROM, it would have to be from the monoarticular muscles that cross the individual joints. Namely, the other three quadriceps (knee flexion), Gmax (hip flexion), and soleus (dorsiflexion).

This also leads to sequencing and homework. Ideal postures would mimic the same joint movement combinations of hip flexion and knee flexion or knee flexion and dorsiflexion, for example, *Balasana* for the former and *Utkatasana* for the latter. Props can also be used to find a workable position. There is not much point having the heels in the air as the balance and foundation are compromised. The body will relax more easily if support is placed under them. If the heels are down but the weight is still going backward, either grab hold of something in front, like a pole or railing, or place the butt against the wall (Figure A2.19). With the balance taken care of, the student can then work on releasing restrictions and gradually reduce the dependence on the support.

I always like to consider whether a pose is strengthening or if a variation could introduce

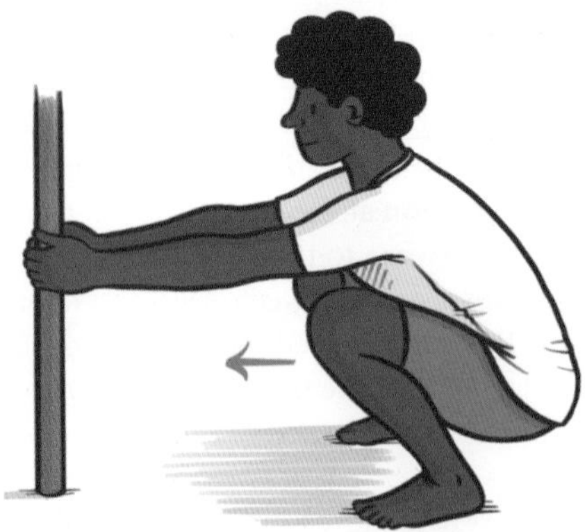

Figure A2.19 Pulling forward to increase the dorsiflexion.

some work. *Malasana* is an ideal example. It reminds me of Down Dog in the way that with the right ROM available, it can be almost effortless. If the backs of the thighs and calves are resting on one another, and enough dorsiflexion is easily available to shift the COG forward, then muscular engagement could be minimal. If, on the other hand, there is a struggle to keep the COG in the right place, then it will be tibialis anterior (an ankle dorsiflexor) that begins to fatigue and burn.

Strength

One way to level out the playing field between the happy and not so happy squatters is to lift out of the bottom position by about 1 to 2 in (2 to 5 cm) (Figure A2.20). Now, everyone will be working as the leg muscles will have to support the body weight against the force of gravity. The quadriceps will be resisting knee flexion and the hamstrings and Gmax resisting hip flexion. If you can remember contraction modes, they would initially be working concentrically to perform the lift up, then isometrically to maintain the position. Lowering back down would be eccentric contractions, but not for very long because hopefully you only lifted up a few centimeters. Actually, the tendency will be to lift too high, as it makes it easier, so watch out for that cheat.

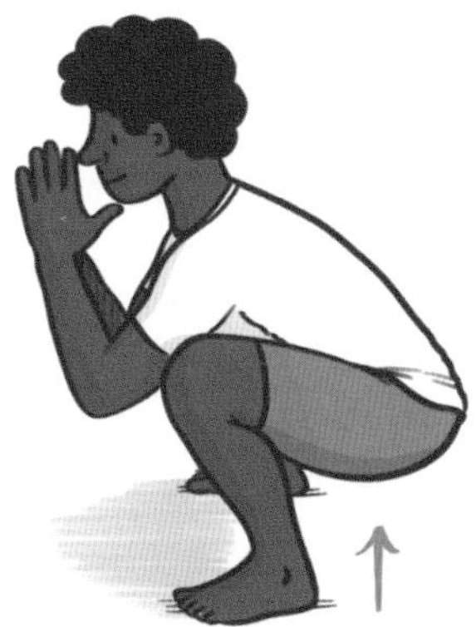

Figure A2.20 Only lift a few centimeters.

Adho Mukha Vrksasana

For those students who did handstands as a kid or trained in gymnastics, they may well not give flipping over and doing a Handstand a second thought, but for others, it can be terrifying (Figure A.21). Much of this trepidation can be extinguished with the use of an immovable object to rest on, like a wall, or learning of how to fall safely. If someone has had an unfortunate accident in the past, a lot more coaxing may be necessary. The individual's mental fortitude toward challenging situations, inversions in general, and dealing with fear, will make a considerable difference to the most suitable learning strategy.

Psychology

Inversions

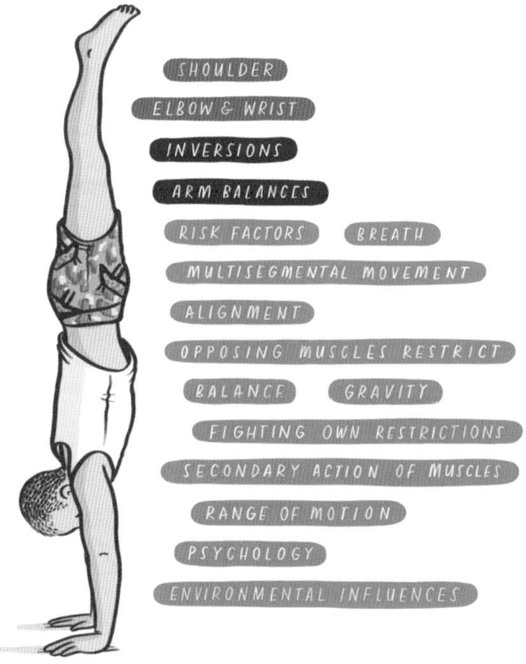

Figure A2.21 Adho Mukha Vrksasana.

If we forget for the moment that this is done upside down balancing on the hands, then what could be simpler than creating a straight line with the body? Well, from the chest down, there are no worries, but when it comes to the shoulders, many people will struggle. The ROM required is shoulder flexion and elevation of the shoulder girdle (Figure A2.22). Due to the proliferation of computer-based working practices, a lot of students will have a degree of restriction in this movement. An easy way to assess this would be lying face up on the floor and recreating the shape. Legs together, toes pointed, ribcage pulled toward the pelvis, which is slightly tucked, straight arms reaching beyond the head, and inner arms touching the ears. It would not be at all surprising to see some space between the hands and the floor.

ROM

Shoulder

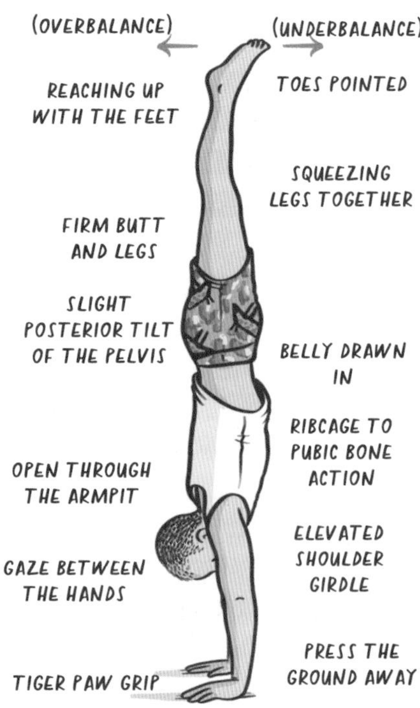

Figure A2.22 Alignment cues in Handstand.

Multi-Segmental Movement

Because a Handstand is a whole-body shape, we know that it is a multi-segmental positioning, and therefore lack of ROM in one place will have to be accommodated somewhere else. In this particular case, that will involve extending the spine, which doesn't present any risk factors but will limit the progressions or variations that will be possible. It is not only the movements at the shoulder that need to be considered but also the amount of wrist extension available. A minimum of 90 degrees is required unless the foundation can be placed at an angle. The raising of the heel of the hand reduces the degree to which the wrist will need to extend. This can be achieved with the use of a block, or if outside, it may be possible to find some ground with a slight camber. The psychological tendency will be to want to set up facing up the slope, as the fall distance is less, and it is probably easier to resist overbalance. However, that would increase the amount of wrist extension rather than reduce it. If fear is a factor, then a spotter should alleviate it.

Elbow and Wrist

Psychology

Alignment

If the desired alignment is to have a straight line from wrist to heel, then this can be achieved by working on the flexibility of the wrist (Figure A2.23), shoulder, or both. Passive stretches could be used to target the movement of shoulder flexion and wrist extension, but as the shoulder flexion will have to be created actively in the pose, it will be hard to overcome any restrictions. Therefore, it is also sensible to include active stretching techniques (Figure A2.24).

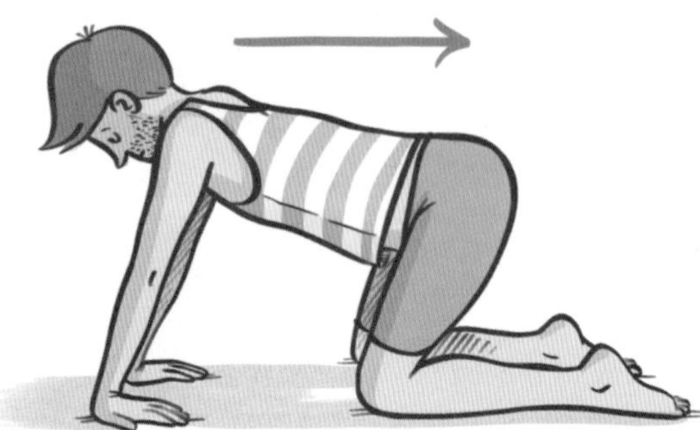

Figure A2.23 Wrist extensor stretch, but if you tend to hyperextend the elbows, keep them slightly bent for this.

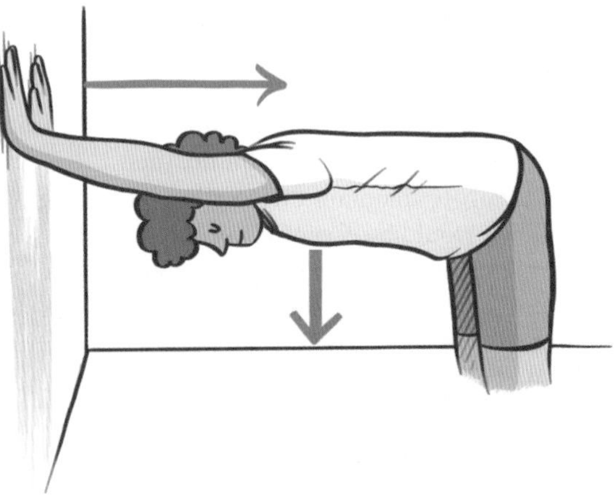

Figure A2.24 Featured in Chapter 17, this is one of my favorite preparatory exercises for Handstands.

When you are new to Handstands, and well, actually for quite some time after, it is hard to sense when the body is straight and a bit of a curve hasn't been allowed to seep in. Using the wall is an ideal way to build up the proprioceptive feedback that can then be tuned into when freestanding. Facing the wall is better than back to the wall because it is stricter, but it will feel scarier to start with. It also requires some additional strength to walk close enough.

Risk Factors

When in a Handstand, the weight of the body will apply a strong force acting on wrist extension, which, if not available, can place the ligamentous and tendinous structures under excessive strain. Initially, the time spent in a Handstand—and the frequency of training—should be kept low and increased gradually as the body adapts to reduce the risk of wrist damage. The use of props, as detailed above, is also advisable if necessary.

Elbow and Wrist

Secondary Action of Muscles

Some of the muscles crossing the shoulder have a secondary action of medial rotation when the joint moves into flexion. This will need to be accounted for by controlling that movement, as we detailed in the butcher's block exercise found in Chapter 17.

One of the main muscles that will oppose shoulder flexion is latissimus dorsi as it is an extensor of the shoulder. It is also a polyarticular muscle attaching to the humerus, passing by the spine to connect with the pelvis via the thoracolumbar fascia. Therefore, to stretch it effectively, there will need to be a combination of shoulder flexion and a side bend.

Opposing Muscles Restrict

Other muscles that influence shoulder flexion are pectoralis major and those of the rotator cuff. A stretch that targets horizontal abduction will help those students who are tighter across the front of the chest as that is the opposite to the major action of the pectoralis major. Working on specific improvements to external rotation will also help to allow clean form in the Handstand.

Strength

Even if the ROM at the shoulders and wrists is sufficient, the student will need the strength to support their body on the arms and to elevate the shoulder girdle when weight-bearing. This can be built up gradually by holding the Handstand for longer times. It is also beneficial to work with isometric static holds in postures like High Plank as well as training the serratus anterior and rhomboids by using exercises such as scapular shrugs.

Gravity

In a straight Handstand, the COG is high, so it makes balancing a challenge. It can help to adopt a split leg position to start with, as this lowers the COG (Figure A2.25). We are not used to balancing on the hands so it will take some time for the body to start to instinctively balance as we do on the feet. Repetition is the key for the body to learn the motor control to achieve the initial balanced position and then to maintain it. I often feel the body acquires skills more quickly when it is constantly challenged. Therefore, as soon as a degree of security in a static position is established, it is a good idea to try adding some movement of the legs and testing out new shapes. Staying still will then become more straightforward.

Balance

Breath

If the arms are bent, and a lot of muscular strength is being used both in the kick up and hold, then the oxygen demand will

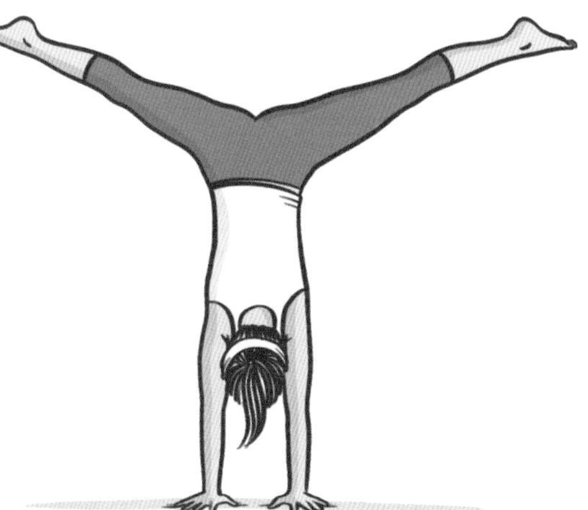

Figure A2.25 Split legs lower the COG and make it easier to balance.

increase, but big ribcage movements are likely to influence balance negatively. It is better, if possible, to breathe more shallowly. I prefer to inhale when entering a Handstand because I feel it gives a certain lightness. At least that is what I thought I did all the time, but I uncovered the truth by paying closer attention. I tend to do the above in a yoga setting as I use a synchronized breath and movement practice. However, when just doing Handstand sessions, I take a short inhale and then hold my breath as I kick up, exhaling when I establish balance. I am also trying to find a solid straight position within two seconds, so it is not a long breath-hold. It seems that this gives more rigidity to the midsection, but experiment for yourselves.

Fighting Down Restrictions

If thinking of placing a Handstand within a broader sequence, it is essential to make sure that the body is ready for the demands that, particularly in the early days, may be considerably more than many other postures.

The wrists should be fully warmed up with mobility drills and poses that replicate the core movements around the shoulder, such as *Ardha Pincha Mayurasana* (Figure A2.26), Active Three-Legged Dog, and *Virabhadrasana C* should be included. Many of the stability poses, such as *Vasishtasana*, Forearm Plank, and High Plank, are also worth fitting in (Figure A2.27). Using multiple floaty kickups without trying to hold the Handstand will start to increase the weight-bearing and load on the joints, improve proprioception, and instill the feeling of using minimal effort in the entry.

Arm Balance

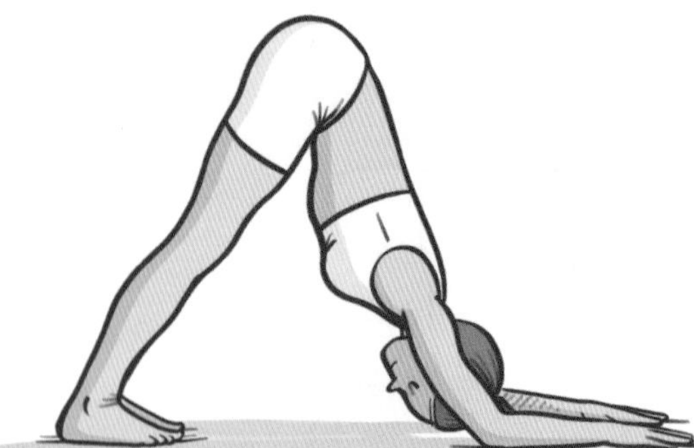

Figure A2.26 I find this pose a killer. It really targets my restriction at the shoulder of external rotation combined with flexion. However, luckily in the Handstand, good shoulder girdle elevation can change the restriction completely.

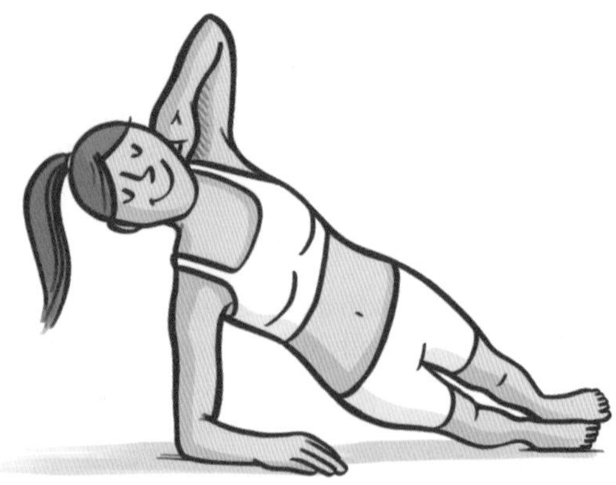

Figure A2.27 Side planks and all sorts of stabilization drills will help the shoulders stay healthy when embarking on Handstands. The shoulders are inherently unstable.

The last two points I will raise, although being simple, made some of the biggest differences to my balancing journey. Firstly, get off your yoga mat. Even that bit of sponginess undermines your foundation. If I want some separation from the floor, I use a travel mat, and for outside, I have a piece of unvarnished wood. It may seem enticing to practice Handstands on the sand or in the park, but that uneven and compressible foundation will place extra strain on the wrists. Happy wrists mean you can practice for longer and more frequently.

Environmental Influences

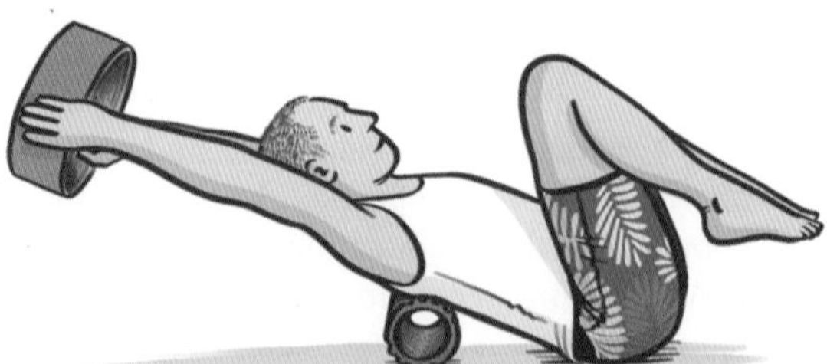

Figure A2.28 Again from Chapter 17, this is one of my go-to stretches to help me find the right ROM at the shoulder.

Strength

The other thing that personally made a significant difference was increasing my wrist flexor strength using the heel of hand raise exercise (Figure A2.29). The technique is to bring your body weight into your hands and then raise the heel of the hand against this load (concentric). Once at the top, slowly lower, now resisting (eccentric), and repeat 10 times. Multiple sets are a splendid idea. Strengthening the wrist flexor muscles helps dramatically to bring you back from overbalance because you need to move from too much to less wrist extension.

Constantly seek calmness of mind even within the struggle of balance, fatigue, and trepidation.

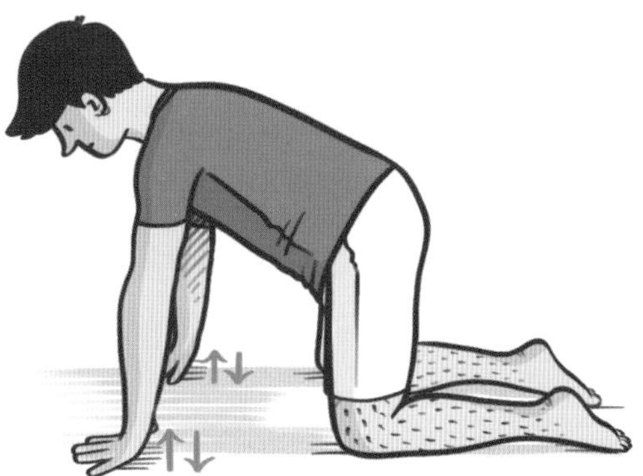

Figure A2.29 Hand raising exercise.

Moving On

As an exercise, you could think of how some of these "Key Concepts" are easily identified as linking together for you personally. Maybe now consider things that might have crossed your mind as positive changes to your practice and how incorporating them might influence other factors.

What I would like you to do is to pick something to work on. It might be strength, balance, breath, or any of the other elements in the model, and choose this time to implement a focus on that area. Write down what your expectations are and how you envisage the new work influencing other areas in the model and your practice in general. After a month, come back to what you have written and see how much of what you expected has come to fruition, what areas didn't change, and were there any areas that experienced a change you were not expecting.

Through self-exploration, you will learn and flourish. Keep this process going until we meet somewhere warm and beautiful.

Names of Poses/Postures (Asanas)

Sanskrit name in italics. "Asana" means "pose" or "posture."

Adho Mukha Svanasana Downward-Facing Dog Pose (Down Dog)	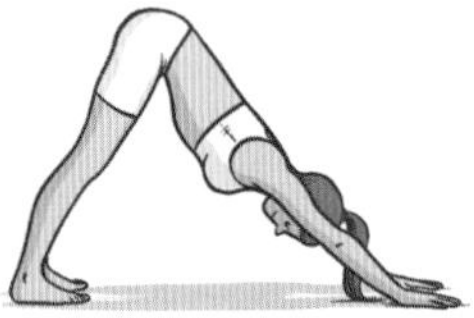
Adho Mukha Vrksasana Downward-Facing Tree Pose (Handstand)	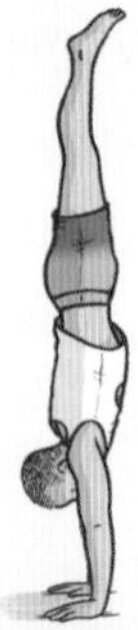
Agnistambhasana Fire Log Pose (Double Pigeon)	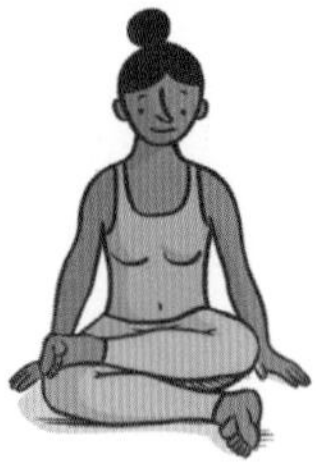
Akarna Dhanurasana Toward-the-Ear Bow Pose (Archer Pose)	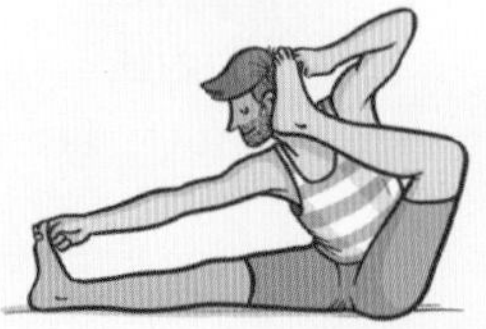

Ananda Balasana Happy Baby Pose	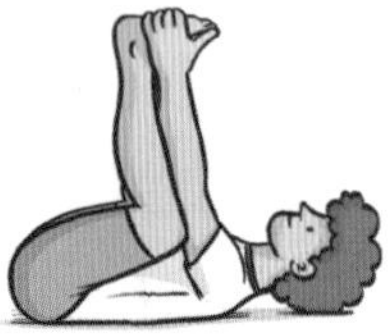
Ardha Ananda Balasana Half Happy Baby Pose	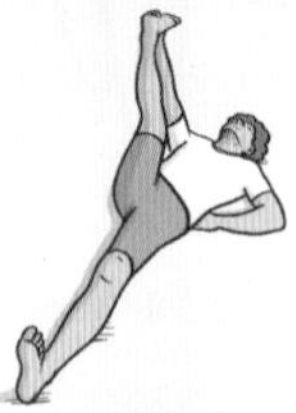
Ardha Baddha Padma Paschimottanasana Half-Bound Lotus Standing Forward Bend Pose	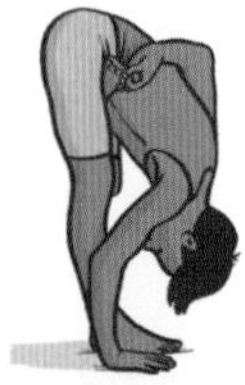
Ardha Baddha Padmottanasana Intense Half-Bound Lotus Pose	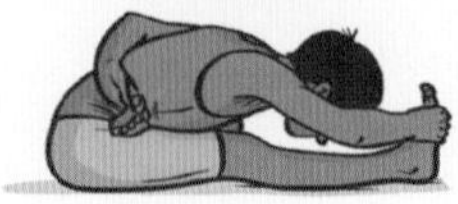
Ardha Chandrasana Half Moon Pose	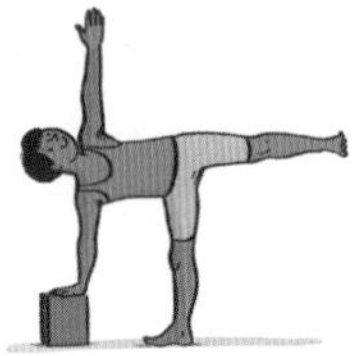

Ardha Matsyendrasana Half Lord of the Fishes Pose (Seated Twist Pose)	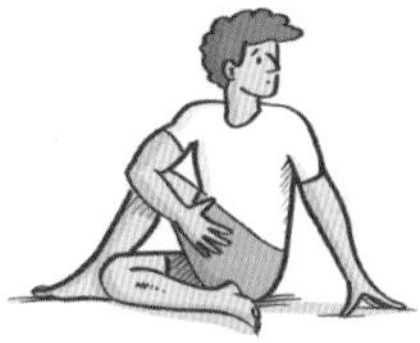
Ardha Padma Prapadasana Half Lotus Tip Toe Pose	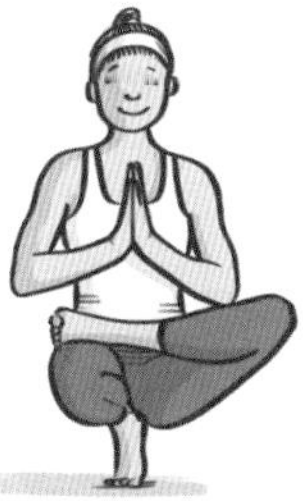
Ardha Padmasana Half Lotus Pose	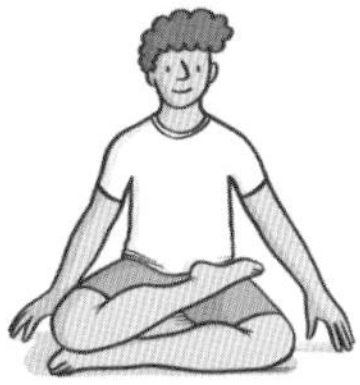
Ardha Pincha Mayurasana Dolphin Pose	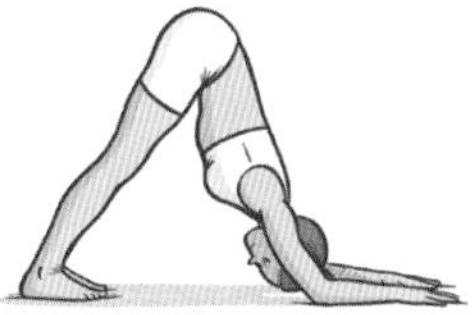
Astavakrasana Eight Angle Pose	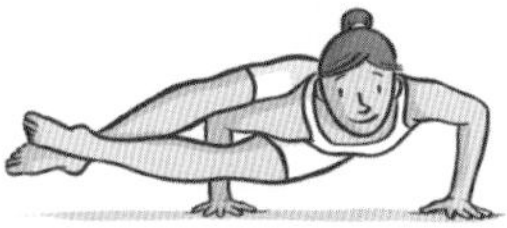
Baddha Konasana Bound Angle Pose	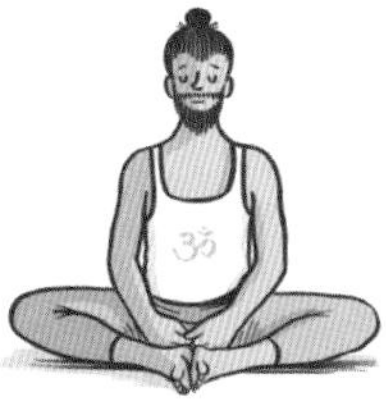
Baddha Konasana B Bound Angle Pose Head to Feet	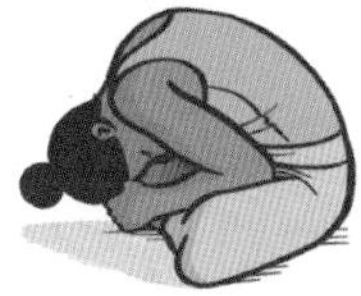
Baddha Parsvakonasana Bound Side Angle Pose	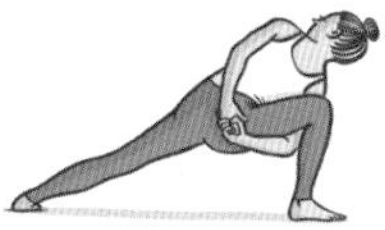

Bakasana Crane Pose	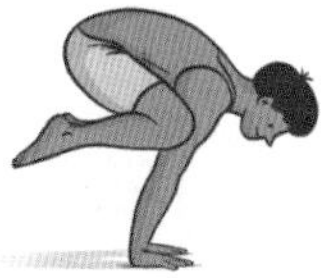
Balasana Child's Pose	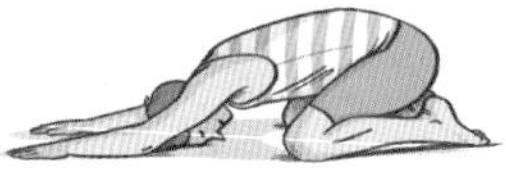
Bhekasana Frog Pose	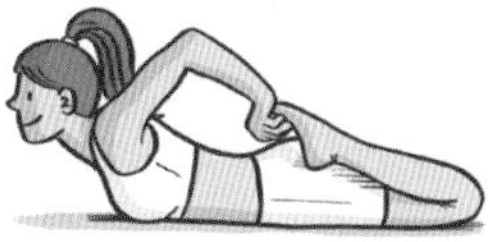
Bhujangasana Cobra Pose	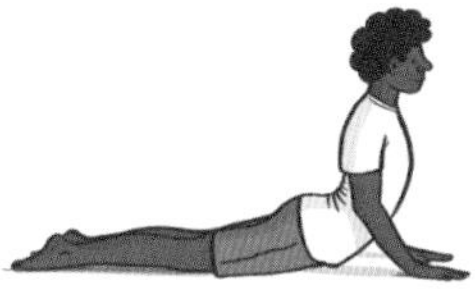
Bhujapidasana Shoulder-Pressing Pose	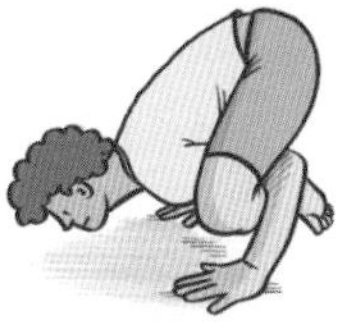
Chaturanga Low Plank	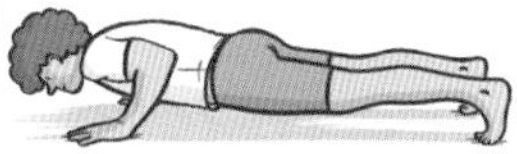
Dandasana Staff Pose	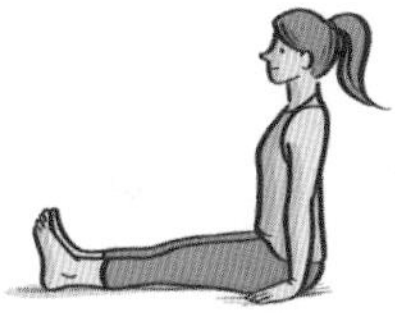
Dhanurasana Bow Pose	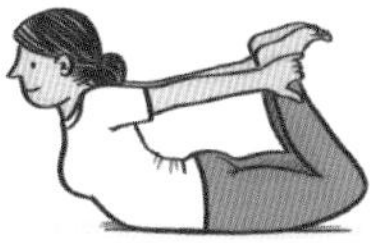
Dwi Pada Koundinyasana Two-Legged Sage Koundinya's Pose	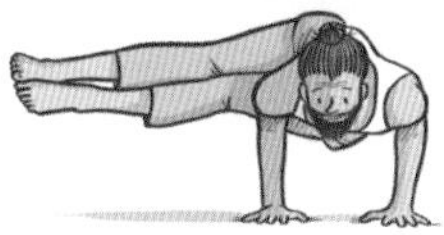
Dwi Pada Sirsasana Both Legs Behind the Head Pose	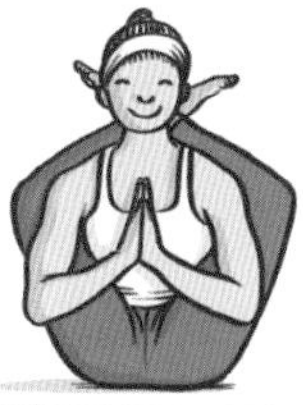

Pose	
Eka Pada Bakasana One-Legged Crane Pose	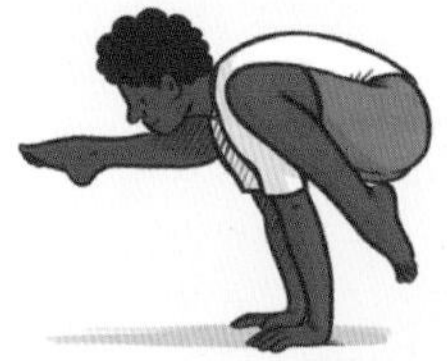
Eka Pada Koundinyasana I One-Legged Sage Koundinya's Pose	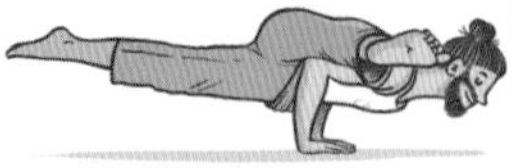
Eka Pada Rajakapotasana One-Legged King Pigeon Pose	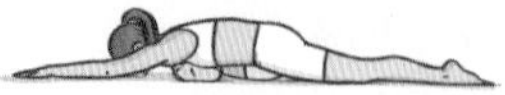
Eka Pada Sirsasana Leg Behind the Head Pose	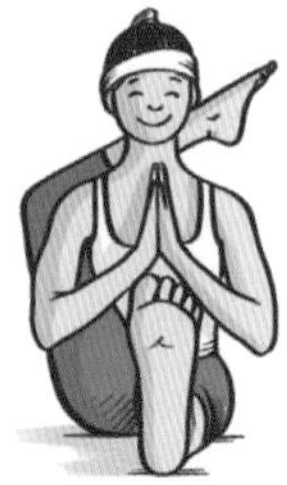
Galavasana Flying Pigeon Pose	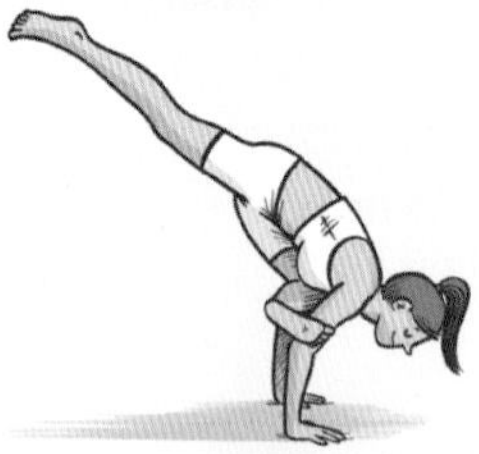
Garudasana Eagle Pose	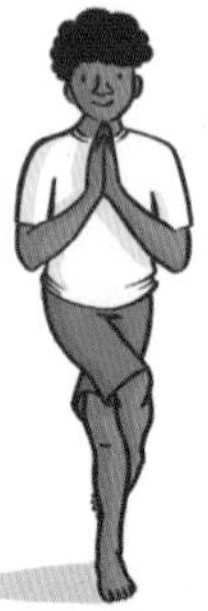
Gomukhasana Cow Face Pose	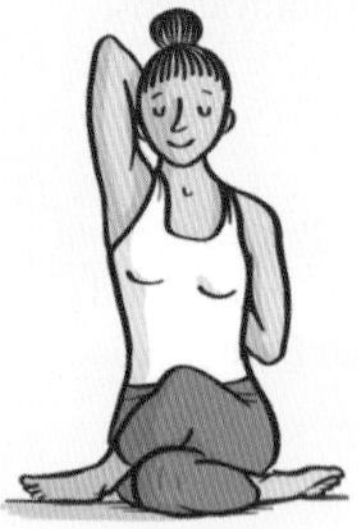

Pose	
Halasana Plow Pose	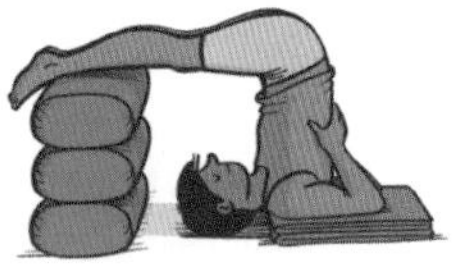
Hanumanasana Monkey Pose	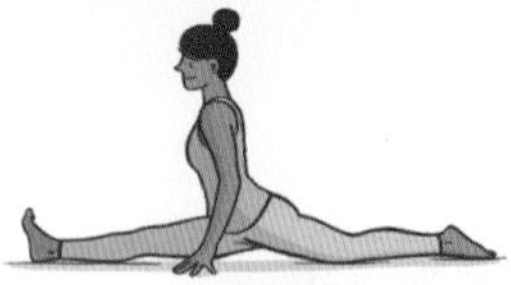
Janu Sirsasana Head-to-Knee Forward Bend Pose	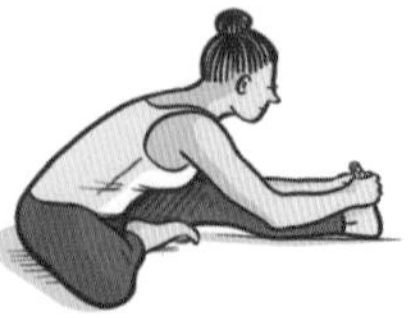
Kapotasana Pigeon Pose	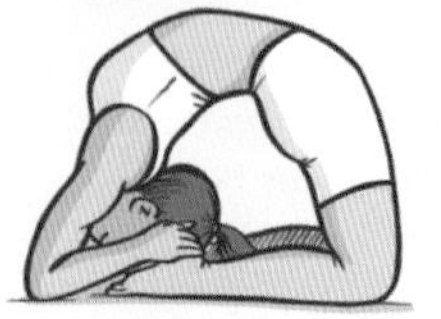
Kapotasana A Pigeon Pose (Straight-Arm Version)	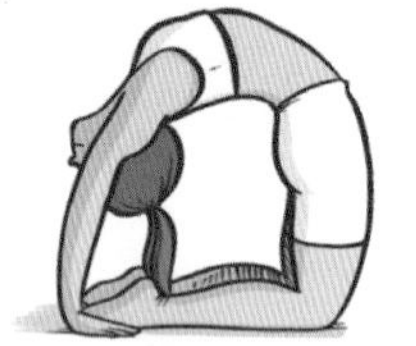
Karnapidasana Ear Pressure Pose (Knee to Ear Pose)	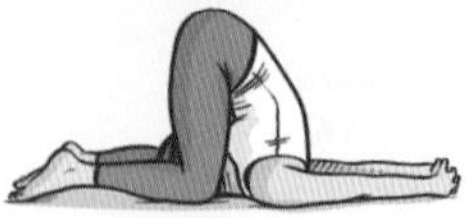
Krounchasana Heron Pose	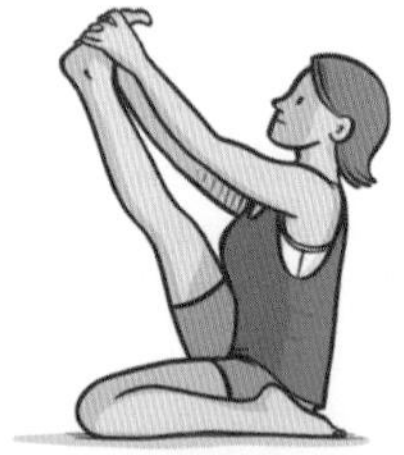
Kurmasana Tortoise (or Turtle) Pose	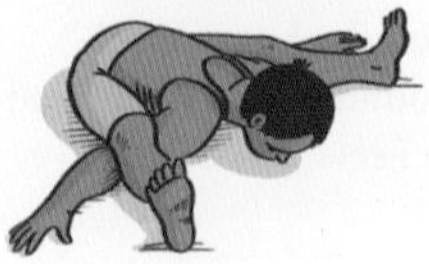
Laghu Vajrasana Little Thunderbolt Pose	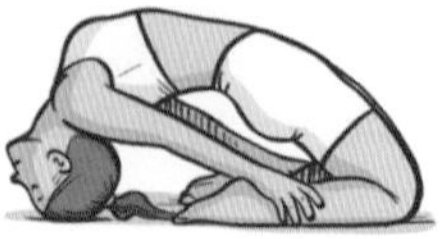

Malasana Garland Pose (Squat)	
Mandukasana Frog Pose	
Marichyasana A, B, C, D Pose of the Sage Marichi I, II, III, IV	
Mayurasana Peacock Pose	
Mukta Hasta Sirsasana A Tripod Headstand	
Nakrasana Crocodile Pose	

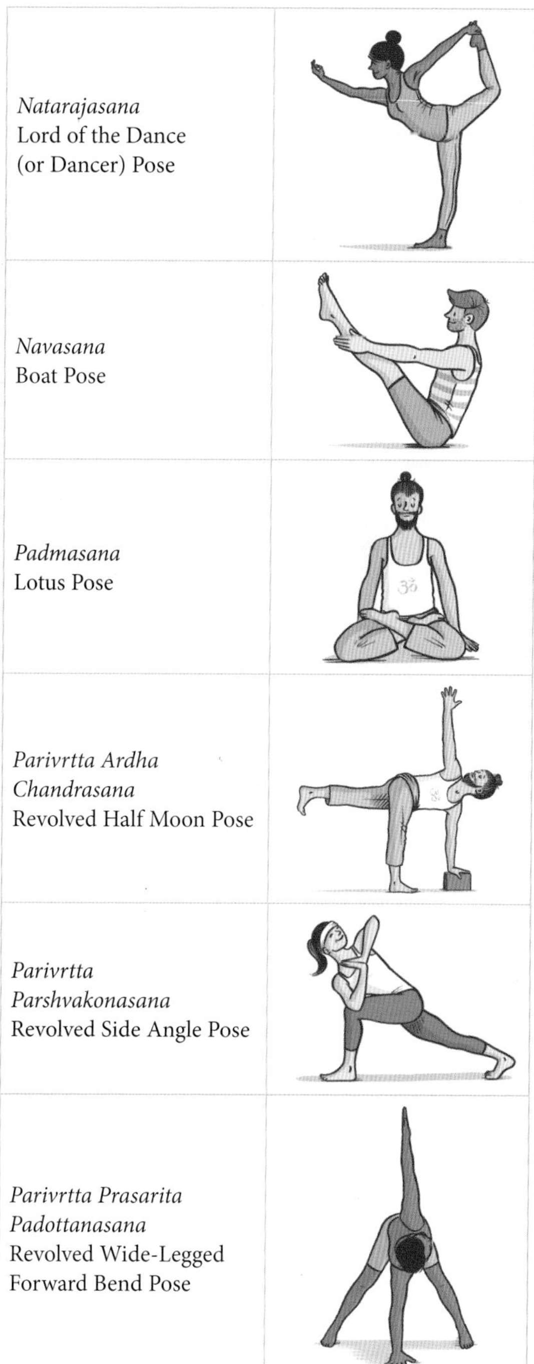

Natarajasana Lord of the Dance (or Dancer) Pose	
Navasana Boat Pose	
Padmasana Lotus Pose	
Parivrtta Ardha Chandrasana Revolved Half Moon Pose	
Parivrtta Parshvakonasana Revolved Side Angle Pose	
Parivrtta Prasarita Padottanasana Revolved Wide-Legged Forward Bend Pose	

Parivrtta Trikonasana Revolved Triangle Pose	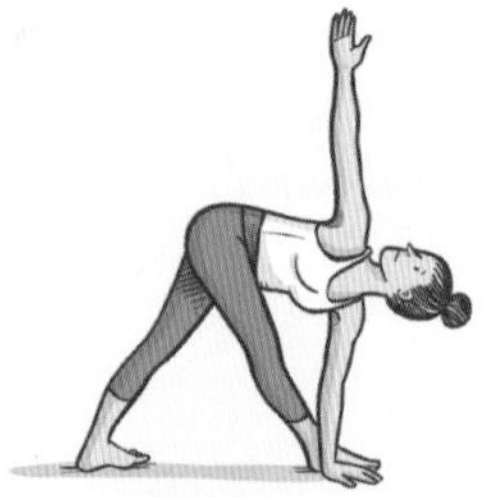
Parsva Bakasana Side Crow Pose	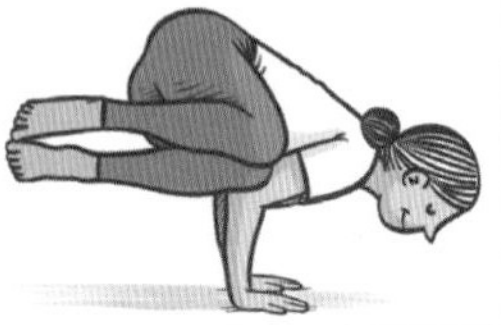
Parsva Bhuja Dandasana Grasshopper Pose	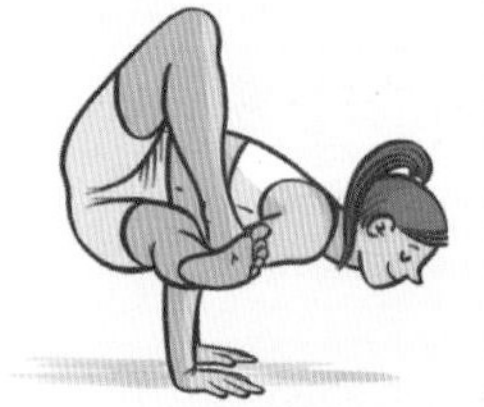
Parsva Dhanurasana Side Bow Pose	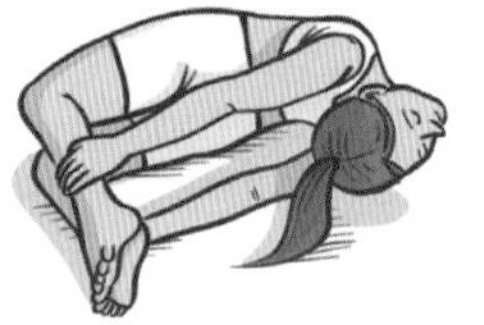
Parsvakonasana Side Angle Pose	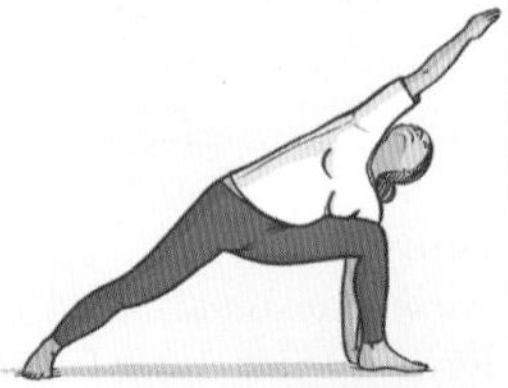
Parsvottanasana Pyramid Pose	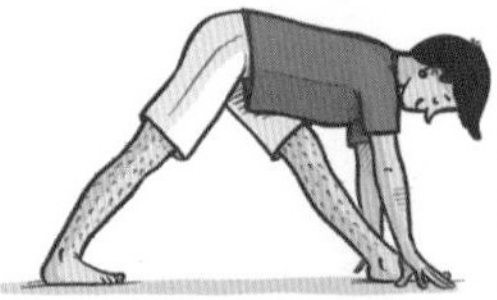
Paschimottanasana Seated Forward Bend Pose	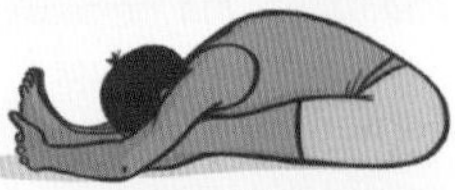
Pashasana Noose Pose	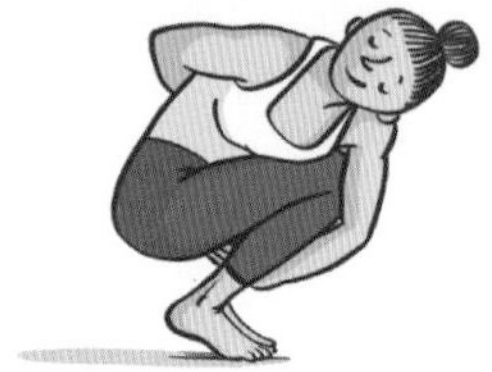

Pincha Mayurasana Feathered Peacock Pose (Forearm Balance)	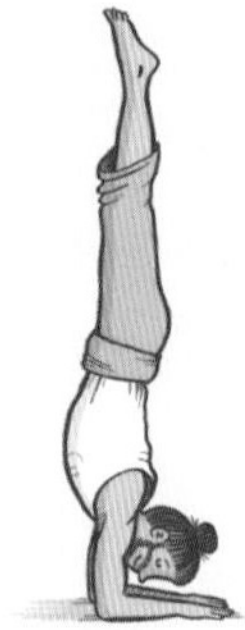
Prasarita Padottanasana C Wide-Legged Standing Forward Bend C	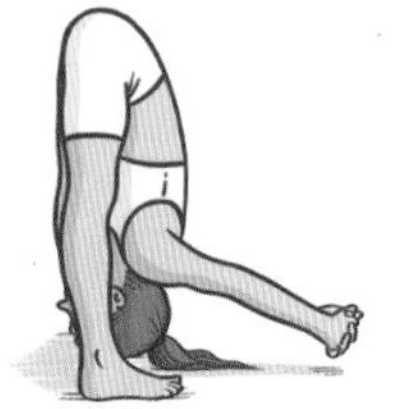
Purvottanasana Upward Plank Pose (Reverse Plank)	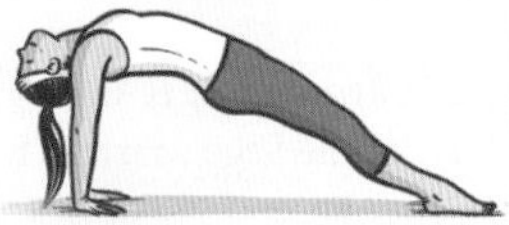
Salamba Bhujangasana Sphinx Pose	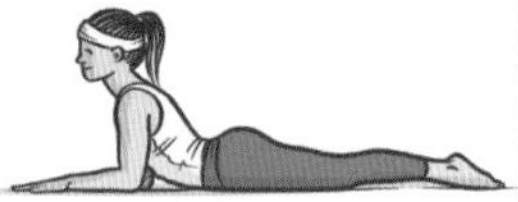
Samakonasana Straight Angle (or Center Splits) Pose	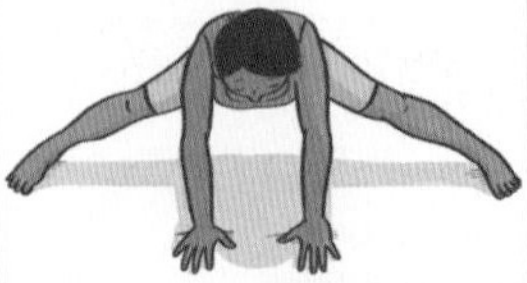
Sarvangasana Shoulderstand	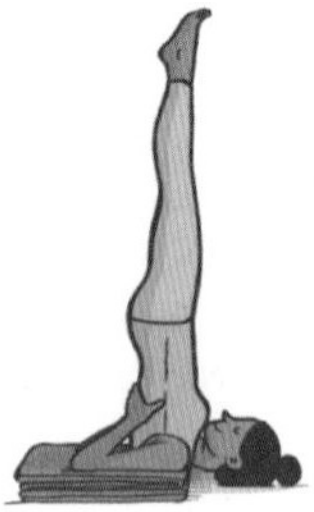
Setu Bandhasana Bridge Pose	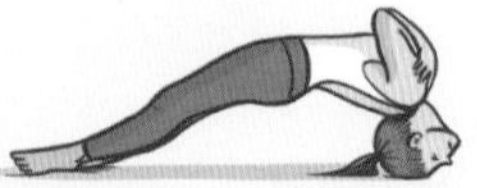
Salabhasana Locust Pose	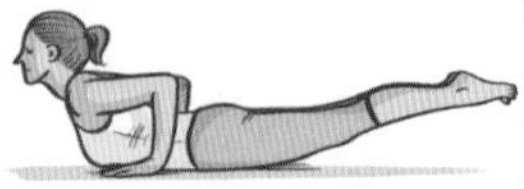
Shavasana Corpse Pose	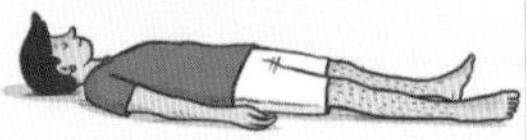

Sirsasana Headstand	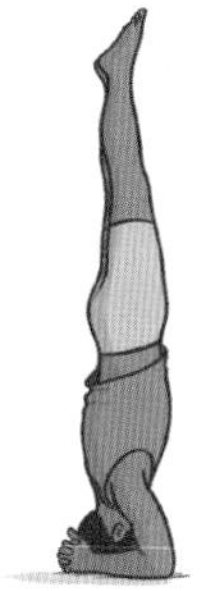
Sucirandhrasana Eye of the Needle (Reverse/Reclined Pigeon) Pose	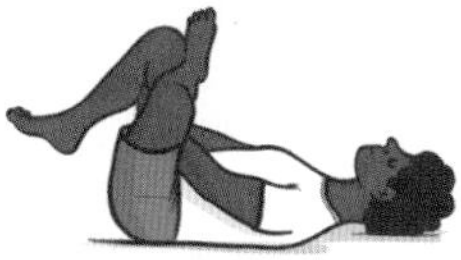
Sukasana Easy Pose	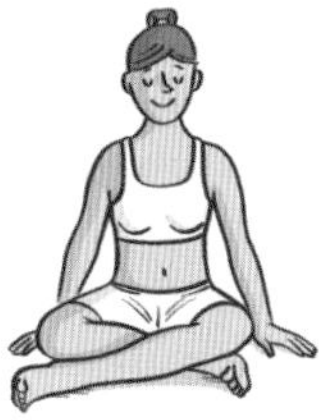
Supta Kurmasana Reclining Turtle Pose	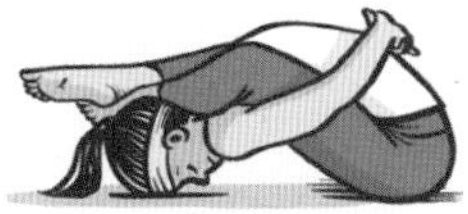
Supta Padangushtasana, B Reclining Hand-to-Big Toe Pose, B	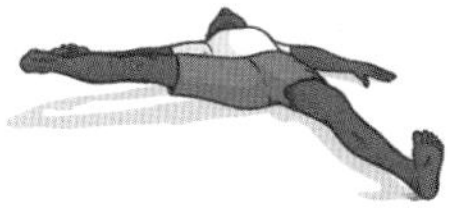
Supta Virasana Reclining Hero Pose	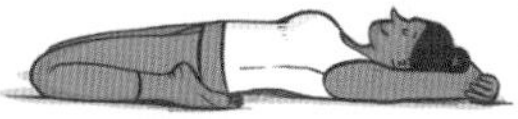
Svarga Dvijasana Bird of Paradise Pose	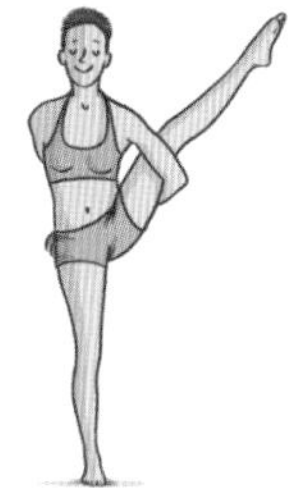
Tadasana Mountain Pose	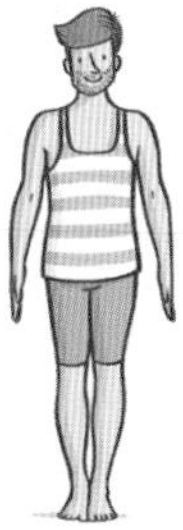

Tittibhasana Firefly Pose	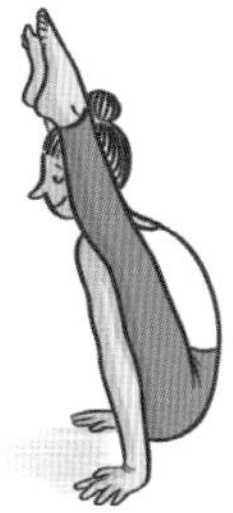
Triang Mukha Eka Pada Paschimottanasana Three-Limbed One Foot Forward Bend	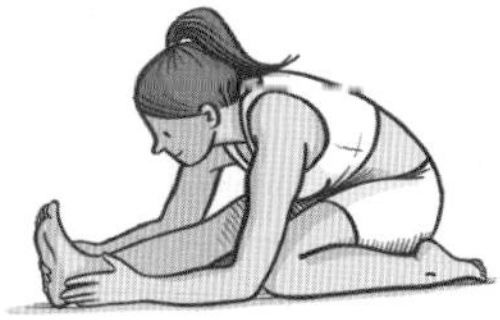
Upavistha Konasana Wide-Legged Seated Forward Bend	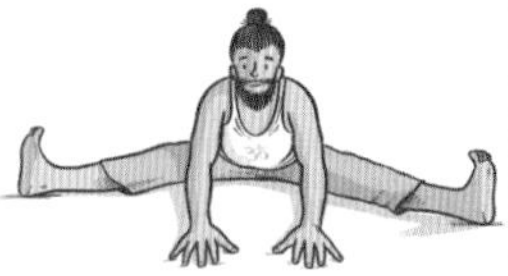
Urdhva Dhanurasana Upward-Facing Bow Pose	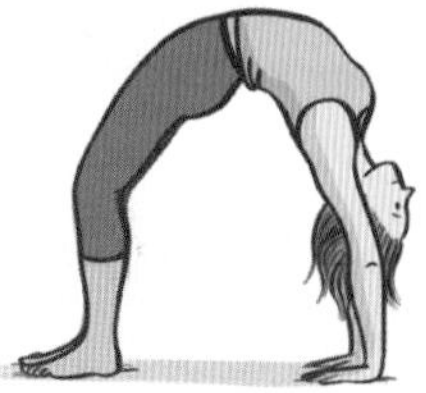
Urdhva Mukha Svanasana Upward-Facing Dog (Up Dog)	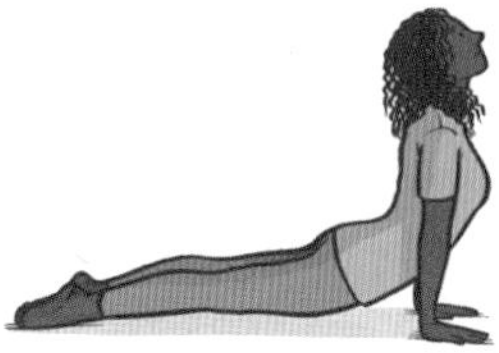
Ustrasana Camel Pose	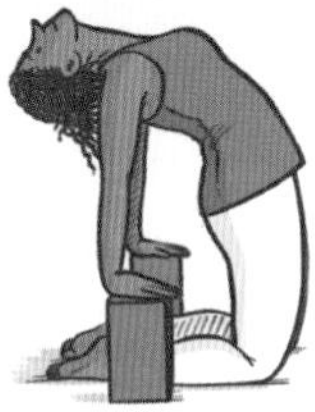
Utkatasana Chair Pose	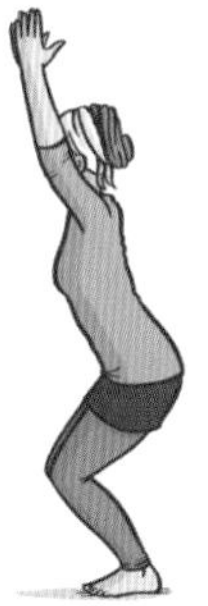

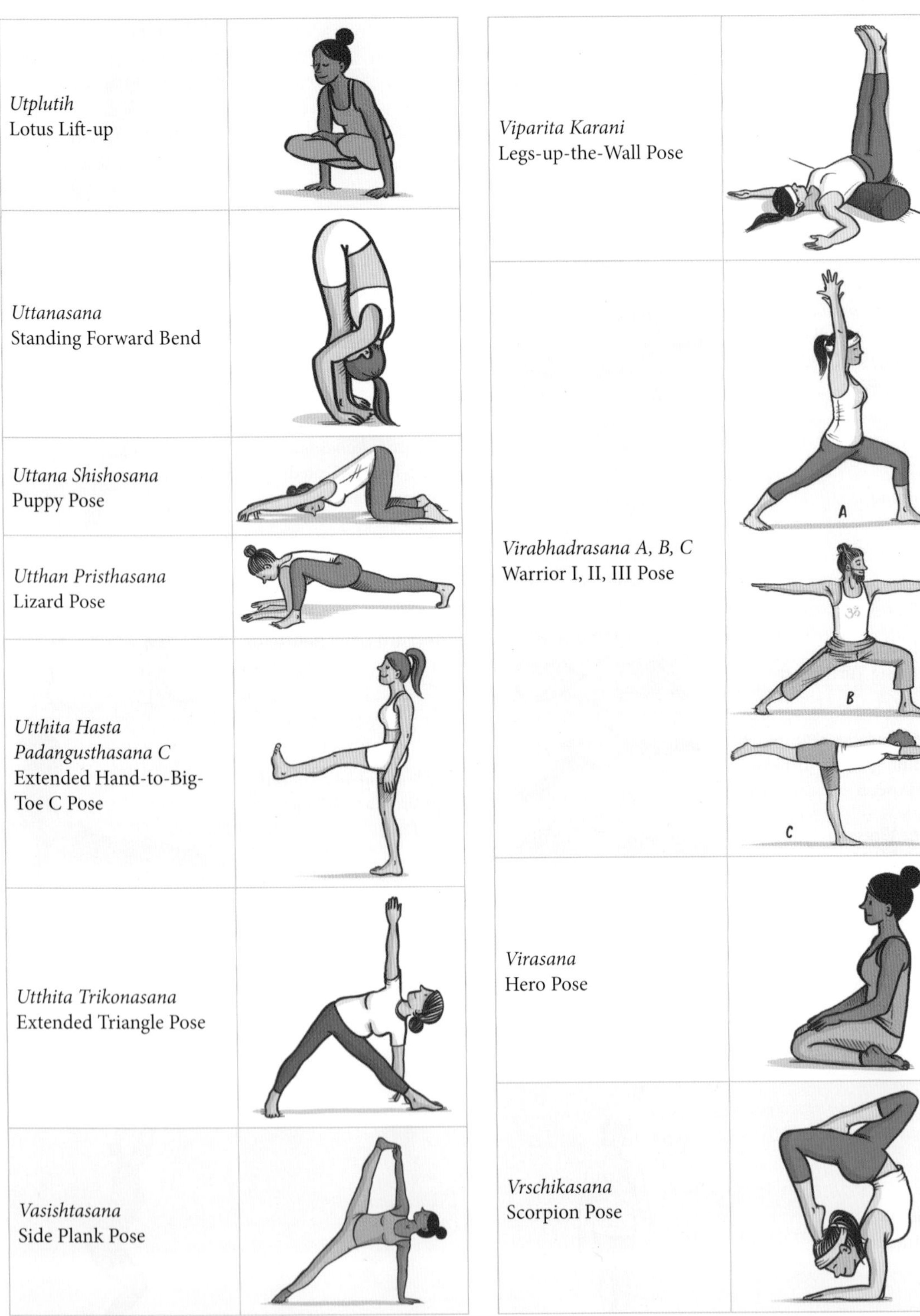

Utplutih Lotus Lift-up	
Uttanasana Standing Forward Bend	
Uttana Shishosana Puppy Pose	
Utthan Pristhasana Lizard Pose	
Utthita Hasta Padangusthasana C Extended Hand-to-Big-Toe C Pose	
Utthita Trikonasana Extended Triangle Pose	
Vasishtasana Side Plank Pose	

Viparita Karani Legs-up-the-Wall Pose	
Virabhadrasana A, B, C Warrior I, II, III Pose	
Virasana Hero Pose	
Vrschikasana Scorpion Pose